J. Schüttler (Ed.)

55 Years German Society of Anaesthesiology and

Intensive Care Medicine

Tradition and Innovation

J. Schüttler (Ed.)

55 Years German Society of Anaesthesiology an Intensive Care Medicine

Tradition & Innovation

Editor:
Jürgen Schüttler
On behalf of the
German Society of Anaesthesiology and Intensive Care Medicine

In collaboration with
M. Goerig, T. Pasch, H. Petermann, J. Schulte am Esch, W. Schwarz

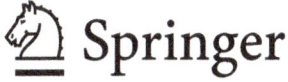 Springer

Schüttler, J., Prof. Dr. Dr. h.c.
Anästhesiologische Klinik,
Universitätsklinikum Erlangen,
Krankenhausstrasse 12, 91054 Erlangen,
Germany

*

ISBN 978-3-540-24257-4 Springer-Verlag Berlin Heidelberg New York

Bibliographic information Deutsche Bibliothek
The Deutsche Bibliothek lists this publication in Deutsche Nationalbibliographie;
detailed bibliographic data is available in the internet at <http://dnb.ddb.de>.

Springer Medizin
Springer-Verlag GmbH
Ein Unternehmen von Springer Science+Business Media

springer.de
© Springer-Verlag Berlin Heidelberg 2012
Printed in Germany

Editor: Diana Kraplow, Heidelberg
Typesetting: TypoStudio Tobias Schaedla, Heidelberg
Cover Design and Layout: deblik Berlin
SPIN: 11374411

Printed on acid free paper: 5 4 3 2 1 0

Preface

In 2003 a book had been published commemorating the 50th anniversary of the German Society of Anaesthesiology and Intensive Care Medicine (DGAI). Since then we have worked hard to realize an English version of this book as many colleagues from abroad had requested for. Now we are pleased to offer you the history of the first 55 years of our Society.

This book presents to our friends and colleagues all over the world historical details and information on the development of anaesthesiology in Germany and the remarkable growth of our Society. At the founding session of the German Society of Anaesthesia in Munich on 10 April 1953 42 persons had signed the founding documents. Today about 12,000 anaesthetists are members of the German Society of Anaesthesiology and Intensive Care Medicine, making the DGAI the biggest national society within ESA.

Well known are the pioneering contributions of German scientists and surgeons to the development of general, regional and local anaesthesia during the 19th and the beginning of the 20th centuries. But less known outside Germany are the reasons for the delayed evolution of anaesthesiology as a specialty of its own in German medicine, far later than in the UK, Scandinavia or the USA. On the following pages you will find answers to this question and detailed information on the successful establishment and development of anaesthesiology especially at the Faculties of Medicine at German universities.

We are greatly indebted to Joseph Rupreht from Rotterdam, the initiator of the International Symposia on the History of Anaesthesia, and other colleagues interested in this field for encouraging us to edit this book. Many thanks go to the authors who worked hard to prepare their chapters for this book in English language. The editor also has to thank those colleagues and native speakers who revised our manuscripts to improve legibility. We very much appreciate the help of Brian Sweeney and Cedric Morris. Special thanks go to Thomas Pasch for shouldering the Sisyphean task to prepare the university chapter for publishing.

The DGAI would not have been able to publish this book without the support of generous sponsors. Gratefully we list the following companies: Abbott GmbH & Co. KG, Baxter Deutschland GmbH, Drägerwerk AG & Co. KGaA, Grünenthal GmbH, Janssen-Cilag GmbH, Maquet GmbH & Co. KG, Pfizer Deutschland GmbH, Smiths Medical Deutschland GmbH. We also thank the officers of the former European Academy of Anaesthesiology for a very generous grant to support printing.

Last but not least we express our gratitude to TypoStudio Tobias Schaedla and the staff of Springer-Verlag Heidelberg for their excellent job and their abundance of patience.

Erlangen, June 2012
Prof. Dr. Dr. h.c. Jürgen Schüttler
Editor

Contents

List of Autors

Ackern, K. van, Prof. Dr. Dr. h.c.
Stiftung Deutsche Anästhesiologie,
Roritzerstrasse 27, 90419 Nürnberg,
Germany

Agarwal, K., Dr.
Therapiezentrum für Integrative
Palliativmedizin und Schmerztherapie,
Medizinisches Versorgungszentrum
Stade, Hohenwedeler Weg 18,
21682 Stade, Germany

Ahrens, P., Dr.
Zentrum Anaesthesiologie, Rettungs-
und Intensivmedizin, Universitätsmedizin Göttingen, Robert-Koch-Strasse 40,
37099 Göttingen, Germany

Aken, H. Van, Prof. Dr. Dr. h.c.
Klinik für Anästhesiologie, operative
Intensivmedizin und Schmerztherapie,
Universitätsklinikum Münster, Albert-
Schweitzer-Campus 1, 48149 Münster,
Germany

Albrecht, D. M., Prof. Dr.
Medizinischer Vorstand, Universitäts-
klinikum Carl Gustav Carus an der
Technischen Universität Dresden,
Fetscherstrasse 74, 01307 Dresden,
Germany

Bahr, J., Dr. rer. biol. hum.
Zentrum Anaesthesiologie, Rettungs-
und Intensivmedizin, Universitätsmedizin Göttingen, Robert-Koch-Str. 40,
37099 Göttingen, Germany

Benad, G., Prof. Dr.
Parkweg 16, 18196 Beselin, Germany

Bender, H.-J., Prof. Dr.
Klinik für Anästhesiologie und Operative Intensivmedizin, Universitätsklinikum Mannheim, Theodor-Kutzer-
Ufer 1-3, 68167 Mannheim, Germany

Boemke, W., Prof. Dr.
Klinik für Anästhesiologie mit Schwer-
punkt operative Intensivmedizin,
Charité – Universitätsmedizin Berlin,
Charité-Platz 1, 10117 Berlin, Germany

Bonhoeffer, K., Prof Dr.
Südliche Auffahrtsallee 40,
80639 München, Germany

Böttiger,B. W., Prof. Dr.
Klinik für Anästhesiologie und Operative Intensivmedizin, Uniklinik Köln,
50924 Köln, Germany

Brandt, L., Prof. Dr.
Ernst-Udet-Strasse 9, 85764 Ober-
schleissheim, Germany

Bucher, M., Prof. Dr.
Universitätsklinik für Anästhesiologie
und operative Intensivmedizin, Martin-
Luther-Universität Halle/Wittenberg,
Ernst-Grube-Strasse 40, 06120 Halle,
Germany

Burchardi, H., Prof. Dr.
Kiefernweg 2, 37120 Bovenden,
Germany

Busch, T., Prof. Dr.
Klinik für Anästhesiologie und Intensivtherapie, Universitätsklinikum Jena, Erlanger Allee 101, 07747 Jena, Germany

Buzello, W., Univ. Prof. Dr.
Peter-von-Fliesteden-Strasse 28, 50933
Köln-Braunsfeld, Germany

Cunitz, G., Prof. Dr.
Trienendorfer Strasse 90A, 58300 Wet-
ter, Germany

Dick, W. F., Prof. Dr. Dr. h.c.
Carl-Orff-Strasse 2, 55127 Mainz,
Germany

Doenicke, A., Prof. Dr.
Hartstrasse 80, 82110 Germering,
Germany

Dudziak, R., Prof. Dr.
Lerchesbergweg 17, 60598 Frankfurt,
Germany

Falke, K. J., Univ. Prof. Dr.
Am neuen Garten 41, 14469 Potsdam,
Germany

Geiger, K., Prof. Dr. Dr. h.c.
Wintererstrasse 22, 79104 Freiburg im
Breisgau, Germany

Georgieff, M., Prof. Dr. Dr. h.c.
Klinik für Anästhesiologie, Universitätsklinikum Ulm, Steinhövelstrasse 9,
89075 Ulm, Germany

Goerig, M., Priv.-Doz. Dr.
Klinik und Poliklinik für Anästhesiologie, Universitätsklinikum Hamburg-
Eppendorf, Martinistrasse 52,
20246 Hamburg, Germany

Goetz, A.E., Prof. Dr.
Klinik und Poliklinik für Anästhesiologie, Universitätsklinikum Hamburg-
Eppendorf, Martinistrasse 52,
20246 Hamburg, Germany

Graf, B.M., Prof. Dr.
Klinik für Anästhesiologie, Universitätsklinikum Regensburg, 93042 Regensburg, Germany

Greim, C.-A., Prof. Dr.
Klinik für Anästhesiologie, Intensiv-
und Notfallmedizin, Klinikum Fulda,
Pacelliallee 4, 36043 Fulda, Germany

Griem, C., Berlin
Klinik für Anästhesiologie mit
Schwerpunkt operative Intensiv-
medizin, Campus Benjamin Franklin,
Charité – Universitätsmedizin Berlin,
Hindenburgdamm 30, 12203 Berlin,
Germany

Hachenberg, T., Prof. Dr.
Universitätsklinik für Anaesthesio-
logie und Intensivtherapie, Universi-
tätsklinikum Magdeburg, Leipziger
Strasse 44, 39120 Magdeburg,
Germany

Heller, A., Prof. Dr.
Klinik und Poliklinik für Anästhesiologie und Intensivmedizin, Universitätsklinikum Carl Gustav Carus an der TU
Dresden, Fetscherstrasse 74,
01307 Dresden, Germany

Hempelman, G., Prof. Dr. Dr. h.c.
Birkenweg 46, 35435 Wettenberg-
Launsbach, Germany

Henrich, M., Priv.-Doz. Dr.
Klinik für Anaesthesiologie und operative Intensivmedizin, Universitätsklinikum Giessen und Marburg, Standort
Gießen, Rudolf-Buchheim-Strasse 7,
35392 Gießen, Germany

Hoeft, A., Prof. Dr.
Klinik und Poliklinik für Anästhesio-
logie und Operative Intensivmedizin,
Universitätsklinikum Bonn, Sigmund-
Freud-Strasse 25, 53105 Bonn,
Germany

Kaisers, U.X., Prof. Dr.
Klinik und Poliklinik für Anästhesiologie und Intensivtherapie, Universitätsklinikum Leipzig, Liebigstrasse 20,
04103 Leipzig, Germany

Kalff, G., Prof. Dr.
Orthstrasse 10, 52072 Aachen,
Germany

Kasper, S.-M., Priv.-Doz. Dr.
Klinik für Anästhesiologie und Operative Intensivmedizin, Uniklinik Köln,
50924 Köln, Germany

Kettler, D., Prof. Dr. Dr. h.c.
Am Weinberg 4 a, 37120 Bovenden,
Germany

Koch, T., Prof. Dr.
Klinik und Poliklinik für Anästhesiologie und Intensivmedizin, Universitätsklinikum Carl Gustav Carus an der
TU Dresden, Fetscherstrasse 74,
01307 Dresden, Germany

Kochs, E. Prof. Dr., Dipl.-Phys.
Klinik für Anaesthesiologie, Klinikum
rechts der Isar der Technischen Universität München, Ismaninger Str. 22,
81675 München, Germany

Koppert, W., Prof. Dr., M.A.
Klinik für Anästhesiologie und Intensivmedizin, Medizinischen Hochschule
Hannover, Carl-Neuberg-Strasse 1,
30625 Hannover, Germany

Kox, W. J., Prof. Dr. Dr.
Institut für Krankenhausmanagement,
Charité – Universitätsmedizin Berlin,
Hindenburgdamm 30, 12200 Berlin,
Germany

Kreimeier, U., Prof. Dr.
Klinik für Anaesthesiologie, Klinikum
der Universität München, Marchioninistrasse 15, 81377 München,
Germany

Krier, C., Prof. Dr.
Klinik für Anästhesiologie und
operative Intensivmedizin am
Katharinenhospital, Klinikum
Stuttgart, Kriegsbergstrasse 60,
70174 Stuttgart, Germany

Larsen, R., Prof. Dr.
Fassanweg 26, 66424 Homburg,
Germany

Laubenthal, H., Prof. Dr.
Klinik für Anästhesiologie, St. Josef-
Hospital der Ruhr-Universität Bochum,
Gudrunstrasse 56, 44791 Bochum,
Germany

Lawin, P., Prof. Dr. Dr. h.c. †

Lennartz, H., Prof. Dr.
Römerweg 12, 35287 Amöneburg,
Germany

Link, J., Prof. Dr.
Klinik für Anästhesiologie mit
Schwerpunkt operative Intensiv-
medizin, Campus Benjamin Franklin,
Charité – Universitätsmedizin Berlin,
Hindenburgdamm 30, 12203 Berlin,
Germany

Martin, E., Prof. Dr.
Klinik für Anaesthesiologie, Universitätsklinikum Heidelberg, Im Neuen-
heimer Feld 110, 69120 Heidelberg,
Germany

Marx, G., Prof. Dr.
Klinik für operative Intensivmedizin
Erwachsene, Universitätsklinikum
Aachen, Pauwelsstrasse 30,
52074 Aachen, Germany

Mildenberger, J., Dr.
Abteilung Anästhesie, Klinik Neustadt,
Paracelsusstrasse 30, 91413 Neustadt
an der Aisch, Germany

Nadstawek, J., Prof. Dr. Dr. h.c.
Klinik und Poliklinik für Anästhesiologie und Operative Intensivmedizin, Universitätsklinikum Bonn,
Sigmund-Freud-Straße 25,
53105 Bonn, Germany

Nöldge-Schomburg, G., Prof. Dr.
Klinik und Poliklinik für Anästhesiologie und Intensivtherapie, Universitätsklinikum Rostock, Schillingallee 35,
18057 Rostock, Germany

Opderbecke, H.W., Prof. Dr.
Kesslerplatz 10, 90489 Nürnberg,
Germany

Palmaers, T., Dr.
Klinik für Anästhesiologie und Intensivmedizin, Medizinischen Hochschule
Hannover, Carl-Neuberg-Strasse 1,
30625 Hannover, Germany

Pannen, B., Prof. Dr.
Klinik für Anästhesiologie, Universitätsklinikum Düsseldorf, Moorenstrasse 5,
40225 Düsseldorf, Germany

Pasch, T., Prof Dr.
Am Meilwald 22, 91054 Erlangen,
Germany

Peter, K., Prof. Dr. Dr. h.c.
Seestrasse 48, 82335 Berg, Germany

Petermann, H., Dr. phil. M.A.
Institut für Ethik, Geschichte und
Theorie der Medizin, Universitätsklinikum Münster, Von-Esmarch-Strasse 62,
48419 Münster, Germany

Peters, J., Prof. Dr.
Klinik für Anästhesiologie und Inten-
sivmedizin, Universitätsklinikum Essen,
Hufelandstrasse 55, 45122 Essen,
Germany

Piepenbrock, S., Prof. Dr.
Birkenweg 19, 30657 Hannover–Isern-
hagen-Süd, Germany

Puchstein, C., Prof. Dr.
Klinik für Anästhesiologie und operative Intensivmedizin, Marienhospital Herne, Universitätsklinik der Ruhr-Universität Bochum, Hölkeskampring 40, 44625 Herne, Germany

Quintel, M. Prof. Dr.
Zentrum Anaesthesiologie, Rettungs- und Intensivmedizin, Universitätsmedizin Göttingen, Robert-Koch-Strasse 40, 37099 Göttingen, Germany

Radke, J., Prof. Dr.
Herzberger Landstrasse 91, 37085 Göttingen, Germany

Reinhart, K., Prof. Dr.
Klinik für Anästhesiologie und Intensivtherapie, Universitätsklinikum Jena, Erlanger Allee 101, 07747 Jena, Germany

Röse, W., Prof. Dr.
Förderstedter Strasse 19, 39112 Magdeburg, Germany

Roewer, N., Prof. Dr. Dr. h.c.
Klinik und Poliklinik für Anästhesiologie, Universitätsklinikum Würzburg, Zentrum Operative Medizin, Oberdürrbacher Strasse 6, 97080 Würzburg, Germany

Rossaint, R., Prof. Dr.
Klinik für Anästhesiologie, Universitätsklinikum Aachen, Pauwelsstrasse 30, 52074 Aachen, Germany

Rüffert, H., Dr.
Klinik und Poliklinik für Anästhesiologie und Intensivtherapie, Universitätsklinikum Leipzig, Liebigstrasse 20, 04103 Leipzig, Germany

Schelling, G., Dr.
Klinik für Anaesthesiologie, Klinikum der Universität München, Marchioninistrasse 15, 81377 München, Germany

Schmucker, P., Prof. Dr.
Klinik für Anästhesiologie und Intensivmedizin, Universitätsklinikum Schleswig-Holstein, Campus Lübeck, Ratzeburger Allee 160, 23538 Lübeck, Germany

Schneeweiss, A., Dr.
Klinik für Anästhesiologie und Intensivmedizin, Universitätsklinikum Schleswig-Holstein, Campus Lübeck, Ratzeburger Allee 160, 23538 Lübeck, Germany

Scholz, J., Prof. Dr.
Vorstandsvorsitzender, Universitätsklinikum Schleswig-Holstein, Arnold-Heller-Strasse 3, 24105 Kiel, Germany

Schüttler, J., Prof. Dr. Dr. h.c.
Anästhesiologische Klinik, Universitätsklinikum Erlangen, Krankenhausstrasse 12, 91054 Erlangen, Germany

Schulte am Esch, J., Prof. Dr. Dr. h.c.
Strassenbahnring 9, 20251 Hamburg, Germany

Schwarz, W.
Zochastrasse 11, 90480 Nürnberg, Germany

Schwilden, H., Prof. Dr. Dr. rer. nat.
Anästhesiologische Klinik, Universitätsklinikum Erlangen, Krankenhausstrasse 12, 91054 Erlangen, Germany

Spies, C.D., Prof. Dr.
Klinik für Anästhesiologie mit Schwerpunkt operative Intensivmedizin, Charité – Universitätsmedizin Berlin, Charité-Platz 1, 10117 Berlin, Germany

Stein, C., Prof. Dr.
Klinik für Anästhesiologie mit Schwerpunkt operative Intensivmedizin, Campus Benjamin Franklin, Charité – Universitätsmedizin Berlin, Hindenburgdamm 30, 12203 Berlin, Germany

Steinfath, M., Prof. Dr.
Klinik für Anästhesiologie und Operative Intensivmedizin, Universitätsklinikum Schleswig-Holstein, Campus Kiel, Schwanenweg 21, 24105 Kiel, Germany

Stoeckel, H., Prof. Dr. Dr. h.c. mult.
Horst-Stoeckel-Museum für die Geschichte der Anästhesiologie, Klinikum der Universität Bonn, Sigmund-Freud-Strasse 25, 53105 Bonn, Germany

Strätling, M., Dr.
Klinik für Anästhesiologie und Intensivmedizin, Universitätsklinikum Schleswig-Holstein, Campus Lübeck, Ratzeburger Allee 160, 23538 Lübeck, Germany

Striebel, J.-P., Prof. Dr.
Ethikkommission II, Medizinische Fakultät Mannheim der Universität Heidelberg, Maybachstrasse 14, 68169 Mannheim, Germany

Taeger, K., Prof. Dr.
Schützenheimweg 19, 93049 Regensburg, Germany

Tarnow, J., Prof. Dr.
Erwin-v.-Witzleben-Strasse 25, 40474 Düsseldorf, Germany

Tempel, G., Univ. Prof. Dr.
Buchenland 5, 82024 Taufkirchen, Germany

Uhlig, T., Dr.
Klinik für Anästhesiologie und Intensivtherapie, Universitätsklinikum Jena, Erlanger Allee 101, 07747 Jena, Germany

Unertl, K., Prof. Dr.
Kleiststrasse 5, 72074 Tübingen, Germany

Volk, T., Prof. Dr.
Klinik für Anästhesiologie, Intensivmedizin und Schmerztherapie, Universitätsklinikum des Saarlandes, 66421 Homburg, Germany

Wappler, F., Prof. Dr.
Lehrstuhl für Anästhesie II, Universität Witten-Herdecke, Klinik für Anästhesiologie und operative Intensivmedizin, Kliniken der Stadt Köln, Krankenhaus Merheim, 51058 Köln, Germany

Wawersik, J., Prof. Dr.
Am Alpengarten 3, 88131 Lindau / Bodensee, Germany

Weigand, M., Prof. Dr.
Klinik für Anaesthesiologie und operative Intensivmedizin, Universitätsklinikum Giessen und Marburg, Standort Giessen, Rudolf-Buchheim-Strasse 7, 35392 Giessen, Germany

Wendt, M., Prof. Dr.
Klinik und Poliklinik für Anästhesiologie und Intensivmedizin, Universitätsmedizin Greifswald, Fleischmannstrasse 42-44, 17475 Greifswald, Germany

Werner, C., Prof. Dr.
Klinik für Anästhesiologie, Universitätsmedizin Mainz, Langenbeckstrasse 1, 55131 Mainz, Germany

Wulf, H., Prof. Dr.
Klinik für Anästhesie und Intensivtherapie, Universitätsklinikum Giessen und Marburg, Standort Marburg, Baldingerstrasse, 35033 Marburg, Germany

Wunder, C., Prof. Dr.
Klinik und Poliklinik für Anästhesiologie, Universitätsklinikum Würzburg, Zentrum Operative Medizin, Oberdürrbacher Strasse 6, 97080 Würzburg, Germany

Zacharowski, K.-D., Prof. Dr.
Klinik für Anästhesiologie, Intensivmedizin und Schmerztherapie, Klinikum der Johann Wolfgang Goethe-Universität Frankfurt am Main, Theodor-Stern-Kai 7, 60590 Frankfurt, Germany

Zenz, M., Prof. Dr.
Henkenbergstrasse 63, 44797 Bochum, Germany

Zindler, M., Prof. Dr.
Himmelgeister Landstrasse 171, 40589 Düsseldorf, Germany

Zwissler, B. Prof. Dr.
Klinik für Anaesthesiologie, Klinikum der Universität München, Marchioninistrasse 15, 81377 München, Germany

Glossary of Terms

Adjunct Professor	Außerplanmäßiger Professor, C2-Professor, W1-Professor
Air rescue helicopter	Rettungshubschrauber, Rettungshelikopter
Assistant (Physician)	Assistent, Assistenzarzt
Associate Professor (with tenure)	Ausserordentlicher Professor, C3-Professor, W2-Professor, Extraordinarius
Association of Emergency Physicians of Germany	Bundesvereinigung der Arbeitsgemeinschaften der Notärzte Deutschlands (BAND)
Association of Hospital Doctors (short form)	Marburger Bund
Association of Salaried and Civil Servant Physicians in Germany	Marburger Bund
Association of the Scientific Medical Societies in Germany	Arbeitsgemeinschaft Wissenschaftlicher Medizinischer Fachgesellschaften (AWMF)
Austrian Society of Anaesthesiology, Resuscitation and Intensive Care Medicine	Österreichische Gesellschaft für Anästhesiologie, Reanimation und Intensivmedizin (ÖGARI)
Central European Anaesthesia Congress	Zentraleuropäischer Anästhesiekongress (ZAK)
Central Working Group on Anaesthesiology and Anaesthesia Technology	Zentraler Arbeitskreis für Anästhesiologie und Anästhesietechnik
Chair (Full = Ordinary, Associate = Extraordinary)	Lehrstuhl (ordentlicher, außerordentlicher)
Chairman, Chairperson	Direktor
Chairmanship	Direktorat
Chief Emergency Physician	Leitender Notarzt
Chief Physician	Chefarzt
Clinic	Ambulanz, Klinik
Collaborative Research Centre of the German Research Foundation	Sonderforschungsbereich der Deutschen Forschungsgemeinschaft
Consultant	(eigenverantwortlicher) Facharzt
Continuing medical education (CME)	(Ärztliche) Fortbildung
Critical care medicine	Intensivmedizin
Day care unit	Tagesklinik
Department	Klinik, Institut
Director	Direktor, Chefarzt, Leiter
Division	Abteilung
Doctor staffed ambulance helicopter	Rettungshubschrauber, Rettungshelikopter
Emergency department, emergency unit	Notfallabteilung, Notaufnahme
Emergency doctor, emergency physician	Notarzt
Emergency doctor's ambulance	Notarztwagen
Emergency medical service (EMS)	Rettungsdienst, Rettungsorganisation
Emergency medical technician (EMT)	Rettungssanitäter
Emergency (rescue) helicopter	Rettungshubschrauber, Rettungshelikopter
Faculty of Medicine	Medizinische Fakultät

Federal Armed Forces (Hospital)	Bundeswehr(krankenhaus)
Federal Council	Bundesrat
Federal Court of Justice	Bundesgerichtshof (BGH)
Federal Ministry of Education and Research	Bundesministerium für Bildung und Forschung (BMBF)
Federal Parliament	Bundestag
Federal Regulation on Doctors	Bundesärzteordnung
Federal state	Bundesland
Full Professor	Ordentlicher Professor, C4-Professor, W3-Professor, Ordinarius
German Academy of Continuing Education in Anaesthesiology	Deutsche Akademie für Anästhesiologische Fortbildung (DAAF)
German Anaesthesia Congress	Deutscher Anästhesiekongress (DAK), Deutscher Anästhesiecongress (DAC)
German Association for the Advancement of Science and Medicine	Gesellschaft Deutscher Naturforscher und Ärzte (GDNÄ)
German Association of Cities	Deutscher Städtetag (DST)
German Association of Senior Hospital Physicians	Verband der Leitenden Krankenhausärzte Deutschlands
German Hospital Federation	Deutsche Krankenhausgesellschaft (DKG)
German Hospital Institute	Deutsches Krankenhausinstitut (DKI)
German Interdisciplinary Association for Pain Therapy	Deutsche Interdisziplinäre Vereinigung für Schmerztherapie (DIVS)
German Interdisciplinary Association of Critical Care and Emergency Medicine	Deutsche Interdisziplinäre Vereinigung für Intensiv- und Notfallmedizin (DIVI)
German Medical Assembly	Deutscher Ärztetag
German Medical Association	Bundesärztekammer (BÄK)
German National Academy of Sciences Leopoldina	Leopoldina Nationale Akademie der Wissenschaften
German Nurses Association	Deutsche Schwesterngemeinschaft, Deutscher Berufsverband für Pflegeberufe
German Pain Association	Schmerztherapeutisches Kolloquium (STK)
German Pharmacological Society	Deutsche Pharmakologische Gesellschaft
German Red Cross	Deutsches Rotes Kreuz (DRK)
German Reich	Deutsches Reich
German Research Foundation	Deutsche Forschungsgemeinschaft (DFG)
German Science Council	Wissenschaftsrat
German Society for the Study of Pain	Deutsche Gesellschaft zum Studium des Schmerzes (DGSS)
German Society for Thoracic and Cardiovascular Surgery	Deutsche Gesellschaft für Thorax-, Herz- und Gefäßchirurgie
German Society of Anaesthesia	Deutsche Gesellschaft für Anaesthesie (DGA)
German Society of Anaesthesia and Resuscitation	Deutsche Gesellschaft für Anaesthesie und Wiederbelebung (DGAW)
German Society of Anaesthesiology and Intensive Care Medicine	Deutsche Gesellschaft für Anästhesiologie und Intensivmedizin (DGAI)

German Society of Clinical Medicine	Deutsche Gesellschaft für Klinische Medizin
German Society of Gynaecology	Deutsche Gesellschaft für Gynäkologie
German Society of Internal Medicine Intensive Care	Deutsche Gesellschaft für Internistische Intensivmedizin und Notfallmedizin (DGIIN)
German Society of Surgery	Deutsche Gesellschaft für Chirurgie (DGCH)
German Working Group on Anaesthesiology	Deutsche Arbeitsgemeinschaft für Anaesthesiologie
Head, Head Physician	Leiter, Chefarzt
Helicopter rescue service	Rettungshubschrauber, Rettungshelikopter
High dependency unit (HDU)	Wachstation, Überwachungsstation
Hospital	Krankenhaus, Klinikum
House Officer	Medizinalassistent
Housemanship	Medizinalassistentenzeit
Institute for Medical and Pharmaceutical Proficiency Assessment	Institut für medizinische und pharmazeutische Prüfungsfragen (IMPP)
Instructor	Lehrbeauftragter
Intensive care	Intensivpflege
Intensive care medicine (ICM)	Intensivmedizin
Intensive care unit (ICU)	Intensivstation
Intensive therapy	Intensivtherapie
Intensive therapy unit (ITU)	Intensivtherapiestation (ITS)
Intensive treatment	Intensivbehandlung
Intermediate care unit	Wachstation, Überwachungsstation
Intern(ship)	Medizinalassistent(enzeit)
Lecturer	Privatdozent, Dozent
Lectureship	Dozentur
Medical Council of the German Reich	Reichsärztekammer
Medical Director	Ärztlicher Direktor
Medical Faculty	Medizinische Fakultät
Medical Licensure Act	Approbationsordnung für Ärzte
Medical Officer	Stabsarzt, Truppenarzt
Miners' Guild	Knappschaft
Miners' Professional Association	Bergbau-Berufsgenossenschaft
Mobile life support unit (MLSU)	Notarztwagen
Municipal Hospital	Stadtkrankenhaus, städtisches Krankenhaus
Order of Merit	Verdienstorden
Order of Merit of the Federal Republic of Germany	Bundesverdienstkreuz
Outpatient pain clinic, pain clinic	Schmerzambulanz, Schmerzsprechstunde
Pain therapy unit	Schmerzklinik
Paramedic	Rettungsassistent
Post-anaesthesia care unit (PACU)	Aufwachraum, Aufwachstation

Postgraduate education, postgraduate training	Weiterbildung zum Facharzt
Postgraduate Training Regulations	Weiterbildungsordnung, bis 1968: Facharztordnng
Preanaesthetic clinic	Anästhesieambulanz, Anästhesiesprechstunde
Professional Association of German Anaesthetists	Berufsverband Deutscher Anästhesisten (BDA)
Professional Association of German Internists	Berufsverband Deutscher Internisten (BDI)
Professional Association of German Surgeons	Berufsverband Deutscher Chirurgen (BDC)
Professional Association of Orthopaedic and Trauma Surgeons	Berufsverband der Fachärzte für Orthopädie und Unfallchirurgie (BVOU)
Professional Code of Conduct	Berufsordnung Deutscher Ärzte
Professorship	Professur
Public Services and Transport Workers' Union	Gewerkschaft Öffentliche Dienste, Transport und Verkehr (ÖTV)
Qualification as Lecturer	Habilitation
Recovery room, recovery unit	Aufwachraum, Aufwachstation
Registrar	Assistenzarzt, Assistent
Research Associate	Wissenschaftlicher Mitarbeiter
Resident	Assistenzarzt, Assistent
Section	Sektion
Senior Consultant	Leitender Oberarzt
Senior House Officer	Assistenzarzt, Assistent
Senior Physician	Oberarzt
Society of Anaesthesiology and Intensive Therapy of the German Democratic Republic	Gesellschaft für Anästhesiologie und Intensivtherapie der DDR (GAIT)
Society of Anaesthesiology and Reanimation of the German Democratic Republic	Gesellschaft für Anästhesiologie und Reanimation der DDR
Society of Clinical Medicine of the German Democratic Republic	Gesellschaft für Klinische Medizin der DDR
Specialist, medical specialist	Facharzt
Specialist in Anaesthesia, Specialist (Physician) Anaesthetist, Specialist in Anaesthesiology	Facharzt für Anästhesie, Anästhesist, Facharzt für Anästhesiologie
Staff physician, staff member	Oberarzt
State Chamber of Physicians, State Medical Association	Landesärztekammer (LÄK)
State Social Insurance Board	Landesversicherungsanstalt (LVA)
Supervision ward	Überwachungsstation
Surgical intensive care medicine	Operative Intensivmedizin
Undergraduate education, undergraduate teaching	Ausbildung der Medizinstudenten, studentische Lehre
Union of Professional Organisations of Medical Specialists	Gemeinschaft Fachärztlicher Berufsverbände (GFB)
University Department, University Clinic	Universitätsklinik, Universitätsinstitut
University Hospital	Universitätsklinikum, Universitätskrankenhaus
University Lecturer	Universitätsdozent
Working Group on Internal Medicine Intensive Care	Arbeitsgemeinschaft für Internistische Intensivmedizin

Development of the Scientific Society

1.1   55 Years of the German Society of Anaesthesiology and Intensive Care Medicine (DGAI)

K. van Ackern, W, Schwarz, J.-P. Striebel

»*In Germany, one also occasionally detects a certain longing for such specialists in anaesthesia, but at the same time, no one has been successful in actually keeping this species alive anywhere*« (Max v. Brunn, 1875–1924; [74])

On 10 April 1953 on the occasion of the 70th Annual Congress of the German Society of Surgery in Munich the German Society of Anaesthesia was founded. In September of the same year, it was decided at the 56th Meeting of the German Medical Assembly in Lindau to recognize the title of »Specialist in Anaesthesia«. The recognition of anaesthesia as an independent specialty in Germany was thus completed. Nearly 60 years after these events it is now fitting to give a brief account of the history of the German Society of Anaesthesiology and Intensive Care Medicine (DGAI), one which is neither an attempt to be comprehensive nor an attempt to place it in a wider historical perspective. Original documents, where possible, either complete or in part, which support certain developments are presented as well as contemporary statements from »pioneers« taken from protocols, letters, reports and publications.

1.1.1   First Steps

The founding of the DGAI in 1953 was later compared with parallel developments in other countries such as the UK and the USA [68]. For example, the Society of Anaesthetists was founded in London in 1883. In 1905 a group of doctors interested in anaesthesia founded the Society of Anesthetists of Long Island, the predecessor of the American Society of Anesthesiology. The delayed establishment of anaesthesia in German medicine is remarkable when one considers that at the end of the nineteenth and beginning of the twentieth centuries important significant contributions were made by German scientists and physicians in both local and regional anaesthesia as well as in general anaesthesia including the technical aspects thereof. It would be a generalization to claim, however, that German surgeons were altogether unreceptive. There were proponents as well as opponents of the independence of anaesthesia. Although in Germany, as in other countries, there was a widely held opinion among surgeons that anaesthesia was an essential component of the medical armamentarium and should be included in the undergraduate curriculum, the idea of establishing an independent specialty could not catch on. It was only after the First World War that contacts between interested surgeons and pharmacologists with established specialist societies in the UK and the USA led to repeated demands for an independent medical specialist in this area of practice.

Among the pioneers for the development of a separate specialty of anaesthesia in Germany was the Hamburg clinician Ernst von der Porten who as early as 1922 described himself as a »professional anaesthetist« [71]. He demanded that anyone who wished to conduct anaesthesia should master the entire spectrum of theory and practice and should have undergone thorough training. His visits in 1923 to specialist colleagues in the UK and especially his participation – as sole representative of the Continent – at a specialist meeting in Nottingham in 1926 allowed him to form links with British as well as American anaesthetists and their societies. Experiences and observations from these contacts led him to the decision to strive towards the establishment in Germany of anaesthesia as a separate discipline with its own mouthpiece in the form of a specialist journal analogous to those abroad.

The recession year 1928 was a significant milestone on the long journey towards the recognition of anaesthesia as an independent speciality in German medicine (► Chaps. 1 and 2). In this year Hans Killian of Freiburg and Helmut Schmidt of Hamburg, both young surgical assistants, upon the invitation of the International Anesthesia Research Society, undertook a lecture and study tour lasting several months, which led them to the USA, Canada and England [35, 41, 65]. In 1928 two specialist journals appeared independently of each other: *Der Schmerz* (Pain) edited by the gynaecologist Carl Joseph Gauß of Würzburg, the pharmacologist Hermann Wieland of Heidelberg, the anaesthetist Ernst von der Porten of Hamburg and the pharmacist B. Behrends of Heidelberg together with *Narkose und Anaesthesie* (Narcosis and Anaesthesia) edited by the gynaecologist H. Franken of Freiburg, the surgeon Hans Killian of Freiburg, the surgeon Helmut Schmidt of Hamburg and the pharmacologist H. Schlossman of Düsseldorf. After the first year of publication, the two journals merged and formed the publication *Schmerz – Narkose – Anaesthesie* (Pain, Narcosis, Anaesthesia) which successfully continued to be published for the next 16 years. Towards the end of 1944 it was compelled – like many other scientific journals in Germany at that time – to cease publication.

In September 1928, at the Annual Meeting of the Gesellschaft Deutscher Naturforscher und Ärzte (German Association for the Advancement of Science and Medicine), a General Meeting of the Sections of Surgery, Pharmacology and Gynaecology took place to discuss the topic of »Inhalational anaesthesia and the anaesthetic problem« [9]. This »First German Anaesthesia Congress« [66], as this meeting is sometimes described, engendered high expectations among the young German proponents of anaesthesia. Hans Killian and Helmut Schmidt announced at their lectures in the USA that at this meeting the formation of a German Society of Anaesthesia had been planned [2]. In order to support this proposal and to gain international recognition the secretary-general of the International Anesthesia Research Society, Francis Hoeffer McMechan, agreed to take part in the Hamburg meeting. In his welcome address [47, 48] at the beginning of the meeting he expressed his wish for mutual co-operation and Hans Killian and Helmut Schmidt strove to achieve political breakthroughs.

Impressed by the professionalism of the American and English anaesthetists they brought back news on developments both technical and professional in these countries [38, 65]. Above all, Helmut Schmidt criticized in his article »Inhalational anaesthesia from the standpoint of the American anaesthetic specialist« [65] the view widely held in German medicine that the »specialization of anaesthesia« was not necessary. He was able to do so because he had first-hand experience of the organizational and professional structures of the anaesthetic framework from his visits to numerous centres in the USA, Canada and England. He was convinced that the value of anaesthesia was not fully appreciated despite representing a higher risk or insult to the patient than the operation itself. Anaesthetic specialists would make the anaesthesia safer and thereby reduce the time in hospital. The introduction of anaesthetic specialists would correspondingly finance themselves. Schmidt pleaded finally for a »moderated specialization in both universities and large hospitals in Germany«. This plea fell however on deaf ears: the Freiburg Chairman and Professor of Surgery, Eduard Rehn, in his closing address viewed the professionalization of anaesthesia as premature [9]. Later H. Schmidt opined that [66] »the 'old fogies' were incensed that someone wanted to place another plenipotentiary at their side«.

Even the scientific lectures of the meeting led to no uniform recommendation for practical anaesthesia [60]. H. Killian expressed the general consternation at the end of the day in an original entry in the guest book of H. Schmidt (�‌ Fig. 1.1): a group of clearly unsettled surgeons surrounds a patient and ask themselves »after this Congress what kind of anaesthetic shall we use?« [66].

While Hans Killian subsequently made no further pronouncements, his surgical colleague Helmut Schmidt decided to undertake, as part of his *Habilitation*, a 2-year intensive theoretical and practical involvement in anaesthesia at the surgical clinic in Hamburg–Eppendorf. On account of the precarious nature of the subsequent professional opportunities he finally settled however on a surgical career [66].

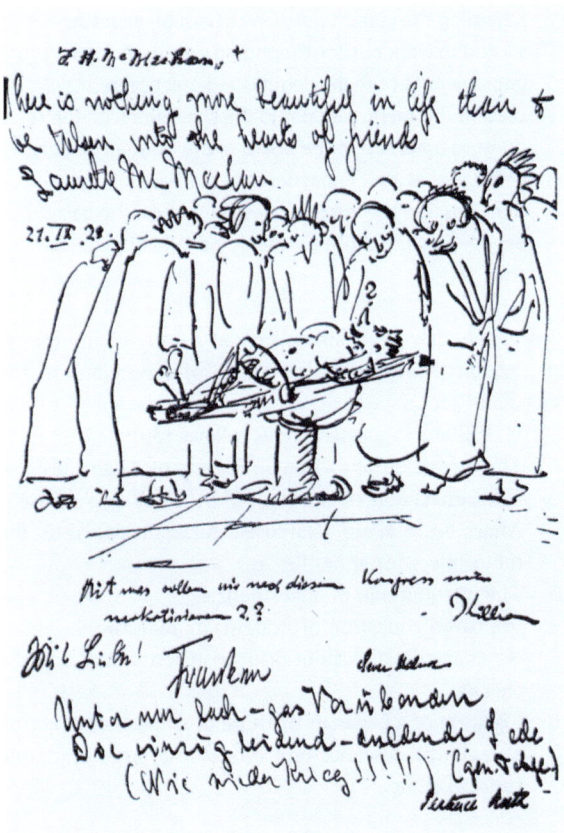

◌ **Fig. 1.1.** Entry on 21 September 1928 in the guest book of Helmut Schmidt [82]

Retrospectively, it is hardly conceivable for us today that the stipulations made by the surgeons in Germany, in contrast to both the UK and the USA, delayed for decades the development of the specialty of anaesthesia which was beneficial for their own work, thus depriving the patients of the advantages of widespread professional anaesthetic care.

Another 11 years elapsed in which there was intense discussion regarding the various anaesthetic agents and techniques but without any substantial change in the education of doctors or any progress in anaesthesia becoming recognized as a medical specialty.

At the yearly Congress of the German Society of Surgery in 1939 Hans Killian, at the end of his presentation on combination anaesthesia, took his concepts regarding the structure of the specialty of anaesthesia including education, research and teaching, to the Board of the Society [36]:

> You all know that from a practical point of view the anaesthetic problem in Germany doesn't seem to have been solved, and I therefore, stimulated by this paper, have felt myself motivated to write a critical overview

regarding the current position of German anaesthesia and to work out corresponding proposals for an improvement both in scientific and practical terms. I present this memorandum to the chairman with the request to present it to the board of the German Society of Surgery, so that it may serve as the basis of discussion. This is in the hope that we can reduce the gap between us and those abroad in the field of practical anaesthesia.

Simultaneously H. Killian also sent a copy of the memo to the Reichsärzteführer (Fuehrer of Physicians of the German Reich).

H. Killian's requests were as follows [36]:

1. The formation of a German Society of Anaesthesia.
2. The conversion of the journal Schmerz – Narkose – Anaesthesie (Pain, Narcosis, Anaesthesia) into the mouthpiece for anaesthesia.
3. The introduction of anaesthetists.
4. Improved education of students in anaesthesia.
5. No anaesthesia without prior instruction and specific checks.
6. Creation of a German Institute of Anaesthesia, acting as a central research unit linked to a large academic surgical clinic.

Six months later Killian received an answer from the Reichsärztekammer (Medical Council of the German Reich) [69] (◘ Fig. 1.2a,b), after the Reichsärzteführer had taken statements through the Central Office of the Ministry of Health from the NS-Dozentenbund (National Socialist League of University Lecturers) and the German Society of Surgery. Based on the objections raised by the NS-Dozentenbund (NS Association of Lecturers and Professors) together with a statement from the Erlangen Professor of Surgery Otto Goetze, the Reichsärztekammer resolutely turned down the request in a written statement on 14 September 1939, despite the clear recognition of insufficient teaching in anaesthesia. A recommendation was made therefore to »submit this important topic for discussion at the next Meeting of German Surgeons, and I am convinced that it will succeed in bringing attention to the important plan which you have in mind to the surgical schools«. Regrettably, the files of the Reichsärztekammer were almost completely destroyed towards the end of World War II, so that it is now virtually impossible to gain insight into the position adopted following Killian's request. However, we can reconstruct the thought processes which led to the decision taken by O. Goetze in the context of his statement to the request for autonomy by the radiologists [25, 26, 42].

An independent surgical specialty is, according to O. Goetze, »characterized by its own comprehensive diagnostics and its own comprehensive therapy«. That

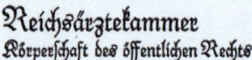

◘ Fig. 1.2a,b. Letter of the *Reichsärztekammer* to Hans Killian on 14 September 1939 (Archive of the DGAI)

»did not apply to X-ray therapy and even less to X-ray diagnostics«. He classified X-ray diagnostics as a »complementary science, which provided us with a diagnostic aid comparable to the microscope, to make visible what we learnt and continue to learn on a daily basis from pathology and pathological anatomy«. We may assume that in his report to the Central Office for Public Health, O. Goetze categorized anaesthesia likewise as complementary science within the bounds of surgery and rejected the move towards its independence as a specialty as well as the creation of an independent specialist in anaesthesia.

Because of the impending Second World War, further discussion, initiated by the Medical Council of the German Reich, did not come about. H. Killian's attempt to stimulate a discussion by publishing his proposals in the December 1941 edition of *Schmerz – Narkose – Anaesthesie* [37] also remained without resonance. During this phase it was not only the dismissive attitude of the surgeons that hindered further developments, but also the increasing isolation of German medicine as a result of the war.

1.1.2 Development After the Second World War

The state of anaesthesia in Germany at the end of World War II was similar to that at the turn of the century. The preferred method was open drop ether anaesthesia, using a Schimmelbusch mask. This was complemented by intravenous barbiturates, either as total intravenous anaesthesia or in combination with open drop ether anaesthesia. There were no trained specialists in anaesthesia. This situation not only led to numerous fatal anaesthetic incidents [58] but also further limited the indications to operate with regard to the patient's condition, age and existing co-morbidity as well as the extent of the operation. For example, a major operation like a gastrectomy would not be considered in a 60-year-old patient.

Very soon however news about medical developments again started arriving in Germany from abroad. German surgeons received news about the enormous advances that were being made – especially for heart and lung operations – with curare (synthesized in 1944), endotracheal intubation, which had become routine, as well as the new anaesthetic machines (▶ Chap. 3.1).

Knowledge of this kind was first available where contacts with foreign anaesthetists existed. Jean Henley, for example, an anaesthesiologist from New York, first reported her experiences in 1949 in Giessen and until 1951 conveyed the new developments to many hospitals of the American-occupied zone in Germany. Karl Mülly, a Swiss colleague trained in Stockholm and Oxford, passed

on his experience in a series of lectures in Düsseldorf, Marburg, Heidelberg and Munich. In this way, new opportunities for the surgical treatment of a great number of patients with tuberculosis also opened up in Germany. Though technical preconditions had considerably improved through availability of the first endotracheal tubes manufactured by Rüsch/Waiblingen in 1947 and the first German anaesthetic machine Model 'F' produced by the Dräger Company in Lübeck in 1948, there was initially a lack in Germany not only of the necessary number of suitable technical instruments but more importantly of doctors who knew how to use them.

Against this background, from 6 to 11 June 1949 the 66th Congress of the German Society of Surgery took place in Frankfurt, the first surgical convention after the Second World War, chaired by Eduard Rehn of Freiburg. At the end of his lecture on »Curare and related substances for the improvement of anaesthesia« [39], Hans Killian asked – 10 years after his historic venture at the Annual Congress of the German Society of Surgery in 1939 – »if it would not be advisable to train specialists in anaesthesia in Germany«. Eduard Rehn commented immediately during the discussion: »I think that the trend in surgery is that we will not be able to avoid specialization in anaesthesia – though perhaps not for all surgical interventions – but for certain operations including major and very extensive surgery. Consequently, I am already in the process of developing a lectureship for anaesthesia at my clinic, evolving out of pharmacology and surgery, with the aim of producing the required manpower.« Some surgeons (including Georg Ernst Konietzny of Hamburg, Emil Karl Frey of Munich, Friedrich Bernhard of Giessen and Ernst Derra of Düsseldorf) also reported at this conference on new surgical possibilities that had come about as a result of endotracheal intubation and artificial ventilation.

1.1.3 Continuing Opposition from the German Society of Surgery [7, 8]

The 52nd German Medical Assembly (General Assembly of the German Medical Association) in Hannover in September 1949 decided, in a move that was forward-looking, to also include the »Specialist in Anaesthesia« as number 18 in the new specialist statutes, along with neurosurgery, bacteriology-serology and bacteriology-microbiology. Three years of training were stipulated, two of which were to be devoted to training in anaesthetics under the guidance of a specialist, a further year could comprise training in surgery, medicine and physiology or pharmacology. Coinciding with the German Medical Assembly, several articles concerning the question of anaesthetic specialists appeared in the journal *Der Krankenhausarzt* (The

Hospital Doctor) – amongst them one by H. Killian with an updated version of his pre-war demands – all generally voicing the same opinion [32, 33, 38, 52]. However, the resolution of the German Medical Assembly was rejected on 22 October 1949 by the Scientific Specialist Societies, among them the German Society of Surgery, referring to their right of co-determination. Leading German surgeons had indeed recognized the value of modern anaesthetic techniques; they believed however that a specialist in anaesthetics was only necessary for special major operations, such as in thoracic surgery, and therefore reasoned that, in contrast to their colleagues in other Western countries, the introduction of a separate specialist was unnecessary. The Board of the German Society of Surgery recommended its discussion of the question of anaesthetic specialists in May 1950 and reinforced its negative attitude in a letter to the President of the German Medical Assembly, Hans Neuffer. Privately the committee decided that an independent central institute for training in anaesthesia was unwanted. More preferable was a lectureship in anaesthesia in conjunction with an anaesthetic group attached to a surgical department within a hospital. Included in the duties which the then President of the German Society of Surgery, Erich von Redwitz (Bonn), set out in a letter to the Secretary of the Society, Arthur Huebner were:

(a) Instruction in both the theory and practice of anaesthesia.

(b) Supervision of all anaesthetics within the hospital. Prior to anaesthesia the indication for an anaesthetic is in each individual case to be decided by the operating surgeon and the anaesthetist together, in accordance with agreements with the chief of surgery, provided the anaesthetist has a full grasp of the history and findings of each individual patient!

(c) Responsibility for the instruction of medical students.

(d) Every opportunity for research should be given.

A request from the German Pharmacological Society for a joint statement about guidelines for anaesthetic training was dealt with as follows:

> It is more appropriate to consider the possibility of training anaesthetic nurses, who are much more suited to German circumstances. According to German law, the surgeon is still responsible for the entire operation; the anaesthetist is his 'proxy'. Therefore the legal requirements would also have to be changed first. 'Specialists in anaesthesia' should be rejected for the time being, but some lectureships in anaesthesia, dedicated to research and training should be created. For this however one would have to demand previous experience in pharmacology (▶ Chap. 2.1).

For the 67th Congress of the German Society of Surgery at the end of May 1950, under the chairmanship of Erich von Redwitz of Bonn, several contributions concerning developments of anaesthetic techniques for surgery were planned and, apart from the main speaker Ernst Derra of Düsseldorf, who reported on »The current state of anaesthetic techniques in surgery« and who also commented on training for anaesthetists [10], several speakers from abroad were invited: Torsten Gordh of Stockholm, Geoffrey Organe of London and Robert Macintosh of Oxford. Despite this contingent no further significant progress was achieved during the detailed discussion. When Fritz Hesse of Saarbrücken, a staunch advocate and promoter of independent specialists in anaesthesia [29] demanded: »that the training of specialists in anaesthesia – or rather, of professional anaesthetists – had to happen on a very broad front, so that they would not be downgraded to mere technicians, but also in the area of research be considered of equal status to all other specialists«, E. Derra replied [30]: »Every little hospital does not need an anaesthetist; five to six schools of anaesthesia with specialists promoting research and teaching are sufficient. Interested trainees can be trained there.« The Chairman E. von Redwitz himself cautioned, in a reply to a statement by Robert Macintosh, in view of the special circumstances in Germany, against the rash creation of a new specialist. He supported lectureships and teaching posts for anaesthesia. That way the question of the requirement for the creation of an independent profession of anaesthetists could be dealt with more calmly and without undue haste. He also announced that the Society would appoint a commission that, together with a group appointed by the German Pharmacological Society, would examine the whole question once again [30].

During the summer term of 1950, three lecturers at the Medical School of Düsseldorf decided to move forward with the limited concessions of the German Society of Surgery for a structured training in anaesthesia. This »three-man course« on »narcosis and anaesthesia« was the first university course of lectures in anaesthesia in Germany after the Second World War and took place within the framework of pharmacology and toxicology and not surgery. The lecturers were: Helmut Weese, chief pharmacologist of the company Bayer and at the time also Professor of Pharmacology in Düsseldorf – he had introduced Evipan in 1932 –, Helmut Schmidt, Remscheid, who under Paul Sudeck in Hamburg earned his *Habilitation* (qualification as Lecturer) for his treatise on nitrous oxide and Ferdinand H. Koss, senior physician at Derra's clinic in Düsseldorf, who was joint author with Wolfgang Irmer of the first textbook on endotracheal anaesthesia in Germany, published in1951.

Immediately after the Surgical Congress in 1950 the North Rhine-Westphalian Ministry of Social Affairs in a letter dated 5 June 1950 also invited as experts the surgical clinical directors of university hospitals of this Federal State to »discuss the problem of training anaesthetic assistants or specialists in anaesthesia and the possible establishment of so-called schools of anaesthesia«. At this meeting Erich von Redwitz, Bonn, managed to push through the German Society of Surgery's opinion that the creation of a specialist in anaesthesia was premature; he declared however, together with his colleague Ernst Derra of Düsseldorf, that they were prepared to work for the creation of lectureships in anaesthesia within their own Faculties of Medicine. The Minister for Social Affairs was asked to approach the Minister of Education and the Finance Minister about the creation of the relevant posts and to provide grants abroad for the training of anaesthetists.

At the 53rd German Medical Assembly in Bonn (1950) the discussion about amendments to the specialist rules was postponed for another year, but meanwhile the Marburger Bund (German Association of Hospital Doctors) announced its intention to found an association of anaesthetists. This fact together with the pressure from the North Rhine-Westphalian Ministry of Social Affairs to recognize anaesthetists – indicators of the virulent nature of this matter – had a demonstrable effect on the Anaesthetic Commission, newly formed together with the German Pharmacological Society, as well as on the Committee of the German Society of Surgery.

Under this pressure, the Anaesthetic Commission, led by Karl Heinrich Bauer, Heidelberg, became convinced that the creation of a specialist in anaesthesia was unstoppable and at the end of November 1950 [17] (◻ Fig. 1.3) it presented its report to the Executive Committee of the German Society of Surgery as well as the following notice

Der Vorstand der Deutschen Gesellschaft für Chirurgie beehrt sich, folgenden Bericht der Narkose-Kommission zu überreichen:

Die von der Deutschen Pharmakologischen Gesellschaft und der Deutschen Gesellschaft für Chirurgie eingesetzte Narkose-Kommission hat am 25. 10. 50 in Heidelberg getagt. Es nahmen daran teil als Pharmakologen: Prof. LENDLE - Göttingen, Prof. WEESE - Elberfeld, als Chirurgen: Prof. K. H. BAUER - Heidelberg und Prof. DERRA - Düsseldorf.

Die Kommission kam zu folgenden Feststellungen bzw. Vorschlägen: Die praktische Ausbildung von Narkosefachärzten ist an chirurgische Kliniken und Krankenhäuser mit entsprechend hohen Operationsziffern (nicht unter 3000 Operationen im Jahr) gebunden, da nur bei großen Operationszahlen genügend zahlreiche und genügend vielseitige Narkosen anfallen. Wegen der Besonderheiten des technischen Vorgehens müssen die betr. Kliniken zugleich auch thoraxchirurgische Abteilungen mit entsprechenden thoraxinneren Operationen aufweisen.

Es besteht ferner Übereinstimmung darin, daß die praktische Ausbildung für die Facharztanerkennung allein nicht als ausreichend angesehen werden kann. Zur Vertiefung des theoretischen Fachwissens werden ein Jahr Physiologie oder Pharmakologie oder innere Medizin, und als praktische Ausbildung ein Jahr Chirurgie und zwei Jahre praktische Anaesthesie gefordert. Entsprechend diesen Forderungen wird die Frage berufsständischer bzw. amtlicher Anerkennung als Narkosefacharzt erst vom Jahre 1952 an aktuell.

Es besteht Einigkeit darüber, daß innerhalb der Kliniken die Narkosefachärzte den Charakter als Oberärzte erreichen sollen, jedoch unter jeweiliger Unterstellung unter den Direktor der betr. Klinik bzw. Krankenhausabteilung. Die Möglichkeit einer Niederlassung als Narkosefacharzt in freier Praxis ist von vornherein vorgesehen.

Eine besondere Förderung der Narkosefacharztfrage wird in der Zulassung von Privatdozenten für das Fach der allgemeinen und örtlichen Betäubung gesehen. Entsprechende Habilitationen sind bereits an mehreren Stellen in Vorbereitung, nachdem die praktische Ausbildung besonderer Narkoseärzte an verschiedenen Kliniken bereits seit bald 3 Jahren in Gang ist.

Vorlesungen für Studierende der Medizin und Zahnheilkunde sollen tunlich von Privatdozenten für allgemeine und örtliche Betäubung gehalten werden.

Narkosepersonal soll aus dem Bestande der betr. Kliniken entnommen werden, wobei Erhöhung des Personalbestandes entsprechend der Zahl der für Narkosezwecke abgestellten Hilfskräfte dringend erforderlich ist.

Fortbildungskurse in Anaesthesiefragen für Fachärzte für Chirurgie, Gynäkologie etc. sind in Aussicht genommen.

Vorstand und Ausschuß der Deutschen Gesellschaft für Chirurgie haben vorstehenden Feststellungen bzw. Vorschlägen in ihrer Münchner Sitzung vom 25. November 1950 zugestimmt.

Die Deutsche Gesellschaft für Chirurgie

Der 1. Schriftführer:

A. Hübner

◻ **Fig. 1.3.** Report of the Anaesthetic Commission in November 1950 (Archive of the DGAI)

to the medical press, which – unanimously approved – was sent to specialist journals and periodicals [16]:

> The question regarding specialists in anaesthesia is in full swing. The 'Anaesthetic Commission', appointed by both the German Pharmacological Society and the German Society of Surgery, has drawn up proposals for the relevant administrative bodies and professional associations. The clinical training of specialists in anaesthesia shall remain tied to hospitals dealing with sufficiently high numbers of operations to guarantee the appropriate number of anaesthetics. Apart from the clinical training (1 year in surgery and 2 years exclusively in anaesthetics) a year in pharmacology, physiology or medicine is required for covering theory. The clinical training of specialists in anaesthesia has already been in progress at a number of hospitals for about 3 years. Opportunities for a habilitation and lectureship in anaesthesia are already being set up at several universities.

With the acceptance of the report of the Anaesthetic Commission, the German Society of Surgery gave up its long resistance to the introduction of specialists in anaesthesia. Apart from the points mentioned in the press release however, its representatives on this commission, in particular Karl Heinrich Bauer, succeeded in pushing through the clause »that within surgical units anaesthetists could achieve the position of senior physicians; however, they were to remain subordinate to the director of the clinic or hospital department«. Thus, for the time being, the development of anaesthesia was predestined to become part of the hierarchical structure of surgery.

While scientific discussions continued at subsequent surgical conferences, increasingly aspects of professional politics – e.g. the »specialist« question, posts in anaesthesia, employment contract, specialist societies – gained in importance after this forced change of direction. A graphic impression of the conflicting views within the German Society of Surgery is revealed by Martin Zindler in his personal reflections about events at this time, which he himself had in part influenced. The following is an extract:

1.1.4 The Fight for Independence

by M. Zindler

An important milestone on the way to recognition as a specialty and to full independence (including university chairs) was the leading presentation by Ernst Derra, Professor of Surgery in Düsseldorf (with whom I later worked) in 1950 at the 67th Conference of the German Society of Surgery about »The current state of anaesthetic techniques in surgery« [10] during which he said in his concluding remarks:

> Modern anaesthesia has become a diverse and difficult art. Abroad, colleges of anaesthesia have been created which train specialists. This is the best solution which will also be unavoidable at our major hospitals. We must not hesitate any longer. A form suiting German circumstances would be the establishment of chairs at several universities with responsibility for the practice of anaesthetics within large clinics as well as for teaching and research.

These were far-sighted, almost prophetic words at a time when there were only about 30 surgical residents with experience in so-called modern anaesthesia, i.e. intubation anaesthesia, who, as it were, dealt with anaesthesia as a side job without prospect of a secure living. Influential surgeons were still decidedly against anaesthesia becoming independent. Robert Macintosh, who received the first Chair of Anaesthesia in Europe in 1934 through an endowment from the car manufacturer Lord Nuffield, was also invited to this conference. He said during the discussion that the choice of anaesthetic technique was without doubt up to the anaesthetist. At that time – 1950 – the surgeons in the audience were very surprised that this natural right, in their opinion, should be taken away from them.

At the end of the meeting, the President of the conference E. von Redwitz announced that the Committee of the German Society of Surgery had considered the problems of anaesthetists and would warn against the rash creation of a Specialist in Anaesthesia [30]. It states in the minutes of this Committee Meeting that it is not the training of anaesthetists that is important but rather the improved tuition of anaesthetic nurses.

The Chairman of the Anaesthetic Commission, K. H. Bauer, Professor of Surgery at Heidelberg University, has hindered the development and independence of anaesthesia in Germany for many precious years. His main objective was that anaesthetists should not achieve independence. Again and again he stressed that in the operating theatre only one could bear responsibility, and this was the surgeon to whom the patient would come. This responsibility would be indivisible and therefore anaesthetists should remain subject to directives.

Again in 1955 – 2 years after introduction of the Specialist Anaesthetist – Bauer addressed this issue at the Congress of the German Society of Surgery: »those of you who want to separate anaesthesia are taking away the core of general surgery«. And he added that it was his opinion that independent anaesthesia departments would not be a matter of interest for the anaesthetists themselves.

1.1.5 Further Steps Towards Independence

The report by the Anaesthetic Commission was published in various journals, including *Medizinische Welt* (Medical World), *Der Krankenhausarzt* (The Hospital Doctor) and *Der Anaesthesist* (The Anaesthetist) [17]. Günter Möller of Wuppertal-Barmen expressed the view of the German Association of Hospital Doctors (Marburger Bund) at the suggestion of the German Society of Surgery and in response to the points raised by Hans Killian [49]. Möller pointed out that the scope of duties of the anaesthetist is substantially more far-reaching than just giving anaesthetics. He proposed a detailed curriculum for their training. However, the education should not be the responsibility of only the universities, but rather mainly of the hospitals. It follows that the German Specialist's Committee was launched through the State Chambers of Physicians and not through the universities.

The following text was adopted unanimously for the introduction of the title »Specialist in Anaesthesia« during a meeting of the Board of Directors of the Working Committee of the West German State Chambers of Physicians on 13 January 1951 in Cologne:

> The final provisions should be defined after discussions with the German Society of Surgery, the German Society of Internal Medicine, the German Pharmacological Society and the German Physiological Society. In the *Ärztliche Mitteilungen* (Information for Physicians) it should be announced that it would be a precondition for the future anaesthetist to work in internal medicine, physiology, pharmacology and surgery as well as spend 2 years of advanced training in anaesthesia which would need to be completed in a large surgical clinic.

Since consultation with the specialty societies had not yet taken place, the Board of the Working Committee of the West German State Chambers of Physicians approved at their meeting on 15 September 1951 in Düsseldorf the Associations' draft of the amendment of the terms of reference for »specialist« approval without reference to anaesthesia. The German Medical Assembly decided therefore to devolve the matter of specialist recognition with respect to anaesthesia to the respective State Chambers of Physicians until a federal template had been established. Regarding this decision a provisional recognition of any individual case in anaesthesia was agreed. The North Rhine Chamber of Physicians proved again to be a forerunner.

In the same year Rudolf Frey of Heidelberg, Otto Mayrhofer of Vienna and Werner Hügin of Basel agreed to assume the traditions of the pre-war journal *Schmerz – Narkose – Anaesthesie* (Pain, Narcosis, Anaesthesia) and to establish their own international German-language journal. In a similar vein to *Der Chirurg* (The Surgeon) the new journal was entitled *Der Anaesthesist* (The Anaesthetist). Despite there being only 17 full-time anaesthetists working at that time in Germany, the publishing house Springer, Heidelberg, agreed to be the publisher. The first issue appeared at the end of April 1952. As subsequent developments have proven, the participation of this publishing house has been worthwhile (► Chap. 1.5.1).

In the year 1952, Ernst Derra stated in »Thoughts on the reorganization of anaesthesia in Germany« [11], published in *Das Krankenhaus* (The Hospital), that an anaesthetist could be a valuable asset not only in thorax surgery, but also in general surgery and the other surgical subspecialties. In his view, the subordination under the surgeon as recommended by the Anaesthetic Commission should be maintained. Furthermore he considered the funding of trainee anaesthetists as a difficult area in view of the unsettled question of specialist recognition.

After the then majority in the *Bundestag* (Federal Parliament) failed to affirm statutory regulations leading to attribution of a specialist medical title – the *Bundesrat* (Federal Council) had not given its approval – the Board of the Working Committee of the West German State Chambers of Physicians decided at the beginning of 1952 to recommend to the various State Chambers to implement the decisions of the respective German Medical Assembly regarding specialist recognition in the future and to guarantee mutual recognition.

The Chamber of Physicians of the Saarland – still under French administration – was the first to follow this recommendation in March 1952 and introduced the specialist title in anaesthesia under the specialist statutes of the Saarland.

The first individual to receive specialist recognition in anaesthesia in Germany was Werner Sauerwein of the Bürgerspital, Saarbrücken, on 27 May 1953 (◘ Fig. 1.4), which was 4 months before the decisive meeting of the German Medical Assembly in Lindau, at which the delegates had decided in favour of the specialist title, i.e. *Facharzt für Anästhesie* (see below).

At the 69th Congress of the German Society of Surgery in April 1952 in Munich the Chairman Karl Heinrich Bauer of Heidelberg discussed in his opening address »the intellectual standing of our specialty« [5] with regard to the problem of the fragmentation of surgery due to specialization and in particular about anaesthesia. He acknowledged the advances in surgery facilitated by modern anaesthesia, which he referred to as the latest surgical specialty. His own receptiveness towards »the anaesthetic problem« was mirrored in the establishment of an anaesthetic department in his own clinic and for the purpose of the congress he had created a new section entitled »Modern Anaesthesia«. He reflected:

The surgeon would never be able to anaesthetize the patient himself and the anaesthetist cannot operate. But surgeon and anaesthetist work in the same hospital, in the same room, at the same time, on the same patient. Serious teamwork is therefore the only possible way forward. So, what is more natural than that the teamwork in the operating theatre is reflected by teamwork during the congress.

However the anaesthetist, like all other specialists in surgery, is restricted, like the surgeon, to the operating theatre, i.e. »under the roof where the operation takes place. Therefore, using this 'under one roof' principle the centrifugal development of the specialization becomes to a considerable degree a centripetal development«. Hence there was no necessity for a totally independent anaesthetic specialty.

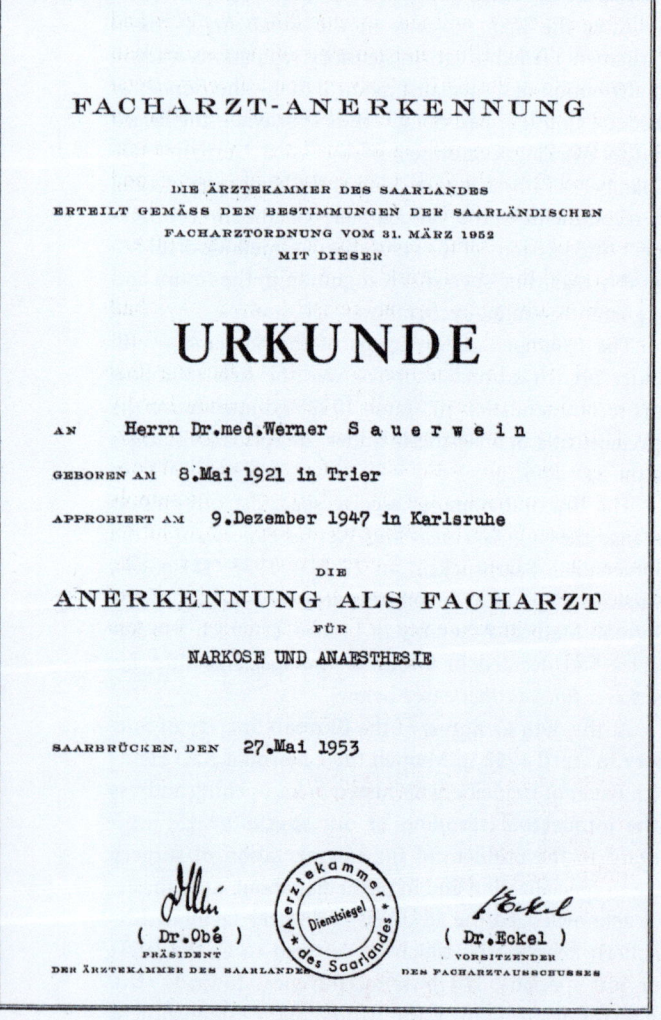

■ **Fig. 1.4.** The first Specialist Diploma for Anaesthesia (courtesy of Dr. Werner Sauerwein, Constance)

Echoing the recommendations of the Anaesthetic Commission he reiterated: »What we can do is to create a confederation of all surgical specialties, to grant the smaller units more independence, but unite them under the umbrella of general surgery. That is our 'Surgical Magna Charta'«. On behalf of the President, Emil Karl Frey of Munich took on the chairmanship of the newly established section »Modern Anaesthesia« [23]. He conceded in his preliminary remarks that just as there are specialists in other areas of surgery, »it cannot be disputed that in the light of the huge importance of modern anaesthesia, that a real expert in his field, who can show that he has the proper credentials should also be accredited as a Specialist in Anaesthesia«. But he also expressed the view that anaesthesia should not be separated from general surgery and that the surgeon should retain sole responsibility, »but involving naturally the appropriate consultation and closest collaboration with the anaesthetist«. There was no apparent objection to the incongruity of this statement. In this regard E. K. Frey alluded to the findings of the Anaesthetic Commission which was set up in conjunction with the pharmacologists. Any relevant questions should be directed to the Head of the Commission, Karl Heinrich Bauer. In addition he announced the imminent appearance of the journal *Der Anaesthesist*, the first issue of which would contain a detailed review of the papers on modern anaesthesia which had been delivered in Munich. In the run-up to the German Medical Assembly in 1952 the decision was made not to deal once again with the statutes of specialization but rather to defer these to the meeting of 1953.

1.1.6 Founding of a German Working Group on Anaesthesiology

In October 1951 the Austrian Society of Anaesthesiology was founded and this was followed by official state recognition of the Specialist in Anaesthesia in June 1952. In September of the same year the first Austrian Congress of Anaesthesiology took place in Salzburg. German representatives who gave talks included Joachim Bark of Todtmoos, Wolfgang Irmer of Düsseldorf, Werner Sauerwein of Saarbrücken, Rudolf Frey of Heidelberg, J. Fischer and J. Hernandez-Richter of Munich, Hans Wilhelm Buchholz of Hamburg and Paul Schostok of Giessen.

At this meeting in Salzburg, and cognizant of the recognition by the Austrian surgeons of their anaesthetic colleagues, the German anaesthetists met on 5 September during the lunch hour and decided upon the establishment of a German Working Group on Anaesthesiology with the purpose of, as stated in the founding statutes, furthering anaesthesia through their joint efforts, the improvement in working conditions as well as striving for the recognition of both the specialist title and specialized training in anaesthesia.

The founding document[1] carries 23 signatures (▫ Fig. 1.5a,b). The founding members elected Heinz-Joachim Bark as Chairman. At this time he was employed at the Grenzlandklinik Wehrawald near Todtmoos in the Black Forest. This working group was conceived as a forerunner of a German Specialist Society whose birth was to be in Munich the following year. The year 1952 was therefore important for anaesthesia in Germany: the **German Working Group on Anaesthesiology** was founded. The journal ***Der Anaesthesist*** appeared and a section of **»Modern Anaesthesia«** was set up as part of the Congress of the **German Society of Surgery**. Recognition of the specialty was at last in sight. With this in mind, a circular was sent out by Heinz-Joachim Bark to all members of the newly founded group which included the following:

1. The Statutes and the conditions of specialization are ready in a provisional form.
2. Contact with the **German Medical Assembly** has been taken up. Professor Neuffer (the then President of the Assembly) endorses the incorporation of the **»Specialist in Anaesthesia«**.
3. The link with the **German Society of Surgery** has been made. The Chairman, Professor Borchers, is sympathetic to our efforts. The anaesthesia session will take place on 11 April 1953.
4. The next business meeting will take place on 10 April 1953 in Munich. The following speakers are invited:
   - L. Zürn: On the organization of our future meetings.
   - R. Frey: Presentation and discussion of the by-laws.
   - M. Zindler: Conditions for recognition as Specialist in Anaesthesia.
   - S. Loennecken: The minimal criteria for a minimum living wage.
   - P. Schostok: Organization of finances.
   - R. Frey: The Society's mouthpiece ***Der Anaesthesist***.
   - W. lrmer and F. H. Koss: The place of the surgical anaesthetist.

[1] The original document has since disappeared. The copy in ▫ Fig. 1.7 comes from a legacy bequeathed by the First Secretary of the Society Rudolf Frey.

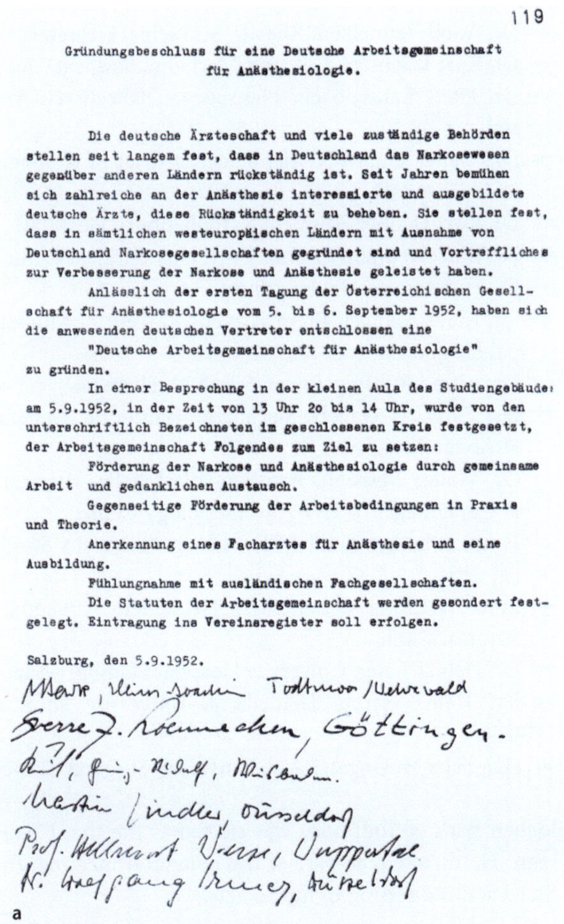

119

Gründungsbeschluss für eine Deutsche Arbeitsgemeinschaft für Anästhesiologie.

Die deutsche Ärzteschaft und viele zuständige Behörden stellen seit langem fest, dass in Deutschland das Narkosewesen gegenüber anderen Ländern rückständig ist. Seit Jahren bemühen sich zahlreiche an der Anästhesie interessierte und ausgebildete deutsche Ärzte, diese Rückständigkeit zu beheben. Sie stellen fest, dass in sämtlichen westeuropäischen Ländern mit Ausnahme von Deutschland Narkosegesellschaften gegründet sind und Vortreffliches zur Verbesserung der Narkose und Anästhesie geleistet haben.

Anlässlich der ersten Tagung der Österreichischen Gesellschaft für Anästhesiologie vom 5. bis 6. September 1952, haben sich die anwesenden deutschen Vertreter entschlossen eine

"Deutsche Arbeitsgemeinschaft für Anästhesiologie"

zu gründen.

In einer Besprechung in der kleinen Aula des Studiengebäudes am 5.9.1952, in der Zeit von 13 Uhr 2o bis 14 Uhr, wurde von den unterschriftlich Bezeichneten im geschlossenen Kreis festgesetzt, der Arbeitsgemeinschaft Folgendes zum Ziel zu setzen:

Förderung der Narkose und Anästhesiologie durch gemeinsame Arbeit und gedanklichen Austausch.

Gegenseitige Förderung der Arbeitsbedingungen in Praxis und Theorie.

Anerkennung eines Facharztes für Anästhesie und seine Ausbildung.

Fühlungnahme mit ausländischen Fachgesellschaften.

Die Statuten der Arbeitsgemeinschaft werden gesondert festgelegt. Eintragung ins Vereinsregister soll erfolgen.

Salzburg, den 5.9.1952.

a

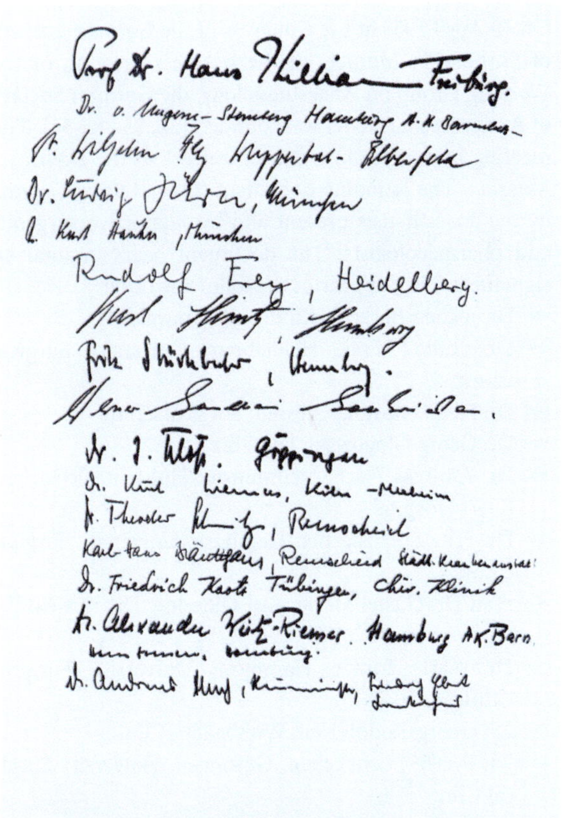

b

▫ **Fig. 1.5a,b.** Certificate of Formation of the German Working Group on Anaesthesiology of 5 September 1952 (Archive of the DGAI)

1

– K. Horatz: The place of the anaesthetist in the public eye.

5. After discussion the foundation of the German Society of Anaesthesia will take place and the Chairman for the coming year will be elected.

6. On 9 April 1953 there will be a dinner meeting of anaesthetists where any remaining questions will be dealt with.

7. The negotiations with State Chambers of Physicians have been either satisfactory or successful.

8. P. Schostok, the Treasurer requests the acceptance of the proposal for immediate payment of the yearly subscription of DM 10.00 which was agreed in Salzburg.

9. Following the efforts of M. Zindler, the North Rhine Chamber of Physicians has recognized the title of Specialist in Anaesthesia and this should determine future developments in the rest of the Federal Republic. It is being discussed whether there should be a written or oral examination at the end of training.

1.1.7 Founding of the German Society of Anaesthesia (DGA)

On 10 April 1953 at the Congress of the German Society of Surgery in Munich, at the business meeting of the Working Group on Anaesthesiology, the German Society of Anaesthesia (DGA) was founded [22, 23, 46, 53]. The meeting took place in lecture theatre 1 in the *Deutsches Museum*. The founding document (◘ Fig. 1.6) was signed by the anaesthetists present and by supportive surgeons and pharmacologists. The document bears in total 46 signatures. They appear in the following order:

- Dr. Jochen Bark, Todtmoos, Wehrawald
- Dr. Rudolf Frey, Heidelberg, University Surgical Clinic
- Dr. Paul Schostok, Giessen, Surgical Clinic
- Dr. Georg Glogowski, Bad Tölz
- Dr. Andreas Flach, Neumünster/Holstein, Friedrich-Ebert Hospital
- Dr. Fritz Stürtzbecher, Hamburg, University Surgical Clinic
- Frau Dr. Gustel Merle, Bad Oldesloe, District Hospital
- Dr. Karl Horatz, Hamburg, University Surgical Clinic
- Dr. Georg-Rudolf Keil, Wiesbaden, Clinic
- Dr. Sverre Loennecken, Göttingen, University Surgical Clinic
- Dr. Friedrich-Wilhelm Koch, Vienna 20, Trauma Hospital
- Dr. Heinz Oehmig, Heidelberg, University Surgical Clinic

- Dr. Otto Just, Berlin-Charlottenburg, University Surgical Clinic, Westend Hospital
- Dr. Friedrich Kootz, Marburg/Lahn, University Surgical Clinic
- Dr. Ludwig Zürn, Munich, Nussbaumstrasse 15
- Dr. Martin Zindler, Düsseldorf, Moorenstrasse 5
- Dr. Wolfgang Irmer, Düsseldorf, Moorenstrasse 5
- Dr. Hans Joachim Harder, Berlin N 65, Rudolf Virchow Hospital
- Dr. Lothar Barth, Berlin-Buch, Lindenberger Weg 76
- Dr. Werner Sauerwein, Saarbrücken, Bürgerhospital
- Prof. Dr. Fritz Hesse, Saarbrücken, Bürgerhospital
- Dr. Günther Möller, Wuppertal-Barmen, Stahlstr. 11
- Dr. Friedrich Körner, Freiburg/Br., Wintererstr. 65
- Prof. Dr. Hellmut Weese, Wuppertal, Doenberger Str. 8
- Prof. Dr. Hans Killian, Freiburg i. Br., Reutestr. 2
- Dr. Josef Schuster, Städt. Krankenhaus, Schweinfurt
- Dr. Horst Wiesebrock, Münster, University Surgical Clinic
- Dr. Robert Enzenbach, Munich, University Surgical Clinic
- Dr. Albert Schürholz, Münster (Westphalia), University Surgical Clinic
- Franz Mathis, Quierschied/Saar, Miner's Hospital
- Dr. Adolf Benoelken, Rheydt, Municipal Hospital
- Dr. Kurt Wiemers, Cologne-Merheim, Surgical Clinic
- Dr. Hans Lautenbach, Flensburg, Diakonissen-Anstalt
- Dr. Walter Quarz, Marienheide, District of Cologne, State Hospital
- Dr. Kurt Hauber, Munich, Nymphenburg Hospital
- Dr. Karl Dietmann, Bonn, University Surgical Clinic
- Dr. Horst Ehren, Ludwigsburg
- Dr. Klaus Mangel, Bremerhaven-M, Central Municipal Hospital
- Dr. Alfred Rohling, Essen, Elisabeth Hospital
- Dr. F. W. v. Ungern-Sternberg, Hamburg, General Hospital Barmbek
- Dr. Walter Massion, Arnsberg/Westphalia, currently at Copenhagen WHO-Anesthesiology Center
- Frau Dr. Esther Krabbe, Heidelberg, University Surgical Clinic
- Frau Dr. Elma v. Lüttichau, Heidelberg, University Surgical Clinic
- Dr. Heiner Lang, University Hospital Homburg/Saar
- Dr. Heinz Georg, Heidelberg, University Surgical Clinic
- (Dr. Felix H. Ungar, Basel, University Surgical Clinic)

Jochen Bark of Todtmoos was elected as the first Chairman. He directed, as part of the inaugural meeting, the first scientific session of the Society.

DEUTSCHE GESELLSCHAFT FÜR ANAESTHESIE

Der Vorsitzende für das Jahr 1953/54:　　Heilstätte Wehrawald, den
DR. J. BARK　　Todtmoos/Schwarzwald

P r o t o k o l l
━━━━━━━━━

über die Gründungsversammlung der Deutschen
Gesellschaft für Anaesthesie
am Freitag, den 10.4.1953
im Vortragssaal 1 des Deutschen Museums in München.

Der Vorsitzende der am 5.September 1952 in Salzburg
gegründeten Deutschen Arbeitsgemeinschaft für Anaesthesiologie,
Herr Dr. J. Bark, berief die deutschen Spezialisten für Anaesthesie auf den 10.April 1953, 9 Uhr vormittags, in das Deutsche
Museum in München ein. Es versammelten sich ca. 70 Anaesthesisten.

Die beiliegenden Satzungen wurden einstimmig angenommen.
Die Annahme wurde durch Unterschrift bestätigt.

Es wurden die Fragen der zukünftigen Kongresse für
Anaesthesie diskutiert, die zusammen mit den oesterreichischen
und schweizerischen Anaesthesie-Gesellschaften abgehalten werden
sollen.

Die von Dozent Dr.R.Frey, Heidelberg, Chir.Univ.Klinik,
redigierte Zeitschrift "Der Anaesthesist" (Springer-Verlag)
wurde zum Organ der Gesellschaft gewählt.

Es wurden gewählt:

1.) Dr. J.Bark, Wehrawald, zum 1. Vorsitzenden,
2.) Dozent Dr.R.Frey, Heidelberg, zum 1. (ständigen) Schriftführer,
3.) Dr. G.Müller, Wuppertal-Barmen, Stahlstr. 11, zum Kassenführer.

In den Ausschuß wurden gewählt:
Dr. O.Just, Berlin, zum 2.Schriftführer, der den ständigen
Schriftführer vertritt und zum Vertreter in Berlin,

a

- 2 -

Dr. K. Zindler, Düsseldorf, zum Sachbearbeiter für Facharztfragen,

Dr. Horatz, Hamburg, zum Sachbearbeiter für Presse und Rundfunk,

Dr. W. Irmer, Düsseldorf, zum Verbindungsmann zu den nebenberuflichen Anaesthesisten.

Im Anschluß an die Gründungsversammlung wurde die
1. wissenschaftliche Sitzung (14 - 19 Uhr) im Hörsaal 1 abgehalten. Die 2. wissenschaftliche Sitzung wurde am Samstag,
den 11.April, gemeinsam mit der Deutschen Gesellschaft
für Chirurgie im Kongreßsaal des Deutschen Museums mit ca.
1 200 Teilnehmern abgehalten.

München, den 10.April 1953
Dr.Fr./Ha

R. Frey.

(Priv.Doz.Dr.R.Frey)
1.(ständiger) Schriftführer

b

S a t z u n g e n
der
Deutschen Gesellschaft für Anaesthesie

§ 1. Name, Zweck und Sitz der Gesellschaft
Die Deutsche Gesellschaft für Anaesthesie (= D.G.A.) bezweckt,
deutsche Ärzte zu gemeinsamer Arbeit am Ausbau und Fortschritt
der Anaesthesie zu vereinen und die Interessen ihrer Mitglieder
zu wahren. Sie ist ein gemeinnütziger eingetragener Verein im
Sinne des § 21 BGB.
Sie hat ihren Sitz am jeweiligen Wohnsitz des Schriftführers.
Die Eintragung ins Vereinsregister erfolgt beim Amtsgericht
Heidelberg.

§ 2. Kongresse
Zur Erreichung dieses Zweckes veranstaltet die D.G.A. jährlich
- in der Regel gemeinsam mit dem Kongress der Deutschen Gesellschaft für Chirurgie - eine Zusammenkunft. Tag, Ort und Programm
der Tagung, sowie die Zahl der Sitzungstage bestimmt der Vorstand
der Gesellschaft.

§ 3. Vermögen
Das Vermögen der D.G.A. setzt sich zusammen aus Kapital und Barver-
mögen, entstanden aus den Jahresbeiträgen und aus Zuwendungen, welche der D.G.A. von Mitgliedern oder von Dritten gemacht werden.
Das Vermögen verwaltet der Kassenführer. Ausgaben außerhalb des
laufenden Geschäftsbetriebes bedürfen der Gegenzeichnung durch den
Vorsitzenden. Der Kassenführer ist verpflichtet, jährlich einen
Kassenbericht zu erstatten. Nach Überprüfung und Richtigbefund
durch zwei von der Vollversammlung gewählte ordentliche Mitglieder
wird ihm von der Vollversammlung Entlastung erteilt.

§ 4. Zusammensetzung und Organe
Die D.G.A. besteht aus ordentlichen, außerordentlichen, korrespon-
dierenden und aus Ehrenmitgliedern, sowie einem wissenschaftlichen
Beirat.
Offizielles Mitteilungsblatt der D.G.A. ist die Zeitschrift
"Der Anaesthesist".

§ 5. Mitglieder
Mitglied der Gesellschaft kann werden, wer sich in anerkannter
Weise praktisch oder wissenschaftlich mit Anaesthesie beschäftigt.
Wer in die Gesellschaft als Mitglied aufgenommen werden will, muß
einen schriftlichen Antrag an den Schriftführer stellen. Über die
Aufnahme entscheidet ein vom Vorstand zu ernennender Ausschuß nach
Anhörung zweier ordentlicher Mitglieder, die den Antragsteller ken-
nen.

c

- 2 -

Ordentliche Mitglieder müssen Fachärzte für Anaesthesie sein gemäß
den beigefügten Facharztbestimmungen.
Pharmakologen, Physiologen, Chirurgen und andere Ärzte und Wissenschaftler, sowie
Anaesthesisten, die noch in Ausbildung begriffen sind oder die Tätigkeit als Anaesthesist nur nebenberuflich ausüben, können als außeror-
dentliche Mitglieder aufgenommen werden. Diese nehmen an den wissenschaftlichen Verhandlungen in gleicher Weise teil, wie die ordentlichen Mitglieder und haben beratende Stimme.
Ausländische Anaesthesisten, die zur Förderung der Anaesthesie in
Deutschland beigetragen haben, können als korrespondierende Mitglieder aufgenommen werden.

§ 6. Ehrenmitglieder
Hervorragende Ärzte, Naturforscher und Gelehrte, die durch ihre Arbei-
ten zur Förderung der Anaesthesie wesentlich beigetragen haben, können
zu Ehrenmitgliedern oder korrespondierenden Mitgliedern ernannt werden.
Hervorragende Vertreter anderer Fachgebiete, die den Problemen der Anaesthesie aufgeschlossen gegenüberstehen, können in den Beirat der Gesellschaft berufen werden. Sie beraten die Gesellschaft in Fragen ihrer Fachgebiete.
Die Ernennung von Ehrenmitgliedern erfolgt auf der Hauptversammlung.
Zur Ernennung von Ehrenmitgliedern bedarf es des einstimmigen Beschlusses des Vorstands und einer Mehrheit von 4/5 der anwesenden Mitglieder;
zur Ernennung korrespondierender Mitglieder und des Beirates des einstimmigen Beschlusses des Ausschusses.

§ 7. Beiträge
Der Jahresbeitrag der ordentlichen und außerordentlichen Mitglieder
wird von der Hauptversammlung festgesetzt.
Ehrenmitglieder und korrespondierende Mitglieder, sowie Mitglieder des
Beirates sind nicht zur Entrichtung von Beiträgen verpflichtet.
Die Zahlung der Beiträge erfolgt in der ersten Hälfte des Jahres an den
Kassenführer.

§ 8. Ausschluß von Mitgliedern
Mitgliedern, welche durch ihr Verhalten die Zwecke und das Ansehen der
Gesellschaft schädigen, kann auf einstimmigen Antrag des Vorstandes der
Rat zum Austritt gegeben werden. Kommen sie dem Rat nicht nach, können
sie durch die Vollversammlung mit 2/3-Mehrheit ausgeschlossen werden.
Ein Mitglied, das trotz zweimaliger Mahnung des Kassenführers mit sei-
nem Beitrag - ohne hinreichenden Grund - länger als ein Jahr in Rück-
stand bleibt, gilt als ausgeschieden und wird in die Liste gestrichen.
Wiedereintritt in die Gesellschaft kann nur mit Genehmigung des Vorstandes erfolgen, sobald die rückständigen Beiträge nachgezahlt worden
sind.
Ein Mitglied, das zum Verlust der Bürgerlichen Ehrenrechte rechtskräf-
tig verurteilt ist, verliert ohne weiteres die Mitgliedschaft.

d

■ Fig. 1.6a–h. Founding documents of the German Society of Anaesthesia of 10 April 1953 (Archive of the DGAI)

- 3 -

§ 9. Vorstand und Ausschuß

Der Vorstand der D.G.A. besteht aus:
1. dem Vorsitzenden,
2. dem ständigen Schriftführer, der die Gesellschaft gerichtlich und außergerichtlich vertritt und zugleich stellvertretender Vorsitzender ist,
3. dem Kassenführer.

Der Vorstand wird unterstützt von einem Ausschuß; dieser setzt sich zusammen aus:
1. den Vorstandsmitgliedern,
2. dem bisherigen Vorsitzenden, der zugleich zweiter stellvertretender Vorsitzender ist,
3. dem 2. Schriftführer, der den ständigen Schriftführer vertritt,
4. dem Sachbearbeiter für Facharztfragen,
5. dem Sachbearbeiter für Presse und Rundfunk,
6. dem Verbindungsmann zu den nebenberuflichen Anaesthesisten,
7. je einem Vertreter in Berlin und in Ostdeutschland.

§ 10. Wahl des Vorstandes und des Ausschusses

Die Wahl der Vorstands- und Ausschußmitglieder erfolgt in der Hauptversammlung nach demokratischen Gesichtspunkten. Ihre Amtsdauer beträgt zwei Jahre.

Zu Vorstands- und Ausschußmitgliedern können nur ordentliche Mitglieder gewählt werden - mit Ausnahme des Verbindungsmannes zu den nebenberuflichen Anaesthesisten, der ein außerordentliches Mitglied sein sollte.

Alle Mitglieder des Vorstandes, mit Ausnahme des Vorsitzenden, sind wiederwählbar.

§ 11. Hauptversammlung

Die Hauptversammlung besteht aus den ordentlichen, außerordentlichen, korrespondierenden und Ehrenmitgliedern der Gesellschaft. Sie ist beschlußfähig, wenn mindestens 20 % der ordentlichen Mitglieder anwesend sind.

Soweit die Statuten nichts anderes bestimmen, faßt die Hauptversammlung durch einfache Stimmenmehrheit der Abstimmenden Beschluß. Bei Stimmengleichheit entscheidet die Stimme des Vorsitzenden.

Vorschläge zur Hauptversammlung sind mindestens 4 Wochen vor der Versammlung beim Vorsitzenden oder den ständigen Schriftführer einzureichen.

Über den Verlauf der Hauptversammlung hat der Schriftführer ein Protokoll anzulegen.

Die Teilnehmer tragen sich in eine Anwesenheitsliste ein.

e

- 4 -

§ 12. Satzungsänderungen

Änderungen der Satzungen können nur durch die Hauptversammlung mit 2/3-Mehrheit beschlossen werden nach vorheriger Mitteilung der vorgeschlagenen Änderung an alle Mitglieder.

§ 13. Auflösung der Gesellschaft

Für die Auflösung der Gesellschaft gelten die gesetzlichen Vorschriften.

Das Gesellschaftsvermögen ist bei der Auflösung oder bei Wegfall der bisherigen Zwecke einer anderen, steuerlich als gemeinnützig anerkannten Gesellschaft zuzuführen, die es im Sinne des § 1 der Satzungen der Deutschen Gesellschaft für Anaesthesie zu verwenden hat.

Jede Zuwendung von Vermögen oder Vermögensvorteilen an Mitglieder der Deutschen Gesellschaft für Anaesthesie kommt nicht in Frage.

Beschlüsse über die Verwendung des Vermögens der Gesellschaft, sowie Beschlüsse über Satzungsänderungen, die die Zwecke der Gesellschaft und Verwendung ihres Vermögens betreffen, sind vor Inkrafttreten dem zuständigen Finanzamt mitzuteilen.

Über die Verwendung in einzelnen und Beachtung der Bestimmungen der vorhergehenden Absätze entscheidet die Generalversammlung.

München, den 10. April 1953

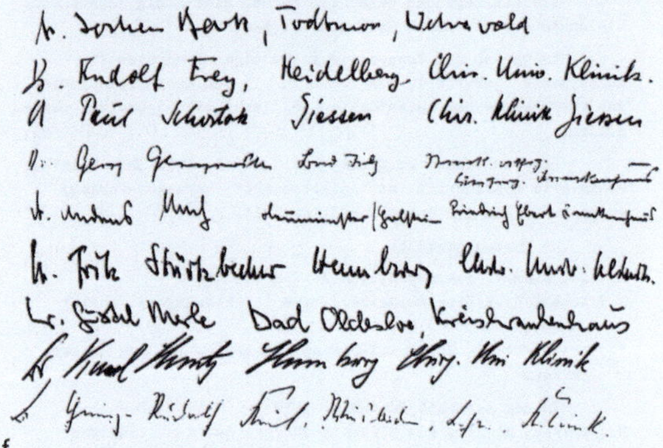

f

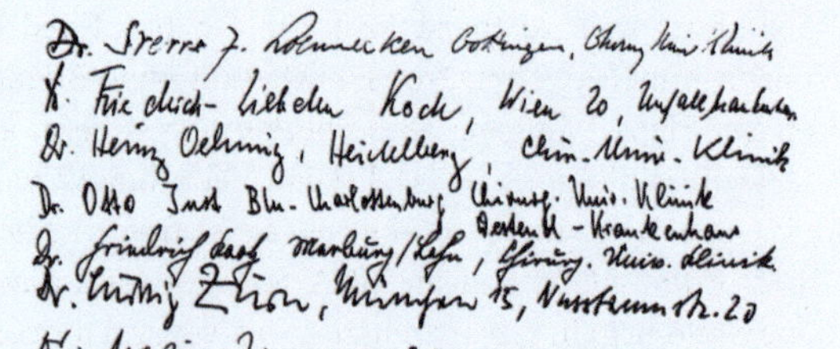

g

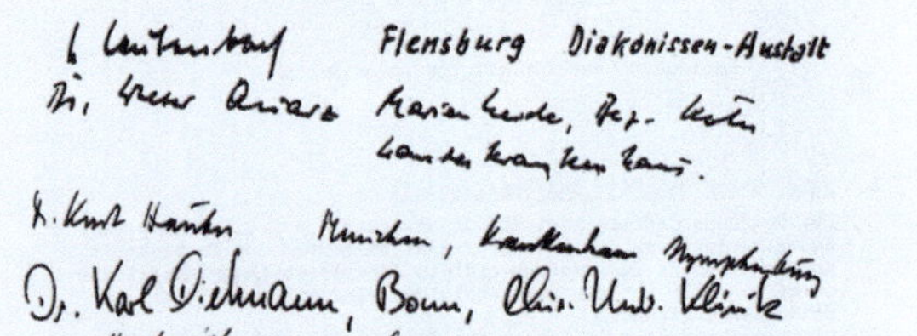

h

■ Fig. 1.6a–h. Continued.

Prof. Dr. Richard Heinz Joachim (Jochen) Bark
(Fig. 1.7)

Born on 23 January 1918 in Weißenborn near Zeitz/Thuringia; deceased on 14 April 1963; 1937–1943 medical studies in Freiburg/Br., Munich and Königsberg, interrupted by military service; 1943 doctorate; 1946 University Surgical Clinic Freiburg (Eduard Rehn) and ENT Clinic (Fritz Zoellner); 1949 thoracic surgery at the Chest Unit Wehrawald, Todtmoos; 1949 anaesthetic training with Sir Robert Macintosh, Oxford; 1949 Anaesthetist at the Chest Unit Wehrawald, Todtmoos; 1952–1954 Founding Chairman of the German Working Group on Anaesthesiology and the German Society of Anaesthesia; 1954 requested by Theodor Naegeli at the Surgical University Clinic of Tübingen to set up an independent anaesthetics department; from 1955 he was obstructed by Theodor Naegeli's successor, Hofrat Walter Dick, for 13 years in his attempts to set up an independent department at Tübingen; 1960–1963 Vice President of the World Federation of Societies of Anaesthesiologists.

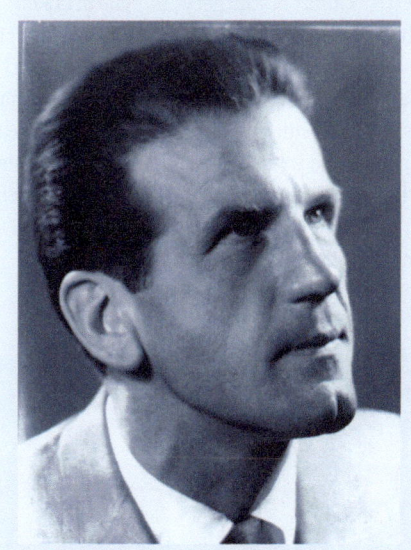

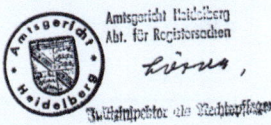 Fig. 1.7. Heinz-Joachim Bark (1918–1963) (Archive of the DGAI)

The journal *Der Anaesthesist*, edited by Rudolf Frey of Heidelberg was earmarked as the Society's official mouthpiece (▶ Chap. 1.5.1). Rudolf Frey was also elected as Permanent Secretary, Günter Möller of Wuppertal-Barmen as Treasurer, Otto Just of Berlin as Vice Secretary and representative in Berlin, Martin Zindler of Düsseldorf was nominated to deal with specialization questions, Karl Horatz of Hamburg was given the portfolio of press and radio and Wolfgang Irmer of Düsseldorf was elected intermediary dealing with avocational anaesthetists. The Society was registered at the Local Court in Heidelberg (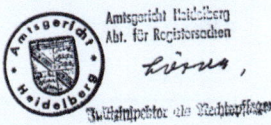 Fig. 1.8).

DEUTSCHE GESELLSCHAFT FÜR ANAESTHESIE

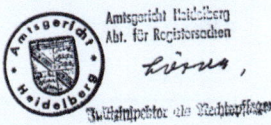 Fig. 1.8. Entry of the DGA into the Register of Societies in Heidelberg (Archive of the DGAI)

The next day a meeting took place with the surgeons represented by the President of the German Society of Surgery Eduard Borchers of Aachen (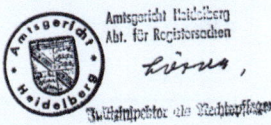 Fig. 1.9). Borchers was the one who had circulated a request made by the DGA through Jochen Bark in August 1953 to the Directors of Academic Surgical Units to set up anaesthetic positions and to consider the creation of »Departments of Anaesthesia« from which surrounding units could be serviced as necessary. He also emphasized that it would be in the interests of the surgeons to work closely with the anaesthetists whose aim was not only recognition but also to be of assistance.

1.1.8 Introduction of the »Specialist Anaesthetist«

At the 56th German Medical Assembly on 19 and 20 September 1953 in Lindau a ballot was proposed to establish the »Specialist Anaesthetist« as a discipline in the Specialist Medical Register. There was almost a historical irony in this, because Otto Goetze, who in his 1939 report had spoken out against the »Specialist Anaesthetist«, was in 1953 President of the German Society of Surgery when this question – 14 years after his statement – was again up for discussion. He did not personally present the vote of his specialist society for health-related reasons, but sent a representative who in the name of the German Society of Surgery wholeheartedly approved the proposal [4]. One justification he put forward was that in current practice the responsibility for the anaesthetic given by nurses and junior doctors lay with the surgeons. This was no longer possible with modern complex operations, as these required the surgeon's undivided attention. Therefore the anaesthetist needed to be on an equal standing with the surgeon and take total responsibility for his actions. »The prerequisite for such a transfer of responsibility to the anaesthetist is dependent on the relevant theoretical training, which is based on specialist subjects that are distinct from surgery and are totally foreign to the surgeon. I am thinking particularly of pharmacology. There is still need for research in this area. Not only their experience, but also the aforementioned considerations demand that the anaesthetist is given the status equivalent to a specialist doctor« [4]. The German Society of Gynaecology also endorsed the proposal to introduce the »Specialist Physician Anaesthetist«, in the run-up to the Medical Assembly. The proposal was accepted by a large majority of the delegates.

To complete the specialist training a 5-year higher postgraduate curriculum was anticipated, comprising 1 year of higher training in surgery, 6 months higher training in pharmacology or physiology, 6 months higher training in general medicine and 1 year in general medical duties – then usual for all postgraduate training programmes. The practical and theoretical postgraduate training in anaesthesia would then take 2 years [3].

Major contributors to this achievement included the surgical mentors Hans Killian (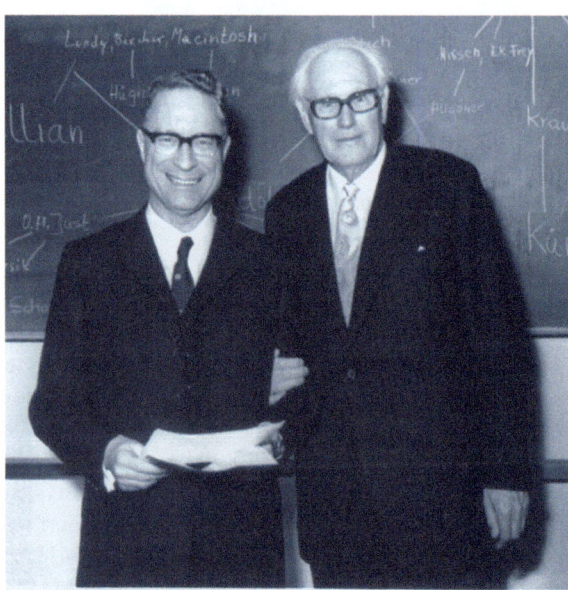 Fig. 1.10) of Donaueschingen, Helmut Schmidt, Chief of Surgery in Remscheid, and Fritz Hesse, Chief of Surgery in Saarbrücken, as well as the pharmacologist Helmut Weese of Wuppertal, who with the help of Ernst Derra secured the support of the Social Welfare Ministry of North Rhine-Westphalia for his request. As a result, 1953 saw the decisive breakthrough for anaesthesia in Germany: the German Society of Anaesthesia was founded and the Specialist Physician Anaesthetist included in the Specialist Medical Discipline Register.

120

EINLADUNG

zur gemeinsamen wissenschaftlichen Sitzung der Deutschen Gesellschaft für Chirurgie und der Deutschen Arbeitsgemeinschaft für Anaesthesiologie am 11. April 1953 im Deutschen Museum in München. Die Sitzung findet statt im Rahmen und im Anschluß an den 70. Deutschen Chirurgenkongreß.

PROGRAMM:

Donnerstag (9. April 1953):

Gemeinsames Abendessen im Regina-Palasthotel, Beginn 18.00 Uhr.

Freitag (10. April 1953):

9—13 Uhr Geschäftssitzung der Deutschen Arbeitsgemeinschaft für Anaesthesiologie im Hörsaal des Deutschen Museums. Vorsitz: J. Bark, Wehrawald.

Samstag (11. April 1953):

9—13 und 14—17 Uhr gemeinsame wissenschaftliche Sitzung der Deutschen Gesellschaft für Chirurgie und der Deutschen Arbeitsgemeinschaft für Anaesthesiologie im Kongreßsaal des Deutschen Museums. Vorsitz: Prof. E. Borchers, Aachen.

Der Vorsitzende, Prof. Borchers, Aachen: Eröffnung der gemeinsamen Sitzung.

R. Frey, Heidelberg: Fortschritte und Erfahrungen mit der künstlichen Blutdrucksenkung.

O. Mayrhofer, Wien: Für und wider die Intubation bei der Anwendung der Muskelrelaxantien.

W. Hügin, Basel: Die Wirkungen der Anaesthetica auf den Stoffwechsel.

K. Mülly, Zürich: Bronchoskopische Technik für den Anaesthesisten, bronchiale Intubation und Blockade.

J. Bark, Wehrawald: Die Anaesthesie bei endobronchialen Eingriffen.

Anmeldungen weiterer Vorträge und Vorführungen (mit kurzer Inhaltsangabe in doppelter Ausfertigung) werden an Professor Dr. E. Borchers, Aachen, Luisenhospital, bis zum 30. Januar 1953 erbeten. Die zugebilligte Sprechzeit darf nicht überschritten werden. Die Zahl der Vorträge ist beschränkt. Der Vorsitzende muß sich deshalb die Aufnahme in das Tagungsprogramm und die Einordnung der Anmeldung vorbehalten. Die weiteren Bedingungen bitten wir dem beiliegenden Einladungsschreiben zum Deutschen Chirurgen-Kongreß entnehmen zu wollen.

Die Mitgliedskarte der Deutschen Gesellschaft für Chirurgie oder der Deutschen Arbeitsgemeinschaft für Anaesthesiologie dient als Teilnehmerkarte. Eintrittskarten für Nichtmitglieder sind außerdem zum Preis von 10.— DM im Kongreß-Büro erhältlich. Quartierbestellung bis 20. März 1953 beim Amtlichen Bayrischen Reisebüro in München, Stachuskiosk, erbeten.

Aachen, im Dezember 1952.   Todtmoos (Schwarzwald), im Dezember 1952.

Der Vorsitzende der Deutschen   Der Vorsitzende der Deutschen Arbeits-
Gesellschaft für Chirurgie   gemeinschaft für Anaesthesiologie

E. Borchers   J. Bark
Luisenhospital Aachen.   Grenzlandheilstätte Wehrawald.

■ Fig. 1.9. Invitation to the general scientific meeting of the German Society of Surgery on 11 April 1953 (Archive of the DGAI)

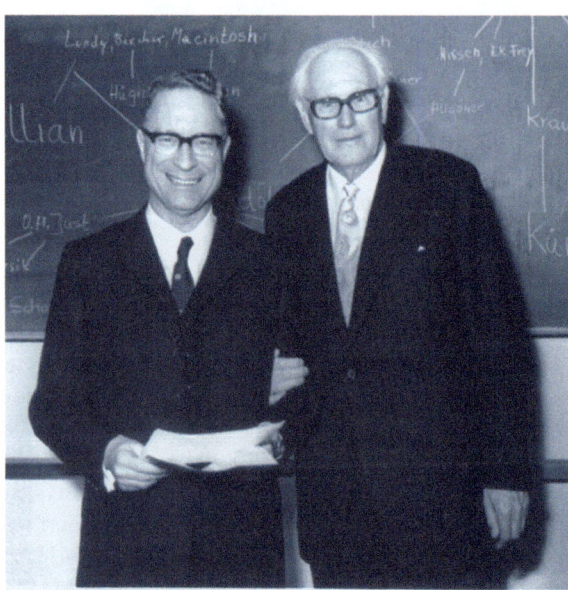

■ Fig. 1.10. Two pioneers of German anaesthesia: Rudolf Frey (left) and Hans Killian (right), on the occasion of the celebration of Hans Killian's 80th birthday on 6 April 1972 in Mainz

1.1.9 The Hierarchical Separation of the Specialties of Surgery and Anaesthesia

The establishment of a specialist society and the introduction of a Specialist Anaesthetist did not mean that anaesthesia, as an independent discipline, was at once of equal ranking to other medical specialties. The anaesthetists continued to remain employees of the hospital department in which they were already working and therefore under the control of the surgical department. It took more than 10 years until a partnership with the surgeons was really achieved with anaesthesia as an independent and autonomous discipline. However, the situation gradually improved: the first anaesthetists reached specialist status and were given their own divisions within the surgical department.

Two years after the introduction of the Specialist Physician Anaesthetist, Karl Heinrich Bauer lectured at the 1955 Annual Meeting of the German Society of Surgery on »The transformation of anaesthesia from the surgeon's perspective« [6] and reiterated his opinion about the status of anaesthesia. His recognition of the achievements of anaesthetists from the surgical viewpoint was more explicit than in his Presidential Address at the 1952 Annual Congress of the German Society of Surgery. We stand »today in the operating theatre before the irretrievable division of labour: the surgeon devotes himself fully to his operation, while the anaesthetist monitors and controls all the patient's vital functions. Those who like paradoxes could express it as follows: the anaesthetist is the specialist for everything non-operative, for everything non-specialist, to a certain extent for everything perioperative, while the surgeon is the specialist for the specific operation«. As a guideline for the collaboration in the operating theatre he proposed: »collaboration through division of labour, a prerequisite for better results and reduced risks.« Naturally the anaesthetist must have the potential to achieve a reasonable career position. However, he also held the view that it was too soon for a professorial »Chair of Anaesthesia« or anaesthesia as an examination subject. He strongly advised against the trend to »separate anaesthesia from general surgery and to expand it in its own right as a specialty for all areas of surgery«. In his opinion, anaesthesia still belonged under the department of general surgery: »those of you who want to separate anaesthesia are taking away the core of general surgery.« The anaesthetist might be legally responsible as a specialist for his anaesthetic but not totally responsible for the patient. That lay with the surgeon who had the contract with the patient. From this arose the transcendence of the operation and therefore the surgeon. K. H. Bauer, representing the surgeons, was still not prepared to give anaesthesia its full independent responsibility, even though he was using flawed logic: the anaesthetist, albeit as a specialist,

was legally responsible for his anaesthetic but the overall responsibility of the surgeon was not negotiable.

In 1961 he tried to reinforce this view with an expert legal opinion. During a period of intensive negotiations between the Anaesthetic Commission of the German Society of Surgery and representatives of the German Society of Anaesthesia, he commissioned a report from the Professor of Criminal Law at the University of Heidelberg and renowned expert for medical law, Karl Engisch, which he presented in 1961: »How is the responsibility of surgeons in relation to the responsibility of anaesthetists during operations to be legally determined and defined?« [19]. At the time that this opinion was being drawn up, co-operation, based on the division of labour between doctors of different disciplines, was long accepted as routine, and the term »principle of trust« in relation to the Road Traffic Act had already been introduced in the context of division of labour during operations. Günther Stratenwerth, an eminent criminal lawyer with his noteworthy commentary, further reinforced this opinion from the standpoint of the physician's duty of care [70]. G. Stratenwerth concluded that the physician should be able to trust the professional co-operation of others in view of their own autonomy, »unless there are special circumstances which raise the risk of negligence«. Otherwise a real division of labour would not be possible. The relevance and consequence of this principle of trust was precisely the subject of Karl Engisch's opinion [19]. Reinforcing Karl Heinrich Bauer's view, Engisch [19] at the Congress of the German Society of Surgery in 1955 carefully examined the concept of mutual trust whilst discussing the criminal implications of the necessary patient-centred teamwork between surgeon and anaesthetist: »The responsibility of the surgeon in the current legal climate is still all-encompassing; therefore, despite recognizing the concept of 'principle of trust', this responsibility can never be abrogated to any other discipline«. With this legal opinion he confirmed the view of Karl H. Bauer that there could not be a divided responsibility between the surgeon and the anaesthetist.

> Because 'division' of responsibility would mean that there is an area about which the surgeon never has to concern himself, in which the anaesthetist carries the sole responsibility. However there is no such area. There are only areas within which, to fulfil the surgeon's overriding duty of care, he engages a trustworthy anaesthetist and leaves the details of his actions to him.

The patient has entrusted himself to the surgeon; on this basis the general duty of care remains solely with the surgeon.

This unequivocal confirmation, by an eminent lawyer, of the hierarchical subordination of the anaesthetist as »proxy« to the all-powerful surgeon was a bitter disappointment for the members of the new specialty. The clinical independence, which they had just won, was again brought into question. The future of scientific research also seemed threatened. In the previous year – 1960 – the **Wissenschaftsrat** (German Science Council), in its recommendations for the development of postgraduate education [80], had just given the impetus to creating professorships (chairs) of anaesthesia in the medical schools, which would serve as the **»seed crystals«** for the establishment of **»anaesthetic departments to serve all surgical specialties«** (▶ Chap. 3.1). The specialty, 12 years after Hans Killian's question during the first post-war German Surgical Congress, was facing an enormous challenge, despite being firmly established in other Western countries.

If this legal opinion could not be adequately »parried«, there was a risk that anaesthetics as a career would be less attractive and the further development of the specialty hindered.

Initially, opinions were sought from law professors specialized in medical law. This proved difficult, as nobody wanted to challenge the renowned Karl Engisch. Before any progress was made, Charlotte Lehmann, the Second Secretary at the DGA's Committee Meeting on 2 December 1961, reported that during a discussion at the Bavarian State Chamber of Physicians Walther Weißauer from the Bavarian Ministry of Justice had been recommended as a highly competent lawyer on medical matters. She added that her source's opinion was that **»a legal opinion by Weißauer would counter any professor's opinion«**. Charlotte Lehmann was then asked by the Committee to contact Weißauer and persuade him to write a counter report. Several days before the next Committee Meeting of the DGA on 2 June 1962, the Committee Members already had the first draft of his comprehensive report **»Division of labour and delimitation of responsibility between anaesthetist and surgeon«** [76]. The author attended this meeting and the final amendments were incorporated in his paper.

Walther Weißauer succeeded in his report in transferring the question of interdisciplinary co-operation from the level of personal authority of one specialist back to that of the overriding importance of the actual task, and therefore developing a horizontal, rather than a hierarchical division of labour. Besides the principles of strict division of tasks and that of trust, he regarded the following as elements of the equality and independence of Anaesthetic Specialists; the reciprocal duty of co-ordination, the overriding importance of the actual task through conflict resolution as well as – and this was an important clarification – the surgeon's competence to »decide to operate«. Constructive work was only possible in the operating theatre when both partners could devote themselves, autonomously and free of supervision, to their own specialist area, and could trust the other's expertise and care. The report was published in *Der Anaesthesist* [76] and was widely distributed as a special edition. This report was the deciding factor in independence of the »mother specialty« of surgery.

It is a credit to Charlotte Lehman's far-sighted commitment that she not only commissioned Walther Weißauer to produce the first judicial review but also kept him as an advisor to the developing specialty and its organizations. Walther Weißauer, later also legal counsel to the DGAI and the **Professional Association of German Surgeons**, became the pre-eminent medico-legal expert in the German-speaking world.

Prof. Dr. med. h.c. Walther Weißauer (◨ Fig. 1.11) was born on 10 November 1921 in Freising. In 1948 he completed his law studies, qualifying as a lawyer and barrister and took up an appointment in the Bavarian State Ministry of Justice. From 1952 to 1954 he was a judge at the Munich County Court. From 1954 to 1984 he held an appointment in the Bavarian State Ministry of Justice focussing on constitutional affairs and international law. The year 1962 saw the beginning of his advisory role in German anaesthesia with his judicial review: »Division of labour and delimitation of responsibility between anaesthetist and surgeon« (*Arbeitsteilung und Abgrenzung der Verantwortung zwischen Anaesthesist und Operateur*). He was made an Honorary Member of the DGAI in 1966 and of the BDA in 1973. The Medical Faculty of the Friedrich-Alexander-University Erlangen-Nuremberg made him an Honorary Doctor of Medicine in 1975. In 1987 he received an honorary professorship from the Minister for Arts and Science in the State of Baden-Württemberg. In 1991 he received the Distinguished Service Medal of the Order of Merit the Federal Republic of Germany.

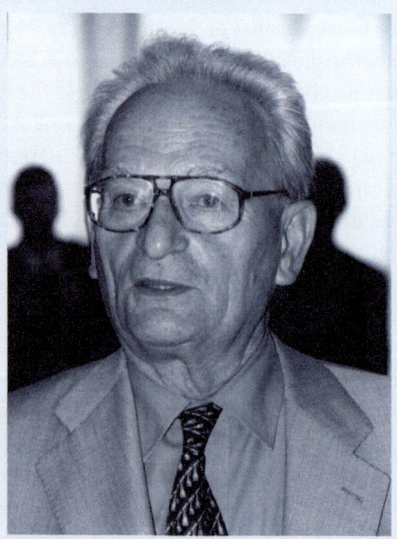

◨ **Fig. 1.11.** Walther Weißauer (Archive of the DGAI)

His profound interest in the concepts and problems in anaesthesia enabled him during 40 years to resolve numerous professional issues. Two items proved to be crucial in shaping the further development of anaesthesia: his expert opinion on anaesthesia given by nurses and his part in Hans Wolfgang Opderbecke's initiative on reaching basic agreements with the other specialties. With hindsight, it is no exaggeration that the new specialty owes him a great debt for its establishment and development. Several years of tedious and occasionally impassioned negotiations with the Anaesthetic Committee of the German Society of Surgery concerning the standing of anaesthetists were settled in the first instance in November 1964 thanks to the objectivity of the argument in Weißauer's judicial review. The two specialist societies jointly published »Guidelines on the position of the managerial anaesthetist« (*Richtlinien für die Stellung des leitenden Anaesthesisten*) [12]. The document was signed by Kurt Wiemers, President of the German Society of Anaesthesia and H. Kraus, President of the German Society of Surgery. It not only details the general principles defining the specialty and the limits of competence and authority of surgeon and anaesthetist point by point, but also explicitly determines the status of the anaesthetist in the university hospital and the district hospital, from departmental director, integration into the medical faculty, independent practice to the billing of private patients. Under point 6 of these guidelines comes the visionary statement:

> The managerial anaesthetist is in charge of the *Aufwach-räume* (recovery rooms) in which patients remain after their operations until they return to the ward. The post-operative and acute care unit is generally managed by the surgeon in close co-operation with the anaesthetist.

This wording, attributable to the then President Kurt Wiemers was pivotal in developing the subsequent competence of anaesthesia in the field of intensive care medicine. The term »recovery room« was included in parentheses in the German text because K. Wiemers' had only just returned from an extended period in the USA before becoming president.

These guidelines finally brought equal status with every other specialty within the German medical faculties and hospitals, 11 years after establishing the Specialist in Anaesthesia. The stringently objective legal clarification of the concept and the principles of the relationship between anaesthetist and surgeon in Walther Weißauer's judicial review made it possible to overcome the vehement resistance of many surgeons to treating anaesthetists as their equals in the operating theatre once and for all.

In the subsequent years, interdisciplinary agreements were negotiated and agreed with the surgeons and thereafter with other operating specialties and the internists on co-operation in surgical patient care and intensive care medicine based on the above guidelines, thus forming what might be termed the foundation agreement [56].

Contributing to the success of this legal framework and the development of the fledgling specialty was the admission of Hans Wolfgang Opderbecke to the board of the specialist society in 1964, a doctor with a legal mind and great diplomatic skill, who complemented the legal counsel W. Weißauer. It was particularly fortunate that these two men met one another through anaesthesia. They worked harmoniously deliberating the precise nature of medical responsibility in anaesthesia and the medico-legal implications of interdisciplinary relations between anaesthetists and members of other specialties. They furthered the anaesthetic specialty significantly not only with their pragmatism and sense of what is possible but also with their ideas and visions, leaving their mark. Giving a lecture in 1993 entitled »Anaesthesiology and the law – a conducive affair?« to mark the 30th anniversary of the Chair of Anaesthesia at Heidelberg University, the well-known Heidelberg forensic expert, A. Laufs, called the pair the »Dioscuri (The Twins) of Medicine«. The success of their co-operation is seen in the unusually large number of co-authored publications. For over three decades, the hard-working and purposeful Opderbecke, with his unique combination of decisiveness and charm, had various roles in the specialist society and later also in the professional association and other organizations furthering German anaesthesia [81].

Prof. Dr. med. Hans Wolfgang Opderbecke
(◘ Fig. 1.12)

was born 5 June 1922 in Düsseldorf. From 1943 to 1950 he studied medicine, first at the University of Cologne and then at the Medical Academy in Düsseldorf – now the Heinrich-Heine University – where he completed the state medical examination and his thesis becoming a doctor of medicine in 1950. He undertook his compulsory basic training in general medicine at the City Hospitals in Düsseldorf-Benrath from 1950 to 1951 and in 1952 started his postgraduate training in pulmonary medicine and surgery at the Surgical Lungenheilstätte Holsterhausen. This awakened his interest in the then relatively new specialty of anaesthesia. In 1956 he transferred to

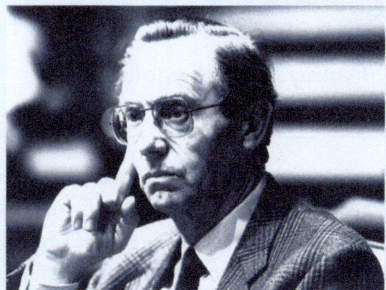

◘ **Fig. 1.12.** Hans Wolfgang Opderbecke (Archive of the DGAI)

the Surgical Clinic of the Municipal Hospital in Nuremberg. In 1957 he became a specialist in pulmonary medicine and he completed specialist training in anaesthesia in 1960. In 1962 he became the Head Anaesthetist at the Department of Anaesthesiology in the Municipal Hospital in Nuremberg. In 1977 he completed his habilitation thesis entitled »Anaesthesia and medical duty of care« at the Medical Faculty of the Friedrich-Alexander University Erlangen-Nuremberg. He was made a Professor (personal title) in 1982 and retired in 1987.

1967–1968	President of the DGAW
1972–1977	Deputy Honorary Secretary DGAW
1973–1993	Editor of the journal *Anästhesiologische Informationen;* renamed *Anästhesiologie & Intensivmedizin* in 1978
1977–1993	Secretary General of the DGAI
1983–1993	Honorary Director of the joint offices of BDA and DGAI in Nuremberg

Opderbecke is an Honorary Member of the DGAI, the BDA, the Association of Clinical Directors in Germany and the German Interdisciplinary Association of Critical Care and Emergency Medicine, in which he was the Honorary Secretary from 1977 to 1990. He is the recipient of many further honours and medals such as the Ernst-von-der-Porten Medal from the BDA and the Wolfgang-Mueller-Osten Medal from the Association of German Surgeons. The President of the Federal Republic of Germany awarded him the Federal Order of Merit, First Class, in 1988.

Probably the most succinct definition of anaesthesia ever found in the postgraduate training regulations for doctors is mainly due to Hans Wolfgang Opderbecke:

> Anaesthesiology comprises general and local anaesthesia including pre- and postoperative therapy, maintenance of vital functions during surgery, resuscitation and intensive care therapy and pain management in co-operation with the doctors treating the underlying disease.

1.1.10 Establishing Anaesthesiology as an Academic Entity

The year 1960 saw the establishment of the first personal Chair of Anaesthesiology in the Medical Faculty of the University of Mainz, taken up by Rudolf Frey (▶ Chap. 3.3.27). A recommendation by the Wissenschaftsrat (German Science Council) [80] in the same year reinforced establishing anaesthesiology as an independent academic specialty in German universities, which progressed rapidly after the

agreement on the joint guidelines with the surgeons. Already in 1966, when not all universities in Germany even had a personal Chair, Karl Horatz was appointed to the first Full Chair of Anaesthesiology at the University Hospital in Hamburg-Eppendorf. Embedding anaesthesiology in academia is an important aspect in establishing the specialty (▶ Chap. 3). A medical specialty can only survive in the long term if it is scientifically sound and continues to develop.

1.1.11 The Involvement of Nursing Staff in Anaesthesia

The acute shortage of anaesthetists in the late 1950s caused a major problem. A survey by Martin Zindler, President of the DGA from 1958 to 1959, highlighted the magnitude of the demand for doctors in anaesthesia. In 1959 Germany had by far the lowest number of anaesthetists per million population (◘ Table 1.1). With only 80 anaesthetists this meant in actual numbers that there was a shortage of 720 anaesthesia specialists at that time compared with Austria. Here a quote on this topic by Martin Zindler:

> This catastrophic deficit (which had existed for some time before and many years after) had disastrous consequences. Missing some 720 specialists (in comparison to Austria) meant that many operations, e.g. those with high risks or serious co-morbidity, and those on the elderly or the very young, simply could not be done. It is difficult to estimate how many complications and deaths could have been avoided considering that it took decades to make up this deficit.

Under these circumstances, Martin Zindler, as President of the DGA, convened a meeting of the clinical directors (chairs) of the German university departments in Göttingen to discuss this crisis. The result of this conference in the Göttingen Medical Centre on 1 February 1959 was a joint memorandum documenting precisely the serious deficit in anaesthesia specialists. It appealed to those responsible in politics, health administration, universities and fund

◘ **Table 1.1.** Number of anaesthetists per million inhabitants in 1959

USA	>50
UK	50
Denmark	23
Belgium	15
The Netherlands	15
France	14
Austria	14
Germany	1.3

holders to help tackle this shortage in human resources. Calculations showed a deficit of at least 2,000 anaesthetic specialists in comparison to other countries. It would take at least another two decades to achieve this goal.

How should one proceed in the mean time? It had been determined that doctors should practice anaesthesia, but who was to anaesthetize when there was no doctor available? There were still nurses who, up till very recently, had been administering anaesthetics. Could these be authorized by a surgeon to give an anaesthetic? The German Nurses Association published a resolution [18] in 1958 stating that »it is not a part of nursing to give an inhalational anaesthetic, intravenous anaesthetic, to intubate or give any anaesthetic requiring the use of apparatus. Such anaesthesia should be performed by doctors and nursing staff cannot be requested to do it«. Surgeons disagreed and demanded specialist training for nurse anaesthetists to fill the gap until there were sufficient anaesthesia specialists [20]. In a reply, Werner Hügin [31] in Basel opined that although anaesthesia was indeed the realm of doctors, the current deficit demanded the support of nurse anaesthetists. He was also in support of quality specialist anaesthetic training for nurses. To clarify the issue the Board of the DGA asked Walther Weißauer for a judicial review, which he provided in 1963 entitled: »The dilemma of anaesthetics delivered by nurses and the training of nurse anaesthetists« [77].

He demonstrated that there were compelling legal reasons why nurses should only ever give an anaesthetic when supervised by a doctor, whether it be an anaesthetist or a surgeon. An anaesthetic could not be given by a nurse if the surgery were likely to demand the surgical team's full concentration or the anaesthetic procedure were to require the doctor's undivided attention during crucial phases of the operation to monitor and maintain vital functions. The same would apply if the anaesthetic technique were to require medical knowledge and experience. He concluded with the question whether it would pay to only train nurse anaesthetists with limited scope given the current shortage of nurses rather than concentrate on postgraduate training of specialists in anaesthesia when a surplus of doctors was beginning to develop.

The legal framework had been established, but this problem was to occupy the Society until the 1970s. The scientific specialist society became active and independently developed a concept for the training of specialized nurse assistants in anaesthesia and intensive care medicine guided by Friedrich Wilhelm Ahnefeld, Ulm. This was based on the legal principles developed by W. Weißauer. It was finally implemented together with the German Hospital Federation (DKG) [15, 56]. With the establishment of specialist nurse training for anaesthesia and intensive care medicine, anaesthetics set a precedent for high quality nurse specialization in medicine in the Federal Republic of Germany.

The legal problem regarding the position of nurse anaesthetists arose once again at the beginning of the 1980s under the heading of »parallel anaesthesia«. This time the question was whether and under what conditions the anaesthetist could assume the medical and legal responsibilities for two simultaneous procedures, for which anaesthetic nurses/technicians or indeed insufficiently qualified anaesthetists were available. In their contribution »The permissibility and limits of parallel anaesthesia« [79] Walther Weißauer and Hans Wolfgang Opderbecke discussed the problems regarding a Federal Supreme Court's decision and proposed various solutions. Thereafter parallel anaesthesia could only be considered as an emergency solution in the face of acute lack of personnel and only after fulfilling strict conditions. Finally, some years later, a resolution of the Professional Association of German Anaesthetists (BDA) was published entitled »Permissibility and limits of parallel procedures in anaesthesia« [56]. Similar resolutions had to be publishedin 2005 and 2007 [83] because the problem of delegated nurse anaesthesia was repeatedly raised, in particular by private hospital companies [6a].

1.1.12 Support of the Scientific Society Through a Professional Organization

In the early 1960s it was deemed necessary, in order to deal with numerous and diverse challenges, to establish a professional organization, which could offer support to the scientific society in the ever more complex areas of professional politics, representation of financial interests and also offer practical services to its members (e.g. help with setting of professional fees, contractual advice, legal advice, continuing education, professional liability, etc.). Up until then the DGA had made every effort in trying to answer those questions. Therefore, in December 1959, the DGA began publishing its own newsletter (outside the framework of the scientific publication *Der Anaesthesist*) [55] in order to pass on this kind of information to its members. The *Informationen der DGA* was published initially in the form of a newsletter and later as a journal. On the initiative of Jürgen Stoffregen, Göttingen, it was possible at the end of October 1959 to win over the medical journalist Karl Heise as spokesperson of the organization and editor of the information newsletter. It is hard for us to understand today, but it was this political initiative of the DGA that put a strain on the negotiations with the Anaesthetics Commission of the German Society of Surgery. The spokesperson of the surgeons, Karl Heinrich Bauer, considered the employment of a journalist and such a publication as »academically worthless, without precedent and distracting« and not befitting of a scientific professional organization. At the meeting of the DGA on 19 November 1960, chaired by the then President Otto

Just, Heidelberg, this opinion was discussed and it was concluded »that with the establishment of a professional organization within the framework of the DGA being responsible for public relations and information it was perfectly possible to counter the verbal attacks of the surgeons«. The idea of establishing a »Division of Professional Issues« found general support. The title of the bimonthly publication was initially changed to *Informations from the Division of Professional Issues in the DGA* and after foundation of the Professional Association of German Anaesthetists (BDA) in 1961 was again changed to *Informations of the DGA and BDA*.

Charlotte Lehmann, who was already heavily involved, took over as editor in 1968. In 1970 the Demeter Verlag was secured as publisher and distributor of the magazine, which now bore the »catchy« title *Anaesthesiological Informations*. The magazine has had its current title of *Anaesthesiology and Intensive Medicine* since September 1978. In 1973 Hans Wolfgang Opderbecke took over from Charlotte Lehmann as editor. In 1994 this was passed on to Bernd Landauer, Munich, and in 2002 to Kai Taeger, Regensburg. Since 2006 Jürgen Schüttler, Erlangen, is the editor-in-chief.

A total of 22,500 copies are printed, distributed and made available to all members of DGAI and BDA (▶ Chap. 1.5.4).

The intended establishment of a »Division for Professional Concerns« was abandoned 3 months later (other than in the title of the magazine), after the legal implications had been discussed and after resolution by the DGA Executive Committee on 23 February 1961. In order to answer the surgeons' accusations it was decided to establish a professional organization and a magazine, the purpose of which was information. Charlotte Lehmann as Second Secretary of the DGA was given the job of preparing for this and at the next Committee Meeting in April, she was able to present not only proposed statutory regulations, but also a proposed personnel structure for the committee and council of the new association. The determining factor was to ensure a tightly knit relationship between the DGA and the new organization, so that the respective goals of the two organizations would not inevitably lead to a rift. Therefore, in accordance with German legislation, the Professional Association of German Anaesthetists (BDA) was founded and registered.

Since 1964 contractual advice is provided for its members by the BDA as a specialist service. This was previously carried out by the representative of hospital anaesthetists in the Committee of the DGA. Much later, this was taken over, in connection with the establishment of its own »contract advice bureau« in co-operation with the legal profession, by the office of Prof. Dr. Dr. Klaus Ulsenheimer, Munich. Since 1966 this service has been extended on the initiative of Hans Wolfgang Opderbecke and Walther Weißauer by providing sample contracts with variables for different situations [78]. These sample contracts have had in many ways a very positive influence on the design of contracts for chief anaesthetists.

Thanks to the involvement and determination of their often long-term Presidents Karl Horatz, Karl-Hans Bräutigam, Walther Henschel, Karl Hutschenreuter, Peter Uter, Klaus Zinganell and Bernd Landauer as well as other prominent figures, the BDA very quickly gained momentum and its own dynamism and over the five decades since then has contributed to the long-term success in consolidating and widening the professional field of anaesthetics. The intention and realization of a close relationship between the DGA and BDA proved to be particularly fruitful. Right from the beginning the President of the DGA, in line with the statutory regulations, had a voice in the Committee of the BDA and after appropriate change in the regulations in 1963 the President of the BDA has the same voice in the Committee of the DGA. An important part of this reciprocal interconnection is the long-term union of the position of Secretary (till 2000 H. W. Opderbecke and Klaus Fischer, Bremen). The synergy, resulting from this dynamic interconnection of the two organizations, has played an important part in the success and high status that anaesthetics enjoy amongst German medical specialties.

1.1.13 Competence in Emergency Medicine – from DGA to DGAW

Anaesthetists have played – as demonstrated in ▶ Chap. 2.3 – a significant part in the conceptual and structural development of emergency medicine in post-war Germany. Notably, Rudolf Frey, together with his students (namely Friedrich Wilhelm Ahnefeld and Wolfgang Dick), showed particular involvement in this area and emphasized again and again that the anaesthetist because of his experience in perioperative patient care had a natural aptitude in the field of emergency medicine and resuscitation.

It was he who, during the Presidency of Karl Horatz, at a Executive Committee Meeting of the DGA on 21 April 1965 introduced the proposal, together with Martin Zindler, to rename the German Society of Anaesthesia the German Society of Anaesthesia and Resuscitation. The anaesthetist deals on a daily basis with the unconscious patient or patient in respiratory arrest and is therefore the most suitable and experienced specialist in resuscitation. This is made clear by the anaesthetist's contribution to the advancements achieved in resuscitation.

It was at the same time stressed that the name change did not mean a monopolization in the area of emergency medicine, »in the same way as non-members of the Ger-

man Society of Blood Transfusion would not have problems in carrying out blood transfusions«. And further:

> We would like to take a special interest in developing and looking after resuscitation. This has become apparent by this subject appearing repeatedly on conference agendas and, in particular, through training of doctors in anaesthetic departments (in Düsseldorf over 2,000 doctors have already been trained).

Furthermore, anaesthetists have been asked on many occasions to give presentations as experts at conferences of other specialties. On the basis of the agreement with the surgeons, the name change seemed justified and if any objections were expected, it would be from the field of internal medicine. It was discussed whether to use the term »reanimation« or »resuscitation« and include it in the name. After lengthy discussion »**Wiederbelebung (resuscitation)**« was decided upon, as Horatz explained at the General Assembly on 17 September 1965 in Zurich: it was felt that »**Wiederbelebung (resuscitation) would be better understood than reanimation by the lay person**«. The proposed name change to **German Society of Anaesthesia and Resuscitation (DGAW)** was unanimously approved by those members present and came into force in 1966.

During the four decades since this decision the organization has been able to successfully contribute (through agreements, recommendations and endorsements) – and since 1979 within the framework of the **German Interdisciplinary Association of Critical Care Medicine** – to the further development and steady renewal of the structures within emergency medicine and indeed further education in this area [56]. Many of these were initiated by anaesthetists. Anaesthetists have always held key positions in the fields of emergency medicine and disaster management and will continue to do so.

1.1.14 Anaesthetics and Intensive Care Medicine – from DGAW to DGAI

The development of intensive care medicine was similar to that of emergency medicine (► Chap. 2.2). The work of the anaesthetist in the intensive therapy unit (ITU) has always been regarded as an extension of his daily activity in the operating theatre. During an anaesthetic the anaesthetist practices acute medicine. The anaesthetist has been and continues to be, like virtually no other specialist colleague, in tune with continuing observation and assessment of his patient's vital functions and their maintenance. The **DGAW** recognized early on that their involvement in intensive care medicine had a positive influence on the anaesthetist's work and working conditions and therefore made it a more attractive career path for young colleagues. The subject of

intensive care medicine when setting guidelines for the position of lead anaesthetist was originally touched upon at a Committee Meeting on 29 September 1964. It was concluded that the anaesthetist should be offered the unique opportunity of extending his knowledge and skill beyond the operating theatre. He would be able to deepen his »pathophysiological« knowledge and gain experience and accuracy in diagnosing/assessing a vast number of clinical situations. This would be an opportunity not to be underestimated in a health service system, which was becoming ever more divided into specialties and subspecialties.

Since the mid-1960s the DGAW wholeheartedly supported the development of acute/intensive care medicine. From the beginning of the 1970s the DGAW was able (after at times gruelling negotiations and a long list of agreements with the societies of internal medicine and later with surgery) to establish the anaesthetists' justifiable interest in »division of labour« and co-operation in intensive care medicine (► Chap. 2.2.1). Over the years that followed, particularly in the hospital environment, these recommendations and agreements formed the basis for the far-reaching organizational establishment and structure of intensive care medicine. We must also remember the productive cooperation with the **German Hospital Federation (DKG)**.

Even during the first tentative contact between representatives of the DGAW and the BDA under the lead of the then President of the DGAW Hans Wolfgang Opderbecke and the delegation from the DKG at the end of March 1967 in Düsseldorf, the main areas of cooperation over the coming decades were touched upon: (1) the position of chief anaesthetist in a hospital, (2) the role of the anaesthetist in the recovery room, high dependency unit (HDU) and ITU and (3) questions of staffing levels.

The anaesthetist was able to, again and again, not least because of good personal connection with the organization, offer his expertise in formulating recommendations for the DKG and in this way received support for their causes like the vital question of staffing levels [56].

As demonstrated in ► Chap. 2.2.1 the international activities in the area of intensive care medicine in the early 1970s led in 1974 to the question of who should nationally and internationally represent German intensive care medicine. The following year Peter Lawin, Münster, submitted a request to the then President of the DGAW, Walter Henschel, to form a working group on acute/intensive care medicine within the Society and to discuss whether the name should be changed to include the term »acute/intensive care medicine«.

This proposal was discussed repeatedly, initially without a concrete result. In the time leading up to the 25th anniversary of the Society, Walther Weißauer – during a discussion on necessary changes in statutory regulations – at a meeting of the Executive Committee on 21 January 1977 appealed emphatically in favour of including the term

»intensive therapy« or »intensive medicine« in the by-laws. He raised the question of whether an appropriate change of name would be useful to the Society. After intense discussion over two meetings with Karl-Heinz Weis, Würzburg, as President it was suggested on 6 May 1977 to scrap the term »resuscitation« as the words »anaesthesiology and intensive care medicine« would suffice. However, at the second meeting on 7 May 1977, without having reached a definite decision, three variations of names were again presented for discussion and resolution: (1) German Society of Anaesthesiology, Resuscitation and Intensive Care Medicine, (2) German Society of Anaesthesiology and Intensive Care Medicine and (3) German Society of Anaesthesiology. In the minutes it was initially recorded that »the term 'anaesthesiology' was an essential component of the name of the Society and should so remain«. Furthermore:

> An extensive and lively discussion revealed the desire to definitely include the term 'intensive care medicine' in the name, not least because there is a 'German Society of Internal Medicine Intensive Care'. Intensive care medicine is an intrinsic part of the anaesthetist's work and therefore it should be included in the name. The general public should be aware that 'the anaesthetist does more than anaesthetize'.

Afterwards different opinions on inclusion or exclusion of the term »resuscitation/reanimation« (*Wiederbelebung/ Reanimation*) were heard. It was felt, for example, that leaving out the term »would give the impression that a previously staked claim had been relinquished and this could, retrospectively, have consequences for rescue services and emergency medicine«. It was therefore voted unanimously to approve the proposed name German Society of Anaesthesiology and Intensive Care Medicine, shortened to DGAI. Both proposals, together with proposals on further changes in the by-laws, were agreed upon at the General Assembly of the DGAW on 19 November 1977 in Saarbrücken. The Society has used the new name since 1978.

1.1.15 Founding of the German Interdisciplinary Association of Critical Care and Emergency Medicine

Before this change of name, the Working Group on Internal Medicine Intensive Care had been renamed the German Society of Internal Medicine Intensive Care. For scientific and organizational development in the field of paediatrics, the Working Group on Neonatology and Paediatric Intensive Care Medicine was formed. In order to document the multidisciplinary approach to intensive care medicine in Germany representatives of this organization together with representatives of the Professional Association of German Anaesthetists and the Professional Association of German Internists founded the

German Interdisciplinary Association of Critical Care and Emergency Medicine (DIVI) as an umbrella organization on 29 January 1977 in Frankfurt/Main in order to thwart the attempts – stimulated by developments abroad – to also form a German Society of Intensive Care Medicine in the Federal Republic of Germany.

The DIVI quickly formed links with other specialist organizations in the field of intensive care medicine, establishing a successful tradition of interdisciplinary cooperation within intensive care medicine. In addition it also acted as a conduit for communication with official bodies and with scientific organizations abroad, which deal with the science and practice of intensive care; it set up a National Congress and represents concerns regarding intensive care medicine on an international level. Several members of the DGAI were members of the Executive Committee of the DIVI for many years and left a long-lasting impression on this association: Hans Wolfgang Opderbecke, Secretary between 1977 and 1990, thanks to whose presence of mind the intended founding of an independent German Society of Intensive Care Medicine did not come about. Credit should be given to Peter Lawin of Münster, as President of the DIVI in 1991, for organizing and steering the first German Interdisciplinary Congress for Intensive Care Medicine in Hamburg. This Congress took place every 2 years, annually since 2010.

1.1.16 Founding of the German Academy of Continuing Education in Anaesthesiology (DAAF)

On 16 November 1977 members of the DGAW and the BDA founded in Saarbrücken a German Academy of Continuing Education in Anaesthesiology (DAAF). The statutory aim of the group was to promote the continuance and broadening of education in anaesthesia and intensive care medicine by organizing targeted learning, providing teaching aids and finding experts through both technical and financial support of meetings, congresses and other events proposed by the DGAW or the BDA.

Anaesthetists were ahead of the game in this respect; their professional Society was the first and for a long time the only one which had an Academy of Medical Education. Only later did others follow this example such as radiologists, cardiologists and surgeons. The work of the DAAF deals primarily with the field of maintaining the accreditation of anaesthetists and their continuing medical education (CME) and continuous professional development (CPD) [73].

Central to the various initiatives of the DAAF are the yearly refresher courses at the German Anaesthesia Congresses, the 1-week intensive course for anaesthesia and intensive care medicine and a structured educational series in the journal *Anästhesiologie & Intensivmedizin* with the opportunity for self-evaluation to confirm one's progress. The respective President of the DAAF is a member of the Executive Board of the DGAI. The Founding President was Karl Hutschenreuter of Homburg-Saar and the current President is Thea Koch of Dresden.

1.1.17 Pain Management – the »4th Pillar« of Anaesthesiology

Whilst the pillars of emergency medicine and intensive care medicine had already become firmly anchored in German anaesthesiology during the 1960s and 1970s, the principle of pain management as an anaesthetic discipline was a more peripheral activity – apart from a few centres, notably Mainz (spearheaded by Hans-U. Gerbershagen) – as demonstrated by Michael Zenz in ▶ Chap. 3.4. Only with the advent of neuraxial opioid-mediated analgesia did the anaesthetists move quite swiftly into a more central role of leadership in pain management.

This increased level of activity also had an impact within the Society, and the year 1989 saw the establishment of the DGAI's Scientific Working Group on Pain Therapy, following the formation of a similar body in the German Democratic Republic in 1982. It was made clear from the outset that anaesthetists would not be involved exclusively in this field. Starting in 1991 a multidisciplinary approach was formalized in negotiations with the BDA. Pending the design of a formal qualification in pain management within anaesthetic training, the DGAI, in conjunction with the Scientific Working Group, introduced an interim certificate of training, designed to be valid until pain management was officially integrated into the teaching syllabus. This ambition was realized in 1996 with the introduction of an additional qualification in »special pain management«, unveiled at the 99th German Medical Assembly.

This integration was taken further in 1995 with the establishment of the German Interdisciplinary Association for Pain Management (DIVS), a project driven significantly by the DGAI, to serve as an umbrella organization for all specialties involved with pain management, analogous to the DIVI in intensive care medicine.

As such a relatively young specialty there remains room for development with regard to the infrastructure required to satisfactorily address patient needs. Thus, a reasonable request was made at the General Assembly of the DGAI in 1998 that in areas where demand for such a service could be demonstrated, an outpatient clinic and inpatient beds dedicated to pain management should be piloted. It is clear that the pillar of pain management is well on its way to becoming similarly anchored just as its more established neighbours.

1.1.18 25 Years DGAI – »We Leave Würzburg in Better Spirits«

On the occasion of its 25th anniversary, the DGAI assembled under its new name at the Annual Meeting in Würzburg on 12 October 1978 to celebrate under the direction of that year's President, Karl-Heinz Weis. An extract of the report entitled »We leave Würzburg in better spirits« [28] reads thus:

> The autumn sun shone on the Annual Meeting of the DGAI in Würzburg, perhaps a gift on this 25th anniversary of its founding. An address at the start, delivered in the *Kaisersaal* of the *Residenz*, was dedicated to reminiscing over the years gone by, full of pride and happiness, but without the pathos of tradition. Since 1953 we have grown into a modern and dynamic specialist body, counting to date around 2,300 members. In his speech, Professor Weis stated that now that the goals have been identified, it was necessary to follow them up with the provision to the community of a seamless service staffed by well-trained anaesthetists. In response to the increasing criticism in the media of the inhumane hospital, Professor Weis said it was now the aim of the anaesthetists to contribute to that debate by providing best practice analgesia in surgery and relieving suffering amongst the very sick in the intensive care environment.

The presence of the Presidents of the various medical societies representing surgery, ENT and head and neck surgery, pharmacology and that of legal medicine as well as the good wishes from the Presidents of the societies of ophthalmology, obstetrics, neurosurgery, orthopaedics and urology confirmed the standing and the recognition of this new field amongst the other specialties at that time. International recognition of the DGAI came in the shape of congratulations from the President of the American Society of Anesthesiologists, Jack Moyers, and the President of the Japanese Society of Anaesthesiologists, Tsutomu Oyama [50, 57]. The President Karl-Heinz Weis pointed out with a certain satisfaction that the international recognition of the DGAI came with the honour of »hosting, in the name of the World Federation of Societies of Anaesthesiologists, the World Congress of 1980 in the Federal Republic of Germany« [75].

The Würzburg Congress saw the first of the now traditional Hellmut-Weese Memorial Lectures in honour of this important pioneer in German anaesthetic research [14]. The pharmacologist Hellmut Weese had always been in touch with clinical problems and had expressed his affiliation with anaesthetics and anaesthetists by co-signing the founding document of the DGA (see above and ▶ Chap. 2.1). The first lecture was delivered by the medical historian Hans Schadewaldt of Düsseldorf University [62].

A special edition of the journal *Anästhesiologie & Intensivmedizin* on the occasion of the 25th anniversary of the DGAI, which was published to coincide with the congress, reiterated in 11 sections the journey from the early days of the foundation of the specialty, via the expansion of the role of anaesthetists, the problems and development of postgraduate training to visions of the future of anaesthesiology [24]. Rudolf Frey gratefully concluded in a reflection on his years as Secretary of the Society that the head start enjoyed by other countries in the field of anaesthetics and intensive care medicine was fast diminishing; indeed, some were in danger of being overtaken [23]. Significant contributions towards this were made by selfless collaboration and support from colleagues the world over, which the German anaesthetists had received from the outset. Without the help and advice of leading international specialists, for example Sir Robert Macintosh (Oxford), Jean Henley (New York), Benjamin H. Robbins (Nashville, TN), Ernst Kern and Jean Lassner (Paris), Harold Griffith (Montreal), Enrico Ciocatto (Turin), Cornelis R. Ritsema von Eck (Groningen), Werner Hügin (Basel), Otto Mayrhofer (Vienna) and Hideo Yamamura (Tokyo), to name but a few, this development would not have been possible. The latter specifically had a strong link with the foundation of the Society, as Japanese medicine, heavily influenced by Germany, had experienced similar teething problems on its introduction of the new speciality. In the closing paragraph of this special journal edition, entitled »From narcosis to homeostasis« [61], Erich Rügheimer developed, from a critical analysis of former days, with reference to what had been achieved, as had been outlined in other contributions, basic perspectives on the ever changing concept of the essence of German anaesthesiology. He showed a degree of foresight by including aspects that had hitherto been less obvious, but were clearly emerging: »Plans to reduce the number of training posts, inadequate numbers of teaching posts, reduced research facilities, economical restrictions, etc., are buzzwords which will cast a shadow over our future«. These topics are further examined elsewhere (▶ Chap. 2.5).

1.1.19 Founding of the European Academy of Anaesthesiology (EAA)

An important event in the jubilee year of the DGAI, on a European level, was the founding of the European Academy of Anaesthesiology (EAA) on the occasion of the 5th European Congress in September 1978 in Paris [44]. After a Steering Committee chosen from the national associations had completed the preparatory work, the respective General Assembly was able to take place: 21 of 27 European Associations sent representatives to this meeting while 4 Societies from Eastern Europe took part as observers and only 2 were opposed to the formation. The German delegation was led by Karl-Heinz Weis. The assembled members elected the first Senate and an Executive Committee with Jean Lassner of Paris as the first President. The Academy saw itself not as a national representation or a representation of national societies but rather as an amalgamation of individual members who, having fulfilled the criteria for membership, had been duly elected. The Academy has achieved the significant objective of creating a European Diploma in Anaesthesiology, which has a valued role in the quality assurance and quality improvement in continuing education in anaesthesiology in Europe. The Academy ran in addition certified international continuing education courses in selected centres and published the *European Journal of Anaesthesiology (EJA)*. The first German »Academicians«, who were appointed to the office of President were Wolfgang Dick of Mainz (1991–1994), following his term as Secretary which he took up in 1983. Hugo van Aken of Münster was President from 2000 until 2003 and was followed by Thomas Pasch of Zurich. During the latter's period of office the EAA merged with the European Society of Anaesthesiologists and the Confederation of European National Societies of Anaesthesiologists resulting in the formation of the European Society of Anaesthesiology (ESA) in 2005.

1.1.20 The 7th World Congress of Societies of Anaesthesiologists in Hamburg (1980) – International Recognition of German Anaesthesia

Two years after the anniversary Congress in Würzburg, the DGAI was the host for the 7th World Congress in Hamburg. From 14 to 21 September 1980, 5,655 anaesthetists from 69 countries in addition to 300 invited scientists and official representatives of the World Federation of Societies of Anaesthesiologists (WFSA) met in the Congress Centre in Hamburg. In the words of Erich Rügheimer in his final report to the Extended Executive Committee of the DGAI on 14 September 1981 in Berlin [62], which dealt with the activities of the Organizing Committee, the Hamburg World Congress was:

> a great success in two ways for our Society: first of all it was pleasing that the level of the multifaceted scientific program was exceptionally high, offering varied stimuli to the specialists. The impression which the scientific program left was complemented by the fact that the proceedings were printed in a suitable format 6 months after the end of the congress. Thanks for this should be accorded to Martin Zindler, the Chairman of the Scientific Committee, for his considerable

work and his continuing flow of original ideas. On the other hand, we had set as our objective, as generous and attentive hosts, to accord our guests, arriving from all over the globe, a hospitality and kindness that was without parallel. That we reached our objective and that in this regard the World Congress was a huge success for our Society was, as I have repeatedly emphasized, merely the sum of the combined efforts of the members of this Society.

As a lasting token – not only for German anaesthesia – the idea arose to offer a prize for the best artistic design of a congress poster. It was possible to acquire the services of the Huber Gallery in Offenbach to help with the realization of this project. Seven sketches were presented with the theme »Anaesthesia« by Klaus Böttger, Bruno Bruni, Simon Dittrich, Rudolf Hausner, Bernhard Jäger, Peter Paul and Paul Wunderlich. The Committee of the DGAI decided to choose the convincing design by Paul Wunderlich to be adopted as a logo for the World Congress in Hamburg (◘ Fig. 1.13). The DGAI obtained the right

to use this picture, not only for the poster, but also for all printed matters used in conjunction with the World Congress. Seldom has the visualization of a medical theme spontaneously found so much positive resonance. The source of several later poster designs could be traced back to the original design of Paul Wunderlich. The Huber Gallery made a folder available at the World Congress entitled »Art and anaesthesia« with all the seven original designs.

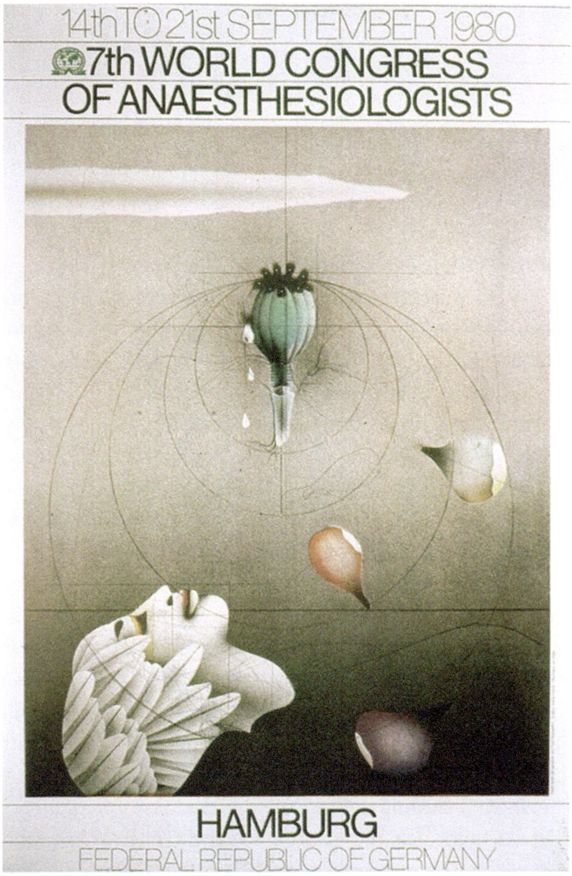

1.1.21 A Look Back at What Has Been Achieved – an Interim Appraisal

The development of anaesthesia into an independent specialty was an unremitting struggle which lasted for decades. Looking back from a current perspective it is only partially understandable:

- The struggle started at the beginning of the 1930s, after countless scientists and doctors in Germany spearheaded pioneering work in the field of anaesthesia.
- This struggle began when anaesthesia had already been established to a great extent in other Western countries.
- The struggle continued after the establishment in 1953 of the Society of Anaesthesia and after the recognition of the specialist title in anaesthesia.

First of all the strength of the argument in favour of the inescapable fact, and on this point everyone was singing from the same hymn sheet, that anaesthesia was an indispensable tool in the operative setting and secondly legal placing anaesthesia on the same level as other specialties led the discussions on anaesthesia to a favourable outcome.

There is one question which emerges at this point: did the prolonged discussion and delays, at times painful for those fighting for the recognition of the specialty, have any positive aspects?

Some of these beneficial aspects are considered here:

Having to assert oneself in order to win contentious and delicately balanced arguments achieves that most precious of possessions, solidarity, which our specialty enjoys until the present day. The unity of anaesthesia in all its diversity is certainly a consequence of these tribulations.

The challenges which the specialty had to overcome have resulted in attracting tough, resilient individuals with a well-defined innovative streak, individuals who were able to make their mark by meeting these challenges head on. The protracted wranglings which lasted several decades has led to German anaesthesia having, in contrast to other countries, both its independence and its clinical roles being more clearly established and legally defined. Anaesthesia has unlike any other country defined its position vis-à-vis other specialties and in particular the surgical disciplines through legally binding agreements [56].

◘ **Fig. 1.13.** Poster of the 7th World Congress 1980 in Hamburg (courtesy of Department of Anaesthesiology, University of Erlangen-Nuremberg, Erlangen)

1.1.22   The Era of Consolidation – The DGAI Undergoing Change

The aim of comprehensive anaesthetic care in Germany had been all but achieved [34, 59, 64]. The skills of the anaesthetist in intensive care, emergency medicine and pain therapy were generally recognized and the scientific basis of the discipline had been established through the setting up of chairs in every German university. F.W. Ahnefeld recorded in a New Year's greeting at the beginning of his Presidency in 1983: »We have left the years of development behind and now find ourselves in the era of consolidation«. He went on »we have become a recognized and independent specialty within medicine. It is wrong, however, to think that we have achieved the most important goal«. Consolidation and change – with these contrasting ideas in mind, some aspects of the further development of the DGAI will be considered.

Consolidation is mirrored in the increasing professionalisation of the infrastructure of the DGAI. Among the members of the Executive Committee of the Society, the Secretary in particular with the help of the office staff has paid particular attention to the necessary continuity of the Society's work. In the first By-Laws both a Permanent Secretary and an Acting Vice Secretary had been created. While the Permanent Secretary – Rudolf Frey held this post for nearly 25 years without interruption – acted more in a strategic role as a representative of the President, Charlotte Lehmann who took over the post of the Vice Secretary in 1958 extended this office into more of a »logistic HQ« where for example the list of members was held, the agendas for meetings were organized, the journal was edited and where proceedings and documents were systematically archived. It should be mentioned that Dr. Lehmann received invaluable support and help from her secretary Marianne Winter whose contributions by far exceeded her contractual obligations. Hans Wolfgang Opderbecke took over this office in 1972.

Dr. med. Charlotte Lehmann (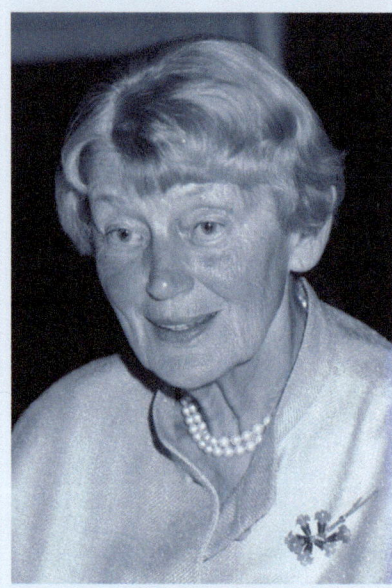 Fig. 1.14)

born 6 February 1922 in Pyritz/Pomerania; medical studies at Breslau, Vienna and Kiel; voluntary Assistant in the District Hospital Neustadt in Holstein and at the University Hospital in Kiel; doctorate awarded in Kiel; 1948 Resident at the Pathology Institute of the University of Munich; 1949–1952 Resident at the Surgical Unit of the Municipal Hospital Rechts der Isar; 1952–1953 studies in Switzerland, England, France, USA; 1953 Specialist in Anaesthesia; starting in 1954 organization of the Anaesthetic Department at the Municipal Hospital rechts der Isar; 1958–1971 Second Secretary

---

of the *DGA/DGAW*; 1961–1971 Secretary of the *BDA*; 1968–1972 Editor of *Anästhesiologische Informationen*; 1972 Department Head at the Municipal Hospital Neuperlach, Munich; 1973 Editor of *Wissenschaftliche Informationen Fresenius-Stiftung – Anästhesie, Wiederbelebung, Intensivbehandlung*; Honorary Member of the *BDA* and the *DGAI*.

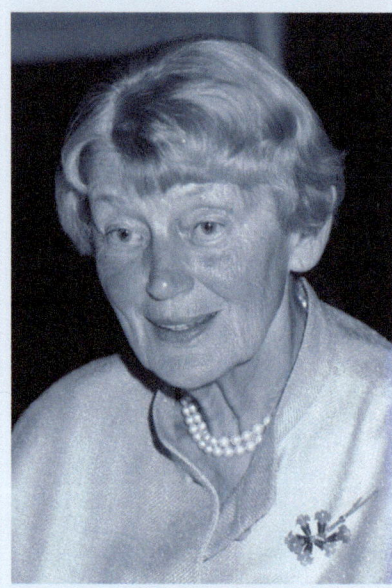

◻ Fig. 1.14. Charlotte Lehmann (Archive of the DGAI)

When Rudolf Frey announced at the General Assembly in 1976 in Travemünde that »25 years of struggle are enough!« and that he would no longer be standing for election to the office of Permanent Secretary, Hans Wolfgang Opderbecke, Nuremberg, was appointed as his successor. After the election the then President of the DGAW, Walter Henschel, announced that the Executive Committee had decided that henceforth the First Secretary would be known as General Secretary while the Second Secretary would be known as Secretary of the Society.

The Committee thus took into account the new distribution of responsibilities effective as of 1977 whereby the General Secretary supported the President in matters of interest to the Society concerning authorities, associations and scientific societies as well as current business, while the Secretary was responsible for correspondence with members and especially for matters concerning membership, including setting up the database of members' details, and also the agenda for the General Assembly as well as the meetings of the Executive Committee and the Extended Executive Committee. The office and the function of the General Secretary proved itself to be an important element of continuity in the Society in the

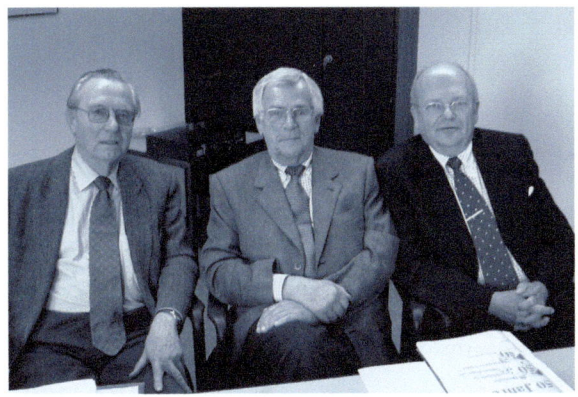

Fig. 1.15. The General Secretaries of the DGAI (*from left to right*): Hans Wolfgang Opderbecke, Friedrich Wilhelm Ahnefeld, Klaus van Ackern (courtesy of Prof. Dr. Jens-Peter Striebel, Mannheim)

ensuing 25 years. During this period there have only been three General Secretaries: Hans Wolfgang Opderbecke (until 1992), Friedrich Wilhelm Ahnefeld (1993–1996) and from 1997–2010 Klaus van Ackern (■ Fig. 1.15).

With the passing of time, the increasing volume of work could no longer be accomplished merely as a »sideline« by co-workers in the respective departments; where needed, additional paid manpower was hired, for example the long-serving secretary to the General Secretary in Nuremberg, Gertraud Mulligan, who was awarded the Society's Franz-Kuhn Medal in 1994 in honour of her exemplary dedication and in recognition of the esteem in which she was held by both the Executive Committee and the members of the DGAI and the BDA [13].

1.1.23 End of the Period of Activity as Honorary Body – Establishing Headquarters

The period of almost exclusive honorary activity of the Society came to a definitive end in 1979 with the decision of the Extended Executive Committee in Nuremberg to establish business headquarters. Property was acquired – for the first time in the history of the Society – at Obere Schmiedgasse 11 (■ Fig. 1.16) at the foot of the fortress in Nuremberg, which served for several years as a meeting place for officials, members and guests of both the DGAI and BDA (■ Fig. 1.17).

The headquarters also provided the required space for the archives of both organizations, dating from 1982, which consisted not only of the business proceedings but also documents from the early pioneering days of the Society. Unfortunately there is only patchy documentation covering the very early years, i.e. immediately after the founding of the DGA. For this reason members were asked to help »fill the gaps« by contributing any old documents which they possessed [54].

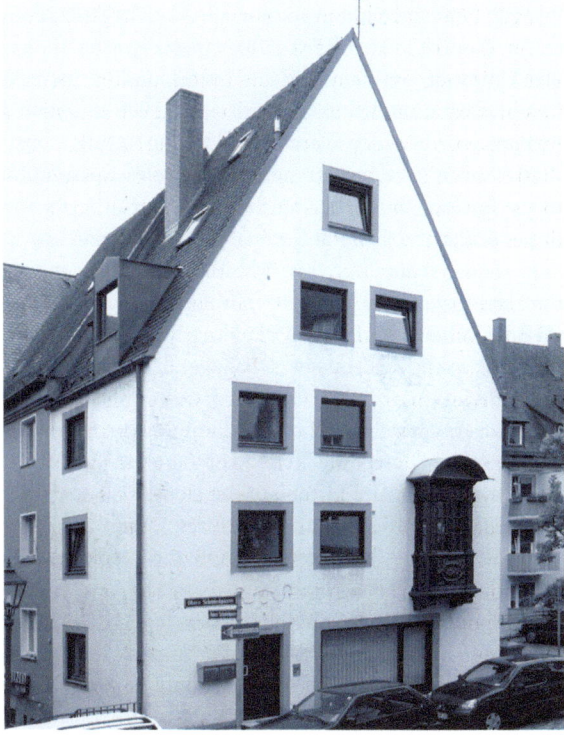

Fig. 1.16. The first headquarters of the DGAI and BDA in Nuremberg, Obere Schmiedgasse 11 (© Bischof + Broel, Bayreuther Str. 21, 90409 Nuremberg)

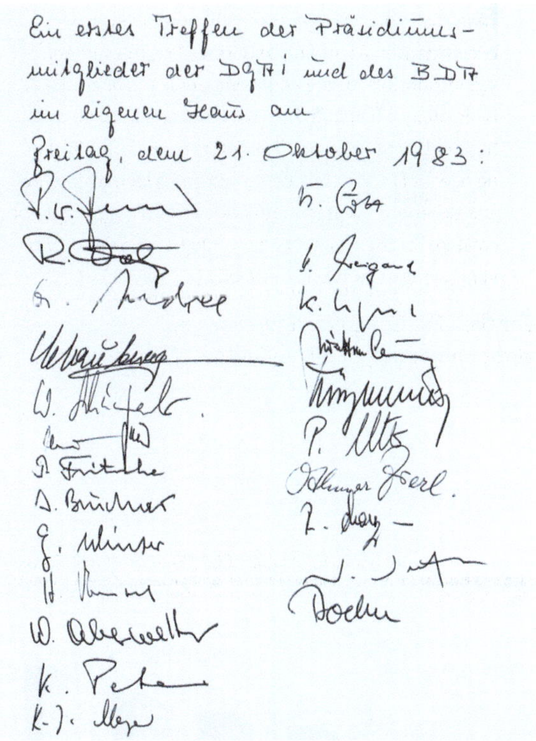

Fig. 1.17. Entry in the guest book in the HQ on the occasion of the first meeting of the Executive Committee of the DGAI und BDA »in its first home« on 21 October 1983 (DGAI/BDA headquarters, Nuremberg)

The rapid increase in numbers in both organizations in the ensuing years (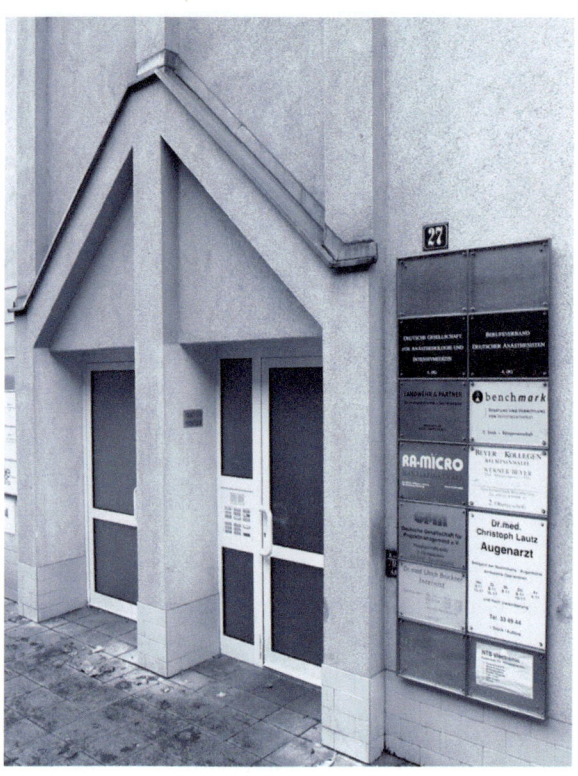 Fig. 1.18), especially after the re-unification of Germany and the corresponding increase in administration, led to the decision in 1990 to obtain a further floor of office space as well as appointing a business manager as a further step in the professionalization of the Society, thus relieving the appointed officials and in particular the General Secretary of their heavy workload. Three years after this decision the Society moved into larger premises at Roritzerstraße 27 in Nuremberg (Fig. 1.19) and on 1 June 1993 Holger Sorgatz assumed his duties as the head business manager of both the DGAI and BDA.

A further step toward consolidating the professionalization of the Society was heralded by the decision of the Executive Committee to replace the Congress Secretariat located at the offices of the Treasurer Jürgen Brückner in Berlin starting in May 1985. On the recommendation of the Executive Committee of the DGAI, the BDA formed the **Medizinische Congressorganisation Nürnberg (MCN)** as a limited joint-stock company that would henceforth offer their services not only to the DGAI, BDA and DAAF but also to a number of other national associations and societies. Within a few years under the direction of Walther Weißauer and Bernd Gottesmann, the MCN would become a key player in the field of medical congress management.

Fig. 1.19. The current headquarters of the DGAI and BDA in Nuremberg, Roritzerstraße 27 (© Bischof + Broel, Bayreuther Str. 21, 90409 Nuremberg)

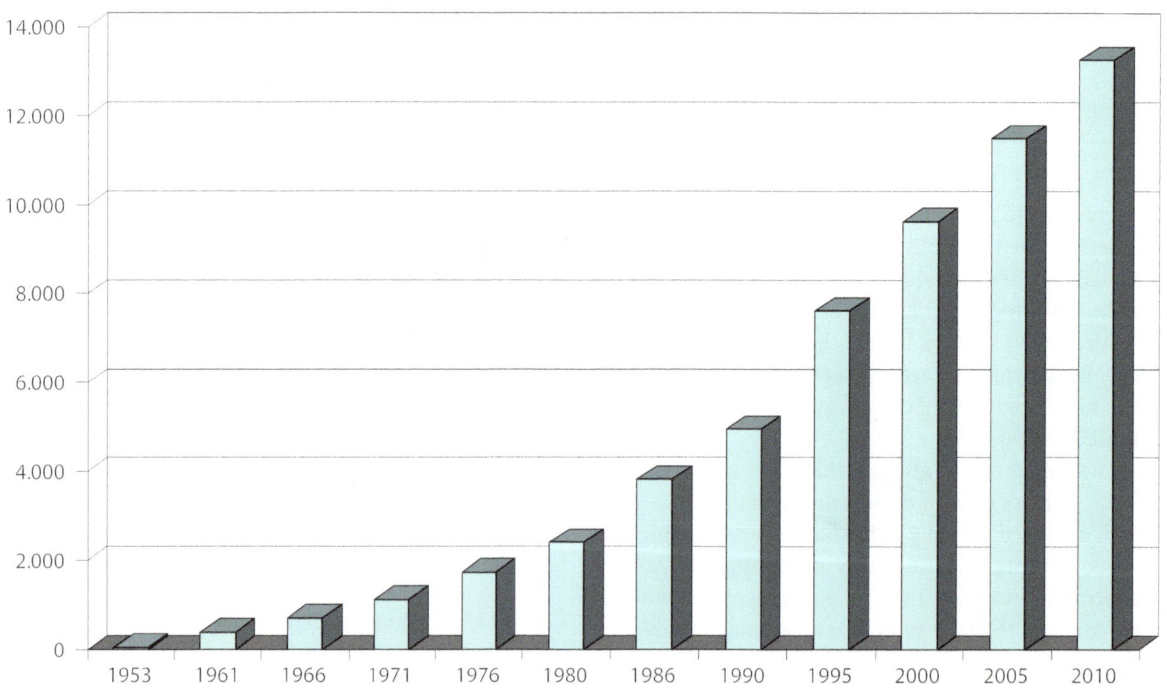

Fig. 1.18. Development of membership of the DGAI (courtesy of Prof. Dr. Jens-Peter Striebel, Mannheim)

1.1.24 A Museum for the History of Anaesthesia

While the archives provided an introspective look at the activities of the Society, the opening of the Horst Stoeckel Museum for the History of Anaesthesia in the year 2000 represented a step towards the public domain (☐ Fig. 1.20). Around 1,000 exhibits and a library with over 12,000 volumes, which Horst Stoeckel assembled, graphically capture the historic development of anaesthesia as a scientific discipline and as a clinical specialty [51] (a comprehensive treatise can be found in ▶ Chap. 1.6).

1.1.25 The Unity of the Specialty – New Paths

Advances and continuing development are based essentially on specialization. The importance of a discipline depends on its unity and solidarity. How is it possible on the one hand to permit the necessary specialization, while on the other hand to ensure the precious unity which has only been achieved with great effort over several decades? The ideal way is by nurturing and promoting this special-

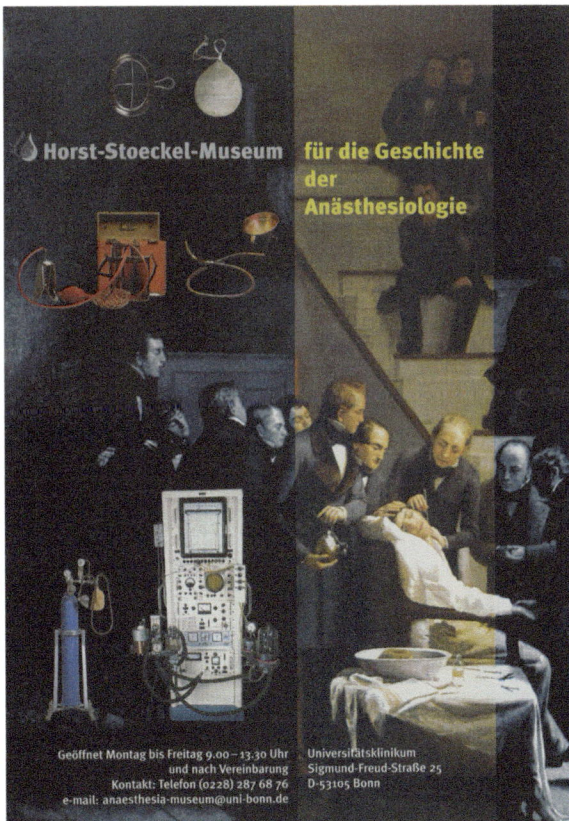

☐ **Fig. 1.20.** Poster of the Horst-Stoeckel Museum for the History of Anaesthesia in Bonn (courtesy of Horst Stoeckel Museum for the History of Anaesthesiology, Bonn)

ization while simultaneously providing a protective roof over the specialty.

Time and time again in private meetings – regardless of the agenda of the day – thought was given to strategies for the current situation as well as medium- and long-term prospects for the specialty in order to anticipate foreseeable developments and, where appropriate, to steer a suitable course rather than merely reacting to pressures as they occurred. These closed meetings (1979, 1981, 1993, 1997, 2000, 2001, 2003, 2005, 2006, 2007) were a fertile source of inspiration for the work of the Executive Committees. Besides the consolidation of the Society therefore, there was also a process of continuous adaptation; innovation and incessant effort to counter the fluctuating environment and meet the ever-present challenges which emerged.

1.1.26 Scientific Working Groups – Diverse Structures of the One Discipline

In recent decades the surgical specialties have developed and become diversified. Hence, for example, the so-called mother of the operative specialties, namely general surgery, has become divided into numerous professional societies. Anaesthesia therefore has had to meet the challenge of subspecialization within its own specialty as well as in surgery.

Because of this, in 1987 the DGAI decided to set up Scientific Working Groups, whose agendas would reflect the aims of the various committees of the DGAI »for the promotion of scientific and medico-political progress as well as for mutual exchange of experiences in specialized areas of anaesthesiology«. In hindsight this succeeded in engaging committed colleagues with special interests, knowledge and experiences in their own field, providing them with the necessary scope for specialization. Through the active support and integration of specialists (and therein lies the strength of anaesthesia – »unity through diversity«), it was possible to preserve this most cherished of possessions, allowing the DGAI to become the envy of other scientific medical specialty groups.

The first working groups were those on paediatric and cardiac anaesthesia, followed in 1989 by the previously mentioned study group on chronic pain and in 1991 by the study group on neuroanaesthesia. In the spring of 1993 the Executive Committee of the DGAI initiated discussions with the speakers of the existing working groups and the previously mentioned concept of continuing professional development within the DGAI was jointly developed.

In the meantime four more scientific working groups of the DGAI have been established besides intensive care medicine, emergency medicine and regional anaesthesia:

a working group on history of anaesthesia was founded at the ZAK (Central European Anaesthetic Congress) in Dresden in 1993, two working groups affiliated with the BDA (anaesthesia and economics and anaesthesia and the law) were formed, and an interdisciplinary group for dental anaesthesia was created. The working groups have proved to be a successful model for focussing on specialist issues of different interest groups among the membership and simultaneously for co-ordinating the personal commitment of the members in the best interests of the specialty as a whole.

1.1.27 The German Anaesthesia Congress – the Unity of the Specialty Becomes Visible

The much-laboured concept of unity of the specialty is by no means merely an idealistic notion. The unity of the specialty also appears today, as the synopsis of individual knowledge, be it in a textbook or recurrently at a congress. Because of this the German Anaesthesia Congress is of central importance in the life of our scientific community as an event in the mutual interests of German anaesthetists. The contemporary German Anaesthesia Congress (DAK) has developed from, among other things, the special sessions on »Modern Anaesthesia« inaugurated by Karl Heinrich Bauer at the German Surgery Congress of 1952. This situation was advantageous for the young specialty, as the infrastructure and synergy of an event which had an established tradition could be used.

The first German Anaesthesia Congress arranged independently of other organizations, with its own preliminary Executive Committee Meeting followed by a General Assembly of the members of the Society, took place on 5 and 6 November 1966 in Munich in the lecture theatre of the Rechts der Isar Hospital. The theme was »Long-term ventilation«. The Congress Director was the then DGAW President, Karl Horatz, and the conference itself was organized by the Second Secretary, Charlotte Lehmann. From then on, an Annual Congress of the DGAW took place independently, at a time of year between the two ZAKs; from 1989 onward this congress also took place in the years in which the ZAK did not take place in Germany. Before this, between 1967 and 1985, the ZAK years were utilized for medico-politically oriented meetings organized by the BDA. Starting in 1986 the DAK hosted the Annual Meeting of the DGAI, the BDA and the DAAF, under whose auspices the DAK annual refresher course took place. On account of the extreme importance of the Annual Congress for the scientific aspects of the specialty, the Executive Committees of the DGAI have always been keenly involved in the structure and content of the meetings.

In 1983 an Industry Advisory Committee was founded for liaison between the DGAI and the captains of industry in order to improve co-operation between industry and the Society in relation to exhibitions and other congress issues; industry already makes a fundamental contribution to the financing of the Annual Meeting by providing exhibition premises. The rapid increase, since the end of the 1970s, in the number of events for continuing educational development in anaesthesia, coupled with failure to agree on dates for these events, has led repeatedly to clashes in both timing and topics. The Society therefore established a co-ordinating centre to handle enquiries and applications for meeting dates. The collected event dates were entered into the current congress calendar in the journal.

Until the 1980s, it was usual to provide an abbreviated summary of the proceedings at the congress and after the event to publish a more detailed version of the proceedings. The publication of these proceedings proved to be increasingly difficult, such that its contemporary significance was lost due to the delayed appearance of the information. At the 1981 General Assembly, this practice was criticized and the Executive Committee invited opinions on how to proceed in order to improve on the unsatisfactory state of affairs. The drive for change was followed up and the abstracts were produced in a supplementary publication of one of the scientific journals. The abstract publications appeared mainly as a supplement to *Der Anaesthesist*, published by Springer-Verlag. In 1988 the Council resolved for financial reasons not to publish congress proceedings any longer, but to publish only the abstracts from then on. Since the journal *Anästhesiologie & Intensivmedizin* is owned exclusively by the anaesthesia fraternity (DGAI, BDA, DAAF) – the owners of *Der Anaesthesist* and *AINS* are the respective publishing houses – and also has a high impact factor and a wide circulation, the Executive Committee decided in 1999 to produce a publication of abstracts only in this journal in future.

At the same time the increasing size of the DAK meant that no longer could all work submitted be accepted either as a lecture or poster presentation. Primarily affected by this were the younger anaesthetists at the start of their academic careers, for whom it was important to discuss their investigations with others. In 1986, on the mutual instigation of Dietrich Kettler (Göttingen) and Karl-Heinz Weis (Würzburg), annual scientific working sessions of the DGAI were set up. This annually occurring event has proved itself to be an important instrument in promoting the recruitment of scientists to anaesthesia. The work presented by the candidates was considered by a committee and the best work was honoured with the DGAI research grant. This scholarship, which was created by an initiative of Dr. Manfred Specker (Bad Homberg), the then Chairman of the Board of the Fresenius Foundation, is presented at the subsequent German Anaesthesia Congress.

Against the background of increasing internationalization, of increasing European unification, and the opening up of Eastern Europe, in 1995 the Executive Committee also discussed the internationalization of the work of the DGAI. As a visible indication of this, the decision was taken that future annual DAKs would be held as the International German Anaesthesia Congress (DAK International), initially focussing on former Eastern Block countries. As Klaus van Ackern expressed in his opening address at the DAK International 1996 [72], the epithet »international« should also henceforth signal that the DGAI as the largest professional anaesthetic body in Europe would be prepared to assume responsibility in the wider sense, as for example had been borne out by the DGAI fellowship programme. At the DAK International 1996, Eastern Europe was introduced as the main focal point. In 1997, under the Presidency of Jochen Schulte am Esch (Hamburg), the topic »Standards between tradition and renewal« [67] in its international setting was put up for discussion (▪ Fig. 1.21). At the same time the »4th International Symposium on the History of Anaesthesia« also took place in connection with the DAK International 1997 in Hamburg. At the DAK International 1998 in Frankfurt, the DGAI, under the Presidency of Gunter Hempelmann (Giessen), was at the same time hosting the »8th Euro-

pean Congress of Anaesthesiology« [27]. Finally, it was possible to incorporate the five Scandinavian anaesthesia societies into the programme of the DAK International 1999, on the occasion of the 50th anniversary jubilee of the founding of those anaesthetic societies; these societies had themselves given willing and generous support to German anaesthesiology during its pioneering and developmental years [63]. In this context, it may also be mentioned as an expression of this increasing international awareness that from members of the DGAI associations of German and Russian as well as German and Turkish anaesthetists have been formed. The same applies to the Association of Anaesthesia and the Third World.

Over many years the abbreviated form DAK had become synonymous with »German Anaesthesia Congress«. No thoughts had been given to the fact that this abbreviation was already protected under patent law by a well-known German health insurance company. Having grown into one of the biggest German medical congresses, the company then claimed to have a monopoly on the logo amid corresponding media hype. The solution was simple; instead of the German word Kongress, the English word Congress was used and hence DAK became DAC: this was implemented at the 2003 jubilee congress (▪ Fig. 1.22).

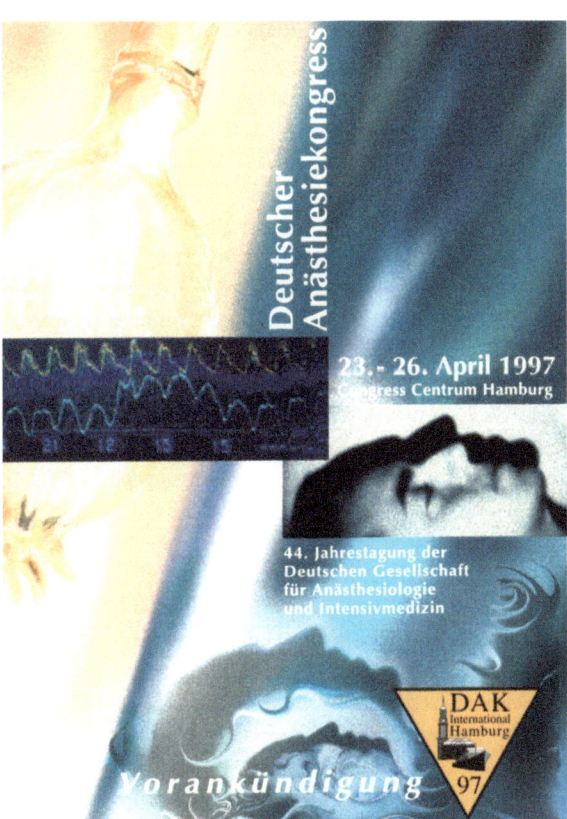

▪ **Fig. 1.21.** Poster of the DAK International 1997 in Hamburg (© MCN, Nuremberg)

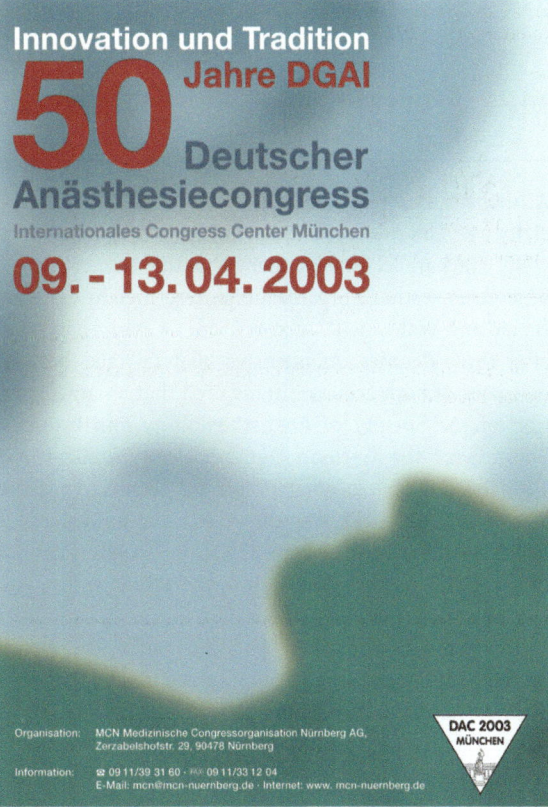

▪ **Fig. 1.22.** Poster of the Jubilee Congress DAC 2003 in Munich (© MCN, Nuremberg)

1.1.28   The Central European Anaesthesia Congress

Joint annual meetings with the Austrian and Swiss Societies of Anaesthesiology were already being organized at the founding meeting of the German Society of Anaesthesia in Munich in 1953. In the early years, the meetings took place simultaneously with the Annual Congress of the German Society of Surgery and at first had a particular theme of interest. At the Second Austrian Congress of Anaesthesia in Velden in 1953, the representatives of the three societies decided to name future joint conferences the Central European Anaesthesia Congress (ZAK). Following the first two Austrian meetings, the third was so named in Munich in 1954. The joint meetings were organized annually on a rotational basis until 1957 and thereafter every 2 years alternating with the European Congress and the World Congress. Over the intervening 40 years the ZAK developed into a highly successful event. However, increasing internationalization of the congress in the 1990s, followed by the appearance of the meetings of the European Academy of Anaesthesiology (EAA) and the European Society of Anaesthesiology (ESA) led to the end of this long tradition which culminated at the 24th ZAK in Vienna in 1995; this followed the first meeting involving a reunified Germany at the 23rd ZAK in Dresden in 1993.

1.1.29   German Reunification and the Unity of the Specialty

A further and unexpected aspect of the unity of the specialty was a by-product of the reunification of Germany in 1990. The parallel establishment in both German States of separate anaesthesia organizations, described by Gottfried Benad and Wolfgang Röse in ▶ Chap. 1.4, had a happy end after three decades. At intensive bilateral talks between delegates of both groups it transpired that an amalgamation of the Society of Anaesthesiology and Intensive Therapy of the German Democratic Republic (GAIT) with the DGAI was not possible for technical reasons. Therefore, the GAIT was dissolved unanimously at its General Meeting in Gera on 23 October 1990. Members of the GAIT were invited to join the DGAI as the pan-German Society of Anaesthesia.

In April 1953 the DGA – 2 months before the popular uprising on 17 June – had been founded as a pan-German Society. Lothar Barth of Berlin had participated at the inaugural meeting in Munich and had signed the Decree of Inauguration. In the early days all East German colleagues were members of the Society with equal rights and privileges. They were all listed in the annual reports of the Second Secretary which dealt with membership matters.

Even during the period when membership fees could not be transferred as a result of inequality between the currencies, Lothar Barth was able to set up an account in 1960 in East Berlin, so that East German colleagues could pay their subscriptions.

After the Berlin Wall was built on 13 August 1961 the East German Government severed direct travel and communication links with the West and thereby increased the existing pressure on their scientists to establish their own structures and to abandon all unified German scientific organizations based in West Germany. In 1960 Lothar Barth founded a Central Working Group on Anaesthesiology and Anaesthesia Technology, which included anaesthetists as well as representatives of the medical-technical industry as members. Following this, on 7 March 1964, anaesthetists set up their own society, the Section of Anaesthesiology of the German Society of Clinical Medicine. The then President of the DGA Kurt Wiemers together with Charlotte Lehmann was able to travel to East Berlin for the Inaugural Ceremony. Lehmann published a detailed report on this event, in which she declared that »The membership in the DGA will not be affected by members joining the Section of Anaesthesiology«. Subsequently, it was discussed whether the Chairman of the Section of Anaesthesiology should be a member of the Executive Committee of the DGA. On 4 November 1966 the Committee of the DGA decided against this possibility »due to recent unfortunate developments and the fact that the Section of Anaesthesiology had made no move to reciprocate«.

Within a few months of inclusion of the East German Society into the WFSA (1968) 60 of 140 anaesthetists resigned from the DGA with a standardized letter, which had been pre-written by the authorities. The Executive Committee then decided to freeze the membership of the East German anaesthetists, but to continue to send them informations. In retrospect the decision to freeze the membership turned out to be prescient; these colleagues only had to reactivate their DGAI membership once GAIT was dissolved. They had remained deferred members of the DGAI even in times of forced separation.

At the first General Assembly following reunification on 21 March 1991 as part of the DAK Meeting in Mannheim, one of these reactivated members, Gottfried Benad of Rostock, was elected to the Presidency of DGAI for the year 1993. In his acceptance speech he expressed his thanks for the trust given to him during the election and emphasized the symbolic importance of this decision which reinforced the feeling of solidarity amongst all German anaesthetists. The only wrinkle in these developments was that according to constitutional rules, anaesthetic and intensive care nurses who had previously been associate members of the GAIT were unable to become associate members of the DGAI.

1.1.30 Current Responsibilities, Organization and Structure of the DGAI – The Armamentarium for the Future

Purpose of the Society

The Society motivates doctors to combine their efforts in developing and advancing anaesthesiology, intensive care medicine, emergency medicine and pain therapy to achieve the highest standard for their patients.

Aims

According to the statutes of the DGAI the aims are:
- Development of the science and practice of anaesthesiology
- Represent anaesthetic interests in teaching and research
- Preserve the specialty's interest with regard to other medico-scientific societies; additionally uphold these interests together with the Professional Association of German Anaesthetists with regard to ministries, authorities and organizations
- Define the main topics of postgraduate and continuing medical education in anaesthesiology
- Develop and promote standards for quality control
- Organize and promote scientific meetings and manage continuing professional education
- Participate in development and structuring of postgraduate medical training in co-operation with the 17 State Chambers of Physicians and their umbrella organization, the German Medical Association
- Public relations work on behalf of anaesthetists
- Organize the German Anaesthesia Congress and regional as well as international meetings
- Publish the journal *Anästhesiologie & Intensivmedizin*

Divisions and Institutions of the Society

- The Board
- The Executive Committee
- The Extended Executive Committee
- The General Assembly
- The Regional Assemblies
- The Scientific Advisory Council
- Scientific Working Groups
- Commissions
- Regional appointees for quality assurance
- German Academy of Continuing Education in Anaesthesiology (DAAF)
- The joint office of the DGAI and BDA

The Board

The Board consists of the President and the Vice-President. Both are entitled to represent the Society officially and unofficially.

The Executive Committee

The Executive Committee consists of the President, the Vice-President, the General Secretary, the Secretary, the Treasurer, the representative of the regional assemblies, the respective Presidents of the BDA and DAAF, and the representative of the trainees, and the speakers of the Scientific Working Groups on Intensive Care Medicine, Pain Therapy and Emergency Medicine. The Executive Committee has to prepare and carry out decisions made by the General Assembly and the Extended Executive Committee. It supervises the daily business and has to attend to all responsibilities of the Society, which have not been allocated to any committee.

The President runs the daily business in conjunction with the Vice-President; he calls board meetings in writing including the agenda of the day and upon the justifiable request of two members the Board has to convene within 4 weeks. During the first year of Presidency the President's predecessor is the Vice-President and the President elect is Vice-President during the second year of Presidency. In the case of the President's absence the Vice-President supervises the responsibilities.

The General Secretary supports the President in representing the Society's interests vis-à-vis the authorities, organizations and scientific societies as well as the daily running of the business. In conjunction with the Treasurer he signs financial transfers.

The Secretary is responsible for the correspondence with the members, especially in matters concerning the DGAI and the membership. He sets up the agenda for the General Assembly in the absence of the General Secretary as well as meetings of the Executive Committee and Extended Executive Committee.

The Treasurer manages the accounts of the Society and is responsible for bookkeeping involving money received and expenditures. The General Secretary may deputize for him in his absence. All expenditures, especially bank drafts, have to be countersigned by the General Secretary; in the case of absence of either one the President countersigns. Payments outside the usual sphere of business require the prior agreement of the President. The Treasurer must supply a receipt when any payment for the Society is received. He must deliver an annual summary of accounts to the General Assembly. After scrutiny and approval of the accounts by two members in good standing chosen by the members, the accounts will be deemed to have been accepted by the Committee.

The Representative of the Regional Chairmen informs the Executive Committee and other organs of the Society regarding events in the Regional Sections and about proposals made to them. He in turn informs the respective sections regarding outcomes of the meetings of the Executive Committees and about current business.

The Extended Executive Committee

The Extended Executive Committee consists of the members of the Executive Committee itself, the last three Presidents of the DGAI, who held this position before the incumbent Vice-President and the Chairpersons of the Regional Sections.

The General Assembly

Once a year an ordinary General Assembly will take place, normally in conjunction with the Congress. An extraordinary meeting may be called when the interests of the Society are involved or when this is requested either by one-third of the ordinary members or by the Executive Committee.

The Scientific Advisory Panel

Experts from other clinical areas may be called to act as scientific advisors for a period of up to 5 years.

Regional Sections

In recognition of regional activities of the DGAI, Regional Sections will be established (*Landesverbände*). They are legally not independent subdivisions of the DGAI. The General Assembly of the DGAI may decide that in States where more than one branch of the *Landesärztekammer* (State Chamber of Physicians) exists, that a Regional Sections may be set up for each *Landesärztekammer*. The membership of the DGAI can determine that in each *Land* (State) where there is more than one Chamber a Regional Sections can be set up for the area of the respective Chamber.

The Publications of the Society

The journals *Anästhesiologie & Intensivmedizin*, *Der Anaesthesist* and *Anästhesiologie, Intensivmedizin, Notfallmedizin, Schmerztherapie (AINS)* are the official mouthpieces of the DGAI (▶ Chap. 1.5).

The Commissions (status in 2008)

Commissions have been set by the Executive Committee of the DGAI to deal with questions of a general or professional nature. Their objective is to provide suggestions to the Executive Committee and where necessary documents and to support the Executive Committee in specialized matters.
- Commissions
  - Airway Management
  - Postgraduate and Continuing Medical Education
  - Standards and Technical Safety
  - Pregraduate and Simulator Training
  - Guidelines
  - Transoesophageal Echocardiography
- Joint Commissions (DGAI and BDA)
  - Congress Programme
  - Working Group on Blood Transfusion

The Scientific Working Groups (status in 2008)

The scientific working groups deal with specific scientific questions relating to particular areas of anaesthesia and intensive care medicine. Any member of the DGAI is free to participate in any of the working groups.
- Scientific Working Groups of the DGAI:
  - History of Anaesthesia
  - Intensive Care Medicine
  - Cardiac Anaestesia
  - Paediatric Anaesthesia
  - Neuroanaesthesia
  - Emergency Medicine
  - Regional Anaesthesia
  - Pain Therapy
  - Anaesthesia for Thoracic Sugery
  - Ultra Sound in Anaesthesiology and ICM
  - Palliative Medicine
  - Young Scientists
- Joint Working Groups (DGAI and BDA):
  - Anaesthesia and the Law
  - Forum for Quality Management and Economics
- Interdisciplinary Working Group:
  - Dental Anaesthesia

Scientific Prizes and Honours of the German Society of Anaesthesiology and Intensive Care Medicine

The DGAI bestows a number of scientific prizes and honours. Lists of honoured individuals can be found in the Appendix (▶ Chap. 1.3).

German Academy of Continuing Education in Anaesthesiology (DAAF)

The German Academy of Continuing Education in Anaesthesiology is supported by both the DGAI and BDA and organizes courses for advanced and continuing medical education for anaesthetists. Tried and proven instruments of CME are refresher courses, revision courses as well as training courses with the anaesthetic simulator designed to refresh and update existing knowledge of topical and important issues in the specialty.

Recently Launched Projects

2005 »e-Learning«: an internet-based platform for CME in anaesthesiology, intensive care medicine, emergeny medicine, and pain therapy. A joint project of DGAI and BDA.

2005 QUIPS (Quality Improvement in Postoperative Pain Therapy): a web-based feedback system for assessing, analyzing, benchmarking and improving postoperative pain treatment. A joint project of DGAI and BDA in cooperation with the German Society of Surgery and the Professional Association of German Surgeons [48a].

2006 PaSOS (Patient Safety Optimisation System): a national anaesthesia incident reporting system. A joint project of DGAI and BDA [59b],

2006 »Young Anaesthesia«: a continous initiative aimed at integrating young doctors in training into the activities of the DGAI [59a].

2007 »Resuscitation Registry«: of the DGAI: collects data of CPR patients in Germany according to the »Utstein-Style« recommendations [26a].

2008 NTA (Regional Anaesthesia Safety Network in Germany): prospective recording of data on the safety of regional anaesthesia in order to identify of risk factors for complications and develop safety improvement strategies. A joint project of DGAI and BDA [73a].

1.1.31 The Future: the Anaesthetist on Track to Becoming a Perioperative Physician?

At the end of our passage through 55 years of the German Society of Anaesthesiology and Intensive Care Medicine, one question remains: where is the journey of the anaesthetist and his scientific association going to? Right at the beginning of this journey Rudolf Frey, the visionary of the fledgling specialty in Germany, in his article »The place of the anaesthetist between surgery and general medicine« [21] outlined the anaesthetist's activity as primarily based in the operating theatre, but extending beyond that and involving general medicine: from preoperative preparation of the patient, postoperative care, acute and emergency medicine to interaction with other specialties. His expert knowledge of resuscitation, shock, pain relief and parenteral nutrition are all required. Frey saw anaesthetics as a cross section of medicine equally encompassing applied internal medicine, physiology and pharmacology. In this way the anaesthetist is qualified for a variety of activities, which instead of isolating him – particularly in the operating theatre – rooted him firmly within the team. One cannot help thinking that Rudolph Frey envisaged 40 years ago what we mean today when we speak of the anaesthetist as a physician in perioperative medicine.

Apart from that, where the journey will lead us depends largely – and Rudolf Frey and his colleagues have stressed this repeatedly – on what kind of basic attitude and ethos we apply to our work. Therefore, in conclusion, to quote a paragraph from Frey's contribution to the 25th anniversary of the DGAI, which is as topical today as ever:

> The history of German anaesthetics mirrors the principles which have existed since Hippocrates: excellence in clinical practice, teaching and research are not achieved by dogma or by the use of power or status or by intrigue, but via the free and voluntary cooperation of independent individuals who desire to achieve progress governed by humanitarian and ethical motives with the objective of achieving a common goal: the well-being of the patient. By that we mean not only the individual patient, but also the well-being of the community as a whole, which we seem to jeopardize today more than ever before, despite, or maybe because, of all our technical and material progress and advances [22].

Acknowledgements

The authors wish to thank Prof. Dr. Dr. h.c. Friedrich Wilhelm Ahnefeld, Ulm, Prof. Dr. Klaus Fischer, Bremen, Prof. Dr. Hans Wolfgang Opderbecke, Nuremberg, and Prof. Dr. Erich Rügheimer (†), Erlangen, for their valuable advice. Special thanks go to the colleagues from the head offices of the DGAI and the BDA for their enthusiastic support and help in researching the archives and for compiling the appendix.

References

Verbatim quotations from minutes and other documents in the archives of the DGAI are marked in the text.

1. Ahnefeld FW (1983) Neujahrsaufruf des Präsidenten der DGAI. Anästh Intensivmed 24:1
2. Anonymous (1928) Germany on the way to organized professional anesthesia. Curr Res Anesth Analg 7:195–196
3. Arbeitsgemeinschaft der Westdeutschen Ärztekammern (ed) (1953) 56. Deutscher Ärztetag. Geschlossene Sitzung am 19. September 1953 im Stadttheater Lindau. Ärztl Mitt 38:532–534
4. Arbeitsgemeinschaft der Westdeutschen Ärztekammern (ed) (1953) Stenographischer Bericht des 56. Deutschen Ärztetages am 19. und 20. September 1953, Lindau/Bodensee. Ärzte-Verlag, Cologne, pp 22–24 und Appendix pp 60–61
5. Bauer KH (1952) Zur geistigen Situation unseres Faches. Langenbecks Arch Chir 273:9–14
6. Bauer KH (1955) Die Wandlungen der Anästhesie vom Standpunkt des Operateurs. Langenbecks Arch Chir 282:163–207
6a. Biermann E, Landauer B (2008) Anästhesie durch Nichtanästhesisten – »Des Kaisers neue Kleider?« Anästh Intensivmed 49:552–554
7. Bräutigam K-H (1993) 40 Jahre »Facharzt für Anästhesie«. Anästh Intensivmed 34:259–268
8. Bräutigam K-H (1997) Die Entwicklung des Fachgebietes. In: Brandt L (ed) Illustrierte Geschichte der Anästhesie. Wissenschaftliche Verlagsgesellschaft, Stuttgart, pp 176–203
9. Brütt H, Kümmel H (1929) 90. Versammlung der Gesellschaft Deutscher Naturforscher und Ärzte in Hamburg am 16.-22. September 1928. Zentralbl Chir 56:143–185, 217–241
10. Derra E (1951) Der heutige Stand der Anästhesieverfahren in der Chirurgie. Langenbecks Arch Klin Chir 267:231–256
11. Derra E (1952) Gedanken zur Neuordnung des Narkosewesens in Deutschland. Krankenhaus 44:49–51
12. DGA und Deutsche Gesellschaft für Chirurgie (1965) Richtlinien für die Stellung des leitenden Anästhesisten. Anaesthesist 14:31–32
13. DGAI (1994) Franz-Kuhn-Medaille an Frau Gertraud Mulligan verliehen. Anästh Intensivmed 35:296
14. DGAI (1978) Hellmut-Weese-Gedächtnisvorlesung. Anästh Intensivmed 19:601

15. DGAW (1973) Entschließung der Deutschen Gesellschaft für Anästhesie und Wiederbelebung über die Weiterbildung von Fachschwestern und Fachpflegern. Anästh Inf 14:28-33

16. Deutsche Gesellschaft für Chirurgie (1950) Notiz für medizinische Presse. Berlin-Grunewald

17. Deutsche Gesellschaft für Chirurgie (1952) Bericht der Narkosekommission. Anaesthesist 1:32

18. Elster R (1958) Hinweis der Schwesterngemeinschaft. Ärztl Mitt 43:1213

19. Engisch K (1961) Wie ist rechtlich die Verantwortlichkeit des Chirurgen im Verhältnis zur Verantwortlichkeit des Anästhesisten bei ärztlichen Operationen zu bestimmen und zu begrenzen? Langenbecks Arch Klin Chir 297:236-254

20. Fischer AW (1959) Wieweit können Schwestern oder Pfleger an Narkosen beteiligt werden? Chirurg 30:535-536

21. Frey R (1963) Die Stellung des Anaesthesiologen zwischen Chirurgie und innerer Medizin. Anaesthesist 12:270-271

22. Frey R (1978) Die Gründung der Deutschen Gesellschaft für Anästhesie. Anästh Intensivmed 19:373-376

23. Frey R, Bauer M, Krabbe E (1953) Bericht über die erste Tagung der Deutschen Gesellschaft für Anaesthesie am 10. und 11. April 1953 im Deutschen Museum in München. Anaesthesist 2:149-156

24. Frey R, Henschel WF, Horatz K, Hutschenreuter K, Just OH, Lawin P, Rügheimer E, Weis KH, Wiemers K, Zindler M (1978) Zum 25jährigen Bestehen der Deutschen Gesellschaft für Anästhesiologie und Intensivmedizin. Anästh Intensivmed 19:369-453

25. Goetze O (1939) Allgemeinchirurgie und Spezialfach. Langenbecks Arch Klin Chir 196:129-133

26. Goetze O (1940) Das Problem der Universalität in der modernen Heilkunst. Zentralbl Chir 67:204-210

26a. Gräsner JT, Messelken M, Scholz J, Fischer M (2006) Das Reanimationsregister der DGAI. Anästh Intensivmed 47:630-631

27. Hempelmann G (1998) 10. Europäischer Anästhesiekongress/ 45. Deutscher Anästhesiekongress 1998. Anästh Intensivmed 39:286

28. Henke W (1978) »Wir verlassen Würzburg heiterer«. Anästh Intensivmed 19:610-611

29. Hesse F (1951) Das Aufgabengebiet des Facharztes für Narkose und Anästhesie. Med Welt 20:356-358

30. Hesse F, Derra E, Macintosh R, Redwitz Ev (1951) Aussprache zu 2-8. Langenbecks Arch Chir 267:24-60

31. Hügin W (1960) Wie weit können Schwestern oder Pfleger an Narkosen beteiligt werden? Chirurg 31:200

32. Hunter AR (1949) Die Narkose als ärztliches Spezialfach. Krankenhausarzt 22:8-11

33. Junghanns H (1949) »Narkosearzt« als neue Facharztmöglichkeit. Krankenhausarzt 22:19-20

34. Kettler D (1985) Grußwort des Präsidenten der DGAI zum Neuen Jahr. Anästh Intensivmed 26:1

35. Killian H (1928) Über amerikanische Narkoseverhältnisse. Narkose Anaesth 1:448-463

36. Killian H (1939) A.C.E. Narkosegemische. Langenbecks Arch Klin Chir 196:211

37. Killian H (1941) Plan zur Neuordnung des Narkosewesens in Deutschland. Schmerz Narkose Anaesth 14:73-87

38. Killian H (1949) Reorganisation des Narkosewesens. Krankenhausarzt 22:15-19

39. Killian H (1950) Die Verwendung des Curare und verwandter Substanzen für die Verbesserung der Narkose. Langenbecks Arch Klin Chir 264:241-246

40. Killian H (1950) Gedanken und Vorschläge zur Frage des Narkosespezialisten. Dtsch Med Wochenschr 75:9-741

41. Killian H (1964) 40 Jahre Narkoseforschung. Erfahrungen und Erlebnisse. Verlag der Deutschen Hochschullehrer-Zeitung, Tübingen

42. Kirschner M (1939) Die Stellung der Röntgenologie zu den Kliniken. Chirurg 11:361-368

43. Kremer K (1951) Sondersitzung: Moderne Anästhesie. Zentralbl Chir 77:948-955

44. Lassner J, Frey R (1979) Bericht über den Europäischen Anästhesiekongress vom 4.-8. September 1978 in Paris und die Gründung der Europäischen Akademie für Anästhesiologie. Anästh Intensivmed 20:205-207

45. Lehmann C (1964) Bericht über die Gründungsversammlung der Sektion Anaesthesiologie der Deutschen Gesellschaft für Klinische Medizin am 7. März 1964 in Berlin 13:395-396

46. Lehmann C (1967) Die Deutsche Gesellschaft für Anaesthesie und Wiederbelebung. Gründung und Entwicklung. Anaesthesist 16:259-268

47. McMechan FH (1928) Zur 90. Versammlung deutscher Naturforscher und Ärzte, Hamburg, September 1928. Narkose Anaesth 1:529-530

48. McMechan FH (1929) Invitation to Germany to join the ranks of international anesthesia during the Hamburg congress. Curr Res Anesth Analg 8:196

48a. Meißner W (2007) QUIPS – ein interdisziplinäres Benchmarkprojekt zur Qualitätsverbesserung in der postoperativen Schmerz-therapie. Anästh Intensivmed 48:715-718

49. Möller G (1951) Gedanken zur Entwicklung des Narkose-Fachwesens in Deutschland. Westfäl Ärztebl 5:167-169

50. Moyers J (1978) Greetings on the occasion of the 25th Anniversary of the DGAI. Anästh Intensivmed 19:613

51. Nadstawek J (2000) Eröffnung des Horst-Stoeckel-Museums für die Geschichte der Anästhesiologie. Anästh Intensivmed 41:714

52. Niedermayer F (1949) »Der Narkosearzt«. Krankenhausarzt 22:20-22

53. Opderbecke HW (1978) Zum 25jährigen Bestehen der Deutschen Gesellschaft für Anästhesiologie und Intensivmedizin. Anästh Intensivmed 19:369-371

54. Opderbecke HW (1983) Gründung eines Archivs der Deutschen Anästhesie. Anästh Intensivmed 24:379

55. Opderbecke HW (2001) Als der Berufsverband laufen lernte. Anästh Intensivmed 42:819-827

56. Opderbecke HW, Weissauer W (Hrsg) (1999) Entschließungen, Empfehlungen, Vereinbarungen, Leitlinien, 3rd. edn. Aktiv Druck & Verlag, Ebelsbach

57. Oyama T (1978) Congratulations 25th anniversary. Anästhesiol Intensivmed 19:455

58. Pribilla O (1964) Der Tod in der Narkose. Anaesthesist 10:340-345

59. Purschke R (1995) Anästhesie auf dem Weg ins 3. Jahrtausend. Anästh Intensivmed 36:41

59a. Radke J, Hahnenkamp K (2006) Junge Anästhesie – eine Initiative der DGAI. Anästh Intensivmed 47:244-245

59b. Rall M, Diekmann P. Stricker ER et al. (2006) Patientensicherheits-Optimierungssystem (PaSOS). Anästh Intensivmed 47 (Suppl 2): S20-S24

60. Rieder W (1929) Gasnarkose. Chirurg 1:83-84

61. Rügheimer E (1978) Zukunftsperspektiven der Anästhesiologie. Vom Narkotiseur zum Homöostatiker. Anästh Intensivmed 19:450-453

62. Rügheimer E (1981) Schlussbericht des Kongresspräsidenten über die Tätigkeit des Organisationskomitees für den 7. Weltkongress für Anästhesiologie vom 14. bis 21. September 1980 in Hamburg vor dem Erweiterten Präsidium der DGAI am 14. September 1981 in Berlin. Anästh Intensivmed 22:411-412

63. Schadewaldt H (1978) Von Galens »Nárkosis« zur modernen »Balanced anaesthesia«. Anästh Intensivmed 19:589-601

64. Schara J (1981) Grußwort. Anästh Intensivmed 22:1

65. Schmidt H (1928) Die Gasnarkose vom Standpunkt des amerikanischen Narkosespezialisten. Narkose Anaesth 1:530-540

66. Schmidt H (1972) Gruß an Hans Killian. In: Frey R, Bonica JJ, Foldes FF et al (eds) Erlebte Geschichte der Anästhesie. Festsitzung zum 80. Geburtstag von Hans Killian am 6. April 1972 in Mainz. Eigenverlag, Mainz, pp 23–26

67. Schulte am Esch J (1997) Ansprache des Präsidenten der DGAI anlässlich der Eröffnung des Deutschen Anästhesiekongresses – DAK '97 – International. Anästh Intensivmed 38:448–450

68. Schwarz W (1989) Attempts to establish anaesthesiology as a specialty in German medicine. In: Atkinson RS, Boulton TB (eds) The history of anaesthesia. Royal Society of Medicine Services, London, pp 170–175

69. Sperling F (1939) Schreiben XI-Dr.Sp./Gd. zu Akte Nr. 3133/92.07. vom 14.9.1939

70. Stratenwerth G (1961) Arbeitsteilung und ärztliche Sorgfaltspflicht. In: Bockelmann, P, Gallas W (eds) Festschrift für Eberhard Schmidt zum 70. Geburtstag. Vandenhoeck & Ruprecht, Göttingen, pp 383–400

71. Tschöp M (1986) Ernst von der Porten 1884-1940 in der Geschichte der deutschen Anästhesiologie. Springer, Berlin

72. van Ackern K (1996) Eröffnungsansprache des Präsidenten der DGAI anlässlich des Deutschen Anästhesiekongresses – DAK '96 – International. Anästh Intensivmed 37:617–620

73. Van Aken H (2002) 25 Jahre DAAF. Anästh Intensivmed 43:577–580

73a. Volk T et al. (2008) Ein Netzwerk zur Sicherheit der Regionalanästhesie in Deutschland. Eine Initiative der DGAI und des BDA. Anästh Intensivmed 49:55–61

74. von Brunn M (1913) Die Allgemeinnarkose. Enke, Stuttgart

75. Weis K-H (1978) Ansprache des Präsidenten der DGAI zum 25jährigen Gründungsjubiläum. Anästh Intensivmed 19:581–588

76. Weißauer W (1962) Arbeitsteilung und Abgrenzung der Verantwortung zwischen Anästhesist und Operateur. Anaesthesist 11:239–271

77. Weißauer W (1963) Zur Problematik der Schwesternnarkose und die Ausbildung von Anaesthesieschwestern. Anaesthesist 12:156–161

78. Weißauer W, Opderbecke HW (eds) (1980) Anästhesist und Krankenhaus. Perimed, Erlangen

79. Weißauer W, Opderbecke HW (1983) Zulässigkeit und Grenzen der »Parallelnarkose«. Anästh Intensivmed 24:214–218

80. Wissenschaftsrat (1960) Empfehlungen des Wissenschaftsrates zum Ausbau der wissenschaftlichen Einrichtungen. Teil 1: Wissenschaftliche Hochschulen. Mohr, Tübingen

81. Zinganell K (1993) Der Lotse geht von Bord. Anästh Intensivmed 34:383–384

82. Ruprecht J, van Lieburg MJ, Lee JA et al (eds) (1985) Anaesthesia: essays on its history. Springer, Berlin, p 280

83. Erneute gemeinsame Stellungnahme des Berufsverbandes Deutscher Anästhesisten (BDA) und der Deutschen Gesellschaft für Anästhesiologie und Intensivmedizin (DGAI) zu Zulässigkeit und Grenzen der Parallelverfahren in der Anästhesiologie (Münsteraner Erklärung II 2007) (2007) Anästh Intensivmed 48: 223–229

1.2 History of the Society of Anaesthesiology and Intensive Therapy of the German Democratic Republic (GAIT)

G. Benad and W. Röse

The development of anaesthesiology started in Germany only after the end of World War II and was strongly influenced by the subsequent division of Germany, which lasted for 40 years. In the 1950s, the development of anaesthesiology was still comparable in East and West Germany and had a great deal in common.

The »German Working Group on Anaesthesiology«, which was founded by J. Bark/Todtmoos in Salzburg in 1952 corresponded to the »Central Working Group on Anaesthesiology and Anaesthesia Technology«, which was founded by Lothar Barth in East Berlin in 1960 [2]. Both institutions were the precursors of the West and East German societies of anaesthesiology, respectively.

The title of »Specialist in Anaesthesia« was introduced in West Germany in 1953 and »Specialist in Anaesthesiology« in East Germany in 1956. The establishment of anaesthesiology as a new, independent medical discipline was accomplished, only after certain conditions common to both parts of Germany and expressed by the representatives of the traditional medical specialties, particularly by its »mother discipline« surgery, had been fulfilled.

Nevertheless, there were great differences between East and West Germany regarding the foundation of a separate anaesthesiological society, which had not existed either in East or in West Germany at the beginning of the 1950s. In West Germany, the »German Society of Anaesthesia« (DGA) was founded at a meeting of its precursor, the »German Working Group on Anaesthesiology«, at a Congress of the »German Society of Surgery« in Munich on 10 April 1953. First and foremost, the DGA was an all-German society [19], which was founded by 46 medical practitioners working in anaesthesia. Among these was the pioneer of anaesthesiology in East Germany, Lothar Barth/Berlin-Buch (◻ Figs. 1.23 and 1.24).

Before the wall was built by the East German government in 1961, many anaesthetists from East Germany could also become members of the DGA, because their membership in a West German society was at first still tolerated by the government. Thus, during the early years of its development, the DGA was able to preserve its character as an all-German society. After the complete division of Germany into East and West Germany, however, East German medical doctors of all disciplines – including anaesthesiology – were forced to withdraw their membership from all West German societies. The DGA, however, regarded the membership of the East German anaesthetists as merely in abeyance, although for many years none

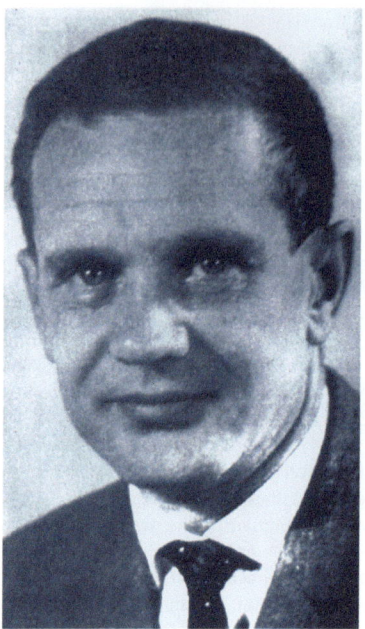

◻ **Fig. 1.23.** Lothar Barth (1921–1979) co-founder of the all-German Society of Anaesthesia (DGA)

◻ **Fig. 1.24.** Part of the founding document of the DGA 1953

of them was allowed to participate in congresses of the DGA. Thus, relations between East and West German anaesthetists were reduced merely to contact by letter, or in some cases, to private visits of West German anaesthetists to East Germany.

This situation together with the fact that in 1962 the number of specialists in East Germany in anaesthesiology had increased to 80, necessitated formation of their own scientific anaesthesiological organization [6, 9]. Furthermore, the other traditional medical fields including surgery and internal medicine had already created their own scientific sections, under the umbrella of the »German Society of Clinical Medicine« later called »Society of Clinical

Medicine of the German Democratic Republic«. Therefore, the existence of an independent »Section of Anaesthesiology« (SA) was regarded as one of the prerequisites for the further development of anaesthesiology within an interdisciplinary framework covering all medical specialties in the German Democratic Republic (GDR).

1.2.1 Foundation of the »Section of Anaesthesiology« of the »German Society of Clinical Medicine«

The head of the »Central Working Group on Anaesthesiology and Anaesthesia Technology«, Lothar Barth/Berlin-Buch, formed a committee consisting of the following specialists of anaesthesiology: Gottfried Benad/Rostock, Wolfgang Bucklitsch/Berlin-Friedrichshain, Karl-Heinz Martin/Halle-Saale, Manfred Meyer/Berlin-Buch, Hartwig Ferdinand Poppelbaum/Berlin-Buch, Manfred Schädlich/Berlin, Ulrich Strahl/Berlin-Buch and Lisa Wilken/Magdeburg. This committee founded the »Section of Anaesthesiology« (SA) in Berlin on 25 October 1963 and Lothar Barth applied for its admission to the »German Society of Clinical Medicine«. The President of this society, F. H. Schulz/Berlin, accepted this application with pleasure on 29 October 1963 [6].

The first meeting of the SA was held in Berlin on 7 March 1964. Of the 116 anaesthetists invited from all parts of East Germany, 86 accepted the invitation of the Founding Committee and its leader Lothar Barth. In addition, an official guest of the East German Ministry of Health, L. Rohland, Director of the »General Secretariat of the Medico-Scientific Societies of the German Democratic Republic« (GS), observed this meeting very carefully. Two surgeons from Berlin-Buch, H. Gummel and T. Matthes, the President of the German Society of Anaesthesia, Kurt Wiemers/Freiburg, and the Secretary of the DGA, Charlotte Lehmann/Munich, who reported on this meeting in the West German journal »Der Anaesthesist« [17] also participated in this meeting as honorary guests of the SA. In a secret ballot, which was the last one in the history of the SA for many years, 86 East German anaesthetists elected 5 anaesthetists out of a group of 14 nominees to set up the Executive Committee of the SA. This election was observed very spectically and critically by the representative of the Ministry of Health, L. Rohland, because, although democratic, the procedure was different from the norm of East German elections at that time, which were only based on a unified list of candidates. Lothar Barth/Berlin-Buch (83 votes) was the winner of this election. He was followed by Manfred Meyer/Berlin-Buch (59 votes), Lisa Wilken/Magdeburg (50 votes), Ulrich Strahl/Berlin-Buch (44 votes) and Gerhard Endres/Jena (40 votes). These five anaesthetists constituted the

Executive Committee of the SA. Their first meeting was also monitored by L. Rohland, who declared emphatically that the leader of the »Central Working Group on Anaesthesiology and Anaesthesia Technology«, Lothar Barth, could not simultaneously be President of the SA as well. Thus Manfred Meyer became the first President of the SA. Ulrich Strahl became Secretary and Lisa Wilken Treasurer, while Gerhard Endres was a member of the Executive Committee without special function. The other nine elected candidates who received fewer votes formed the »Extended Executive Committee«: G. Benad/Rostock, W. Bucklitsch/Berlin-Friedrichshain, G. Gmyrek/Leipzig, H. Hartmann/Leipzig, L. Klimpel/Greifswald, K.-H. Martin/Halle-Saale, H.F. Poppelbaum/Berlin-Buch, M. Schädlich/Berlin and R. Schmerso/Stralsund.

During the meetings of the Executive Committee and Extended Executive Committee, which took place in Berlin-Buch in June and August 1964, respectively, G. Benad presented the first draft of the statutes of the SA [6], against which repeated objections were raised by the GS and the Executive Committee of the »Society of Clinical Medicine of the German Democratic Republic«. Only after agreement was reached between the »Section of Anaesthesiology« (SA) – [renamed »Society of Anaesthesiology and Reanimation of the German Democratic Republic« (SAR) in 1967] – and the controlling institutions could the definite »Statute of the SAR« [22], which finally took into account the rights and duties of the members of the SAR [8], be published in January 1975 and sent to all members of the SAR [10].

According to § 5 of the Statute, a difference was made between full and extraordinary membership. Anaesthetists and scientists from other specialities closely related to anaesthesiology could become full members. Extraordinary membership was given to »Specialized Anaesthetic Nurses«. Although they were not allowed to give anaesthesia themselves in East Germany, their inclusion in the SAR proved to be advantageous for them and the further development of anaesthesiology in the German Democratic Republic.

In October 1965, the first issue of the »Information Sheet of the SA« was published. Because of difficulties in providing a sufficient amount of printing paper, it was only possible to regularly publish four issues per year of the later renamed »Bulletin of the GAIT« between 1973 and 1986 (◻ Fig. 1.25). In 1986, the GS even ordered a complete halt to its publication because of a shortage of paper [23].

Another major problem arose when R. Frey and H. Kronschwitz [13] published the »Register of the Specialists in Anaesthesiology in Germany, Austria and Switzerland«. This register was published in agreement with the anaesthetic societies of both parts of Germany, Austria and Switzerland and it contained the personal and scientific data of all specialists for anaesthesiology of these

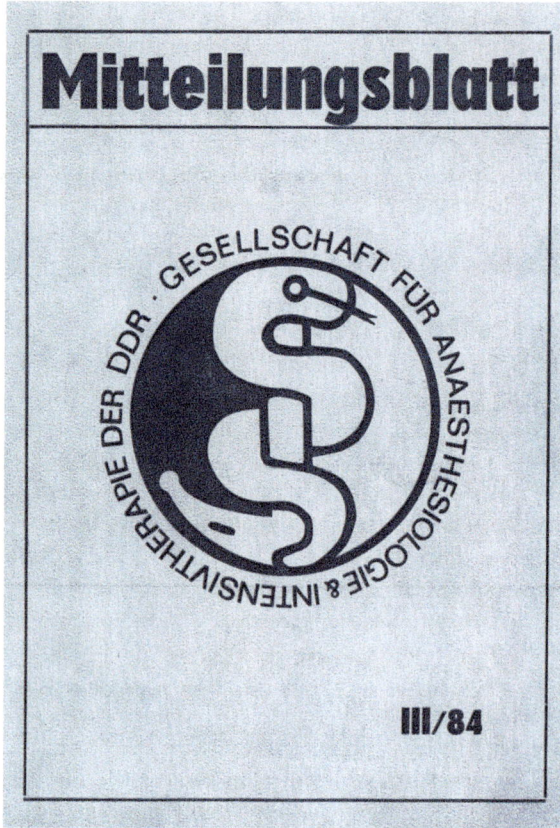

Fig. 1.25. Issue III/1984 of the Bulletin of the GAIT

countries. The 351 specialists for anaesthesiology from West Germany and 68 from East Germany were simply designated as »Germans« rather than »East Germans« or »West Germans«. The Executive Committee of the SA was severely criticized for this by the Director of the GS, L. Rohland.

Forced Resignation of East German Anaesthetists from the West German Society

Publication of the »Register of the Specialists in Anaesthesiology in Germany, Austria and Switzerland« was probably the decisive reason for increasing political pressure on East German members of the West German anaesthesiological society, which had changed its name to »German Society of Anaesthesia and Resuscitation« (DGAW) in 1965. The GS took the view that citizens of the German Democratic Republic could not be members of West German scientific societies. Based on this opinion, all East German members of West German societies were forced to withdraw from these societies in the late 1960s. Thus, the GS forced East German anaesthetists who were still members of the DGAW to give up their membership in the West German society [23]. The large number of resignations which arrived simultaneously at the office of

the DGAW demonstrated clearly that they were the result of political pressure. As a result, the DGAW introduced a so-called »silent membership« for all East German members, which proved to be a wise and far-sighted decision regarding further political developments.

On the one hand, separation from the West German society, which had resulted from political pressure by the East German government during the »Cold War«, was a painful process for all German anaesthetists – in particular for those in East Germany – but on the other hand, the creation of a separate anaesthesia society was absolutely necessary for the further development of this specialty into an independent medical field in East Germany. In addition, the SA was also able to contribute to the further international development of anaesthesiology.

1.2.2 Further Development of the East German Society of Anaesthesiology

Two Name Changes

Analogous to the West German society, which in 1978 made a second change to its name from »German Society of Anaesthesia and Resuscitation« (DGAW) to »German Society of Anaesthesiology and Intensive Care Medicine« (DGAI), the East German »Section of Anaesthesiology« (SA) also changed its name twice. In 1967 it was changed to »Society of Anaesthesiology and Reanimation of the German Democratic Republic« (SAR) and in 1977 to »Society of Anaesthesiology and Intensive Therapy of the German Democratic Republic« (GAIT) in order to demonstrate that the »interdisciplinary intensive therapy«, which had already led to the founding of a »Working Group on Interdisciplinary Intensive Therapy« of the SAR under the leadership of G. Baust/Halle-Saale in 1972, was an integral part of anaesthesiology.

Congresses

A scientific congress was usually held every second year. The series of congresses started with the congress »anaesthesia '66«, which was led by the first President of the SA, Manfred Meyer/Berlin-Buch, and organized by W. Bucklitsch/Berlin-Friedrichshain (■ Fig. 1.26). The topics of »anaesthesia '66«, which was held in East Berlin 26–29 June 1966, were:
- Pre- and postoperative period
- Cardiac arrhythmias in anaesthesia
- Blood transfusion and blood substitutes

The first anaesthesia congress of the GDR, in which also the President of the West German Society (DGAW) Karl Horatz/Hamburg and the Secretary Rudolf Frey/Mainz (■ Fig. 1.27) were still allowed to participate (participants from West Germany were later not allowed to attend East

German anaesthesia congresses), aroused international attention [18]. Anaesthetists from Austria, Australia, Belgium, Brazil, Bulgaria, Czechoslovakia, Finland, Greece, Holland, Hungary, India, Ireland, Japan, Nigeria, Soviet Union, Switzerland, UK and USA attended this congress – among them many well-known anaesthetists, such as H. Bergmann/Linz, G. Corssen/Ann Arbor/MI, St. Couremenos/Athens, A. B. Dobkin/New York, G. Hossli/Zurich, M. Johnstone/Manchester, Sir R. R. Macintosh/Oxford, W. W. Mushin/Cardiff, G. Organe/London (President of the WFSA), E. M. Papper/New York, J. P. Payne/London, J. Pokorny/Prague, W. N. Rollason/Aberdeen, I. S. Shorow/Moscow, N. P. Singh/New Delhi and G. J. van Weerden/Rotterdam.

The »anaesthesia '66« was followed by nine further congresses [15], but in none of them were so many anaesthetists from the so-called Western countries allowed to participate.

The further congresses were as follows:

»anaesthesia '68« – Berlin, 3–5 September 1968

- Scientific Director: H. F. Poppelbaum/Berlin-Buch
- Organizing Director: M. Schädlich/Berlin
- Topics:
  - Acute life-threatening states and limits of resuscitation
  - Hypothermia
  - Security measures in anaesthesia

»anaesthesia '70 – Berlin, 7–10 September 1970

- Scientific Director: H. F. Poppelbaum/Berlin-Buch
- Organizing Director: M. Schädlich/Berlin
- Topics:
  - Paediatric anaesthesia and paediatric intensive therapy
  - Anaesthesia in emergencies
  - Medical technology

»anaesthesia '72« in conjunction with the »5th International Symposium of Anaesthesiology« – Dresden, 4–6 July 1972

- Scientific Director: M. Schädlich/Berlin
- Organizing Director: H. Hache/Dresden
- Topics:
  - Cerebral function and anaesthesia
  - Electronic measurements and data processing
  - Training of the anaesthetist

»anaesthesia '74« – Dresden, 18–21 November 1974

- Scientific Director: G. Benad/Rostock
- Organizing Director: H. Hache/Dresden
- Topics:

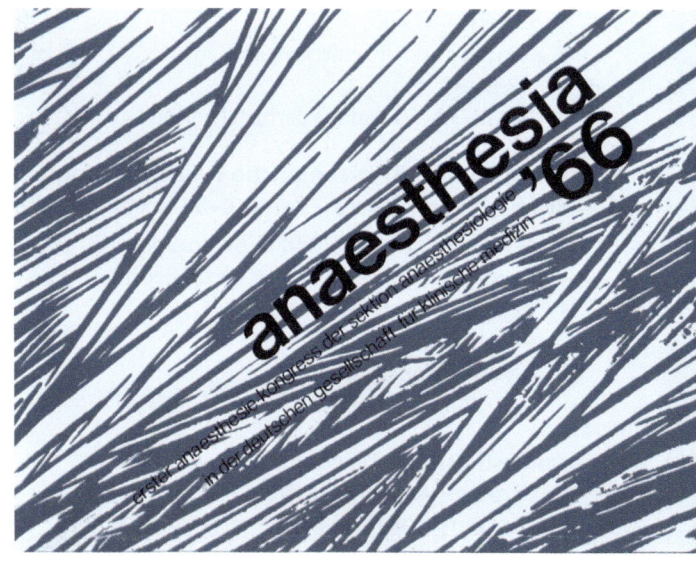

■ **Fig. 1.26.** Cover of the programme of »anaesthesia '66« (background shows crystal modifications of phenobarbital)

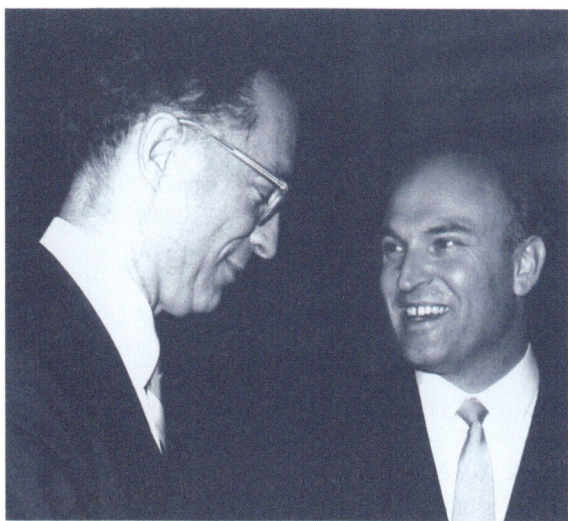

■ **Fig. 1.27.** Congress President of »anaesthesia '66«, M. Meyer/Berlin-Buch, in conversation with R. Frey/Mainz, Secretary of the DGAW

  - Problems in anaesthesia encountered in cardiac diseases
  - Head injuries
  - Haemotherapy

»anaesthesia '77 in conjunction with the Congress of Anaesthetic Nurses – Karl-Marx-Stadt (Chemnitz), 11–13 May 1977

- Scientific Director: W. Röse/Magdeburg
- Organizing Director: V. Burkhard/Karl-Marx-Stadt (Chemnitz)

1

- Topics:
  - Anaesthesia in emergencies
  - Shock
  - Anaesthesia and the perinatal period

»anaesthesia '78« in conjunction with the Congress of Anaesthetic Nurses – Berlin, 6–8 December 1978

- Scientific Director: U. Strahl/Berlin-Buch
- Organizing Director: G. Gottschalk/Berlin
- Topics:
  - Acute poisoning
  - Ambulatory anaesthesia
  - Artificial ventilation

»anaesthesia '81« in conjunction with the Congress of Anaesthetic Nurses – Berlin, 6–8 January 1981

- Scientific Director: M. Lüder/Berlin-Buch
- Organizing Director: H. J. Wilke/Berlin
- Topics:
  - The dangers of and complications due to:
    - Technical equipment
    - Drugs
    - Anaesthetic procedures

»anaesthesia '83« in conjunction with the Congress of Anaesthetic Nurses – Berlin, 5–8 December 1983

- Scientific Director: Ingrid Hörning/Cottbus
- Organizing Director: H. J. Wilke/Berlin
- Topics:
  - Anaesthesia for abdominal diseases
  - Blood substitution and blood coagulation
  - Nerve blocks

During the presidency of K. Borchert/Greifswald, »anaesthesia '87« in conjunction with the Congress of Anaesthetic Nurses was due to take place in Berlin in January 1987. Although this congress had already been prepared (◘ Fig. 1.28), the Minister of Health cancelled it because of heavy snowstorms which led to a traffic chaos in East and West Germany [15]. Some of the papers prepared for this congress were presented at a Workshop in Schwerin in September 1987.

»anaesthesia '90« in conjunction with the Congress of Anaesthetic Nurses – Dresden, 4–7 February 1990

- Scientific Director: H. Hache/Dresden
- Organizing Director: Helga Schiffner/Dresden
- Topics:
  - The septic patient
  - Treatment of chronic pain
  - Microelectronics and anaesthesia
  - Anaesthesia for the geriatric patient

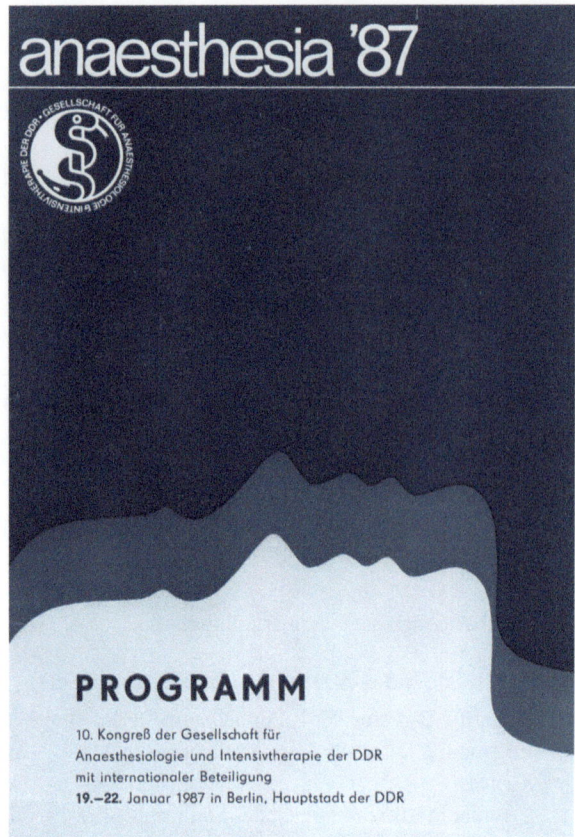

◘ Fig. 1.28. Cover of the programme of the cancelled »anaesthesia '87«

From the congresses held between 1966 and 1981, proceedings edited by E. Danzmann/Berlin-Buch in close cooperation with the shorthand Secretary of the Society, Bärbel Poppe/Berlin-Buch, were published by the Society. They consisted of two volumes with approximately 1,200 pages and contained the speeches presented at the opening ceremonies, the encomium for Honorary Members and the full text of all papers presented. Before the East German anaesthesiological journal *Anaesthesiologie und Reanimation* was created in 1976, the proceedings were the only way for East German anaesthetists to publish scientific papers because they were not allowed to publish papers in journals of so-called Western countries from the end of the 1960s onwards [4].

All anaesthesia congresses took place with international participants. Before the Society could invite foreign guests, however, permission had to be sought from the GS of the Ministry of Health. After 1966 invitations of West German anaesthetists were not allowed by the GS for nearly 15 years and invitations of East German anaesthetists to participate in national congresses of the West German Society or »Central European Congresses« (ZAK) held in West Germany could not be accepted. Only on a few occasions were East

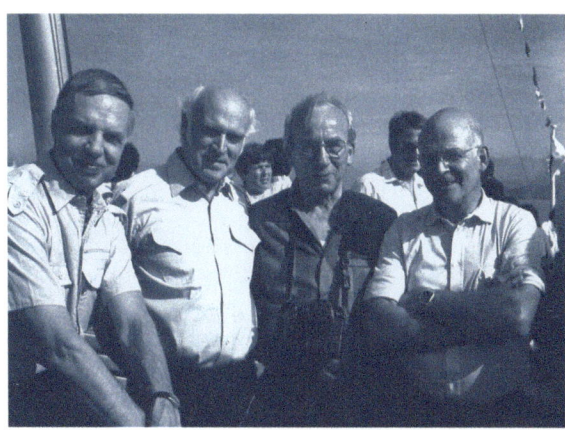

◘ Fig. 1.29. A rare meeting of former Presidents of the two German anaesthesiological societies at the Central European Congress 1983 in Zurich (*from left to right:* W. Röse/Magdeburg, M. Meyer/Berlin-Buch, K. Hutschenreuter/Homburg and K. Wiemers/Freiburg)

German anaesthetists allowed to participate in a Central European Congress, as long as they were not held in West Germany but in Austria or Switzerland (◘ Fig. 1.29).

The first exception to this draconian rule was made at the »7th World Congress of Anaesthesiology« which was held by the German Society of Anaesthesiology and Intensive Care Medicine (DGAI) in Hamburg in 1980. The government of the German Democratic Republic was extremely interested in gaining international recognition and therefore, 17 East German anaesthetists were allowed to accept invitations to this congress as guests of the DGAI. This was the first time East German anaesthetists had participated in a congress in West Germany since the building of the wall in 1961 and it was followed by a few visits by West German anaesthetists to East Germany, among them the Congress President of the 7th World Congress of Anaesthesiology, E. Rügheimer/Erlangen, who participated in the congress »anaesthesia '81« in East Berlin.

International Symposia

Apart from the national congresses, the East German society held two »International Symposia«. One of them was led by M. Lüder/Berlin-Buch and organized by the East German Society in close co-operation with the Academy of Sciences of the German Democratic Republic on the topic »Future trends in anaesthesia« in Berlin-Buch in 1978. The second one, which was held in Potsdam in 1980, was led by M. Meyer/Berlin-Friedrichshain and organized by the Research Department of Intensive Care Medicine of the City Hospital Berlin-Friedrichshain on the problem of »Acute respiratory failure«. Both Symposia were attended by scientists from 14 European and non-European countries, but the GS of the Ministry of Health of the German Democratic Republic did not allow invitations to be sent to anaesthetists from West Germany.

Workshops

Between national congresses, the East German Society held ten workshops, at which the Presidents of the Society and the leaders of various »Working Groups« (◘ Table 1.2) and later the editor-in-chief of the journal Anaesthesiologie und Reanimation [5] reported on their activities. In addition, elections of the new President and the members of the Executive Committee and Extended Executive Committee took place.

The »1st Workshop« was held in Oberhof/Thuringia on 19–22 April 1971. It was headed by M. Schädlich/Berlin and was of special importance for the further development of anaesthesiology in the German Democratic Republic. Prior to this »1st Workshop«, the Extended Executive Committee of the Society had worked out a document at a closed meeting in Lubmin on 14–17 January 1971, which was published in »Information Sheet of the SAR« [1], in which basic data for the further development of anaesthesiology were summarized. Based on this document, the General Assembly of the SAR adopted the so-called Oberhof Programme [7], in which the profession of »Specialist in Anaesthesiology«, including the official training programme and characteristics of postgraduate teaching, were described in detail. In each rural hospital a »Department of Anaesthesiology« should be established, to which an »Intensive Observation Ward« should be assigned. In bigger hospitals, such as city hospitals and university clinics, »Clinics of Anaesthesiology and Intensive Therapy« should be established, to which an »Interdisciplinary Intensive Care Unit« should be affiliated. Finally, anaesthesiology should become a compulsory medical field in the education of medical and dental students, who had to pass a final examination in anaesthesiology. The result of this examination should be included in the final state examination as a special mark in anaesthesiology. Furthermore, it was decided to establish a »Working Group on Teaching Medical and Dental Students« and some other working groups, which are summarized in ◘ Table 1.2.

The »Oberhof Programme«, which was approved by the General Assembly of the SAR and passed on to the Ministry of Health [10], was an important document for the development of anaesthesiology in the German Democratic Republic. It was very helpful for the further work of the SAR, but it was also used by the Ministry of Health [23], which was relatively open to the members' demands.

After this first workshop nine further workshops were held [15]:

2nd Workshop in Gera, 3–5 October 1972

- Scientific Director: M. Schädlich/Berlin
- Organizing Director: L. Lieb/Gera
- Topics:
  - Anaesthesiology – an integrating factor
  - Postgraduate teaching

1

3rd Workshop in Kühlungsborn, 11–14 October 1973

- Scientific Director: G. Benad/Rostock
- Organizing Director: G. Benad/Rostock
- Topics:
  - Emergency medicine
  - Water rescue service

4th Workshop in Eisenach, 19–22 March 1975

- Scientific Director: G. Benad/Rostock
- Organizing Director: F. Seidel/Arnstadt
- Topic:
  - Problems of postgraduate teaching

5th Workshop in Wernigerode, 10–13 November 1977

- Scientific Director: W. Röse/Magdeburg
- Organizing Director: V. Thiele/Wernigerode
- Topic:
  - Anaesthesia care in smaller hospitals

6th Workshop in Neubrandenburg, 11–13 November 1979

- Scientific Director: U. Strahl/Berlin-Buch
- Organizing Director: G. Grünewald/Neubranden- burg
- Topic:
  - Limits of reanimation:
    - Apallic syndrome
    - Brain death

7th Workshop in Neubrandenburg, 8–11 November 1981

- Scientific Director: M. Lüder/Berlin-Buch
- Organizing Director: G. Grünewald/Neubranden- burg
- Topic:
  - Problems of hygiene in anaesthesiology

8th Workshop in Magdeburg, 26–28 November 1984 (◻ Fig. 1.30)

- Scientific Director: Ingrid Hörning/Cottbus
- Organizing Director: W. Röse/Magdeburg
- Topic:
  - New developments in medical technology

9th Workshop in Schwerin, 23–25 September 1987 (in conjunction with »anaesthesia 87«, which had to be cancelled in Januar 1987 because of snow)

- Scientific Director: K. Borchert/Greifswald
- Organizing Director: J. Mesewinkel/Schwerin
- Topics:
  - Postoperative period
  - Cardiopulmonary and cerebral resuscitation

10th Workshop in Gera, 23–25 October 1990

- Scientific Director: H. Hache/Dresden
- Organizing Director: Uta Weiser/Gera
- Topic:
  - Paediatric anaesthesia and intensive therapy

◻ **Table 1.2.** Survey of the Working Groups of the East German Society (year of foundation in parentheses)

- Working Group on Working and Living Conditions (1970)
- Working Group on Information and Documentation (1970)
- Working Group on Research and Technology (1971)
- Working Group on Teaching Medical and Dental Students (1972)
- Working Group on Interdisciplinary Intensive Therapy (1972)
- Working Group on Paediatric Anaesthesia and Intensive Therapy (1972)
- Working Group on Medico-legal Problems (1973); in 1982 renamed Working Group on Ethics and Law
- Working Group on Hospital Building and Reconstruction (1977)
- Working Group on Specialized Anaesthetic Nurses (1978)
- Working Group on Hospital-Acquired Infection in Anaes- thesiology, Intensive Therapy and Emergency Medicine (1978)
- Working Group on Pain (1982); in 1988 transferred to the status of a »Section of Pain Therapy«

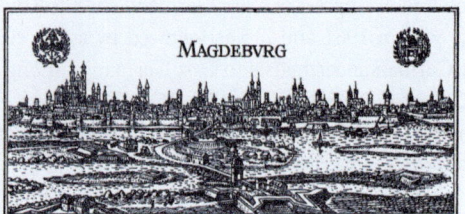

Gesellschaft für Klinische Medizin der DDR

MAGDEBVRG

8. Arbeitstagung
der
Gesellschaft für Anaesthesiologie und Intensivtherapie
der DDR

Magdeburg, 26. – 28. November 1984

Programm

◻ **Fig. 1.30.** Cover of the programme of the 8th Workshop in Magde- burg, 26–28 November 1984

Consultant Medical Doctors in Anaesthesiology and Intensive Therapy

In every district of the German Democratic Republic, »Consultant Medical Doctors« were appointed by the respective »District Physician« for each medical field. According to the development of our specialty, these »Consultant Medical Doctors « were first called »Consultant Medical Doctors in Anaesthesiology« and later on »Consultant Medical Doctors in Anaesthesiology and Intensive Therapy«. They gave advice to the »District Physicians« regarding the structural development of anaesthesiology and intensive therapy, the technical equipment in the departments and clinics of anaesthesiology and intensive therapy and the course of postgraduate teaching in the respective district of the German Democratic Republic. Since they had certain influence on the development of anaesthesiology and intensive therapy in their districts, they were included in meetings of the Extended Executive Committee of the GAIT [24], to which they were invited once a year.

Advisory Role of Members of GAIT's Executive Committee Vis-á-Vis the Ministry of Education and the Ministry of Health

Members of the Executive Committee of the GAIT were repeatedly asked for consultations by both ministries regarding special problems of anaesthesiology and intensive therapy. For the Ministry of Education, the »Working Group on Teaching Medical and Dental Students« of the GAIT not only elaborated the educational programmes of medical and dental students in anaesthesiology, intensive therapy, emergency medicine and pain therapy, but also prepared a »Concept of anaesthesiology and intensive therapy at University Hospitals«.

In the early 1980s, the Executive Committee of the GAIT prepared a »Recommendation for the diagnosis of brain death« and a »Concept for anaesthetic care in the event of disasters«, and in 1985 a »Recommendation for conditioning of donor organs for kidney transplantation« was formulated in co-operation with the »Society of Nephrology«.

In 1987 a »Commission for Anaesthesiology and Intensive Therapy-Related Problems« was created by the Ministry of Health in order to co-ordinate the work of the »Consultant Medical Doctors for Anaesthesiology and Intensive Therapy«. This board of six included four members of the Executive Committee of the GAIT and designed a »General concept of anaesthesiology and intensive therapy«. Besides positive elements of the development of anaesthesiology and intensive therapy, it also showed the deficiencies regarding the personal and technical working conditions of this specialty in the German Democratic Republic, where there was a deficit of more than 1,000 medical doctors and 3,000 nurses.

International Activities of the GAIT

Since its foundation in 1963, the East German anaesthesiological society has had good contacts to the anaesthesiological societies of the so-called »socialist countries«, with which they had a great deal in common, including very similar political structures, as well as a limited financial scope due to the lack of »hard currencies« together with severely restricted access to new medications and modern technical equipment. Due to the shortage of monitoring devices, greater emphasis was placed on clinical signs as well as on training and postgraduate education. Travelling activities of East European anaesthetists, which were already extremely limited for political reasons, were further reduced by the shortage of foreign exchange. Therefore, new ways for the exchange of information and personnel had to be found.

Under these restricted conditions, intimate contact between the GAIT and the »Czechoslovak Society of Anaesthesiology and Resuscitation in the Medical Society of J. E. Purkinje« was intensified by holding five Bilateral Anaesthesiological Symposia of the CSSR and the GDR [15]:

1st Bilateral Anaesthesiological Symposium CSSR/GDR in Karlovy Vary (Karlsbad), 23–24 April 1975

- Scientific Directors: J. Pocta/Prague and G. Benad/Rostock
- Topic:
  - Working and living conditions in anaesthesiology and intensive therapy

2nd Bilateral Anaesthesiological Symposium CSSR/GDR in Leipzig, 25–26 May 1978

- Scientific Directors: G. Benad/Rostock and J. Pocta/Prague
- Topic:
  - Obstetric anaesthesia

3rd Bilateral Anaesthesiological Symposium CSSR/GDR in Usti nad Labem (Aussig), 2–4 June 1982

- Scientific Directors: J. Pocta/Prague and H. Hache/Dresden
- Topic:
  - Resuscitation

4th Bilateral Anaesthesiological Symposium CSSR/GDR in Greifswald, 28–29 April 1985

- Scientific Directors: K. Borchert/Greifswald and V. Trávnicek/Prague
- Topic:
  - Neuroanaesthesia

5th Bilateral Anaesthesiological Symposium CSSR/GDR in Hradec Kralove (Königgrätz), 21–23 September 1988

- Scientific Directors: Jarmila Drabková/Prague and H. Hache/Dresden
- Topics:
  - Poisoning
  - Balanced anaesthesia

These bilateral meetings of anaesthetists from both countries were supplemented by three »Bilateral Symposia of Anaesthetic Nurses from the CSSR and GDR«, which were held in Bad Schandau (1984), Usti nad Labem (Aussig) (1986) and Cottbus (1989).

Contact with the anaesthesia societies of other socialist countries of Eastern Europe was not only maintained by reciprocal invitations to anaesthetists from these countries to national congresses, but also through the organization of joint »International Anaesthesiological Symposia«. The 1st International Anaesthesiological Symposium was held in Prague/Czechoslovakia in 1965 and it was followed by further symposia in Poznań (Posen)/Poland (1967), Varna/Bulgaria (1970), Dresden (1972) in conjunction with »anaesthesia '72, and in Balatonfüred/Hungary (1975). Later on these »International Anaesthesiological Symposia« were called »International Anaesthesiological Congresses« and were held in Bratislava (Pressburg)/Czechoslovakia (1977), Wroclaw (Breslau)/Poland (1979), Bucharest/Romania (1981) and Kiev/Soviet Union (1986).

In contrast to congresses in the German Democratic Republic, these »International Anaesthesiological Symposia or Congresses« could also be attended by West German anaesthetists and so these events became very welcome meeting points for East and West German colleagues and friends.

Very close and cordial contacts also existed between the GAIT and anaesthesiological societies of »West« European and non-European countries, such as the »Austrian Society of Anaesthesiology, Resuscitation and Intensive Care Medicine« (ÖGARI). Not only were Austrian anaesthetists frequent participants in the congresses of the GAIT, but in 1978 an agreement was concluded between the two societies, which regulated an exchange of members without any foreign money exchange. Members of the Executive Committee of the ÖGARI, such as O. Mayrhofer/Vienna, K. Steinbereithner/Vienna, H. Bergmann/Linz and W. List/Graz very often lectured at various clinics of anaesthesiology and intensive therapy in the German Democratic Republic and were invited guests at the congresses of the GAIT. In 1988 a »Joint Symposium of the Anaesthesiological Societies of the German Democratic Republic and the Republic of Austria« was held in Dresden under the scientific leadership of H. Hache/Dresden and O. Mayrhofer/Vienna. It dealt with:

- Problems of premedication
- Monitoring in anaesthesiology and intensive therapy
- Problems and tasks of anaesthesiology in teaching and postgraduate education
- Development of new muscle relaxants

Very good relations also existed between the GAIT and the »Association of Anaesthetists of Great Britain and Ireland«. Even in the early 1950s, long before an anaesthesiological society had been founded in East Germany, internationally renowned British anaesthetists, such as W. W. Mushin/Cardiff and J. P. Payne/London were guest lecturers at postgraduate courses organized by Lothar Barth at the Department of Anaesthesiology of the Robert-Rössle Clinic in Berlin-Buch [2] (Fig. 1.31). East Germany anaesthetists were invited to anaesthetic departments in Oxford, Cardiff and London. Later on Sir Robert Macintosh/Oxford, H. G. Epstein/Oxford, D. D. C. Howat/London, C. Franklin/Manchester and R. Eltringham/Gloucester lectured at various anaesthesiological departments of the German Democratic Republic. In 1981 an agreement between these two societies was concluded which regulated the further exchange programme of anaesthetists from the two sides.

The GAIT also had close relations to the »World Federation of Societies of Anaesthesiologists« (WFSA) to which it was admitted at the 4th World Congress of Anaesthesiology in London in 1968. East German anaesthetists had close contacts to various Presidents, the Executive Committee and to some other Committees of the WFSA. Very often Presidents of the WFSA participated in congresses of the GAIT, such as G. Organe/UK (1966), O. Mayrhofer/Austria (1974), Q. Gomez/Philippines (1977) and J. J. Bonica/USA (1983) (Fig. 1.32). C. P. Parsloe/Brazil visited several clinics of anaesthesiology and intensive therapy of East Germany in 1984. Some East German anaesthetists held various posts in the WFSA: H. F. Poppelbaum/Berlin-Buch (Vice President 1972–1976); W. Röse/Magdeburg (Member of the Executive Committee 1980–1988, Vice President 1988–1992, Head of the Committee on Cardiopulmonary Resuscitation 1988–1996), M. Lüder/Berlin-Buch (Founder and Head of the Committee on Safety in Anaesthesia 1984–1992); M. Meyer/Berlin-Buch (Member of the Committee on Education and Scientific Affairs 1984–1988); G. Benad/Rostock (Member of the Statutes and Bylaws Committee 1988–1992 and Head of the Statutes and Bylaws Committee 1992–1996).

Furthermore, M. Meyer/Berlin-Buch was a member of the Council of the »World Federation of Societies of Intensive and Critical Care Medicine« (WFSICCM) and Head of the Committee on International Relations of the WFSICCM between 1981 and 1985.

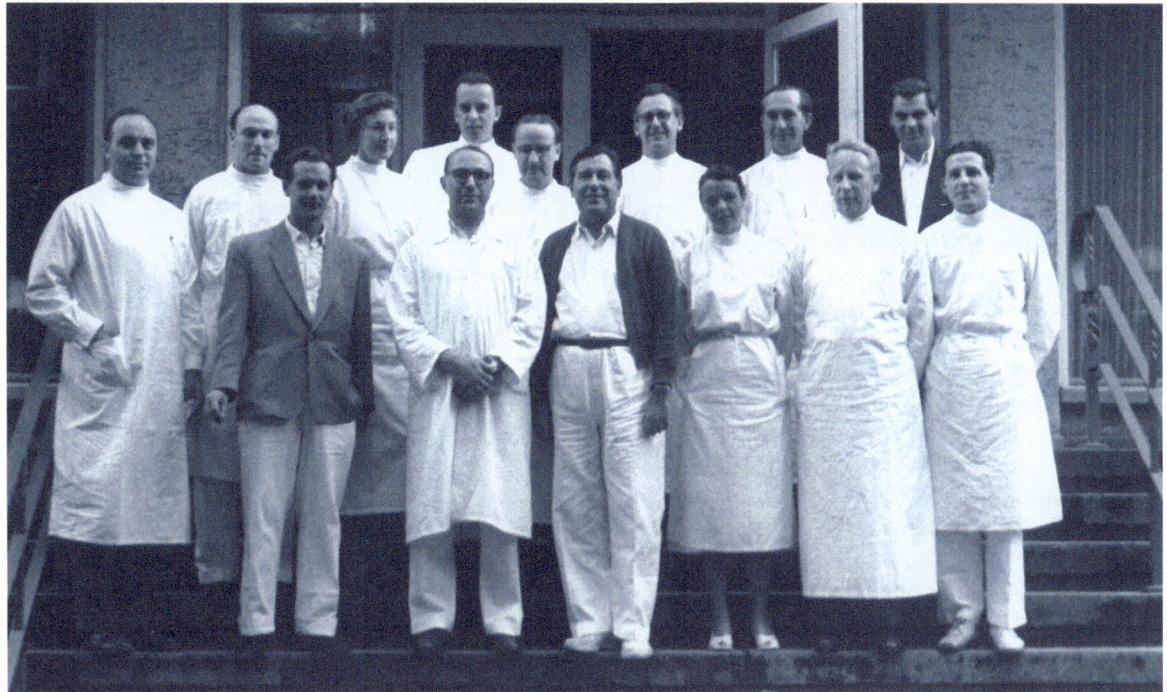

Fig. 1.31. First postgraduate course held in 1957 at the Department of Anaesthesia of the Robert-Rössle Clinic in Berlin-Buch, led by L. Barth/ Berlin-Buch, W. W. Mushin/Cardiff and H. Gummel, Head of the Surgical Clinic, Berlin-Buch (*first row from left to right*). Among the participants in the course: (*second row from left to right*) M. Meyer/Berlin-Buch, Lisa Wilken/Magdeburg, M. Schädlich-Halle/Saale and (*second row, second from the right*) G. Endres/Jena

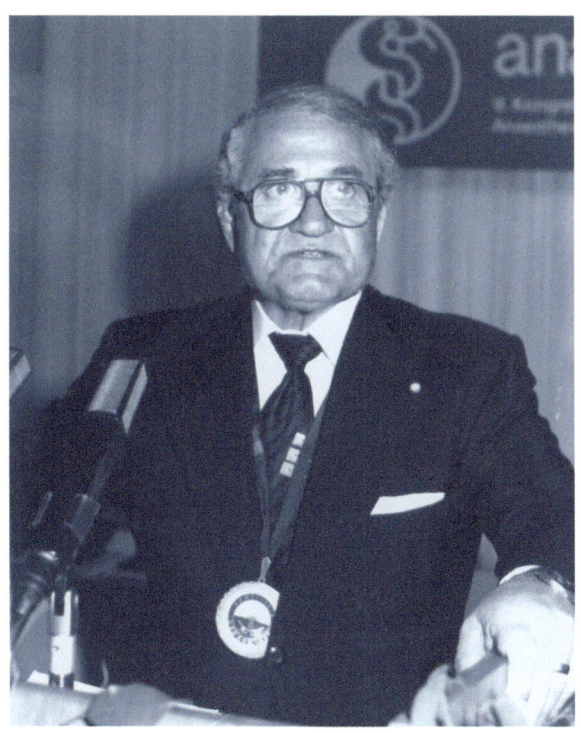

Fig. 1.32. J. J. Bonica/USA during his speech as President of the WFSA at »anaesthesia '83« in East Berlin

W. Röse/Magdeburg was one of the founding members of the »European Academy of Anaesthesiology« (EAA) in 1978.

1.2.3 Honours

Several members of the GAIT were honoured with national and international awards. The title »Fellow of the Faculty of Anaesthetists of the Royal College of Surgeons (FFARCS)« was awarded to L. Barth/Berlin-Buch in 1965, H. F. Poppelbaum/Berlin-Buch in 1972 [11] and M. Meyer/Berlin-Buch in 1982.

The »National Prize Second Class for Science and Technology of the German Democratic Republic« was awarded to Helga Schiffner/Dresden for her anaesthesiological contributions as a member of »Liver Transplantation Team« at the Medical Academy Dresden and to M. Schädlich and D. Olthoff/Berlin for their work in developing cardiac anaesthesia and extracorporeal circulation as members of the Cardiac Surgery Team at the Charité University Hospital/Berlin.

As the first German anaesthetist, G. Benad/Rostock was elected a member of the »German Academy of Sciences Leopoldina« in 1985.

Furthermore, some foreign anaesthesiological societies appointed members of the GAIT Honorary or Corresponding Members.

Honorary Memberships of East German Anaesthetists

- Czechoslovak Society of Anaesthesiology and Resuscitation in the Medical Society of J. E. Purkinje: M. Schädlich/Berlin (1974), U. Strahl/Berlin-Buch (1979), H. Hache/Dresden (1984), G. Benad/Rostock (1985) and M. Meyer/Berlin-Buch (1988)
- Polish Society of Anaesthesiology and Intensive Therapy: M. Schädlich/Berlin (1976)
- Romanian Society of Anaesthesiology and Intensive Therapy: M. Lüder/Berlin-Buch (1981)
- Bulgarian Society of Anaesthesiology and Reanimation: M. Meyer/Berlin-Buch (1980) and G. Benad/Rostock (1985)
- Society of Anaesthesiologists and Reanimatologists of the Soviet Union: M. Schädlich/Berlin (1986) and W. Röse/Magdeburg (1989)
- Hungarian Society of Anaesthesiology and Intensive Therapy: L. Barth/Berlin-Buch (1968), W. Röse/Magdeburg (1977) and K. Borchert/Greifswald (1989)

Corresponding Memberships of East German Anaesthetists

- Czechoslovak Society of Anaesthesiology and Resuscitation in the Medical Society of J. E. Purkinje: G. Baust/Halle-Saale (1977)
- Austrian Society of Anaesthesiology, Resuscitation and Intensive Care Medicine: G. Benad/Rostock (1989) and W. Röse/Magdeburg (1989)
- German Society of Anaesthesiology and Intensive Care Medicine: G. Benad/Rostock (1990) and D. Olthoff/Leipzig (1990)

Honours Awarded to Scientists by the »Society of Anaesthesiology and Intensive Therapy of the German Democratic Republic« (◘ Fig. 1.33)

Honorary Members

H. Gummel †	German Democratic Republic	1966
Sir R. R. Macintosh †	UK	1966
W. W. Mushin †	UK	1966
W. Negowski †	Soviet Union	1966
H. G. Epstein †	UK	1968
T. Gordh	Sweden	1968
S. Pokrczywnicki †	Poland	1968
J. Hoder †	Czechoslovakia	1970
K. Scheidler	German Democratic Republic	1970
L. Shorow †	Soviet Union	1970
O. Mayrhofer	Austria	1974
E. Stojanov	Bulgaria	1977
Q. Gomez †	The Philippines	1981
J. Pocta	Czechoslovakia	1981
M. Meyer	German Democratic Republic	1983
H. Bergmann	Austria	1983
W. Jurczyk	Poland	1983
W. Lembcke †	German Democratic Republic	1983
Elena Damir	Soviet Union	1987
J. Pokorný	Czechoslovakia	1987
M. Schädlich †	German Democratic Republic	1987
K. Steinbereithner †	Austria	1987
G. Ugoscai	Hungary	1990
H. F. Poppelbaum †	German Democratic Republic	1990

Corresponding Members

D. Kettler	Federal Republic of Germany	1990
H.-W. Opderbecke	Federal Republic of Germany	1990
V. V. Suslov	Soviet Union	1990

The »Honorary Badge of the Society of Anaesthesiology and Intensive Therapy of the German Democratic Republic« [20] was awarded to W. Bucklitsch/Berlin-Friedrichshain (1981), W. Röse/Magdeburg (1981), Ingrid Hörning/Cottbus (1987), M. Lüder/Berlin-Buch (1987), D. Fröhlich/Zwickau (1990) and K.-H. Pickart/Bad Saarow (1990) for their contribution to the development of anaesthesiology and intensive therapy in the German Democratic Republic.

The »Heinrich-Braun Prize of the Society of Anaesthesiology and Intensive Therapy of the German Democratic Republic« [21] was awarded to E. Friis/Berlin (1981), Helga Schiffner/Dresden (1983), Lina Wild/Leipzig (1990) and K. Siegismund/Dresden for their excellent postdoctoral theses.

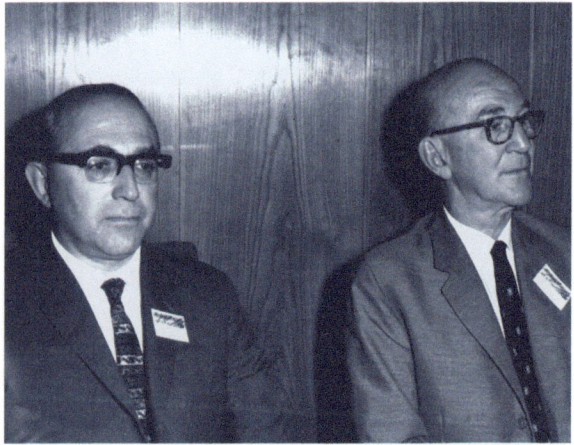

◘ Fig. 1.33. W. W. Mushin/Cardiff and Sir Robert Mactintosh/Oxford (*from left to right*), two of the first Honorary Members of the East German Society, who received their honour at »anaesthesia '66« in East Berlin

1.2.4 The Last Congress of the GAIT »anaesthesia '90« in Dresden, 4–7 February 1990, and the Official Re-establishment of Contact Between the Two German Societies DGAI and GAIT

This congress was a milestone in the history of relations between the DGAI and the GAIT. The »wall« had been opened 3 months earlier and so many colleagues from West Germany were able to participate in this congress without any restrictions (Fig. 1.34). The separation of East and West German anaesthetists, which had lasted for 25 years, was overcome. During an unforgettable meeting of the members of both societies it was decided that the DGAI and the GAIT should immediately establish close contact with the aim of unification. On the same day, the Presidents and members of the Executive Committees of the two societies arranged a first meeting at the Bellevue Hotel. This resulted in a »Common Declaration of the DGAI and the GAIT«, which was published in journals of the two societies. It clearly showed that the members of the Executive Committees of the two societies were of the opinion »....that the amalgamation into a single German anaesthesiological society will take place in the foreseeable future« [16].

The process of unification, which had begun at »anaesthesia '90« in Dresden, was continued during the following Congress of the DGAI in Mannheim in 1990. In discussions between members of the two Executive Committees it became obvious that the West German »Law on Associations« did not allow unification of the two societies [14]. The unification of West and East German anaesthetists into one society could only be achieved on the same basis as the unification of East and West Ger-

many: the GAIT had to dissolve itself and then East German anaesthetists could become members of the DGAI. Under these circumstances, it was a great advantage that the »silent membership« of East German members in the former DGA only had to be reactivated.

1.3.5 Dissolution of the GAIT

In a historically meaningful circular from the President, H. Hache/Dresden, dated 23 July 1990 [16], the members of the GAIT were invited to Gera on 23 October 1990 in order to participate in the last General Assembly and to vote on the recommendation of the Executive Committee to dissolve the Society according to § 19, section 1 of the Statute of the GAIT.

In addition to a large number of East German anaesthetists, members of the Executive Committee of the DGAI attended this meeting and were witnesses to the dissolution of the GAIT, which had begun with 86 founding members and grown up in its 26-year history into a society of 2,201 members – 1,264 of them were ordinary members, 874 extraordinary members (Specialized Anaesthetic Nurses) and 63 secondary members on 1 January 1989.

In agreement with the Executive Committee of the DGAI, the »Heinrich-Braun Award of the GAIT« was replaced by the »Heinrich Braun Commemorative Medal« and was declared the highest honour of the DGAI [14].

The journal *Anaesthesiologie und Reanimation*, which had been the organ of the East German Society since 1976, was published as of 1 January 1991 as an organ of the DGAI [12].

According to § 19, section 3 of the Statute of the GAIT, the Society's assets, in the event of its dissolution, were to be transferred to the head society of the GAIT, the »Society of Clinical Medicine of the German Democratic Republic«. Since this Society had already been dissolved on 2 April 1990, the assets of the GAIT, which after conversion into West German currency and payment of open bills amounted to more than 60,000 German marks, were transferred to the DGAI [14].

Retrospectively it was recognized that, despite adverse external conditions, the unique political circumstances and shortages in many areas, which hindered the sustained development of the material and technical basis of anaesthesiological institutions in the German Democratic Republic, the GAIT had made essential contributions to the national and international development of anaesthesiology, intensive therapy, emergency medicine and pain therapy.

From our point of view, it would have been desirable if we could have taken into the DGAI three positive elements of East German anaesthesiology, which were achieved by the resolute work of the GAIT [3]:

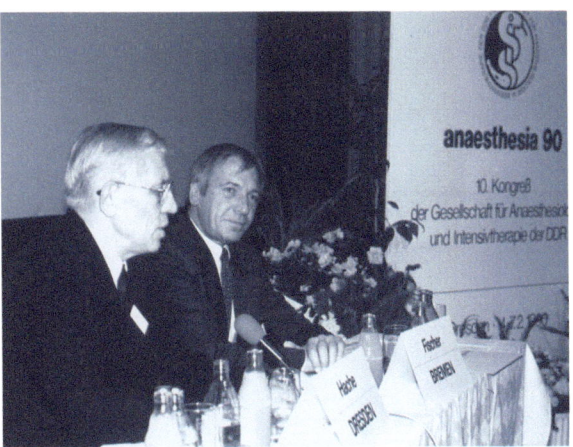

 Fig. 1.34. »Bringing together what belongs together«: H. Hache/ Dresden, President of the GAIT and K. Fischer/Bremen, President of the DGAI (*from left to right*) at »anaesthesia '90« in Dresden

First, the full academic recognition of anaesthesiology as a compulsory medical field for medical and dental students with a final examination, the mark for which became part of the final mark of the state examination; this was achieved in East Germany in 1969.

Second, the change of the specialist's title from »Specialist in Anaesthesiology« to »Specialist in Anaesthesiology and Intensive Therapy«, which was achieved in East Germany in 1986.

Third, the transfer of the »Specialized Anaesthetic Nurses«, who had been able to become extraordinary members of the GAIT since 1975, to a comparable status within the DGAI.

Unfortunately these three points could not be achieved [3], but we are grateful for the positive changes both in anaesthesiology and in our personal life that have occurred since the bloodless revolution in 1989, which resulted in freedom returning to East Germany.

References

1. Arbeitsunterlagen der 1. Arbeitstagung der Gesellschaft für Anaesthesiologie und Reanimation der DDR im Panorama-Hotel Oberhof, 19. – 22. 04. 1971, erarbeitet vom Erweiterten Vorstand auf der Klausurtagung in Lubmin 14. – 17. 01. 1971. Information II/1971 des Vorstandes der Gesellschaft für Anaesthesiologie und Reanimation der DDR, 16 pp
2. Barth L (1967) Die Entwicklung der Anästhesiologie in der DDR. Anaesthesist 16:268–269
3. Benad G (1998) Effect of reunification on anaesthesiology in former East Germany. European Academy of Anaesthesiology Newsletter No. 9:4–5
4. Benad G (2000) 25 Jahre »Anaesthesiologie und Reanimation« – Ein historischer Rückblick. Anaesthesiol Reanim 25:4–11
5. Benad G (2003) Entwicklung der Zeitschrift »Anaesthesiologie und Reanimation«. In: Schüttler J (ed) 50 Jahre Deutsche Gesellschaft für Anästhesiologie und Intensivmedizin. Springer, Berlin, p 169 – 174
6. Bucklitsch W (1976) Die Entwicklung der Gesellschaft für Anaesthesiologie und Reanimation der DDR – 1. Mitteilung. Mitteilungsblatt der Gesellschaft für Anaesthesiologie und Reanimation der DDR Nr. I: 5 – 9
7. Bucklitsch W (1976) Die Entwicklung der Gesellschaft für Anaesthesiologie und Reanimation der DDR – 2. Mitteilung. Mitteilungsblatt der Gesellschaft für Anaesthesiologie und Reanimation der DDR Nr. II: 1 – 4
8. Bucklitsch W (1976) Die Entwicklung der Gesellschaft für Anaesthesiologie und Reanimation der DDR – 3. Mitteilung. Mitteilungsblatt der Gesellschaft für Anaesthesiologie und Reanimation der DDR Nr. II: 5 – 7
9. Bucklitsch W (1984) Die Entwicklung der Gesellschaft für Anaesthesiologie und Intensivtherapie der DDR – Eine Bilanz zum zwanzigjährigen Bestehen. Anaesthesiol Reanim 9:67–74
10. Bucklitsch W, Hörning I (1980) 30 Jahre DDR – 15 Gesellschaft für Anaesthesiologie und Reanimation der DDR. Mitteilungsblatt der Gesellschaft für Anaesthesiologie und Reanimation der DDR Nr. I: 3 – 9
11. Bucklitsch W, Röse W (1977) Die Entwicklung der Gesellschaft für Anaesthesiologie und Reanimation der DDR – 4. Mitteilung. Mitteilungsblatt der Gesellschaft für Anaesthesiologie und Reanimation der DDR Nr. I: 2 – 5
12. Fischer K, Benad G (1991) Zum Geleit – Die Zeitschrift »Anaesthesiologie und Reanimation« erscheint ab 1. Januar 1991 als Organ der Deutschen Gesellschaft für Anästhesiologie und Intensivmedizin. Anaesthesiol Reanim 16:3–4
13. Frey R, Kronschwitz H (1966) Verzeichnis der Fachärzte für Anästhesiologie in Deutschland, Österreich und in der Schweiz. Springer, Berlin
14. Hache H (1990) Circular of the President of the Society of Anaesthesiology and Intensive Therapy of the GDR to the Members of the GAIT, 7 July 1990
15. Hache H (1990) Abschlussbericht des Vorstandes der Gesellschaft für Anaesthesiologie und Intensivtherapie der DDR. Anästhesiol Intensivmed 32:8–13
16. Hache H, Fischer K (1990) Gemeinsame Erklärung der Deutschen Gesellschaft für Anästhesiologie und Intensivmedizin und der Gesellschaft für Anaesthesiologie und Intensivtherapie der DDR (GAIT). Anaesthesiol Reanim 15:137.
17. Lehmann C (1964) Bericht über die Gründungsversammlung der Sektion Anaesthesiologie der Deutschen Gesellschaft für Klinische Medizin am 7. März 1964 in Berlin. Anaesthesist 13:395–396
18. Meyer M (1966) Eröffnungsansprache zum 1. Kongress der Sektion Anaesthesiologie der Deutschen Gesellschaft für Klinische Medizin »anaesthesia '66«, 26. Juli 1966 in Berlin. Kongress-Bericht »anaesthesia '66« 1:1–10
19. Röse W (1990) 40 Jahre Anästhesie in Deutschland. Anaesthesiol Reanim 24:19–26
20. Ordnung über die Verleihung der Ehrenplakette der Gesellschaft für Anaesthesiologie und Reanimation der DDR. Mitteilungsblatt der Gesellschaft für Anaesthesiologie und Reanimation der DRR 1979; Nr. I: 4.
21. Ordnung zur Verleihung des Heinrich-Braun-Preises der Gesellschaft für Anaesthesiologie und Reanimation der DDR. Mitteilungsblatt der Gesellschaft für Anaesthesiologie und Reanimation der DDR 1979; Nr. I: 2 – 3
22. Statut der Gesellschaft für Anaesthesiologie und Reanimation der DDR vom 1. Januar 1975
23. Stober H-D, Bucklitsch W (1991) Die Geschichte der Gesellschaft für Anaesthesiologie und Intensivtherapie der DDR. Anaesthesiol Reanim 16:403–411
24. Strahl U (1979) Die Entwicklung der Anaesthesiologie in der Deutschen Demokratischen Republik. Anaesthesiol Reanim 4: 131–134

1.3 Supplementary Material: Presidents of the DGAI and GAIT, Honorary and Corresponding Members, Congresses

Compilation: the Editors with support of the Administrative Office of the DGAI

1.3.1 Contents

1.3.2 Presidents of the DGAI 1953–2006

- 1953–1954: Heinz-Joachim Bark †
  - Todtmoos / Tübingen
  - Curriculum vitae: see p 15
- 1955–1956: Ludwig Zürn †
  - Munich
  - Curriculum vitae: see p 276
- 1957–1958: Martin Zindler
  - Düsseldorf
  - Curriculum vitae: see p 230
- 1959–1962: Otto H. Just
  - Berlin / Heidelberg
  - Curriculum vitae: see p 256
- 1963–1964: Kurt Wiemers †
  - Freiburg im Breisgau
  - Curriculum vitae: see p 238
- 1965–1966: Karl Horatz †
  - Hamburg
  - Curriculum vitae: see p 250
- 1967–1968: Hans W. Opderbecke
  - Nuremberg
  - Curriculum vitae: see p 19
- 1969–1970: Karl Hutschenreuter †
  - Homburg/Saar
  - Curriculum vitae: see p 257
- 1971–1972: Peter Lawin †
  - Hamburg / Münster
  - Curriculum vitae: see p 282
- 1973–1974: Erich Rügheimer †
  - Erlangen
  - Curriculum vitae: see p 233
- 1975–1976: Walter F. Henschel †
  - Bremen

- **Prof. Dr. med. Walter F. Henschel**
  Born 11 January 1926 in Weimar; deceased 7 June 2002; 1948–1953 student of medicine in Jena and Berlin; 1954 doctorate at Jena; 1955 Hufeland-Hospital Berlin-Buch; 1956 Specialist in Surgery. University Hospital Westend University of Berlin; 1961 Specialist in Anaesthesiology; 1961 Head Physician, Dept. of Anaesthesiology of the Central Hospital St.-Jürgen-Strasse, Bremen; 1979 Adjunct Professor at the Medical Faculty of the University of Göttingen; 1991 retirement

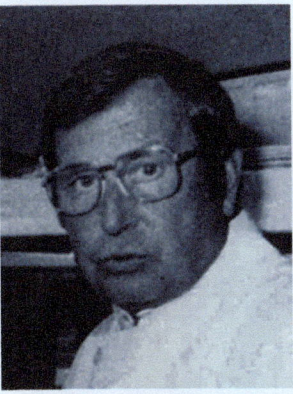

◘ Fig. 1.35. Walter F. Henschel

- 1977–1978: Karl H. Weis
  - Würzburg
  - Curriculum vitae: see p 293
- 1979–1980: Erich Rügheimer †
  - Erlangen
  - Curriculum vitae: see p 233
- 1981–1982: Joachim Schara
  - Wuppertal
- 1983–1984: Friedrich W. Ahnefeld
  - Ulm
  - Curriculum vitae: see p 290
- 1985–1986: Dietrich Kettler
  - Göttingen
  - Curriculum vitae: see p 243
- 1987–1988: Klaus Peter
  - Munich
  - Curriculum vitae: see p 278
- 1989–1990: Klaus Fischer
  - Bremen
- 1991–1992: Klaus Eyrich
  - Berlin
  - Curriculum vitae: see p 221
- 1993: Gottfried Benad
  - Rostock
  - Curriculum vitae: see p 286

▬ Dr. med. Joachim Schara

Born 29 October 1928 in Konstadt/Upper Silesia; 1949–1954 student of medicine in Hamburg; 1955 doctorate in Hamburg; 1955 internship Cincinnati, OH, USA; 1956-1957 anaesthesia training at Albert-Einstein Med. Center Philadelphia, PA (Goldstein); 1958 anaesthesia Lahey-Clinic, Boston, MA; 1958 postgraduate training Philadelphia, PA; 1959–1969 surgery in Bremen (Scheringer, Rieder); 1960 respiratory function in Bremen (Buhr); 1961 Specialist in Anaesthesiology; 1961–1962 Head Physician, Dept. Anaesthesia at the Central Hospital Bremen-Blumenthal; 1963 Head Physician Dept. Anaesthesia of the Hospital Wuppertal-Barmen; 1993 retirement

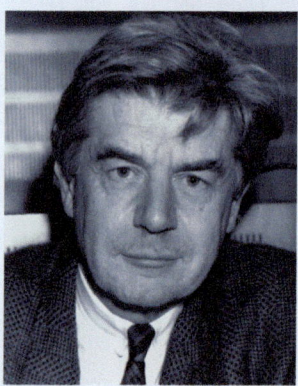

▫ Fig. 1.36. Joachim Schara

▬ Prof. Dr. med. Klaus Fischer

Born 3 May 1936 in Berlin; 1959–1964 student of medicine in Kiel, Göttingen, Innsbruck and Vienna; 1964 doctorate at the Georg August University Göttingen; postgraduate training at the Dept. Anaesthesia of the University Hospital Kiel;1969 Specialist in Anaesthesiology; 1970 und 1971 Interim Head of Dept. Anaesthesia; after the appointment of Prof. Dr. J. Wawersik Deputy Medical Director; 1978 Lecturer in Anaesthesiology; 1978 Head Physician, Dept. Anaesthesia and Surgical Intensive Care Medicine of the Protestant Deaconess Hospital Bremen; 2002 retirement

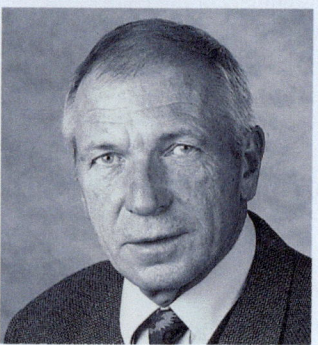

▫ Fig. 1.37. Klaus Fischer

▬ Prof. Dr. med. Reinhard Purschke

Born 16 February 1938 in Kreuzenort/Upper Silesia; 1958–1964 student of medicine in Bonn; 1968 doctorate in Bonn; 1969–1977 postgraduate anaesthesia training at Düsseldorf University (M. Zindler); 1972 Specialist in Anaesthesiology; 1973 Senior Physician, Dept. Anaesthesia, University Hospital Düsseldorf; 1974 Lecturer; 1977 Head Physician, Dept. Anaesthesia, St. Johannes Hospital, Dortmund; 1978 Adjunct Professor; 2003 retirement

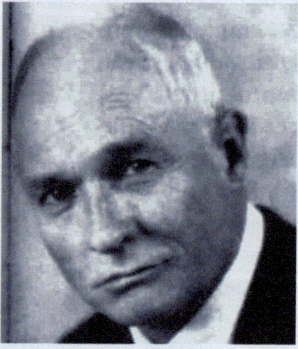

▫ Fig. 1.38. Reinhard Purschke

▬ 1994: Rafael Dudziak
  – Frankfurt
  – Curriculum vitae: see p 237
▬ 1995: Reinhard Purschke
  – Dortmund
▬ 1996: Klaus van Ackern
  – Mannheim
  – Curriculum vitae: see p 273
▬ 1997: Jochen Schulte am Esch
  – Hamburg
  – Curriculum vitae: see p 251
▬ 1998: Gunter Hempelmann
  – Giessen
  – Curriculum vitae: see p 241
▬ 1999: Detlev Patschke
  – Marl
▬ 2000: Klaus Geiger
  – Freiburg
  – Curriculum vitae: see p 239
▬ 2001: Eberhard Götz
  – Darmstadt

▬ Professor Dr. med. Detlev Patschke

Born 13 November 1939 in Königsberg; 1961–1966 student of medicine; 1966 doctorate in Erlangen; 1968 postgraduate anaesthesia training at Erlangen (Rügheimer); from 1969 in Berlin (Eberlein); 1973 Specialist in Anaesthesiology; 1975 Lecurer, Berlin; 1977 Senior Physician, Dept. Anaesthesiology at Giessen; 1980 Head Physician, Dept. Anaesthesia and Surgical Intensive Medicine, Paracelsus Hospital, Marl; 2004 retirement

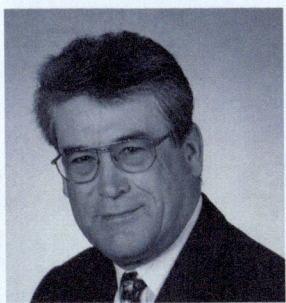

◘ **Fig. 1.39.** Detlev Patschke

▬ Prof. Dr. med. Eberhard Götz

Born 11 May 1930 in Darmstadt; 1958–1963 student of medicine in Mainz, Munich and Tübingen; 1964 doctorate in Tübingen; 1967–1968 medical officer at the Luftwaffenschule Fürstenfeldbruck; thereafter postgraduate training in Tübingen and Munich; 1970 physician in charge of the blood bank of the Surgical Dept. of Munich University Hospital; 1971 Specialist in Anaesthesiology; 1972–1976 Senior Physician at Munich; 1975 Lecturer, Munich; 1976–1981 Deputy Chairman of the Dept. of Anaesthesiology of Münster University; 1978 Professor at Münster University; 1981 Head Physician, Dept. Anaesthesia and Surgical Intensive Care Medicine, Darmstadt Hospital; 2005 retirement

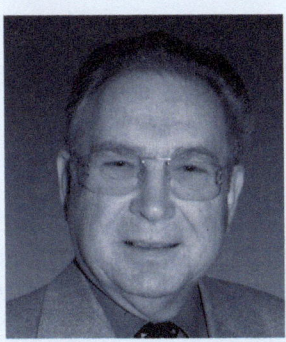

◘ **Fig. 1.40.** Eberhard Götz

▬ Prof. Dr. med. Claude Krier

Born 12 June 1948 in Luxembourg; 1969–1974 student of medicine in Luxembourg, Nancy, Brussels and Heidelberg; 1980 doctorate in Heidelberg; 1980 Specialist in Anaesthesiology; 1980 Senior Physician, Heidelberg; 1986 Lecturer, Heidelberg; 1986–1989 Deputy Chairman of the Dept. of Anaesthesiology of Heidelberg University Hospital; 1989–2008 Head, Dept. of Anaesthesiol. and ICM, Katharine Hospital Stuttgart; since 2006 Medical Director, Municipal Hospitals Stuttgart

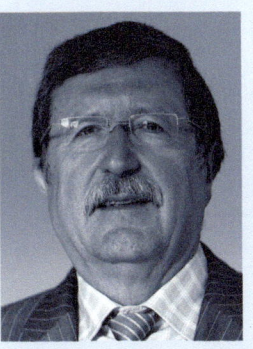

◘ **Fig. 1.41.** Claude Krier

▬ 2002: Jörg Tarnow
  – Düsseldorf
  – Curriculum vitae: see p 231
▬ 2003: Eike Martin
  – Heidelberg
  – Curriculum vitae: see p 256
▬ 2004: Claude Krier
  – Stuttgart
▬ 2005–2006: Joachim Radke
  – Halle
  – Curriculum vitae: see p 249
▬ 2007–2008: Hugo Van Aken
  – Münster
  – Curriculum vitae: see p 283
▬ 2009–2010: Jürgen Schüttler
  – Erlangen
  – Curriculum vitae: see p 233
▬ 2011–2012: Gabriele Nöldge-Schomburg
  – Rostock
  – Curriculum vitae: see p 287

1.3.3 Presidents of the Society of Anaesthesiology and Intensive Therapy of the German Democratic Republic (GAIT) (1964–1990)

▬ 1964–1966: Manfred Meyer
  – Berlin

- 1966–1970: Hartwig Ferdinand Poppelbaum
  - Berlin
- 1970–1972: Manfred Schädlich
  - Berlin
  - Curriculum vitae: see p 216
- 1972–1975: Gottfried Benad
  - Rostock
  - Curriculum vitae: see p 286
- 1975–1977: Wolfgang Röse
  - Magdeburg
  - Curriculum vitae: see p 268
- 1977–1979: Ulrich Strahl
  - Berlin
- 1979–1981: Manfred Lüder
  - Berlin
- 1981–1984: Ingrid Hörning
  - Cottbus
- 1984–1987: Klaus Borchert
  - Greifswald
  - Curriculum vitae: see p 247
- 1987–1990: Heinz Hache
  - Dresden

- **Prof. Dr. med. habil. Manfred Meyer, FFARCS**
  Born 2 August 1928 in Chemnitz; 1946–1952 student of medicine in Leipzig; 1952 doctorate; 1954 post-graduate training in neurosurgery at the Municipal Hospital Berlin-Buch; 1956 postgraduate training in anaesthesia at Robert Rössle Hospital of the Academy of Sciences of the German Democratic Republic (Lothar Barth); 1958 study visits to Great Britain (Mushin, Payne); 1958 Specialist in Anaesthesiology, Senior Physician; 1959–1965 Chief of the Department for Experimental Anaesthesiology; 1965–1971 Head Physician ICU, Robert Rössle Hospital, Berlin, Lecturer; 1972 Head Physician of the Research Division of Intensive Care Medicine; 1974 Professor of Anaesthesiology and Chair of Anaesthesiology at the Academy for Continuous Medical Education of the German Democratic Republic; 1995 retirement; 1983 Fellow of the Faculty of Anaesthetists of the Royal College of Surgeons of England (FFARCS)

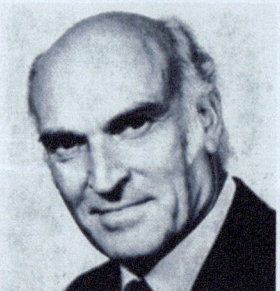

◘ **Fig. 1.42.** Manfred Meyer

- **Prof. Dr. med. habil. Hartwig Ferdinand Poppelbaum**
  Born 28 July 1920 in Frankfurt/Main; 1939–1945 student of medicine in Marburg; 1945 doctorate in Marburg; postgraduate training in anaesthesia in France and surgical training in Biedenkopf/Lahn; 1951–1957 Sund Hospital, Stralsund; 1954 Specialist in Surgery; 1956 Specialist in Anaesthesiology; study visits to Oxford and Moscow; 1957 to Stockholm (Crafoord); 1958 Chief, Dept. Bronchology of the Research Institute of Tuberculosis and Pulmonary Diseases at Berlin-Buch; 1960 Head Physician, Second Dept. of Anaesthesiology, Municipal Hospital Berlin-Buch; 1967–1974 Chairman of Anaesthesiology and of the Central Commission for Anaesthesiology of the Academy of Continuing Medical Education of the German Democratic Republic; 1970 Lecturer; 1976 Honorary Lecturer and 1979 Honorary Professor of Anaesthesiology at the Academy for Continuing Medical Education of the German Democratic Republic; 1988 retirement

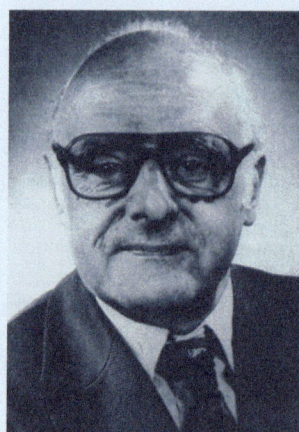

◘ **Fig. 1.43.** H. Ferdinand Poppelbaum

- **Dr. med. Ulrich Strahl**
  Born 9 April 1922 in Berlin; deceased 4 December 1999; 1943–1949 student of medicine in Berlin and Königsberg; 1949 doctorate in Berlin; 1949 training in surgery at the Municipal Hospitals Prenzlauer Berg and Berlin-Buch; 1954 study visit to Basel; 1955 Specialist in Surgery; 1956 Head Physician, Dept. of Anaesthesia; 1957 study visit to Copenhagen; 1958 Specialist in Anaesthesiology; 1958 Head Physician, Dept. of Anaesthesia and Respiratory

Centre, Berlin-Buch; 1959 study visit to Rotterdam; 1987 retirement; 1965 Purkyne-Medal; 1979 Honorary Member of the Czechoslovak Society of Anaesthesiology and Resuscitation

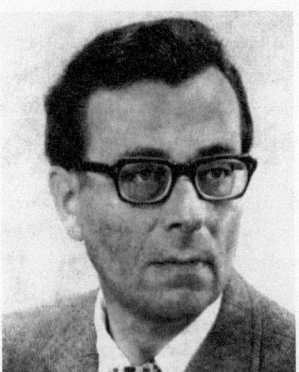

■ **Fig. 1.44.** Ulrich Strahl

▬ Prof. Dr. med. habil. Manfred Lüder

Born 23 November 1930 in Berlin; 1951–1956 student of medicine at Humboldt University Berlin; 1956 doctorate; 1959 postgraduate training in anaesthesia at the Central Institute for Cancer Research of the Academy of Sciences of the German Democratic Republic at Berlin-Buch; 1963 Specialist in Anaesthesiology; 1969 Lecturer, University of Leipzig; 1972 Head Physician of the Dept. of Experimental and Clinical Anaesthesiology at the Central Institute for Cancer Research of the Academy of Sciences of the German Democratic Republic; 1979 Professor of Anaesthesiology at the Academy of Sciences of the German Democratic Republic; 1995 retirement

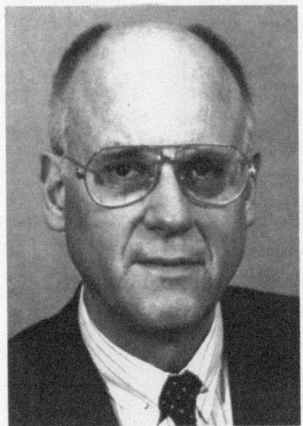

■ **Fig. 1.45.** Manfred Lüder

▬ Dr. med. Ingrid Hörning

Born 19 September 1935 in Naumburg/Saale; 1953–1958 student of medicine at Martin Luther University Halle-Wittenberg; 1958 doctorate; 1961 postgraduate training in anaesthesia at the District Hospital Burg near Magdeburg; 1962–1965 anaesthesia training at the Surgical Dept. of the Medical Academy Magdeburg (Wilken); 1965 Specialist in Anaesthesiology; 1966 Head Physician, Dept. of Anaesthesia at the District Hospital Cottbus; 1998 retirement

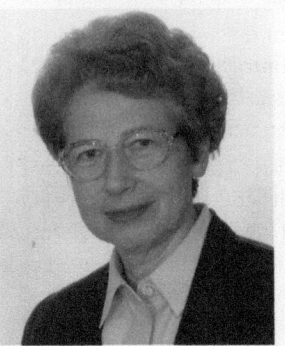

■ **Fig. 1.46.** Ingrid Hörning

▬ Dr. med. habil. Heinz Hache

Born 8 July 1928 in Gleiwitz; deceased 6 December 1991; 1948–1955 student of medicine at Leipzig University; 1955 doctorate; 1956–1957 Resident at the VP-Hospital; 1957 postgraduate training in surgery at the District Hospital Dresden-Friedrichstadt; 1961 Specialist in Surgery; 1961 Senior Physician, Dept. Surgery District Hospital Dresden-Friedrichstadt; 1964 Specialist in Anaesthesiology and Intensive Care Therapy; 1966 Head Physician, Dept. Anaesthesia, District Hospital Dresden-Friedrichstadt, 1983 Lecturer, Dresden University

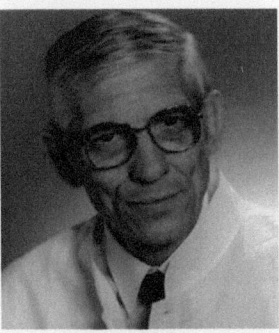

■ **Fig. 1.47.** Heinz Hache

1.3.4 Officers of the Executive Committee of the German Society of Anaesthesiology and Intensive Care Medicine

1953	J. Bark, Tübingen †	President
	R. Frey, Heidelberg †	Permanent Secretary
	G. Moeller, Wuppertal †	Treasurer
1954	J. Bark, Tübingen †	President
	R. Frey, Heidelberg †	Permanent Secretary
	H. Oehmig, Heidelberg †	Treasurer
1955	L. Zuern, Munich †	President
	R. Frey, Heidelberg †	Permanent Secretary
	H. Oehmig, Heidelberg †	Treasurer
1956	L. Zuern, Munich †	President
	R. Frey, Heidelberg †	Permanent Secretary
	H. Oehmig, Heidelberg †	Treasurer
1957	M. Zindler, Duesseldorf	President
	L. Zürn, Munich †	Vice-president
	R. Frey, Heidelberg †	Permanent Secretary
	O. Just, Berlin †	Vice-secretary
	H. Oehmig, Marburg †	Treasurer
1958	M. Zindler, Duesseldorf	President
	L. Zürn, Munich †	Vice-president
	R. Frey, Heidelberg †	Permanent Secretary
	O. Just, Berlin †	Vice-secretary
	H. Oehmig, Marburg †	Treasurer
1959	O. Just, Berlin †	President
	M. Zindler, Duesseldorf	First Vice-president
	J. Bark, Tuebingen †	Second Vice-president
	R. Frey, Heidelberg †	Permanent Secretary
	Ch. Lehmann, Munich	Vice-secretary
	H. Oehmig, Marburg †	Treasurer
1960	O. Just, Berlin †	President
	M. Zindler, Duesseldorf	First Vice-president
	J. Bark, Tuebingen †	Second Vice-president
	R. Frey, Heidelberg †	Permanent Secretary
	Ch. Lehmann, Munich	Vice-secretary
	H. Oehmig, Marburg †	Treasurer
1961	O. Just, Berlin †	President
	M. Zindler, Duesseldorf	Vice-president
	R. Frey, Mainz †	Permanent Secretary
	Ch. Lehmann, Munich	Vice-secretary
	H. Oehmig, Marburg †	Treasurer
1962	O. Just † / K. Wiemers †	President
	M. Zindler, Duesseldorf	Vice-president
	R. Frey, Mainz †	Permanent Secretary
	Ch. Lehmann, Munich	Vice-secretary
	R. Beer, Munich †	Treasurer
1963	K. Wiemers, Freiburg †	President
	O. Just, Heidelberg †	Vice-president
	R. Frey, Mainz †	Permanent Secretary
	Ch. Lehmann, Munich	Vice-secretary
	R. Beer, Munich †	Treasurer
	K. Horatz, Hamburg †	President BDA
1964	K. Wiemers, Freiburg †	President
	O. Just, Heidelberg †	Vice-president
	R. Frey, Mainz †	Permanent Secretary
	Ch. Lehmann, Munich	Vice-secretary
	R. Beer, Munich †	Treasurer
	K. H. Bräutigam, Stuttgart †	President BDA
1965	K. Horatz, Hamburg †	President
	K. Wiemers, Freiburg	Vice-president
	R. Frey, Mainz †	Permanent Secretary
	Ch. Lehmann, Munich	Vice-secretary
	R. Beer, Munich †	Treasurer
	K. H. Bräutigam, Stuttgart †	President BDA
1966	K. Horatz, Hamburg †	President
	K. Wiemers, Freiburg †	Vice-president
	R. Frey, Mainz †	Permanent Secretary
	Ch. Lehmann, Munich	Vice-secretary
	R. Beer, Munich †	Treasurer
	W. F. Henschel, Bremen †	President BDA
1967	H. W. Opderbecke, Nuremberg	President
	K. Horatz, Hamburg †	Vice-president
	R. Frey, Mainz †	Permanent Secretary
	Ch. Lehmann, Munich	Vice-secretary
	R. Beer, Munich †	Treasurer
	W. F. Henschel, Bremen †	President BDA
1968	H. W. Opderbecke, Nuremberg	President
	K. Horatz, Hamburg †	Vice-president
	R. Frey, Mainz †	Permanent Secretary
	Ch. Lehmann, Munich	Vice-secretary
	R. Beer, Munich †	Treasurer
	W. F. Henschel, Bremen †	President BDA
1969	K. Hutschenreuter, Homburg †	President
	H. W. Opderbecke, Nuremberg	Vice-president
	R. Frey, Mainz †	Permanent Secretary
	Ch. Lehmann, Munich	Vice-secretary
	R. Beer, Munich †	Treasurer
	W. F. Henschel, Bremen †	President BDA
1970	K. Hutschenreuter, Homburg †	President
	H. W. Opderbecke, Nuremberg	Vice-president
	R. Frey, Mainz †	Permanent Secretary
	Ch. Lehmann, Munich	Vice-secretary
	R. Beer, Munich †	Treasurer
	W. F. Henschel, Bremen †	President BDA
1971	P. Lawin, Hamburg †	President
	K. Hutschenreuter, Homburg †	Vice-president
	R. Frey, Mainz †	Permanent Secretary

	H. W. Opderbecke, Nuremberg	Vice-secretary
	R. Beer, Munich †	Treasurer
	W. F. Henschel, Bremen †	President BDA
1972	P. Lawin, Hamburg †	President
	K. Hutschenreuter, Homburg †	Vice-president
	R. Frey, Mainz †	Permanent Secretary
	H. W. Opderbecke, Nuremberg	Vice-secretary
	R. Beer, Munich †	Treasurer
	W. F. Henschel, Bremen †	President BDA
1973	E. Ruegheimer, Erlangen †	President
	P. Lawin, Hamburg †	Vice-president
	R. Frey, Mainz †	Permanent Secretary
	H. W. Opderbecke, Nuremberg	Vice-secretary
	R. Beer, Munich †	Treasurer
	W. F. Henschel, Bremen †	President BDA
1974	E. Ruegheimer, Erlangen †	President
	P. Lawin, Hamburg †	Vice-president
	R. Frey, Mainz †	Permanent Secretary
	H. W. Opderbecke, Nuremberg	Vice-secretary
	R. Beer, Munich †	Treasurer
	K. Hutschenreuter, Homburg †	President BDA
	J. Schara, Wuppertal	Representative of the Regional Chairmen
1975	W. F. Henschel, Bremen †	President
	E. Ruegheimer, Erlangen †	Vice-president
	R. Frey, Mainz †	Permanent Secretary
	W. F. Henschel, Bremen †	Vice-secretary
	R. Beer, Munich †	Treasurer
	K. Hutschenreuter, Homburg †	President BDA
	H. Kronschwitz, Frankfurt	Representative of the Regional Chairmen
1976	W. F. Henschel, Bremen †	President
	E. Ruegheimer, Erlangen †	Vice-president
	R. Frey, Mainz †	Permanent Secretary
	W. F. Henschel, Bremen †	Vice-secretary
	R. Beer, Munich †	Treasurer
	K. Hutschenreuter, Homburg †	President BDA
	H. Kronschwitz, Frankfurt	Representative of the Regional Chairmen
1977	K.-H. Weis, Würzburg	President
	W. F. Henschel, Bremen †	Vice-president
	H. W. Opderbecke, Nuremberg	Generalsekretär
	K. Eyrich, Würzburg	Schriftführer
	J. B. Brueckner, Berlin	Treasurer
	K. Hutschenreuter,	President BDA

	Homburg †	
	H. Kronschwitz, Frankfurt	Representative of the Regional Chairmen
1978	K.-H. Weis, Würzburg	President
	W. F. Henschel, Bremen †	Vice-president
	H. W. Opderbecke, Nuremberg	Generalsekretär
	K. Eyrich, Würzburg	Schriftführer
	J. B. Brueckner, Berlin	Treasurer
	K. Hutschenreuter, Homburg †	President BDA
	H. Kronschwitz, Frankfurt	Representative of the Regional Chairmen
1979	E. Ruegheimer, Erlangen†	President
	K.-H. Weis, Würzburg	Vice-president
	H. W. Opderbecke, Nuremberg	Generalsekretär
	K. Eyrich, Würzburg	Schriftführer
	J. B. Brueckner, Berlin	Treasurer
	K. Hutschenreuter, Homburg †	President BDA
	W. F. Henschel, Bremen †	Representative of the Regional Chairmen
1980	E. Ruegheimer, Erlangen †	President
	K.-H. Weis, Würzburg	Vice-president
	H. W. Opderbecke, Nuremberg	Generalsekretär
	K. Eyrich, Würzburg	Schriftführer
	J. B. Brueckner, Berlin	Treasurer
	P. Uter, Hannover †	President BDA
	W. F. Henschel, Bremen †	Representative of the Regional Chairmen

Year	President	1st Vice-President	2nd Vice-President	General Secretary	Secretary	Treasurer	Representative of the Regional Chairmen	President BDA	President DAAF
1981	J. Schara, Wuppertal	E. Ruegheimer, Erlangen †		H. W. Opderbecke, Nuremberg	K. Eyrich, Berlin	J. B. Brueckner, Berlin	J. Wawersik, Kiel	P. Uter, Hannover	K. Hutschenreuter, Homburg †
1982	J. Schara, Wuppertal	E. Ruegheimer, Erlangen †		H. W. Opderbecke, Nuremberg	K. Eyrich, Berlin	J. B. Brueckner, Berlin	J. Wawersik, Kiel	P. Uter, Hannover	K. Hutschenreuter, Homburg †
1983	F. W. Ahnefeld, Ulm	J. Schara, Wuppertal		H. W. Opderbecke, Nuremberg	K. Eyrich, Berlin	J. B. Brueckner, Berlin	J. Wawersik, Kiel	P. Uter, Hannover	K. Hutschenreuter, Homburg †
1984	F. W. Ahnefeld, Ulm	J. Schara, Wuppertal		H. W. Opderbecke, Nuremberg	K. Eyrich, Berlin	J. B. Brueckner, Berlin	J. Wawersik, Kiel	P. Uter, Hannover	K. Hutschenreuter, Homburg †
1985	D. Kettler, Goettingen	F. W. Ahnefeld, Ulm		H. W. Opderbecke, Nuremberg	K. Eyrich, Berlin	J. B. Brueckner, Berlin	K. Fischer, Bremen	P. Uter, Hannover	K. Hutschenreuter, Homburg †
1986	D. Kettler, Goettingen	F. W. Ahnefeld, Ulm		H. W. Opderbecke, Nuremberg	K. Eyrich, Berlin	J. B. Brueckner, Berlin	K. Fischer, Bremen	P. Uter, Hannover	K. Hutschenreuter, Homburg †
1987	K. Peter, Munich	D. Kettler, Goettingen		H. W. Opderbecke, Nuremberg	K. Eyrich, Berlin	K.-H. Weis, Wurzburg	K. Fischer, Bremen	P. Uter, Hannover	K. Hutschenreuter, Homburg †
1988	K. Peter, Munich	D. Kettler, Goettingen		H. W. Opderbecke, Nuremberg	K. Eyrich, Berlin	K.-H. Weis, Wuerzburg	K. Fischer, Bremen	K. Zinganell, Kassel	K. Hutschenreuter, Homburg †
1989	K. Fischer, Bremen	K. Peter, Munich		H. W. Opderbecke, Nuremberg	K. Eyrich, Berlin	K.-H. Weis, Wuerzburg	D. Patschke, Marl	K. Zinganell, Kassel	K. Hutschenreuter, Homburg †
1990	K. Fischer, Bremen	K. Peter, Munich		H. W. Opderbecke, Nuremberg	K. Eyrich, Berlin	K.-H. Weis, Wuerzburg	D. Patschke, Marl	K. Zinganell, Kassel	K. Hutschenreuter, Homburg †
1991	K. Eyrich, Berlin	K. Fischer, Bremen		H. W. Opderbecke, Nuremberg	K. Fischer, Bremen	K.-H. Weis, Wuerzburg	D. Patschke, Marl	K. Zinganell, Kassel	G. Hempelmann, Giessen
1992	K. Eyrich, Berlin	K. Fischer, Bremen	G. Benad, Rostock	H. W. Opderbecke, Nuremberg	K. Fischer, Bremen	K.-H. Weis, Wuerzburg	D. Patschke, Marl	K. Zinganell, Kassel	G. Hempelmann, Giessen
1993	G. Benad, Rostock	K. Eyrich, Berlin	R. Dudziak, Frankfurt	F. W. Ahnefeld, Ulm	K. Fischer, Bremen	K.-H. Weis, Wuerzburg	D. Patschke, Marl	K. Zinganell, Kassel	G. Hempelmann, Giessen
1994	R. Dudziak, Frankfurt	G. Benad, Rostock	R. Purschke, Dortmund	F. W. Ahnefeld, Ulm	K. Fischer, Bremen	K.-H. Weis, Wuerzburg	D. Patschke, Marl	B. Landauer, Munich	G. Hempelmann, Giessen
1995	R. Purschke, Dortmund	R. Dudziak, Frankfurt	K. van Ackern, Mannheim	F. W. Ahnefeld, Ulm	K. Fischer, Bremen	K.-H. Weis, Wuerzburg	D. Patschke, Marl	B. Landauer, Munich	G. Hempelmann, Giessen

Year	President	1st Vice-President/ Vice-President	2nd Vice-President	General Secretary	Secretary	Treasurer	Representative of the Regional Chairmen	President BDA	President DAAF
1996	K. van Ackern, Mannheim	R. Purschke, Dortmund	J. Schulte am Esch, Hamburg	F. W. Ahnefeld, Ulm	K. Fischer, Bremen	K.-H. Weis, Wuerzburg	D. Patschke, Marl	B. Landauer, Munich	G. Hempelmann, Giessen
1997	J. Schulte am Esch, Hamburg	K. van Ackern, Mannheim	G. Hempelmann, Giessen	K. van Ackern, Mannheim	K. Fischer, Bremen	K.-H. Weis, Wuerzburg	D. Patschke, Marl	B. Landauer, Munich	R. Purschke, Dortmund
1998	G. Hempelmann, Giessen	J. Schulte am Esch, Hamburg	D. Patschke, Marl	K. van Ackern, Mannheim	K. Fischer, Bremen	K.-H. Weis, Wuerzburg	D. Patschke, Marl	B. Landauer, Munich	R. Purschke, Dortmund
1999	D. Patschke, Marl	G. Hempelmann, Giessen	K. Geiger, Freiburg	K. van Ackern, Mannheim	K. Fischer, Bremen	G. Hempelmann, Giessen	E. Kochs, Munich	B. Landauer, Munich	R. Purschke, Dortmund
2000	K. Geiger, Freiburg	D. Patschke, Marl	E. Götz, Darmstadt	K. van Ackern, Mannheim	K. Fischer, Bremen	G. Hempelmann, Giessen	E. Kochs, Munich	B. Landauer, Munich	R. Purschke, Dortmund
2001	E. Götz, Darmstadt	K. Geiger, Freiburg	J. Tarnow, Duesseldorf	K. van Ackern, Mannheim	J. Schüttler, Erlangen	K. Taeger, Regensburg	J. Radke, Halle	B. Landauer, Munich	H. Van Aken, MMuenster
2002	J. Tarnow, Duesseldorf	E. Götz, Darmstadt	E. Martin, Heidelberg	K. van Ackern, Mannheim	J. Schüttler, Erlangen	K. Taeger, Regensburg	J. Radke, Halle	B. Landauer, Munich	H. Van Aken, Muenster
2003	E. Martin, Heidelberg	J. Tarnow, Duesseldorf	C. Krier, Stuttgart	K. van Ackern, Mannheim	J. Schüttler, Erlangen	K. Taeger, Regensburg	J. Radke, Halle	B. Landauer, Munich	H. Van Aken, Muenster
2004	C. Krier, Stuttgart	E. Martin, Heidelberg	J. Radke, Halle	K. van Ackern, Mannheim	J. Schüttler, Erlangen	K. Taeger, Regensburg	J. Radke, Halle	B. Landauer, Munich	H. Van Aken, Muenster
2005	J. Radke, Halle	C. Krier, Stuttgart		K. van Ackern, Mannheim	J. Schüttler, Erlangen	K. Taeger, Regensburg	J. Radke, Halle	B. Landauer, Munich	H. Van Aken, Muenster
2006	J. Radke, Halle	H. Van Aken, Muenster		K. van Ackern, Mannheim	J. Schüttler, Erlangen	K. Taeger, Regensburg	J. Radke, Halle	B. Landauer, Munich	H. Van Aken, Muenster
2007	H. Van Aken, Muenster	J. Radke, Halle		K. van Ackern, Mannheim	J. Schüttler, Erlangen	N. Roewer, Würzburg	J. Scholz, Kiel	B. Landauer, Munich	Th. Koch, Dresden
2008	H. Van Aken, Muenster	J. Schüttler, Erlangen		K. van Ackern, Mannheim	J. Schüttler, Erlangen	N. Roewer, Würzburg	J. Scholz, Kiel	B. Landauer, Munich	Th. Koch, Dresden
2009	J. Schüttler, Erlangen	H. Van Aken, Muenster		K. van Ackern, Mannheim	J. Scholz, Kiel	N. Roewer, Würzburg	W. Schaffartzik, Berlin	B. Landauer, Munich	Th. Koch, Dresden
2010	J. Schüttler, Erlangen	G. Nöldge-Schomburg, Rostock		K. van Ackern, Mannheim	J. Scholz, Kiel	N. Roewer, Würzburg	W. Schaffartzik, Berlin	B. Landauer, Munich	Th. Koch, Dresden
2011	G. Nöldge-Schomburg, Rostock	J. Schüttler, Erlangen		K. van Ackern, Mannheim	J. Scholz, Kiel	N. Roewer, Würzburg	W. Schaffartzik, Berlin	B. Landauer, Munich	Th. Koch, Dresden

1.3.5 Honorary Members of the German Society of Anaesthesiology and Intensive Care Medicine 1953–2008

1953	Prof. Dr. E. K. Frey, Germany †
1953	Prof. Dr. Friedrich Hesse, Germany †
1953	Prof. Dr. Hans Killian, Germany †
1953	Prof. Dr. Helmut Schmidt, Germany †
1953	Prof. Dr. Helmut Weese, Germany †
1954	Prof. Dr. Dr. h. c. Ernst Derra, Germany †
1963	Prof. Dr. Sir Robert Macintosh, Großbritannien †
1963	Prof. Dr. Dr. h. c. Rudolf Nissen, Switzerland †
1966	Prof. Dr. h. c. Walther Weissauer, Germany
1971	Prof. Dr. Ludwig Zukschwerdt, Germany †
1978	Prof. Dr. Rudolf Frey, Germany †
1978	Prof. Dr. Werner Hügin, Switzerland †
1978	Prof. Dr. Dr. h. c. mult. Otto Mayrhofer, Austria
1980	Prof. Dr. Martin Holmdahl, Sweden
1980	Prof. Dr. Jean Lassner, France †
1980	Prof. Dr. Emanuel M. Papper, USA †
1980	Prof. Dr. Hideo Yamamura, Japan
1981	Prof. Dr. Francis Foldes, USA †
1981	Prof. Dr. Jean Henley, USA †
1986	Prof. Dr. Hans-Jürgen Bretschneider, Germany †
1986	Prof. Dr. Gertie Marx, USA †
1987	Prof. Dr. Hans Bergmann, Austria
1987	Prof. Dr. Olof Norlander, Sweden †
1987	Prof. Dr. Hans Wolfgang Opderbecke, Germany
1993	Prof. Dr. Sir Malcolm Keith Sykes, Great Britain
1994	Prof. Dr. Erich Rügheimer, Germany †
1995	Prof. Dr. Otto H. Just, Germany †
1995	Prof. Dr. Kai Rehder, USA
1995	Prof. Dr. Kurt Wiemers, Germany †
1995	Prof. Dr. Martin Zindler, Germany
1996	Prof. Dr. Dr. h. c. Friedrich Wilhelm Ahnefeld, Germany
1996	Prof. Dr. Dr. h. c. mult. Antoni Aronski, Poland †
1996	Prof. Dr. Witold Jurczyk, Poland
1996	Prof. Dr. Dr. Cedric Prys-Roberts, Great Britain
1996	Prof. Dr. Dr. h. c. Karl Steinbereithner, Austria †
1996	Prof. Dr. Marek H. Sych, Poland †
1997	Prof. Dr. Richard Kitz, USA
1997	Prof. Dr. Georg Litarczek, Romania
1997	Prof. Dr. Jean-Claude Otteni, France
1997	Prof. Dr. Dr. h. c. mult. Horst Stoeckel, Germany
1998	Prof. Dr. David Richard Bevan, Canada
1998	Dr. T. C. Kester Brown, Australia
1998	Prof. Dr. Dr. h. c. Peter Lawin, Germany †
1998	Prof. Dr. Werner F. List, Austria
1998	Prof. Dr. Dr. Georges Rolly, Belgien
1998	Prof. Dr. Karl-Heinz Weis, Germany
1999	Prof. Dr. Gottfried Benad, Germany
1999	Prof. Dr. Dr. Harald Breivik, Norway
1999	Prof. Dr. Wilhelm Hartel, Germany
2000	Prof. Dr. Dr. Pierre Foëx, Great Britain
2000	Prof. Dr. John Hedley-White, USA
2001	Prof. Dr. Elena A. Damir, Russia
2001	Prof. Dr. Joachim Eckart, Germany
2001	Prof. Dr. Dag B. A. Lundberg, Sweden
2002	Prof. Dr. Dr. h.c. Wolfgang F. Dick, FRCA, Germany
2002	Prof. Dr. Klaus Fischer, Germany
2003	Dr. oec. publ. Christian Dräger, Germany
2003	Prof. Dr. Dr. h.c. Dietrich Kettler, Germany
2003	Prof. Sten Lindahl, MD, PhD, FRCA, Sweden
2003	Prof. Dr. Dr. h.c. Klaus Peter, Germany
2004	Prof. Dr. Alfred Doenicke, Germany
2004	Prof. Dr. Heinz Oehmig, Germany †
2005	Prof. Dr. Hilmar Burchardi, Germany
2005	Prof. Dr. Ronald D. Miller, USA
2005	Prof. Dr. Dr. h.c. Jochen Schulte am Esch, Germany
2006	Prof. Dr. Iurie Acalovschi, Romania
2006	Dr. Charlotte Lehmann, Germany
2006	Dr. rer. nat. Manfred Specker, Germany
2007	Prof. Dr. Dr. h.c. Klaus van Ackern, Germany
2007	Prof. James E. Cottrell, MD, FRCA, USA
2007	Sir Peter Jeffrey Simpson, MD, FRCA, FRCP, FRCS, FCARCSI, Great Britain

1.3.6 Corresponding Members of the German Society of Anaesthesiology and Intensive Care Medicine 1953–2008

Foreign colleagues, having essentially contributed to the development of anaesthesiology by their scientific work are eligible for corresponding membership (from the bylaws).

	Prof. Dr. L. A. Boeré, The Netherlands
	Dr. Jacques Boureau, France
	Dr. B. John Dillon, USA
	Prof. Dr. Erick Nilsson, Sweden
	Sir Geoffrey Organe, Great Britain †
	Prof. Dr. R. Rizzi, Italy
1966	Prof. Dr. Bruno Haid, Austria †
1966	Prof. Dr. Georg Hossli, Switzerland
1966	Prof. Dr. Werner Hügin, Switzerland †
1966	Prof. Dr. Dr. h. c. mult. Otto Mayrhofer, Austria
1967	Prof. Dr. Jean Lassner, France †
1968	Prof. Dr. Henning Poulsen, Denmark
1968	Prof. Dr. Martin Holmdahl, Sweden
1971	Prof. Dr. Peter Safar, USA †
1978	Dr. Alfredo Arias, Spain
1978	Prof. Dr. Dr. h. c. mult. Antoni Aronski, Poland †
1978	Prof. Dr. William K. Hamilton, USA
1978	Prof. Dr. Tigran M. Darbinyan, Russia
1978	Prof. Dr. Witold Jurczyk, Poland

1978	Prof. Dr. Richard J. Kitz, USA
1978	Prof. Dr. Jack Moyers, USA †
1978	Dr. E. S. Siker, USA
1978	Dr. Dr. John F. Nunn, Great Britain
1978	Prof. Dr. Hideo Yamamura, Japan
1981	Prof. Dr. Marcel Gemperlé, Switzerland
1981	Prof. Dr. Dr. h. c. Karl Steinbereithner, Austria †
1981	Prof. Dr. Bruno Tschirren, Switzerland †
1981	Prof. Dr. Herbert Benzer, Austria †
1981	Dr. Franz Kern, Switzerland †
1981	Prof. Dr. Hans Bergmann, Austria †
1982	Prof. Dr. Josef Hoder, Czech Republic †
1983	Prof. Dr. Zeno Filipescu, Romania †
1983	Prof. Dr. Marek H. Sych, Poland †
1983	Prof. P. A. Foster, South Africa
1983	Prof. Dr. Miquel A. Nalda Felipe, Spain
1985	Thomas B. Boulton, T.D., M.B., B. Chir, Great Britain
1985	Michael T. Inman, M.B., B.S., Great Britain
1985	Prof. Dr. Graham Smith, B.S., Great Britain
1986	Dr. Gyula Ugocsai, Hungary
1987	Prof. Dr. Tapani Tammisto, Finland
1987	Prof. Dr. Dr. Burnell R. Brown, USA †
1990	Prof. Dr. habil. Gottfried Benad, Germany
1990	Prof. Dr. Dr. h. c. Joachim Stefan Gravenstein, USA
1990	Prof. Dr. habil. Derk Olthoff, Germany
1997	Prof. Dr. Dag B.A. Lundberg, Sweden
1997	Prof. Dr. Iurie Acalovschi, Romania
1997	Prof. Dr. Philippe André Scherpereel, France
1997	Prof. Dr. Georgs Andrejevs, Latvia
1998	Prof. Dr. Pierre Coriat, France
1998	Prof. Dr. Dr. Maria Janecskó, Hungary
1998	Prof. Dr. Anneke E.E. Meursing, The Netherlands
1998	Prof. Dr. Per Henrik Rosenberg, Finland
1998	Dr. Richard George Walsh, Australia
1999	Prof. Dr. Kutay Akpir, Turkey
1999	Prof. Dr. Karel Cvachovec, Czech Republic
1999	Prof. Dr. Simon de Lange, The Netherlands
2000	Prof. Dr. Uður Oral, Turkey
2000	Prof. Dr. Dr. Miklós Tekeres, Hungary
2001	Prof. Dr. Armen A. Bunatian, Russia
2001	Prof. Dr. Gian P. Novelli, Italy †
2001	Prof. Dr. Peter M. Suter, Switzerland
2001	Prof. Dr. Dick A. Thomson, Switzerland
2002	Prof. Dr. Leonardus H. D. J. Booij, FRCA, The Netherlands
2002	Prof. Dr. Luciano Gattinoni, Italy
2002	Prof. Dr. C. Göran Hedenstierna, FRCA, Sweden
2003	Prof. Zeljko J. Bosnjak, Ph.D., USA
2003	Prof. James E. Cottrell, MD, FRCA, USA
2003	Prof. Adrian W Gelb, MB, ChB, D.A., FRCPC, Canada
2003	Prof. Shigeto Morita, MD, Ph.D., Japan
2004	Prof. Dr. Maurice Lucien François Joseph Lamy, FRCA, Belgium
2004	Prof. Dr. Donat Rudolf Spahn, FRCA, Switzerland
2005	Prof. Dr. Leon Drobnik, Poland
2005	Prof. Jørgen Viby-Mogensen, MD, DA (Hafnia), DMSc, Sweden
2006	Prof. Dr. Antonino Gullo, Italy
2006	Prof. Dr. Ali Resat Moral, Turkey
2006	Sir Peter Jeffrey Simpson, MD, FRCA, FRCP, FRCS, FCARCSI, Great Britain
2007	Prof. Henrik Kehlet, MD, PhD, Denmark
2008	Dr. René Heylen, Belgium
	Prof. Dr. M. J. Yuke Tian, China

1.3.7 Congresses of the German Society of Anaesthesiology and Intensive Care Medicine

	Congress	Year	Date	Location	President German Society
	1st Austrian Congress of Anaesthesiology (together with the Swiss Society of Anaesthesiology and the German Working Group on Anaesthesiology)	1952	September 5-6	Salzburg	Jochen Bark, Todtmoos
	Scientific Session of the German Society of Anaesthesia within the framework of the Congress of the German Society of Surgery	1953	April 10-11	Munich	Jochen Bark, Todtmoos
1.	2nd Austrian Congress of Anaesthesiology (together with the Swiss Society of Anaesthesiology and the German Society of Anaesthesia)	1953	May 17-19	Velden	Jochen Bark, Todtmoos / Tübingen
2.	3rd Joint Meeting of the German Society of Anaesthesia, the Austrian Society of Anaesthesiology and the Swiss Society of Anaesthesiology (Central European Anaesthesia Congress, ZAK)	1954	April 24-26	Munich	Jochen Bark, Tübingen

	Congress	Year	Date	Location	President German Society
3.	4th Central European Anaesthesia Congress (ZAK)	1956	August 23-25	Scheveningen	Lutz Zürn, Munich
4.	5th Central European Anaesthesia Congress (ZAK)	1957	June 13-15	Vienna	Martin Zindler, Düsseldorf
5.	6th Central European Anaesthesia Congress (ZAK)	1959	September 9-12	Düsseldorf	Martin Zindler, Düsseldorf
6.	7th Central European Anaesthesia Congress (ZAK)	1961	September 8-10	Geneva	Otto Just, Berlin/Heidelberg
7.	8th Central European Anaesthesia Congress (ZAK)	1963	September 12-14	Freiburg	Kurt Wiemers, Freiburg
8.	9th Central European Anaesthesia Congress (ZAK)	1965	September 16-18	Zürich	Karl Horatz, Hamburg
9.	Meeting of the German Society of Anaesthesia an Resuscitation	1966	November 5-6	Munich	Karl Horatz, Hamburg
10.	10th Central European Anaesthesia Congress (ZAK)	1967	September 21-23	Salzburg	H.W. Opderbecke, Nuremberg
11.	German Anaesthesia Congress (DAK)	1968	November 15-16	Nuremberg	H.W. Opderbecke, Nuremberg
12.	11th Central European Anaesthesia Congress (ZAK)	1969	September 3-6	Saarbrücken	Karl Hutschenreuter, Homburg/Saar
13.	German Anaesthesia Congress (DAK)	1970	November 5-7	Nuremberg	Karl Hutschenreuter, Homburg/Saar
14.	12th Central European Anaesthesia Congress (ZAK)	1971	September 1-3	Bern	Peter Lawin, Münster
15.	German Anaesthesia Congress (DAK)	1972	November 23-25	Hamburg	Peter Lawin, Münster
16.	13th Central European Anaesthesia Congress (ZAK)	1973	September 5-8	Linz	Erich Rügheimer, Erlangen
17.	German Anaesthesia Congress (DAK)	1974	October 2-5	Erlangen	Erich Rügheimer, Erlangen
18.	14th Central European Anaesthesia Congress (ZAK)	1975	September 10-13	Bremen	Walter Henschel, Bremen
19.	German Anaesthesia Congress (DAK)	1976	October 7-9	Lübeck-Travemünde	Walter Henschel, Bremen
20.	15th Central European Anaesthesia Congress (ZAK)	1977	September 13-16	Geneva	Karl Heinz Weis, Würzburg
21.	German Anaesthesia Congress (DAK)	1978	October 12-14	Würzburg	Karl Heinz Weis, Würzburg
22.	16th Central European Anaesthesia Congress (ZAK)	1979	September 5-8	Innsbruck	Erich Rügheimer, Erlangen
23.	7th World Congress of Anaesthesiologists	1980	September 14-21	Hamburg	Erich Rügheimer, Erlangen
24.	17th Central European Anaesthesia Congress (ZAK)	1981	September 15-19	Berlin	Joachim Schara, Wuppertal
25.	German Anaesthesia Congress (DAK)	1982	October 2-6	Wiesbaden	Joachim Schara, Wuppertal
26.	18th Central European Anaesthesia Congress (ZAK)	1983	September 13-17	Zürich	Friedrich Wilhelm Ahnefeld, Ulm
27.	German Anaesthesia Congress (DAK)	1984	September 26-30	Wiesbaden	Friedrich Wilhelm Ahnefeld, Ulm
28.	German Anaesthesia Congress (DAK)	1985	May 15-19	Bonn	Prof. Dr. Dietrich Kettler, Göttingen
29.	19th Central European Anaesthesia Congress (ZAK)	1985	September 10-14	Graz	Dietrich Kettler, Göttingen
30.	German Anaesthesia Congress (DAK)	1986	March 4-9	Wiesbaden	Dietrich Kettler, Göttingen
31.	20th Central European Anaesthesia Congress (ZAK)	1987	September 14-19	Munich	Klaus Peter, Munich
32.	German Anaesthesia Congress (DAK)	1988	September 21-25	Mannheim	Klaus Peter, Munich
33.	German Anaesthesia Congress (DAK)	1989	April 26-30	Bremen	Klaus Jürgen Fischer, Bremen
34.	21st Central European Anaesthesia Congress (ZAK)	1989	September 12-16	Innsbruck	Klaus Jürgen Fischer, Bremen
35.	German Anaesthesia Congress (DAK)	1990	March 21-25	Mannheim	Klaus Jürgen Fischer, Bremen
36.	German Anaesthesia Congress (DAK)	1991	March 20-25	Mannheim	Klaus Eyrich, Berlin
37.	22nd Central European Anaesthesia Congress (ZAK)	1991	September 10-14	Interlaken	Klaus Eyrich, Berlin

	Congress	Year	Date	Location	President German Society
38.	German Anaesthesia Congress (DAK)	1992	September 26-30	Berlin	Klaus Eyrich, Berlin
39.	23rd Central European Anaesthesia Congress (ZAK)	1993	September 14-18	Dresden	Gottfried Benad, Rostock
40.	German Anaesthesia Congress (DAK)	1994	June 14-18	Nuremberg	Rafael Dudziak, Frankfurt
41.	German Anaesthesia Congress (DAK)	1995	March 21-25	Hamburg	Reinhard Purschke, Dortmund
42.	24th Central European Anaesthesia Congress (ZAK)	1995	September 4-8	Vienna	Reinhard Purschke, Dortmund
43.	German Anaesthesia Congress (DAK)	1996	June 19-22	Nuremberg	Klaus van Ackern, Mannheim
44.	German Anaesthesia Congress (DAK)	1997	April 23-24	Hamburg	Jochen Schulte am Esch, Hamburg
45.	10th European Congress of anaesthesiology (ECA) / German Anaesthesia Congress (DAK)	1998	June 30 - July 4	Frankfurt	Gunter Hempelmann, Gießen
46.	German Anaesthesia Congress (DAK)	1999	May 5-8	Wiesbaden	Detlef Patschke, Marl
47.	German Anaesthesia Congress (DAK)	2000	May 6-9	Munich	Klaus Geiger, Freiburg
48.	German Anaesthesia Congress (DAK)	2001	June 13-16	Nuremberg	Eberhard Götz, Darmstadt
49.	German Anaesthesia Congress (DAK)	2002	June 22-25	Nuremberg	Jörg Tarnow, Düsseldorf
50.	German Anaesthesia Congress (DAC)	2003	April 9-13	Munich	Eike Martin, Heidelberg
51.	German Anaesthesia Congress (DAC)	2004	June 19-22	Nuremberg	Claude Krier, Stuttgart
52.	German Anaesthesia Congress (DAC)	2005	April 16-19	Munich	Joachim Radke, Halle
53.	German Anaesthesia Congress (DAC)	2006	June 17-20	Leipzig	Joachim Radke, Halle
54.	German Anaesthesia Congress (DAC)	2007	May 5-8	Hamburg	Hugo Van Aken, Münster
55.	German Anaesthesia Congress (DAC)	2008	April 26-29	Nuremberg	Hugo Van Aken, Münster
56.	German Anaesthesia Congress (DAC)	2009	May 9-12	Leipzig	Jürgen Schüttler, Erlangen
57.	German Anaesthesia Congress (DAC)	2010	June 19-22	Nuremberg	Jürgen Schüttler, Erlangen
58	German Anaesthesia Congress (DAC)	2011	May 14-17	Hamburg	Gabriele Nöldge-Schomburg, Rostock

1.4   Development of the Specialist Journals

Co-ordination: K. Taeger and J. Schüttler

1.4.1   *Der Anaesthesist*: a Dynamic, Scientific and Practice-Oriented Journal in Times of Change

A. Doenicke

The first specialist German-language anesthesiological journal *Schmerz-Narkose-Anaesthesie* (Pain, Narcosis, Anaesthesia: 1928–1943) was of great service due to its commitment to pain-related problems and the continual development of anaesthesia. However, the intellectual opening occurring after the Second World War and the renewal of contacts with the leading countries in anaesthesiology, the UK, USA and France, made it possible in a second attempt to found our own journal (1951) for the new specialist area of anaesthesiology.

In 1951, young Austrian, Swiss and German doctors who had been trained in anaesthesiology in Anglo-American countries met with the aim of founding not only a new society but also an appropriate new journal.

This was the birth of *Der Anaesthesist* (The Anaesthetist). In the first editorial on p. 1 of Vol. 1 in 1952 [3], the three Editors R. Frey (Heidelberg), W. Hügin (Basel) and O. Mayrhofer (Vienna) announced their aims and concept for the journal. *Der Anaesthesist* thus became the official organ of the Austrian Society of Anaesthesiology in its year of foundation (◘ Fig. 1.48). Starting in June 1953 (Vol. 2, issue 3), it also became the official organ of the German Society of Anaesthesia upon its foundation and in the same year for the Swiss Society of Anaesthesiology (issue 4). In 1959, one of the founders, W. Hügin, retired in favour of F. Kern, who was then Editor until 1978. From 1979 onwards, H.J. Schaer has been the Swiss Editor.

The driving force during the founding years was, in addition to W. Hügin and O. Mayrhofer, the unforgettable R. Frey, who can be considered the Nestor of German anaesthesiology. He was Editor of the journal until 1969 and Editor-in-Chief until 1981. Frey died in 1981. In 1969, Alfred Doenicke took over the office of Editor and from 1977 onwards that of Editor-in-Chief.

One of these founding members, O. Mayrhofer, had a major influence on the fate of the journal as an Editor until the end of 1991, i.e. for a period of 40 years. This is undoubtedly unique in the history of an international scientific journal. Over the past two decades, Mayrhofer has significantly supported the Editor-in-Chief as a friend and circumspect advisor in the not always easy exercise of making important decisions.

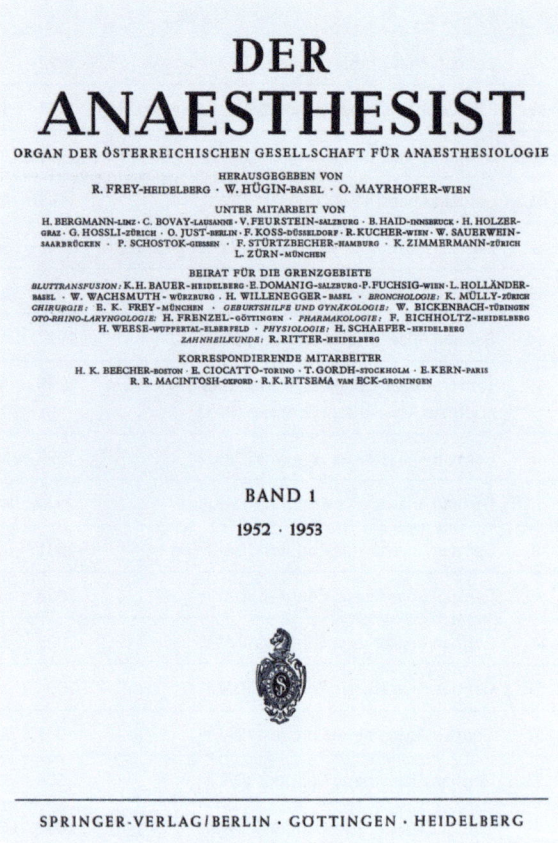

◘ **Fig. 1.48.** Title page of Vol. 1 of *Der Anaesthesist*

The international standing of *Der Anaesthesist* was significantly influenced by Mayrhofer's personality. The scientific achievements and international recognition of this Editor have been praised within the framework of several laudations. Nevertheless, one unique point should be repeated once again: Mayrhofer had a formative influence on the World Federation of Societies of Anaesthesiologists (WFSA) for 12 years – 8 years as secretary (1964–1972) followed by 4 years as president. Thus, the Editor of our journal influenced the development of anaesthesiology worldwide over a long period. Changes in the Editorial Committee and Editors since the journal's foundation in 1952 are listed in ◘ Table 1.5.

Beginning in 1953, members of the Editorial Committee and the Advisory Council have predominantly been chosen equally from among the Austrian, German and Swiss societies.

From 1969 to 1974, the Editorial Board was divided into sections (◘ Table 1.6): original papers, reviews, resuscitation and acute care therapy, errors and dangers, letters to the Editor, technical innovations, and conference reports.

Table 1.5. Changes in the Editorial Board and Editor-in-Chief since the founding year of 1952

Der Anaesthesist

Year	Editors
1953–1959	R. Frey, W. Hügin, O. Mayrhofer
1960–1977	R. Frey, F. Kern, O. Mayrhofer
1977–1978	R. Frey, F. Kern, O. Mayrhofer, A. Doenicke
1979–1981	A. Doenicke, R. Frey, O. Mayrhofer, H. Schaer
1982–1990	A. Doenicke, O. Mayrhofer, H. Schaer
1991–1994	A. Doenicke, W. List, H. Schaer
1995–1998	K. Peter
1998–2002	R. Larsen, K. Peter
	Honorary Editors
From 1999	A. Doenicke, O. Mayrhofer

Regional-Anaesthesie

Year	Editors
1978–1988	H.C. Niesel, H. Nolte, O. Schulte-Steinberg
1989–1992	J. Neumark, H.C. Niesel, H. Nolte, O. Schulte-Steinberg
	Editorial Secretary
1967	H. Nolte, M. Halmágyi
1968–1969	M. Halmágyi
	Editors-in-Chief
1970–1994	A. Doenicke
1995–1997	K. Peter
1998–2002	R. Larsen, K. Peter
2008–2009	R. Larsen, B. Zwißler
2010	R. Rossaint, B. Zwißler

Table 1.6. Editorial Committee and Editorial Board from 1969 to 1974

Editorial Committee/Editorial Board

Original papers	H. Bergmann (Linz), R. Frey (Mainz), F. Kern (St. Gallen), O. Mayrhofer (Vienna)
Reviews	A. Doenicke (Munich), D. Langrehr (Bremen)
Reanimation and acute care therapy	H. Halmágyi (Mainz), R. Kucher (Vienna), K. Steinbereithner (Vienna)
Errors and dangers	B. Tschirren (Bern)
Letters to the Editor	F. Kern (St. Gallen)
Technical innovations	H. Bergmann (Linz)
Conference reports	R. Frey (Mainz)

Colleagues who were particularly active in the development of anaesthesiology in Central Europe and had acted as referees were included in the Advisory Council for bordering countries. This interdisciplinary Advisory Council was dropped in 1995.

Table 1.7. Editorial Committee in 1991

Editorial Committee/Editorial board

G. Benad (Rostock), H. Benzer (Innsbruck), H. Bergmann (Linz), W. Dick (Mainz), R. Dudziak (Frankfurt am Main), R. Gattiker (Zurich), M. Gemperle (Geneva), M. Halmágyi (Mainz), D. Kettler (Göttingen), W. List (Graz), T. Pasch (Zurich), K. Peter (Munich), K. Steinbereither (Vienna), J. Tarnow (Düsseldorf), B. Tschirren (Bern), J. Wawersik (Kiel)

Advisory Board

F.W. Ahnefeld (Ulm), K.-H. Altemeyer (Saarbrücken), J.O. Arndt (Düsseldorf), W. Buzello (Cologne), K. Falke (Berlin), U. Finsterer (Munich), S. Fitzal (Vienna), W. Heinrichs (Mainz), G. Hempelmann (Giessen), G. Kreienbühl (St. Gallen), K.A. Lehmann (Cologne), N. Mutz (Innsbruck), H. Nolte (Minden), D. Olthoff (Leipzig), H.-J. Priebe (Freiburg), D. Scheidegger (Basel), E.R. Schmid (Zurich), H. Sonntag (Göttingen), D. Thomson (Bern), K.H. Weis (Würzburg), M. Zenz (Bochum)

With the appearance of Vol. 24 in 1975, the subdivision of the Editorial Board was discontinued, while the Board itself increased continually during the following years, as seen, for example, in a synopsis from 1991 (■ Table 1.7).

The current Editorial Committee, co-ordinated by the Editor-in-Chief and composed of the Rubric Editors supported by a Council, is listed from the July edition 2002 (Vol. 51) (■ Table 1.8).

Der Anaesthesist contributed significantly to recognition of the independence of this specialist area (1952), to the foundation of specialist societies in German-speaking countries (1951 and 1952) as well as to the joint congresses held by these societies. The combined work of W. Hügin (Basel) and the journal also provided a decisive impulse for the production of the Lehrbuch der Anästhesiologie (Textbook of Anaesthesiology): 1955, 1968, 1974 und 1977). The »supranational« character of this journal for German-speaking countries proved to be a blessing from its inception. Thus, *Der Anaesthesist* has made an important contribution to mutual collegial demands as well as to scientific and specialist co-operation between Central European anaesthetists. The scientific reputation achieved in this way was an important factor in the creation of professorships for anaesthesiology at German-language universities from 1959 onwards.

Regional-Anaesthesie (Local Anaesthesia) – a Journal Within a Journal

At the beginning of its 27th year, the editors of *Der Anaesthesist* announced an important innovation. Regular publications in the area of local anaesthesia would appear in the future as a type of »journal within a journal«.

This new journal, which was edited by H.C. Niesel (Ludwigshafen), H. Nolte (Minden) and O. Schulte-Stein-

Table 1.8. Editorial Committee in 2002

Rubric Editors	
Leading themes and casuistics	K. Peter
Original papers and short communications	R. Larsen (Homburg/Saar), T. Fuchs-Buder (Homburg/Saar)
Clinical pharmacology	J. Schüttler (Erlangen)
General anaesthesia	M. Jöhr (Lucerne), C. Werner (Munich), B. Zwissler (Munich)
Local anaesthesia	D.M. Albrecht (Dresden), V. Hempel (Constance)
Pain therapy	C. Stein (Berlin)
Acute care medicine	R. Kuhlen (Aachen), K.E. Unertl (Tübingen)
Emergency medicine	W. Dick (Mainz), H. Lindner (Innsbruck)
Errors and dangers	W. List (Graz), H. Metzler (Graz)
Medical law	R. Dudziak (Frankfurt), K. Ulsenheimer (Munich), W. Weißauer (Nuremberg)
Current medicine	F. Christ (Munich), W. Rößling (Heidelberg)
Trends and medical economics	E. Martin (Heidelberg)
Continuing and advanced education	H.J. Bardenheuer (Heidelberg), H. Forst (Augsburg), R. Rossaint (Aachen), D. Spahn (Lausanne)

Advisory Board

K.-H. Altemeyer (Saarbrücken), M. Bauer (Homburg/Saar), G. Benad (Rostock), H. Benzer (Innsbruck), P. Biro (Zurich), W. Buhre (Aachen), W. Buzello (Cologne), P. Conzen (Munich), K. Falke (Berlin), S. Fizal (Vienna), H. Gerber (Lucerne), B.-M. Graf (Heidelberg), R. Gust (Heidelberg), W. Heinrichs (Mainz), G. Hempelmann (Giessen), A. Hoeft (Bonn), J. Jage (Mainz), J.-P. Jantzen (Hannover), T. Koch (Dresden), E. Kochs (Munich), H.G. Kress (Vienna), K.A. Lehmann (Cologne), C. Maier (Bochum), S.C.U. Marsch (Basel), F. Mertzlufft (Bielefeld), T. Möllhoff (Münster), N. Mutz (Innsbruck), J. Neumark (Vienna), H.C. Niesel (Ludwigshafen), G. Nöldge-Schomburg (Rostock), D. Olthoff (Leipzig), P.M. Osswald (Hanau), T. Pasch (Zurich), J. Plötz (Bamburg), G. Prause (Graz), H.-J. Priebe (Freiburg), M. Ragaller (Dresden), P. Ravussin (Lausanne), M. Schäfer (Berlin), E.R. Schmid (Zurich), M.C. Schneider (Basel), G. Schwarz (Graz), D. Schwender (Friedrichshafen), H. Schwilden (Erlangen), M. Semsroth (Vienna), H.J. Sparr (Innsbruck), K. Taeger (Regensburg), D. Thomson (Bern), M.R. Tramer (Geneva), M. Tryba (Kassel), N. Weiler (Mainz), H. Wissing (Frankfurt), M. Zlalunardo (Zurich), M. Zenz (Bochum), M. Zimpfer (Vienna)

berg (Starnberg) under the leadership of A. Doenicke as Editor-in-Chief, was closely associated with the mother journal and added 20 printed pages to *Der Anaesthesist* every 3–4 months. In 1989, J. Neumark (Vienna) was added to this list of Editors.

Over the previous few decades, local anaesthesia had undoubtedly made great advances and increased in significance. These facts were taken into account by this innovative addition within the framework of the journal in terms of both scientific research and clinical practice.

This branch of anaesthesiology has received full recognition in Austria, Germany and Switzerland over the years. This is due to the resolute publication of practice-related work as well as scientific knowledge, such as, for example, the pharmacokinetics and dynamics of local anaesthesia.

The appearance of *Regional-Anaesthesie* as part of *Der Anaesthesist* was particularly praised by H. Berg-

mann in an editorial in 1978 [1] in which he wrote that historical data testified to the traditional association between German-language anaesthesiology and local anaesthesia. In this regard Bergmann mentioned the names Koller (Vienna: discovery of the local anaesthetic action of cocaine, 1894), Schleich (Berlin: infiltration anaesthesia, 1892), Bier (Kiel: the first to propose spinal anaesthesia as a method for blocking pain during surgery on humans, 1898), Einhorn (Hoechst: discovery of Novocain, 1905) and Braun (Leipzig: the additional use of vasopressors in order to increase the active time of local anaesthetics, 1909).

As indicated by its name, the first specialist German-language journal for anaesthesiology, *Schmerz-Narkose-Anaesthesie* (Pain, Narcosis and Anaesthesia), which was published in Leipzig by Georg Thieme from 1927 until 1944, had already placed emphasis on local methods of anaesthesia for pain control during surgery.

The establishment of a section of the journal devoted to local anaesthesia, and the independence of this section within *Der Anaesthesist*, show that after many years of »vegetating« this method of locally blocking pain, based on advances in modern general anaesthesia and having undergone a renaissance over the last 15 years, had taken an appropriate place in German-language literature on anaesthesiology. That this measure was also quantitatively justified is demonstrated by the fact that no fewer than 56 contributions to the problems of local anaesthesia have been made in the last 10 years in this journal.

The advances made in local anaesthesia, which also make the renewed interest in this area understandable, are:
- The development of new local anaesthetics
- Technical and methodological innovations
- A better understanding of the physiology and pathophysiology of local anaesthesia

It therefore seems appropriate to promote the methods of local anaesthesia with their undoubted advantages and not to neglect them. To teach these in the most modern way brings to fruition a statement made by Heinrich Braun 73 years ago in the introduction to the first edition of his book **Die örtliche Betäubung, ihre wissenschaftlichen Grundlagen und praktische Anwendung** (Local Anaesthesia, Its Scientific Bases and Practical Use: Leipzig 1905) that the extended use of local anaesthesia for the maximum benefit of the surgical patient was previously only possible for those individuals who had the opportunity to study a large number of relevant works and who, through practice and experience, had learnt the limits of this procedure.

He continued: **»It is therefore high time to summarize our current knowledge of local anaesthesia«.**

100 Years of Local Anaesthesia by H. Nolte (1984) *Regional-Anaesthesie* 1:113–114

An historical overview was provided by Hans Nolte, a pioneer of local anaesthesia, in a further editorial from 1984 entitled »100 years of local anaesthesia« [6].

Nolte wrote of an additional discovery which, although less spectacular for the general public, was enthusiastically greeted by medical practitioners. On 14 September 1884, exactly 100 years previously, Dr. Breithard reported on the discovery of Dr. Karl Koller of Vienna at the ophthalmological congress in Heidelberg. After intensive studies, Koller had determined that subsequent to sprinkling the cornea with a cocaine solution, fully conscious patients did not feel any pain. In addition, their eyes showed no reflectory movement after touching the cornea or the sclera, and also that the lid reflex was missing. This presentation left a deep impression, and the news spread rapidly throughout the world among the medical profession.

Thus, 1884 became the year in which local anaesthesia was born.

Within a few years, especially in Germany, France and the USA, a variety of techniques were developed for pain control using cocaine. After about three decades, with the development of new local anaesthetics (Novocain), practically all of the currently used methods for local anaesthesia had been discovered and their clinical use developed. German medicine, and in particular surgery, played a major role in this development. The first 30 years after the discovery of the local anaesthetic effects of cocaine are closely tied to the names Bier, Braun, Härtel, Hackenbruch, Hirschel, Kulenkampff, Läwen, Oberst, Perthes, Schleich and Stöckel. These, as well as many other colleagues, are to be thanked for the considerable number and variety of local anaesthetic procedures available today.

Nolte continued that after these 30 years of pioneer work, the popularity of local anaesthesia received considerable new impetus between 1910 and 1930. Peripheral plexus blockades were further developed, lumbar peridural anaesthesia became a clinically realizable method in the 1920s, and the particular possibilities of spinal anaesthesia enjoyed a great many supporters. During this period, local anaesthesia was a real alternative to general anaesthesia.

Between 1930 and 1960, the popularity of local anaesthesia sank significantly. At this time major advances in general anaesthesia took place. After 1960, however, a slow but continual revival in local anaesthesia was observed. This had various causes: the complications and, in particular, the irremovable side effects of general anaesthesia had been better studied and recognized, long-acting local anaesthetics were introduced into clinical practice and reliable, disposable materials had made their impact, not only in general but also in local anaesthesia.

Nevertheless, the deciding factors leading to the revival of local anaesthesia were our increased knowledge and the better training of anaesthetists.

Finally, realization that postoperative morbidity and mortality were markedly lower for certain operations and patient groups under local compared to general anaesthesia led to a significant increase in the proportion of local anaesthesias in the total number of anaesthesias performed, with 40–50% of all anaesthesias being applied locally in many hospitals.

Nolte wrote that in Germany, in particular, commemoration of the 100th anniversary of local anaesthesia could be made with pride. German medicine had made not only a major contribution to the development and spread of local anaesthesia in its early phase, but it had also been of great service during the renaissance of local anaesthesia in the previous 20 years.

Looking into the future, Nolte asked what could make local anaesthesia even more popular. There seemed to be three critical factors:

- The indications and contraindications for local anaesthesia needed to be more clearly defined.
- The quality of local anaesthesia needed to be increased through better training and greater experience.
- The quantitative use of local anaesthetic techniques should increase in order to offer the patients greater safety and younger colleagues more training possibilities.

Nolte concluded that with 100 years of experience and established procedures, local anaesthesia could enter its second century with assurance.

Ten Years of *Regional-Anaesthesie* in *Der Anaesthesist*

Ten years after the initiation of the special section on local anaesthesia, the Editors, H.C. Niesel, H. Nolte and O. Schulte-Steinberg, could retrospectively take stock.

In the previous 10 years, it had not only been possible to maintain the quarterly issues, but these could be markedly improved due to the increased number of manuscripts submitted.

With a print run of 5,000 per issue in 1992 (in 2008 this has increased to 7,000), *Der Anaesthesist* ranks worldwide behind *Anesthesiology* and the *British Journal of Anaesthesia* as a leading journal in its field. Thus, the distribution of the special section *Regional-Anaesthesie* is particularly noteworthy. Also welcome is the fact that *Regional-Anaesthesie* is also recorded in the Index Medicus through its association with *Der Anaesthesist*.

Of the 250 manuscripts published in the special section on local anaesthesia over the last 10 years, »Letters to the Editor« took second place after original papers, with about 30% of the total contributions. This led the Editors to conclude that not only was there great interest in this work per se, but also that this branch of anaesthesia – local anaesthesia – was followed and discussed in the medical profession with great interest.

From 1982 onwards, this special section on local anaesthesia was no longer produced separately, but was integrated as a component of the main body of *Der Anaesthesist*. After 40 years, the format of the journal was also changed to a more modern concept. Appropriate to the four pillars of anaesthesia, Specialist Editors attend to sections on acute care medicine, local anaesthesia, emergency and disaster medicine as well as pain therapy. Together with the Editors, this should place the journal's scientific and organizational work on a broader foundation.

A New Concept: the Addition of Comprehensively Structured English Abstracts

The international character of the journal has been emphasized by a comprehensively structured English abstract, especially for original papers. In addition to the aims, the abstract contains important results with reference to relevant figures and tables. With a short discussion and conclusions, the scientific knowledge of German anaesthetists is provided to a non-German-speaking, foreign audience. The key contents of German publications can thus be conveyed into English-speaking areas. This concept provides a scientific bridge to foreign anaesthetists; hopefully a promising contribution to overcoming the language barrier.

In the 1980s, the suggestion was frequently made to the Editorial Committee by scientifically active colleagues that English language articles should be published. However, in 1981 the editors R. Frey, O. Mayrhofer, H.J. Schaer and A. Doenicke, together with the Production Committee and the publisher, decided that *Der Anaesthesist*, as German-language journal, should only publish German-language articles. The comprehensive English abstract offered a satisfactory compromise.

Impact Factor

The currently much discussed »impact factor« of a journal can be raised for *Der Anaesthesist* through the citation of its papers by foreign, but especially by German colleagues. In the Citation Report for 1990, *Der Anaesthesist* reached the tenth place for standard journals as the only German-language publication listed.

Continuing Education and Reviews

A new section for questions of anesthesiological continuing education handles important problems, which are also available in refresher courses, in a very compact form.

Relevant themes from the specialist areas of anaesthesia, acute care medicine, emergency and disaster medicine as well as pain therapy are didactically illustrated in a suitably structured way. They are handled by specially invited colleagues who have experience in continuing education. Thus, over the years a catalogue of informative, continuing education texts can be offered to colleagues. This can be seen as a permanent component of our journal. Colleagues involved in primary training as well as continuing education, such as head physicians, should find these a first-class method of providing information to trainees.

In addition, special attention continues to be paid to reviews which illustrate and evaluate particular aspects of anesthesiological practice. In the ideal case, these are paired with an editorial commentary.

Thus, the new concept for *Der Anaesthesist* offers anaesthetists interested in scientific themes, as well as all those involved in continuing and advanced training, diverse and meaningful stimulation [2].

In an editorial in the first issue of *Der Anaesthesist* from 1996, Klaus Peter took a stand on the conceptual changes in the journal's content [7].

»Leitthema«: the Leading Theme

Der Anaesthesist changed its previous conception in the first issue of 1996. In addition to the unchanged extent of the section containing original papers, a new form of review appeared under the title »*Leitthema*« (leading theme), with the Section Editor inviting authors who, in turn, provide their article with a structured bibliography. These bibliographies designate »interesting« and »particularly interesting« articles with one and two dots, respectively. However, not all readers have the time to make a comprehensive literature research, and not all have access to a well supplied library with the corresponding journals. For this reason, the authors of the reviews summarize the essential message of the articles indicated by the dots in a few sentences, providing the reader with the opportunity to select those articles which are of real personal value.

The theme of the first review in this form was adult respiratory distress syndrome or ARDS.

The reader will not find the usual »state-of-the-art« article under the section of continuing education in this issue. Rather, there is a carefully formulated contribution covering one of the central themes of modern medicine: is everything which can be done always medically worthwhile for severely ill patients whose condition is not compatible with survival over a longer time? On the one hand, the prolongation of life at all costs should not be the aim of intensive medical therapy; on the other, there is the danger that not everything medically valuable can be made available to all patients due to ever more limited financial resources. Especially in emergency and acute care medicine, a decision on treatment can often only be made once all aspects of the case have been carefully considered.

In 1996, O. Mayrhofer published his thoughts on the book **Das Jahrhundert der Chirurgen** (The Century of Surgeons, 1956) by J. Thorwald. The article **»The 150th anniversary of anaesthesia: thoughts on a century of surgery«** [4] documents the greatest achievements of anaesthesiologists in the realm of surgery and, in particular, acute care medicine.

Der Anaesthesist: Companion and Promoter of German-Language Anaesthesia

In an editorial from April 2002, Klaus Peter and Reinhard Larsen defined their new concept for the journal on its 50th anniversary [8].

They wrote that 25 years after its founding – the subscription was 3,000 worldwide – the Editors at that time, Rudolf Frey, Otto Mayrhofer and Franz Kern, drew a positive balance for their work: *Der Anaesthesist* had contributed significantly to recognition of the independence of their specialist area, as well as to the foundation of specialist societies in German-speaking countries and scientific and medical co-operation between Central European anaesthesiologists.

The history of anaesthesia was well kind to these Editors as they could write that after these 25 years they could look back on a time of rapid change, to a large extent caused by a process which could be defined by the catchwords globalization or internationalization of medicine. During this process, in which they were more driven than formative, the publication of scientific results in the German language lost more and more in terms of importance and recognition. The language of science is English; its evaluation in publications is called »impact factor«!

The consequences of globalization for German-language journals and scientific work were immense: although the main thrust of publication previously comprised original papers, in the previous 5 years continuing and advanced education had been pushed into the foreground. Original papers in the German language, which had dealt mostly with clinical questions, were becoming less and less common and it seemed possible that they could disappear completely. The results of basic research or animal experiments were almost always published in English-language journals, at least in part due to the pressure from German universities for achieving a high impact factor for publications by younger scientists. The Editors wrote that, though much this development may be deplored, it could not be stopped.

Both the Editorial Board and the publisher were therefore exceptionally pleased with the success of the recently defined new concept for *Der Anaesthesist* as a reaction to these changes, which followed the success story written by the previous Editors. Indeed, the position of the journal had even improved. In particular, one important goal of the Editors was still to provide a bridge between science and clinical practice.

The Editors continued that *Der Anaesthesist* of that time was, also in international comparison, the leading German-language anesthesiological journal, recognizable by its increasing subscriber list – especially over the preceding 6 years – and its high impact factor for a German-language journal.

A Founding Member Recalls [5]

In issue 5 from May 2002, a founding member of the journal, Otto Mayrhofer, recalled the time 50 years ago. He wrote that in 1951 three, by today's standards, young doctors met to finalize a priority project: the foundation of a specialist German-language journal for anaesthesia.

The enormous daring and optimism of these doctors – Otto Mayrhofer, Werner Hügin and Rudolf Frey – can be measured by the fact that at that time the specialist area of anaesthesia was not even officially recognized and the number of specialist practitioners was only about 30. Mayrhofer, the last witness and Co-Editor of the journal until 1991, i.e. from an unimaginably long period of 40 years, recalled the founding year when, exactly 50 years ago in April 1952, the first issue of *Der Anaesthesist* appeared. On the occasion of this golden anniversary, Mayrhofer provided, as long-term and then Honorary Editor, as well as being the last surviving member of the founding trio, a short history of the journal's origin. In the Statutes of the Austrian Society of Anaesthesiology, which was founded in autumn 1951, one of the Society's aims was to publish a specialist scientific journal. As *Der Chirurg* (The Surgeon) was a long-standing journal published by Springer, Mayrhofer took the risk, as the Society's President, of querying this Heidelberg publishing house in 1951. Springer advised him to contact the head of the anaesthesia section of the Heidelberg Surgical Clinic, Dr. Rudolf Frey, who had also recently contacted this publisher with the same idea.

Frey immediately suggested striving for a joint German-language journal. He indicated that he would contact Werner Hügin in Basel, with whom he had completed part of his training, in order to include their Swiss colleagues.

Mayrhofer knew Hügin personally because the latter had written to him after the publication of Mayrhofer's monograph on intratracheal narcosis (1949). Mayrhofer then visited him in Basel on his return from training in New York in 1950. Hügin himself had studied with Professor H.K. Beecher at Harvard University in Boston. Thus, they were working along the same lines. Frey had another discussion with the senior head of the publishing house, Dr. Ferdinand Springer, before Christmas 1951. This went extremely well. Dr. Springer was of the opinion that anaesthesiology, an up-coming and promising specialization, deserved his and the publisher's full support.

Initially, the journal was to be published bimonthly and comprise 36 pages. Mayrhofer, Frey and Hügen would act as joint Editors, with Frey being the direct contact person to the publishers. In analogy with Der Chirurg, the journal would be called *Der Anaesthesist*, and it should become the official publication of the, in part not even founded, specialist societies of the three countries. The subscription requirements on the part of the publisher were very generous from the beginning. How it was possible to print the first issue by the end of April remained a puzzle, but all three Editors were still young (Frey was born in 1917, Hügin in 1918 and Mayrhofer in 1920) and full of enthusiasm. The first contribution came from the Heidelberg Professor for Physiology Hans Schäfer on the theory of the neuromuscular transfer of muscle tone. The second was written by Mayrhofer on his experiences with succinylcholine chloride, a new, quick-acting muscle relaxant, while the third was a shortened version of Frey's just finalized habilitation thesis on »Vergleichende Untersuchung der muskelerschlaffenden Mittel« (Comparative investigations on muscle relaxants).

At the end of this historical perspective, Mayrhofer wished the journal luck and success for its next half century.

In the last 50 years, the Editors of *Der Anaesthesist* from R. Frey, W. Hügin and O. Mayrhofer to R. Larsen and K. Peter (2003) have always modified the journal in terms of their viewpoint and the current situation. They have modernized it and led it to success, with the number of subscribers increasing from 1,000 in 1952 to 7,000 in 2008. In 2008, B. Zwißler replaced K. Peter and R. Rossaint replaced R. Larsen one year later.

The Importance of the Publisher H. Goetze for *Der Anaesthesist*

Special thanks go to the publisher and the responsible individuals from the time of the journal's foundation, F. Springer and H. Goetze, to the present time, as well as to the Editorial Boards of 2003 and after.

That *Der Anaesthesist* has been so successful in the last five decades is especially due to H. Goetze, who, while he lived, benevolently accompanied the anaesthetists from the publisher's stand point, but who in times of crisis (1969/1970) also made decisions which changed the future of the journal and its Editors.

Those who have the opportunity to examine the 57 volumes of *Der Anaesthesist* until 2008 will find not only exceptional scientific studies, but also invaluable editorials, reviews, original papers, leading themes and articles on continuing education. Only a few articles with an historical background have been selected for this commemorative issue. It is also certain that past work published in *Der Anaesthesist* can still be read with benefit, based on current criteria, in the areas of inhalation anaesthesia, i.v. hypnotics and narcotics, and acute care medicine. It is worth advising currently active anaesthetists and scientists to emulate their predecessors and to publish new information in the area of anaesthesiology.

I wish the Editors and members of the publishing house of *Der Anaesthesist* much good fortune and success during the next 50 years.

(Alfred Doenicke)

References

1. Bergmann H (1978) Editorial: Regional-Anaesthesie 1:1–2
2. Doenicke A (1992) Editorial. Anaesthesist 41:238
3. Frey R, Hügin W, Mayrhofer O (1952) Editorial. Anaesthesist 1:1
4. Mayrhofer O (1996) Gedanken zum 150. Geburtstag der Anästhesie. Anaesthesist 45:881–883
5. Mayrhofer O (2002) 50 Jahre *Der Anaesthesist* – ein Gründer erinnert sich. Anaesthesist 51:418–419
6. Nolte H (1984) 100 Jahre Regionalanästhesie.Regional-Anaesthesie 1:113–114
7. Peter K (1996) Editorial. Anaesthesist 45:1
8. Peter K, Larsen R (2002) *Der Anaesthesist* – Begleiter und Förderer der deutschsprachigen Anästhesie. Anaesthesist 51:419

1.4.2　The Journal *Anästhesiologie & Intensivmedizin*

K. Taeger

The first forerunners of the journal *Anästhesiologie & Intensivmedizin* were typed and hectographed pamphlets called *Informationen der Deutschen Gesellschaft für Anaesthesie* (◘ Fig. 1.49). They were edited by the Executive Committee of the Deutsche Gesellschaft für Anaesthesie (DGA), under the Editorship of Dr. phil. K. Heise.

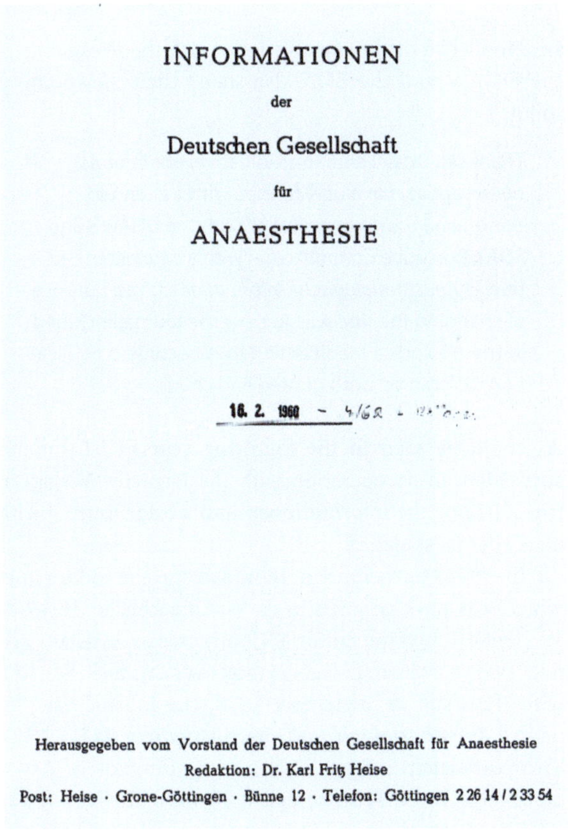

INFORMATIONEN

der

Deutschen Gesellschaft

für

ANAESTHESIE

16. 2. 1960　–　4/62　–

Herausgegeben vom Vorstand der Deutschen Gesellschaft für Anaesthesie
Redaktion: Dr. Karl Fritz Heise
Post: Heise · Grone-Göttingen · Bünne 12 · Telefon: Göttingen 2 26 14 / 2 33 54

◘ **Fig. 1.49.** First issue of the *Informationen der Deutschen Gesellschaft für Anästhesie*

In the pamphlet of 16 February 1960, O. Just outlined the goals of these pamphlets as follows: »For the purely technical we have our journal *Der Anaesthesist*; all other questions, however, like terms of employment, questions concerning invoicing, recognition of specialist titles, etc. are to be discussed here«.

Under the heading »Request for contributions« the following was noted:

> The situation of anaesthesia in the Federal Republic of Germany differs so considerably from that of anaesthesia in the Anglo-Saxon countries that it is about time to analyze this situation thoroughly. Nobody is more called upon for this than the anaesthetists themselves. If the attempt is to be made to raise anaesthesia to the same high standard as in the Anglo-Saxon countries in the next few years, we must realize where we stand and where we want to go. Write to the Editor if you want to comment on the following thoughts:
> — Anaesthesia at the universities
> — Anaesthesia care provided to the population
> — Health insurance
> — Tactical approaches to establishing the specialty of anaesthesia in the Federal Republic of Germany
>
> These are just some suggestions. Surely, you know much more to say about these topics. Please, write to us.

The next pamphlet, most likely published in May 1960, contains interesting information, which is hardly believable today:

> Comparative figures of specialized anaesthetists per 1 million inhabitants: Denmark 23, Belgium 15, Holland 15, France 14, Austria 14, Germany 1.3.
> The number of 50 anaesthetists per 1 million inhabitants can be considered as the normal condition. This number has already been achieved in the UK and USA today [in 1960!]. Comparing the conditions in Germany to the development in other countries like the UK, Denmark, Sweden, Belgium, France and the Netherlands, the need for no less than 2,000 specialized anaesthetists is calculated; but at the moment there are only about 90 specialized anaesthetists in Germany!

Further below the text continues:

> In the USA more than 8,000 specialized anaesthetists are practising. The USSR has recognized the necessity of anaesthesia training and in 1956 already developed a plan, according to which 1 specialized anaesthetist should be available for every 100 surgical beds. In North Rhine-Westphalia there is 1 active specialized anaesthetist per 3,500 surgical beds and in the Federal Republic of Germany there is 1 per 2,700 beds.

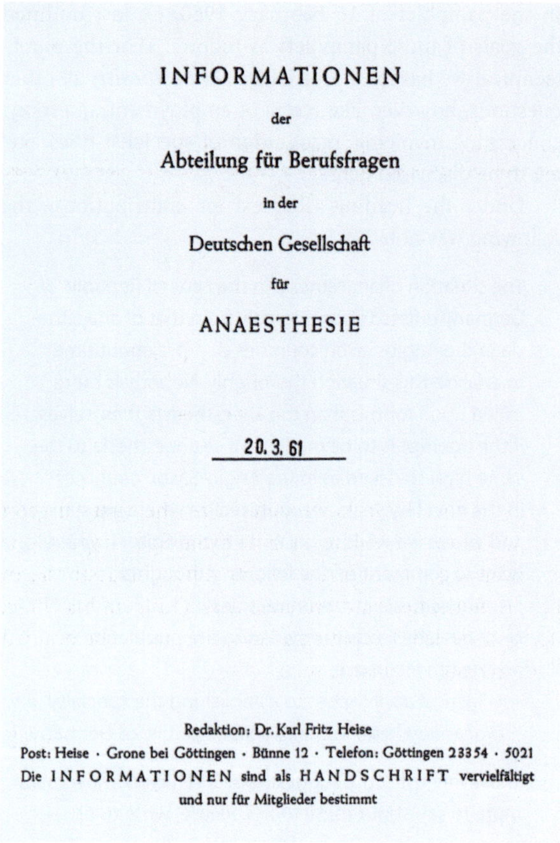

Fig. 1.50. Cover of the »Information of the Division of Professional Issues in the German Society of Anaesthesia«

In addition to the information pamphlets, a paper was published in March 1961 with the title »*Informations of the Division of Professional Issues in the German Society of Anaesthesia*« (◻ Fig. 1.50). Below the editorial data, the following note can be read: »**This information is reproduced as a manuscript and for members only**«.

This pamphlet was further developed and led to the creation in 1962 of a bulletin entitled *Informationen der Deutschen Gesellschaft für Anaesthesie und des Berufsverbandes Deutscher Anästhesisten*, which even then was greatly influenced by Charlotte Lehmann, Munich, who at that time was Second Secretary of the **Berufsverband Deutscher Anästhesisten (BDA)** which had been founded in 1961 [1].

What were anaesthetists informed about at that time? The *Informationen* contained forewords of the Presidents of the DGA, invitations to general meetings, statutes, vacancies, congress calendars, obituaries, press reports, minutes of general meetings (often the entire text), but also much about occupational law and policy, for example guidelines for leading anaesthetist positions in hospitals.

In 1964, K. Heise retired as Editor. W. Reichstein, who published the bulletin, became the new Editor. In 1965, the **Deutsche Gesellschaft für Anaesthesie** was renamed *the* **Deutsche Gesellschaft für Anaesthesie und Wiederbelebung** (DGAW). In 1968, C. Lehmann took over the Editorship.

Until 1970, the *Informationen* were largely filled with association news, professional law and policy. In April 1970, C. Lehmann told the readers:

> The reorganization of the *Anästhesiologische Informationen* [as the bulletin was now called (◻ Fig. 1.51)] makes it possible to include specialized articles and thus contribute to continuing medical education, whose support belongs to the tasks of the *Deutsche Gesellschaft für Anaesthesie und Wiederbelebung* and the *Berufsverband Deutscher Anästhesisten*, according to the statutes. These papers are not intended to compete with our scientific papers [...], but are designed to increase the anaesthetist's knowledge by reporting and describing practical experience. The main focus of the *Informationen* will also in future be on topics concerning professional policy, that is, on reports about the work inside the *Deutsche Gesellschaft für Anaesthesie und Wiederbelebung* and the *Berufsverband Deutscher Anästhesisten*.

In a foreword of the issue in July 1970, the Presidents of the DGAW and the BDA also stated their viewpoint as follows:

> Thanks to Dr. C. Lehmann's initiative, our *Informationen* appears in a new format, with a changed design and – with approval of both the DGAW's and BDA's Executive Committees – with a new extended title as *Anästhesiologische Informationen*. The purpose of changing the title was to have the journal included in the »Periodica Medica« and thus become a publication that can be both quoted and cited.

As could be seen in the following years, C. Lehmann succeeded, in co-operation with the Demeter-Verlag, in transforming the *Informationen* into a trade journal with an academic standard.

In 1973, C. Lehmann retired from the Editorship, which was now assigned to H. W. Opderbecke. In 1976, W. Henke joined the Editorial Committee as Assistant Editor. Two years later, E. Gebert took over this task. Starting with the issue in September 1978, the journal was renamed *Anästhesiologie und Intensivmedizin* (◻ Fig. 1.52). Two years later, E. Bock took over the function of Assistant Editor. In 1981, the so-called *Theme of the Month* was integrated into the part of the journal devoted to continuing medical education, and requested essays on various themes were presented under this heading.

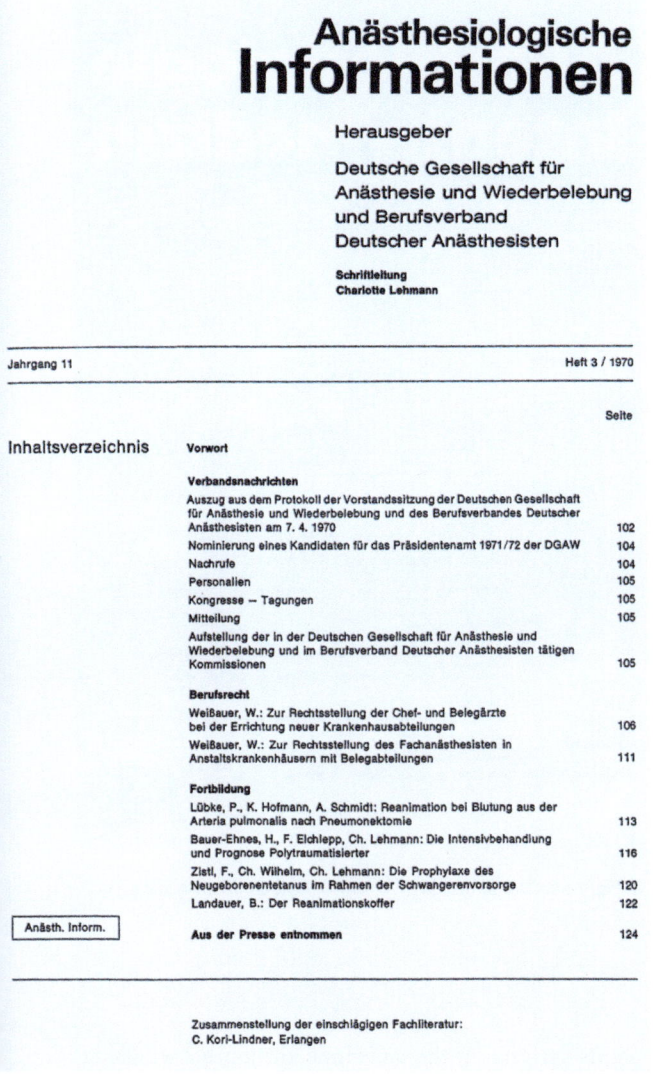

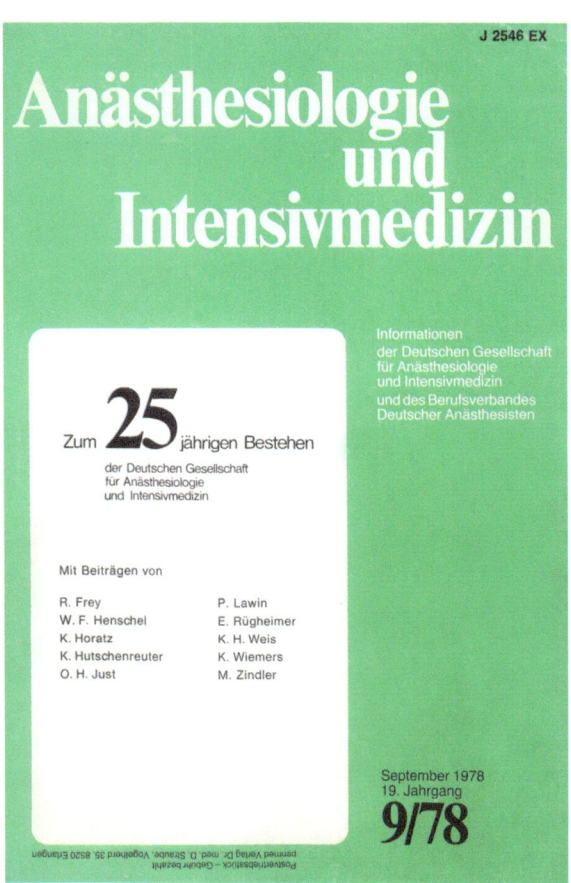

At the beginning of the 1984 volume, the **Deutsche Akademie für Anästhesiologische Fortbildung** signed on as the third group responsible for issuing the journal *Anästhesiologie und Intensivmedizin* in addition to the **Deutsche Gesellschaft für Anästhesiologie und Intensivmedizin** and the **Berufsverband Deutscher Anästhesisten**. At the same time, the Editorship was extended by one member for the section on continuing medical education (K. Peter), one for the section on law (W. Weißauer) and P. Schmucker (Assistant).

In 1985, P. Schmucker was replaced as Editorial Assistant by K. Taeger. From 1986 onwards, the table of contents had to be printed in two languages because the journal had been included in **Current Contents**. In 1987, E. Bock retired as General Editor because of a serious illness.

In 1992, the Editorship was regrouped so that K. Peter and K. Taeger took the responsibility for the continuing medical education part of the journal. In 1994, H. Sorgatz was integrated into the Editorship.

Beginning with issue 4 of the 1994 volume, B. Landauer took over the General Editorship from H.W. Opderbecke. On this occasion, Opderbecke commented under the heading: »On our own behalf« as follows:

In my eyes, the journal *Anästhesiologie und Intensivmedizin* represents the backbone of the association's policy work in our field. It is not only of service to continuing medical education of the members of our associations, but also serves as a forum for discussion of occupational law and policy questions from anaesthesiology's point of view. Beyond informing its circle of readers, it is an organ which can influence medico-legal and public health policy decisions [1].

In 1996, *Anästhesiologie & Intensivmedizin* changed from the Perimed to the Blackwell Publishing House, as evi-

A 2330

Anästhesiologie & Intensivmedizin

Offizielles Organ der Deutschen Gesellschaft für Anästhesiologie und Intensivmedizin, des Berufsverbandes Deutscher Anästhesisten und der Deutschen Akademie für Anästhesiologische Fortbildung

37. Jahrgang 1/96

Editorial

B. Landauer
In eigener Sache

A. Bedürftig
Wechsel des Verlages

Zum neuen Jahr

B. Landauer
„Der Anästhesist im Spannungsfeld zwischen Politik, Operateur und Patient"

Schmerztherapie

R. Sümpelmann, D. Schröder, S. Krohn, J.M. Strauß und J. Hausdörfer
Patientenkontrollierte Analgesie bei Kindern

Klinische Anästhesie

H. Unseld und B. Kähny
Prophylaxe von postoperativem Erbrechen durch Histamin-Rezeptorantagonisten

J. Martin, M. Meßelken, L. Cecconi, U. Hiltenmaier und P. Milewski
Der Aufwachraum
Eine prospektive Analyse der Prozeß- und Strukturqualität in der postoperativen Aufwachphase

Recht

H. W. Opderbecke und W. Weißauer
Grenzen der ärztlichen Behandlungspflicht bei irreversibler Bewußtlosigkeit
- zugleich ein Kommentar zum Urteil des 1. Strafsenats des BGH vom 13. September 1994 - 1 StR 357/94

GOÄ/BMÄ/E-GO – aktuell

H. Weigand
Zur 4. Verordnung zur Änderung der GOÄ

Blackwell Wissenschaft

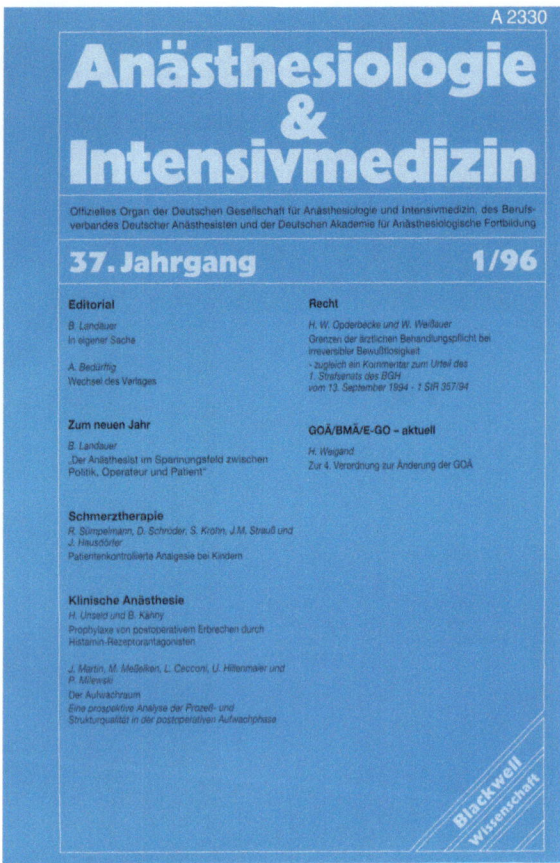

■ **Fig. 1.53.** First issue published by Blackwell

B 2330

Anästhesiologie & Intensivmedizin

CME-Zertifiziert

Offizielles Organ der Deutschen Gesellschaft für Anästhesiologie und Intensivmedizin, des Berufsverbandes Deutscher Anästhesisten und der Deutschen Akademie für Anästhesiologische Fortbildung. Organ der Deutschen Interdisziplinären Vereinigung für Intensiv- und Notfallmedizin

43. Jahrgang Januar 2002

EDITORIAL

B. Landauer
In eigener Sache

B. Landauer und A. Schleppers
Zum neuen Jahr: Die Bedeutung der Anästhesie innerhalb des German Refined DRG-Systems

KLINISCHE ANÄSTHESIE

U.-R. Jahn, A. Reich, H. Van Aken, I. Büche, R. Braun und E. Schäfer
Konzept zur Erstversorgung frakturierter oder luxierter Zähne während der Intubationsnarkose durch den Anästhesisten
Primary care of fractured or dislocated teeth during endotracheal anaesthesia by the anaesthetist

G. Wiesner, K. Schrögendorfer, K. Hörauf, P. Sobczynski, M. Harth, K. Taeger und H.-W. Rüdiger
Eine hohe Arbeitsplatzbelastung mit Inhalationsanästhetika ist mit einer vermehrten Bildung von Schwesterchromatidaustauschen assoziiert – Eine Untersuchung zur Gentoxizität von Inhalationsanästhetika
A high occupational exposure to inhaled anaesthetics is associated with an increased formation of sister chromatid exchanges – A study on the genotoxicity of inhaled anaesthetics

INTENSIVMEDIZIN

M. Krüger, R. Regenthal, R. Böhm, D. Lindner, H. Trauer und P. Caffier
Letale Diethylenglykol-Intoxikation nach mißbräuchlicher Anwendung von Goldgeist® forte – Ein Fallbericht
Fatal diethylene glycol intoxication after misuse of Goldgeist® forte – a case report

NOTFALLMEDIZIN

C. Janke, C. Denz, T. Bertsch, T. Luiz, K. Ellinger und H. Krieter
Effekte hypertoner-hyperonkotischer Infusionslösungen nach kardiopulmonaler Reanimation beim Schwein
Effects of hypertonic-hyperoncotic infusion solutions after cardiopulmonary resuscitation in the porcine model

I. Rummler und C.Uhl
Symptomlose Aspiration eines Zahnprothesenfragmentes nach Airbag-Entfaltung – Ein Fallbericht
Asymptomatic aspiration of a denture fragment after air bag deployment – a case report

RECHT

L. Figgener
Rechtliche Aspekte der zahnärztlichen/anästhesiologischen Minderjährigen-Behandlung

FORT- UND WEITERBILDUNG

S. Münte und H. A. Adams
Anästhesiologisches „Stand-by" und Analgosedierung (CME 1/02)
Monitored anaesthesia care and analgosedation (CME 1/02)

VERBANDSMITTEILUNGEN

Leitlinie zur Therapie der malignen Hyperthermie

DIOmed
http://www.diomed.de

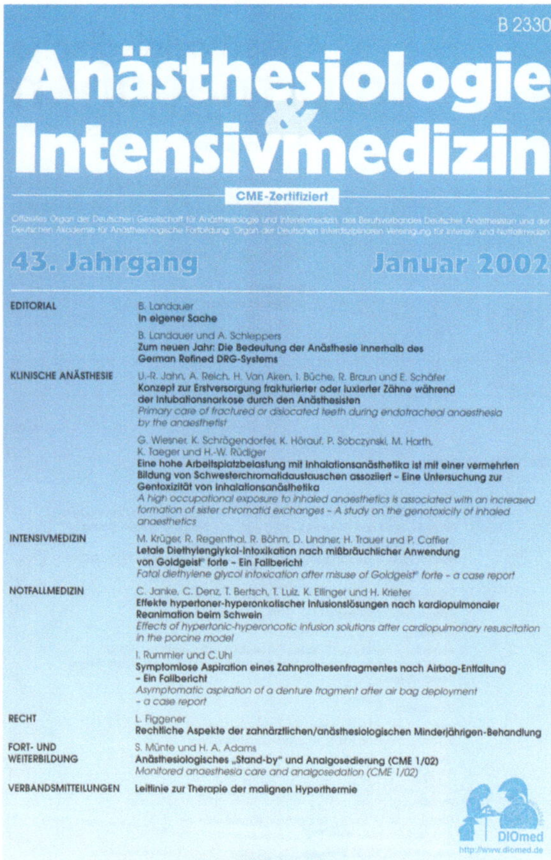

■ **Fig. 1.54.** Current design of *Anästhesiologie & Intensivmedizin*

denced by a new cover design and a change of the colour from green to blue (■ Fig. 1.53). In the same year, K. Peter retired from the Editorship, which was restructured. B. Landauer continued to be the General Editor, supported by K. van Ackern, K. Geiger, G. Hack, A. Hoeft, K. Taeger and W. Weißauer, and H. Sorgatz was the responsible Editor. In 1999, J. Radke was integrated into the Editorship. K. Taeger took charge of the Assistant General Editorship and became Editor-in-Chief in 2002. In 2006 this position was taken over by J. Schüttler.

In 1999, the abstracts of the academic working sessions of the DGAI in Würzburg were published in the journal for the first time, as well as the abstracts of the **Deutscher Anästhesiekongress** from 2000 onwards. Finally in 2002 a new section **Weiter- und Fortbildung** (Postgraduate and Continuing Medical Education) was included, which was supervised by the Deutsche Akademie für Anästhesiologische Fortbildung. It has been officially recognized by the Landesärztekammern (State Chambers of Physicans) as structured interactive training and enables the acquisition of a maximum of 10 CME points per year. At the same time, the journal was taken over by the publishing house DIOmed (■ Fig. 1.54).

In summary we can say that Lehmann and Opderbecke have fully succeeded in making ***Anästhesiologie & Intensivmedizin*** a respected journal with influence on medico-legal and public health developments, a source of information on professional law and policy questions, and a tool for continuing medical education.

Anästhesiologie & Intensivmedizin has the largest circulation among the anaesthesia journals published in the German language. It reaches all members of the DGAI and BDA and has a respectable impact factor. As Just already stated in1960, the active cooperation of the members of the DGAI, the BDA and the DAAF was the driving force behind the enduring success of the journal ***Anästhesiologie & Intensivmedizin***.

Reference

1. Opderbecke HW (1994) In eigener Sache. Anäesthesiol Intensivmed 35:51

1.4.3 History of the Journal *Anästhesiologie Intensivmedizin Notfallmedizin Schmerztherapie*

C. Krier

In the year 1966 a new journal named *Zeitschrift für Praktische Anästhesie und Wiederbelebung* (Practical Anesthesia and Resuscitation) was founded by O.H. Just, Chairman of the Department of Anaesthesiology at the University of Heidelberg (Germany). The journal was issued by Thieme Verlag in Stuttgart, Germany. The main goal of the Founding Editor was to contribute to qualified continuous education focusing on manuscripts dealing with daily anaesthesiological practice. In the following years the focus of the journal changed from mainly practical topics to more scientifically oriented contributions; as a consequence the name of the journal changed several times (Table 1.9).

Since 1991 the journal *Anästhesiologie Intensivmedizin Notfallmedizin Schmerztherapie (AINS)* has covered the four main special fields of anaesthesiology: anaesthesia care for surgical and diagnostic procedures, intensive care medicine, emergency medicine and pain therapy. *AINS* is indexed in Science Citation Index Extended, Index Medicus/MEDLINE and EMBASE/Excerpta Medica and its impact factor was 0.473 in 2003. In the beginning the circulation of the journal was 2,500 copies/year and reached a maximum of over 5,500 subscriptions in the mid-1990.

With full support of the publisher Dr. h.c. G. Hauff (1927–2001), owner of the Thieme Verlag Stuttgart, the first issue of the »blue journal« (the colour of the cover was and still is blue) was published in April 1966 (Fig. 1.55). Since the journal Der Anaesthesist had already begun publication in 1952 it has been a challenging story to publish another third scientific journal in Germany besides *Der Anaesthesist* and the journal *Anaesthesiologische Informationen* – a periodical initially dealing with professional issues. In 1952 O.H. Just, Heidelberg, was Founding Editor and Editor-in-Chief whereas H. Auberger, Cologne, and P. Lawin, Hamburg, and H. Lutz, Heidelberg, were Associate Editors of the new scientific periodical. The Editorial Board included renowned scientists such as A. Dönhardt, Hamburg, M. Gemperle, Geneva, W. Henschel, Bremen, K. Hutschenreuter, Homburg/Saar, H.W. Opderbecke, Nuremberg and E. Rügheimer, Erlangen. Horst Lutz died in 1987 and Horst Stoeckel became a member of the editorial staff in 1987, followed by Klaus Wiedemann, Heidelberg, and Claude Krier, Heidelberg (later Stuttgart). The Editorial Board was enlarged by K. van Ackern, J. Arndt, K. Geiger, J. Hildebrandt, F. Lackner, S. Schwarz, J. Schulte am Esch, P. Suter, J. Tarnow, D. Thomson and M. Zimpfer. The editorial team of the following years is shown in Table 1.10.

 Table 1.9. Title of the journal and number of issues/year

Year	Title	Number of issues/year
1966–1973	*Praktische Anästhesie und Wiederbelebung*	6
1974–1979	*Praktische Anästhesie, Wiederbelebung und Intensivtherapie*	6
1980–1990	*Anästhesiologie, Intensivtherapie, Notfallmedizin*	6
1991–present	*AINS Anästhesiologie Intensivmedizin Notfallmedizin Schmerztherapie*	8 (1991–1995) 10 (1996) 12 (1997–present)

ZEITSCHRIFT FÜR

Praktische Anästhesie und Wiederbelebung

Herausgeber:
O. H. Just, Heidelberg

Redaktion:
H. Auberger, Köln
P. Lawin, Hamburg
H. Lutz, Heidelberg

Wissenschaftlicher Beirat:
W. Becker, Bonn
W. Doerr, Heidelberg
A. Dönhardt, Hamburg
M. Gemperle, Genf
W. Henschel, Bremen
H. Hensel, Marburg
K. Hutschenreuter, Homburg
W. Jaeger, Heidelberg
W. Janssen, Heidelberg
R. Janzen, Hamburg
O. Käser, Frankfurt a. M.
K. Kremer, Essen

R. Kucher, Wien
G. Kuschinsky, Mainz
Ch. Lehmann, München
M. Meyer, Berlin
H. W. Opderbecke, Nürnberg
E. Rügheimer, Erlangen
K. F. Schlegel, Köln
K. Schuchardt, Hamburg
W. Spielmann, Frankfurt a. M.
P. Thurn, Bonn
A. Windorfer, Erlangen
E. Wollheim, Würzburg

1. Jahrgang

125 Abbildungen in 130 Einzeldarstellungen und 31 Tabellen

GEORG THIEME VERLAG · STUTTGART

 Fig. 1.55. Cover of the first issue of *Zeitschrift für Praktische Anästhesie und Wiederbelebung*

1

Table 1.10. Editorial Board of *AINS* from 1996 to 2003

Year	Editors	Co-Editors
1966	O.H. Just	H. Auberger, P. Lawin, H. Lutz
1987	O.H. Just	P. Lawin, H. Stoeckel, K. Wiedemann
1988	O.H. Just	P. Lawin, J. Schulte am Esch, H. Stoeckel, K. Wiedemann
1990	O.H. Just	C. Krier, R. Larsen, P. Lawin, J. Schulte am Esch, H. Stoeckel
1991	P. Lawin, H. Stoeckel	G. Hempelmann, C. Krier, R. Larsen, J. Schulte am Esch
1994	P. Lawin, H. Stoeckel, C. Krier	K. van Ackern, K. Geiger, M. Georgieff, G. Hempelmann, E. Kochs, R. Larsen, E. Martin, J. Schulte am Esch
1995	G. Hempelmann, J. Schulte am Esch, C. Krier	K. van Ackern, W. Buzello, K. Geiger, M. Georgieff, A. Hoeft, E. Kochs, R. Larsen, E. Martin, K. Reinhart, N. Roewer, P. Schmucker, M. Wendt
1996	G. Hempelmann, J. Schulte am Esch, C. Krier	K. van Ackern, W. Buzello, K. Geiger, M. Georgieff, A.F. Hammerle, A. Hoeft, E. Kochs, R. Larsen, E. Martin, K. Reinhart, N. Roewer, Würzburg, P. Schmucker, M. Wendt, M. Zimpfer
1997	G. Hempelmann, J. Schulte am Esch, C. Krier	K. van Ackern, D.M. Albrecht, W. Buzello, K. Geiger, M. Georgieff, A.F. Hammerle, A. Hoeft, E. Kochs, J. Peters, R. Larsen, E. Martin, K. Reinhart, N. Roewer, P. Schmucker, J. Tarnow, M. Wendt, M. Zimpfer
1998	G. Hempelmann, J. Schulte am Esch, C. Krier	K. van Ackern, W. Buzello, S. Fitzal, K. Geiger, M. Georgieff, A.F. Hammerle, A. Hoeft, E. Kochs, K.H. Lindner, T. Pasch, J. Peters, E. Martin, K. Reinhart, N. Roewer, P. Schmucker, J. Tarnow, M. Wendt, M. Zimpfer
1999	G. Hempelmann, J. Schulte am Esch, C. Krier	K. van Ackern, W. Buzello, S. Fitzal, K. Geiger, M. Georgieff, A.F. Hammerle, A. Hoeft, E. Kochs, K.H. Lindner, E. Martin, T. Pasch, J. Peters, K. Reinhart, N. Roewer, P. Schmucker, J. Tarnow, M. Wendt, M. Zimpfer
2000	G. Hempelmann, J. Schulte am Esch, C. Krier	K. van Ackern, D. Balogh, W. Buzello, S. Fitzal, K. Geiger, M. Georgieff, A. Hoeft, Bonn, E. Kochs, G. Nöldge-Schomburg, T. Pasch, J. Peters, K. Reinhart, N. Roewer, P. Schmucker, J. Scholz, J. Tarnow, M. Wendt, M. Zimpfer
2001	G. Hempelmann, J. Schulte am Esch, C. Krier	K. van Ackern, D. Balogh, W. Buzello, S. Fitzal, K. Geiger, M. Georgieff, A. Hoeft, E. Kochs, G. Nöldge-Schomburg, T. Pasch, J. Peters, K. Reinhart, N. Roewer, P. Schmucker, J. Scholz, J. Tarnow, M. Zimpfer
2002	G. Hempelmann, J. Schulte am Esch, C. Krier, H.A. Adams	K. van Ackern, D. Balogh, W. Buzello, S. Fitzal, K. Geiger, M. Georgieff, T. Hachenberg, A. Hoeft, E. Kochs, W.J. Kox, M. Leuwer, W. List, G. Nöldge-Schomburg, T. Pasch, J. Peters, S. Piepenbrock, K. Reinhart, N. Roewer, P. Schmucker, J. Scholz, J. Schüttler, J. Tarnow, K. Ulsenheimer, H. Van Aken, H. Wulf, R. Zander, M. Zimpfer
2008	T. Hachenberg, C. Krier, N. Roewer, J. Scholz, C. Spies, H. Van Aken, H. Wulf	E. Biermann, J. Biscoping, J. Boldt, H. Bürkle, W. Buzello, B. Dirks, K. Ellinger, M. Fischer, H. Gervais, H. Groeben, M.K. Herbert, K.P. Ittner, M. Leuwer, C. Madler, I. Nachtigall, G. Pauser, M. Schäfer, U. Schwemmer, T. Standl, R. Sümpelmann, M. Tryba, K. Ulsenheimer, F. Wappler, E. Weis, K. Wiedemann, M. Zimpfer

In 1990 O.H. Just became Emeritus at the University of Heidelberg and adhering to a general rule of the publishing house Thieme he left the Editorial Board of *AINS* at the end of his active duty in the Department of Anaesthesiology in Heidelberg. Peter Lawin and Horst Stoeckel took over the Editor-in-Chief positions (1991–1994), assisted by Claude Krier and later by Hans-Anton Adams, Hannover. During this period of time the name and the structural design of the journal were totally changed and remodelled. In addition to the section containing original articles, which represent the core of a scientific journal, different sections with specific focus on continuing education were introduced to improve the acceptance of the readers. General articles covering the neighbouring disciplines of internal and surgical medicine, congress reports, case reports, mini-symposia and pro and contra contribu-

tions were included and special issues with a well-defined topic were published. Close co-operation with the Austrian scientific community was established and several Austrian authors assumed Editorial Board positions.

In 1994 Gunter Hempelmann, Giessen, Jochen Schulte am Esch, Hamburg, and Claude Krier, Stuttgart, took charge of the journal as Editors-in-Chief, assisted by H.-A. Adams, who joined the team of Editors-in-Chief in 2002. Again new sections were included and electronic publishing was continuously developed. Since 1999 abstracts in English and German can be accessed at the homepage of the journal (http:/www.thieme.de/ains). In summary the goal of *AINS* is to provide up-to-date and peer-reviewed information on new scientific developments in all fields of interest of anaesthesiology and to actively contribute to high-level continuing education of anaesthesia practioners as well. Along the same lines, between 1999 and 2002 with the support of Thieme Verlag, Stuttgart, G. Hempelman, J. Schulte am Esch and C. Krier issued a **Textbook of Anesthesiology** in four volumes: **Anaesthesiology** (Editors: E. Kochs, C. Krier, W. Buzello, H.-A. Adams; 2nd edn. 2008), **Intensive Care Medicine** (Editors: H. Van Aken, K. Reinhart, M. Zimpfer; 2nd edn. 2006), **Emergency Medicine** (Editors: G. Hempelmann, H.-A. Adams, P. Sefrin; 2nd edn. 2007) and **Pain Medicine** (Editors: H. Beck, E. Martin, J. Motsch, J. Schulte am Esch).

1.4.4 History of the Journal *Anaesthesiologie und Reanimation*

G. Benad

The emergence of the journal *Anaesthesiologie und Reanimation (A & R)* reflects in particular the difficulties of East German anaesthetists who wanted to publish the results of their scientific work [8]. Between 1950 and 1960, East German anaesthetists could still publish papers in journals of West Germany and other »Western« European or non-European countries. However, after the German Democratic Republic built the wall between East und West Germany in 1961, the political pressure on professors, assistants and students was increased by the *Sozialistische Einheitspartei Deutschlands* (SED) mainly by the restrictions of the »Third Reform of the Universities of the German Democratic Republic« [3], which, for instance, led to the constitution of so-called *Departments of International Relations (DIR)* at all universities of the German Democratic Republic, which controlled all international correspondence including that between East and West Germany. All incoming letters were opened by the DIR before reaching their recipients and outgoing letters had first to be presented unsealed to the DIR, which then decided to post or withhold them. Due to these regulations, publications in »Western« anaesthesiological journals were nearly impossible. Only in exceptional cases and after a special application had been made could the »Deputy Rector of Medicine« allow the submission of a paper to a »Western« journal.

Due to this situation, East German anaesthetists were forced to publish their papers on special anaesthesiological problems in surgery or gynaecology in the *Zentralblatt für Chirurgie or Zentralblatt für Gynaekologie*, two traditional German medical journals, published by Ambrosius Barth/Leipzig, since their foundation in the nineteenth century. Besides these two well-established journals, which were also highly regarded in other countries, there were four other medical journals founded in the German Democratic Republic: *Zeitschrift für die gesamte Innere Medizin, Deutsches Gesundheitswesen, Zeitschrift für ärztliche Fortbildung* and *medicamentum*. However,

there was no special journal for anaesthesiology, intensive care medicine, emergency medicine or pain therapy in the German Democratic Republic before 1976. This situation was not only difficult for anaesthetists who wanted to publish their papers in anaesthesiological journals, but was also disadvantageous for the further development of anaesthesiology as an independent medical field in the German Democratic Republic. In order not to interfere in this process that was just beginning, I even rejected a proposal made in 1973 by the Editor-in-Chief of the *Zentralblatt für Chirurgie*, W. Schmitt/Rostock, to devote 2 of the 52 annual issues of this journal to publishing only anaesthesiological papers [26, 27].

Rejecting this proposal, the Executive Committee of the **Society of Anaesthesiology and Reanimation** of the German Democratic Republic (SAR) decided in 1973 to found its own anaesthesiological journal and engaged its President, G. Benad/Rostock, to apply to the »General Secretariat of the Medico-Scientific Societies at the Ministry of Health of the German Democratic Republic«, simply abbreviated as »GS«, for the foundation of a »Journal for Anaesthesiology, Intensive Therapy and Urgent Medical Aid«. However, the President of the East German Society of Internal Medicine, G. Klumbies/Jena [16], did not agree to this title, because his specialty also covered intensive therapy. Therefore, we applied for a journal with the same name as the society *Anaesthesiologie und Reanimation (A & R)*, but we added the subtitle *Journal for Anaesthesiology, Intensive Therapy and Urgent Medical Aid*, which he finally accepted. One year later, the Director of the »GS«, L. Rohland [23], informed us that the application of the SAR for its own journal had not only been confirmed by the Minister of Health, but also by the »Secretariat of the Central Committee of the SED«. It lasted another 1 ¼ years until a printer (Magnus Poser/Jena) with free printing capacity and a sufficient amount of printing paper was found and the lists of the Editorial Board and the Advisory Board, which were proposed by the Executive Committee of the SAR, were eventually confirmed by the Director of the »GS«, L. Rohland, after agreement with the Secretary of the SED group of the SAR (◘ Table 1.11) [2, 5].

After all questions relating to work and to personnel matters had been solved within 2 years, the members of the SAR were informed in an open letter published in the »Information of the SAR« number II/1975 [4] that in January 1976 the SAR would publish its own journal *Anaesthesiologie und Reanimation – Zeitschrift für Anaesthesie, Intensivtherapie und Dringliche Medizinische Hilfe* (Anaesthesiology and Resuscitation – Journal for Anaesthesiology, Intensive Therapy and First Medical Aid), consisting of four issues per year.

The first issue of *A & R* (◘ Fig. 1.56) contained prefaces from L. Mecklinger/Berlin [19], at that time Minister of Health of the German Democratic Republic, O. Mayrhofer/

□ **Table 1.11.** Composition of the Editorial Board and the Advisory Board of *A & R*

Editorial Board:

Editor-in-Chief: G. Benad/Rostock
Editorial Secretary: K. Borchert/Rostock
Members of the Editorial Board:
H. Bekemeier/Halle/Saale (pharmacologist), G. Felsch/Jena (internist), M. Meyer/Berlin (anaesthetist), H. Röding/Potsdam (surgeon), M. Schädlich/Berlin (anaesthetist), Inge Schneider/Berlin (anaesthetist), U. Strahl/Berlin (anaesthetist), H. Winkler/Jena (anaesthetist) and H. Wilken/Wismar (gynaecologist)

Advisory Board:

W. Bethmann/Leipzig (orofacial surgeon), A. Bunatian/Moscow (anaesthetist), T.M. Darbinyan/Moscow (anaesthetist), J. Frenzel/Jena (paediatrician), H. Friedel/Lostau (pulmonologist), T. Jakab/Budapest (anaesthetist), W. Jurczyk/Poznan (anaesthetist), H. Klinkmann/Rostock (nephrologist), K.-E. Krüger/Halle/Saale (ophthalmologist), M. Mebel/Berlin (urologist), H.-G. Niebeling/Leipzig (neurosurgeon), J. Pocta/Prague (anaesthetist), W. Reimann/Dresden (forensic physician), J. Roewer/Rostock (transfusion expert), S.K. Saev/Sofia (anaesthetist), V. Sinz/Dresden (pathophysiologist), W. Tischer/Greifswald (paediatric surgeon), J. Wilke/Erfurt (ENT surgeon)

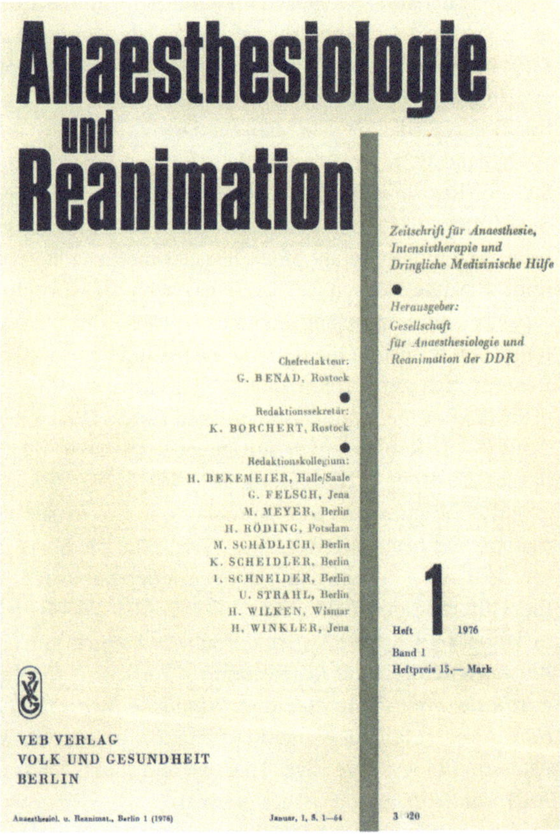

□ **Fig. 1.56.** Cover of the first issue of *Anaesthesiologie und Reanimation*, Vol. 1, issue 1, 1976

Vienna [18], at that time President of the WFSA and W. Röse/Magdeburg, at that time President of the SAR, and the Editor-in-Chief, G. Benad/Rostock [24].

The journal was soon accepted by a great number of East German anaesthetists, but also by anaesthetists from the so-called socialist countries and in some cases also by anaesthetists from the so-called non-socialist countries, such as West Germany and other Western European and non-European countries, who offered papers for publishing on anaesthesiology, intensive care medicine, medical first aid and in some cases also on pain therapy. The number of authors from non-socialist countries accounted for 33% in 1989 [21].

In 1976, the number of copies of this journal amounted to 1,200 and it was mainly subscribed to by anaesthetists of the German Democratic Republic (946 subscribers) and by a few anaesthetists from the non-socialist countries (34 subscribers) and socialist countries (32 subscribers). Over the years, the number of copies had to be increased to 1,600 because there was a further rise in the number of subscribers. In 1989, there were 1,190 subscribers in the German Democratic Republic, 301 in East European countries and 51 in West European countries [21]. The relatively large number of subscribers from East European countries was due to their difficulties in publication and information, which were very similar to those in East Germany, and it was very advantageous that they could pay for A & R in their national currencies.

A & R also received attention in West European countries. In 1978 Foëx [14] published a review on *A & R* in *Anaesthesia* and concluded that »The journal is well presented and makes one more aware of the quality of research carried out in East Germany«. Summaries of papers published in A & R were published in Excerpta Medica–Anesthesiology soon after the foundation of *A & R* and from 1986 on it was also indexed in Index Medicus and MEDLINE [22].

The existence of our own journal also gave us the advantage of being able to ask mainly West German and West European publishers for new editions of various textbooks on anaesthesiology, intensive care medicine, emergency medicine and pain therapy to review them in *A & R*. The reviewers thus had access to modern scientific books, which were often not available even in our libraries because of the chronic shortage of hard currencies in the German Democratic Republic.

With the help of the publishers from West Germany and other Western countries we also organized an exchange of *A & R* with other anaesthesiological journals, such as *Der Anaesthesist, Anästhesiologie & Intensivmedizin, Anästhesiologie • Intensivmedizin • Notfallmedizin • Schmerztherapie (AINS), anaesthesiologische praxis, Acta Anaesthesiologica Belgica, Acta Anaesthesiologica Scandinavica, Anaesthesia and Intensive Care, Anes-*

thesiology, Anesthesia and Analgesia, British Journal of Anaesthesia, Cahiers d'Anesthésiologie and Canadian Anaesthetists' Society Journal. The exchange with »Western« journals was combined with unbelievable difficulties because sometimes the East German customs officials confiscated these journals. Instead of the expected journal, we got only a record of its confiscation. I remember a particularly incomprehensible case, in which an issue of *anästhesiologische praxis* was confiscated, even though I was a member of the Editorial Board of this journal [11]. I objected to this decision and eventually I got the issue, but only a few weeks later.

There were other problems which were typical of the political system of the German Democratic Republic. On one occasion the printers had difficulties in obtaining good paper and had to print one issue on low-quality paper. Only due to my objections and comments on the negative effects of such a loss of quality on the international development of the number of subscribers to the journal was the next issue printed again on high-quality paper [6].

Because of the steadily increasing number of good manuscripts accepted for publishing, we asked the publisher for an extension of the journal from four to six issues per year in 1977. Given the stringent supply of paper [20], however, the »GS« allowed the extension of *A & R* only 4 years later.

On special political occasions, such as the 100th birthday of the first President of the German Democratic Republic, Wilhelm Pieck, the 9th Party Congress of the SED or the 30th anniversary of the foundation of the German Democratic Republic [12], all Editors-in-Chief of East German medical journals were obliged by the »Coordination Council of Medico-Scientific Societies of the German Democratic Republic« and by the »GS« [28] to publish special political contributions. Some Editors-in-Chief, for instance, the Editor of the journal Das Deutsche Gesundheitswesen, W. Schmincke [25], fulfilled this demand. A & R never published such a special political contribution. On the country's 30th anniversary, we got out of it by publishing an article by the President of the SAR U. Strahl on a politically neutral subject: »The development of anaesthesiology in the German Democratic Republic« [29].

The political changes in 1989 led to new conditions for editorial work. The former nationally owned publisher *VEB Verlag Volk und Gesundheit/Berlin* was changed into a private publishing house *Verlag Gesundheit GmbH/Berlin*, but it adapted its working style to the conditions of the free market economy relatively slowly. Thus, the Editor-in-Chief himself had to obtain advertisements from pharmaceutical and medical firms for publishing in the journal [7].

In Dresden in February 1990, at the last Congress of the East German Society, the name of which had been changed since 1981 from Society of Anaesthesiology and Reanimation of the German Democratic Republic (SAR) to Society of Anaesthesiology and Intensive Therapy of the German Democratic Republic (GAIT) [10], the unification process of East and West German anaesthetists began. The last official meeting between East and West German anaesthetists had taken place in Berlin in 1964 [17] and since then no official contacts between the East and West German societies had taken place, although personal contacts between anaesthetists from East and West Germany were never interrupted during the 26 years of separation. At this congress in Dresden in February 1990, a first official meeting of the Presidents and members of the Executive Committee of the two German societies, the GAIT and the German Society of Anaesthesiology and Intensive Care Medicine (DGAI) took place and the official statement culminated in the Presidents' closing remarks that »in the foreseeable future an amalgamation into a joint German society will take place« [15]. After dissolution of the »GAIT« on 23 October 1990 and the reuniting of all German anaesthetists in the »DGAI«, the journal *A & R* became an organ of the »DGAI« on 1 January 1991 [13].

After the publisher *Verlag Gesundheit GmbH/Berlin* was dissolved in 1992, *A & R* was published by *Selecta Verlagsgesellschaft mbH/Munich–Wiesbaden* until 1999 and thereafter by Medical Tribune/Wiesbaden until 2003. On 1 January 2004, *A & R* was bought by Georg Thieme Verlag/Stuttgart, but they published only issues 1–3 of the 29th volume in its original form. As Georg Thieme Verlag/Stuttgart has been publishing another anaesthesiological journal *Anästhesiologie · Intensivmedizin · Notfallmedizin · Schmerztherapie (AINS)* since 1966, the profile of which corresponds completely to that of *A & R*, the publisher decided to amalgamate these two journals on 1 July 2004 [1]. Thus, *Anaesthesiologie und Reanimation (A & R)* came to an end in the original form in which it was published for nearly 30 years, but its name still existed as the subtitle of *AINS*, which has been named *Anästhesiologie · Intensivmedizin · Notfallmedizin · Schmerztherapie– Vereinigt mit Anaesthesiologie und Reanimation* since the amalgamation of these two journals on 1 July 2004 [9]. This subtitle of AINS existed until April 2006.

References

1. Adams HA, Hempelmann G, Krier C, Schulte am Esch J (2004) Editorial in eigener Sache – zur Vereinigung von »ains« mit »A & R«. Anästhesiol Intensivmed Notfallmed Schmerzther 39:455
2. Benad G (1973) Letter to Dr. L. Rohland, Director of the »General Secretariat (GS) of Medico-Scientific Societies at the Ministry of Health of the GDR«, 3 July 1973, referring to the commitment of the GS, that both the president of the »Society of Anaesthesiology and Reanimation of the GDR« (SAR) and the secretary of the »SED group« of the SAR have to present separate lists with proposals for the composition of the Editorial Board of the journal Anaesthesiologie und Reanimation (A & R)

3. Benad G (1998) Effect of reunification on anaesthesiology in former East Germany. European Academy of Anaesthesiology, Newsletter No. 9: 4–5

4. Benad G (1975) Letter to the members of the SAR on the foundation of the journal *Anaesthesiologie und Reanimation*. Mitteilungsblatt der »Gesellschaft für Anaesthesiologie und Reanimation der DDR«, No. II: 6–7

5. Benad G (1985) Letter of the Editor-in-Chief of the journal *A & R* to the GS referring to the extension of the scientific board of *A & R*, 2 January 1985

6. Benad G (1989) Letter of the Editor-in-Chief of the journal *A & R* to Dr. R. Künzel, head of the publisher »VEB Volk und Gesundheit/Berlin« regarding the low paper quality of issue number 3/1989 of *A & R* and the resulting negative effects on the development of subscribers mainly from abroad, 30 October 1989

7. Benad G (1990) Circular of the Editor-in-Chief to the pharmaceutical and medical firms asking for advertisements in the journal *A & R*, 19 February 1990

8. Benad G (2000) 25 Jahre »Anaesthesiologie und Reanimation« – Ein historischer Rückblick. Anaesthesiol Reanim 26:4–11

9. Benad G (2004) Editorial – Vereinigung der Zeitschriften »A & R« und »AINS«. Anaesthesiol Reanim 29:62–63

10. Benad G, Röse W (1999) Strukturelle Entwicklung der Intensivmedizin in der früheren DDR. Anaesthesist 48:251–262

11. Confiscation by the customs of the GDR, Schwerin, 7 May 1973, no. B 171665

12. Coordination Council of the Medico-Scientific Societies of the GDR (1978) Conception of the medico-scientific societies for the preparation of the 30th anniversary of the foundation of the GDR

13. Fischer K, Benad G (1991) Zum Geleit: Die Zeitschrift »Anaesthesiologie und Reanimation« erscheint ab 1. Januar 1991 als Organ der Deutschen Gesellschaft für Anästhesiologie und Intensivmedizin. Anaesthesiol Reanim 15:2–3

14. Foëx P (1978) Book review: »Anaesthesiologie und Reanimation«. Anaesthesia 33:850–851

15. Hache H, Fischer K (1990) Gemeinsame Erklärung der »Deutschen Gesellschaft für Anästhesiologie und Intensivmedizin« und der »Gesellschaft für Anaesthesiologie und Intensivtherapie der DDR«. Anaesthesiol Reanim 15:137.

16. Klumbies G (1974) Letter of the President of the »Society of Internal Medicine of the GDR« to the President of the »Society of Anaesthesiology and Reanimation of the GDR«, Prof. Dr. G. Benad, objecting to the proposed naming of the journal »Anaesthesiologie und Reanimation«, 17 January 1974

17. Lehmann C (1964) Bericht über die Gründungsversammlung der »Sektion Anaesthesiologie« der »Deutschen Gesellschaft für Klinische Medizin« am 7. März 1961 in Berlin. Anaesthesist 13:395–396

18. Mayrhofer O (1976) Grußwort des Präsidenten des »Weltbundes der Anästhesiegesellschaften«. Anaesthesiol Reanim 1:4.

19. Mecklinger L (1976): Zum Geleit. Anaesthesiol Reanim 1:3.

20. Minutes of the meeting of the Editorial Board of the journal *Anaesthesiologie und Reanimation* analysing the problem of reduced paper capacity, Berlin, 2 November 1977

21. Minutes of the meeting of the Editorial Board of the journal *Anaesthesiologie und Reanimation* analysing the origin of authors and the development of subscribers. Berlin, 13 December 1989

22. Rada R (1986) Letter of the Editor of Index Medicus, Department of Health & Human Services of the National Institutes of Health and National Library of Medicine, Bethesda/MD/USA to the Editor-in-Chief of the journal *Anaesthesiologie und Reanimation*, Dr. G. Benad, Rostock, regarding the admission of *Anaesthesiologie und Reanimation* in *Index Medicus* and *MEDLINE*, 23 May 1986

23. Rohland L (1974) Letter of the Director of the »General Secretariat (GS) of the Medico-scientific Societies at the Ministry of Health of the GDR« to the President of the »Society of Anaesthesiology and Reanimation of the GDR«, Prof. Dr. G. Benad, confirming the foundation of the journal *Anaesthesiologie und Reanimation*, 8 October 1974

24. Röse W, Benad G (1976) Anaesthesiol Reanim 1:5.

25. Schmincke W (1976) Wilhelm Pieck – Sohn und Führer der Arbeiterklasse, Präsident der Deutschen Demokratischen Republik. Dtsch Gesundheitswes 31:1–2

26. Schmitt W (1972) Editorial anlässlich der Übernahme der Chefredaktion des »Zentralblattes für Chirurgie« durch Prof. Dr. W. Schmitt, Rostock. Zentralbl Chir 97:2.

27. Schmitt W (1973) Personal information of Prof. Dr. G. Benad regarding the offer of two issues per year containing anaesthesiological publications in the weekly journal »Zentralblatt für Chirurgie«

28. Stiebritz (1976) Circular of the Director of the »General Secretariat (GS) of the Medico-Scientific Societies at the Ministry of Health of the GDR« regarding a medical field-related analysis of the resolutions and documents of the 9th Party Congress of the SED in medical journals of the GDR, 1 December 1976

29. Strahl U (1979) Die Entwicklung der Anästhesiologie in der Deutschen Demokratischen Republik. Anaesthesiol Reanim 4:131–134

1.5 The Horst Stoeckel Museum for the History of Anaesthesia in Bonn

H. Stoeckel

»Whoever does not know the past, will not get a grip on the future« (Golo Mann)

»The beautiful dream of removing pain has become reality«. Anaesthesia was discovered in Boston in 1846 and shortly thereafter the famous Berlin surgeon J.F. Dieffenbach used these poetic words in the same year that the first ether anaesthetic was administered by Heyfelder in Erlangen on 24 January 1847. That same day the Leipzig dentists, H.E. Weickert and C.F.E. Obenaus, carried out a tooth extraction under ether anaesthetic, although this was reported only in a short press item. At last surgeons could perform pain-free operations. Up until that time surgery was almost comparable to torture. True, in previous centuries there had been anaesthetic methods such as the so-called sleep sponges, which were soaked with anaesthetic substances; their effect however was inadequate.

Following the American H. Wells' failed experiment using laughing gas as an anaesthetic in 1845 and his countryman C.W. Long's ether anaesthesia in 1842 (published only in 1849), the first successful demonstration of anaesthesia was carried out on 16 October 1846 by W.T.G. Morton in Boston, MA (◻ Fig. 1.57). This event enabled operative medicine to move from its early stage of development to the modern age of anaesthesia-assisted surgical procedures. This date stands today as the »birth date« of anaesthesia. At that time surgery's two scourges were operative pain and life-threatening wound infection. Anaesthesia conquered the first and news of its discovery spread in a very short time throughout the civilized world.

Almost 150 years later, on 7 October 2000, the Horst Stoeckel Museum for the History of Anaesthesia was opened in Bonn (◻ Fig. 1.58). The museum and at-

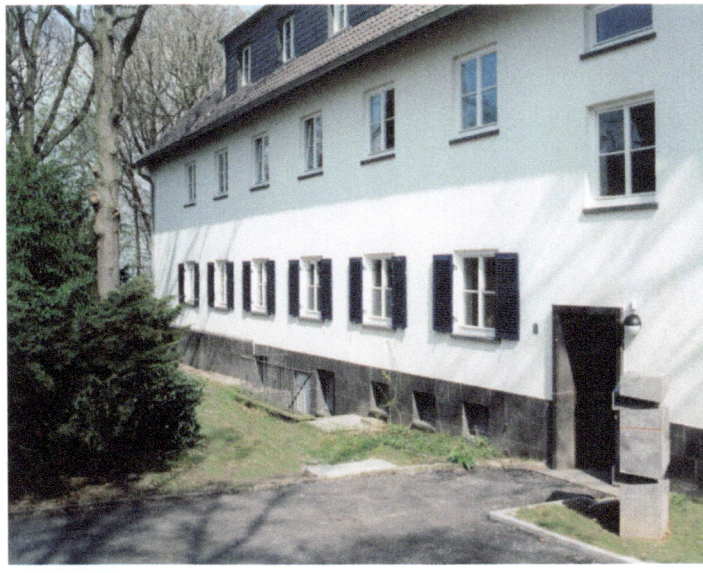

◻ **Fig. 1.58.** The Museum in the University Hospital on the Venusberg

tached library were created from the private collection of H. Stoeckel, retired Professor of Anaesthesiology, and a larger number of exhibits, books and publications donated and loaned in the last several years by about 150 German anaesthetists and industrial firms. During a ceremony attended by representatives of international museums for the history of medicine and anaesthesia, the museum was presented to the Friedrich-Wilhelms University in Bonn. The University had made the 500 m² area available and borne the costs of considerable reconstruction and renovation. The museum's permanent exhibition and library cover the time from the first successful demonstration of ether anaesthesia in 1846 up to the year 2008, the 55th anniversary of the foundation of the German Society of Anaesthesiology and Intensive Care Medicine (originally the German Society of Anaesthesia).

What sparked the idea of creating an anaesthesia museum in Bonn?

In 1994, about 1.5 years before his retirement, its initiator and founder, always interested in the history of anaesthesia, was presented with two anaesthesia artefacts from the pioneer period on the occasion of the dedication of a new hospital building. It was this gift that provided the original spark: if such almost 100-year-old »trophies« could be obtained »at one go«, then it should be possible to create an entire museum. Other plans for the forthcoming retirement were abandoned and an intensive and successful search for apparatus, drugs, books and publications was launched.

Now, more than 10 years after opening, the museum has become well known both in Germany and abroad, particularly amongst specialists, but also amongst the general public, to which the number of visitors can attest.

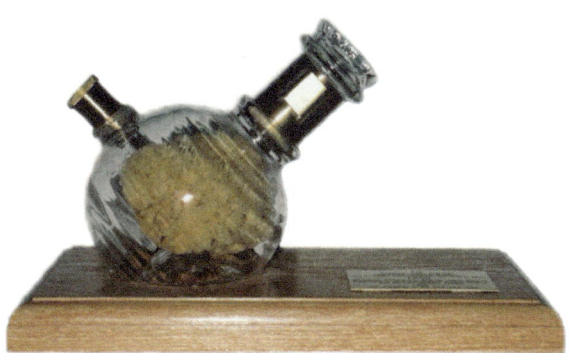

◻ **Fig. 1.57.** The Boston Glass Ball, the apparatus with which the first successful demonstration of ether anaesthetic was carried out in 1846 (replica)

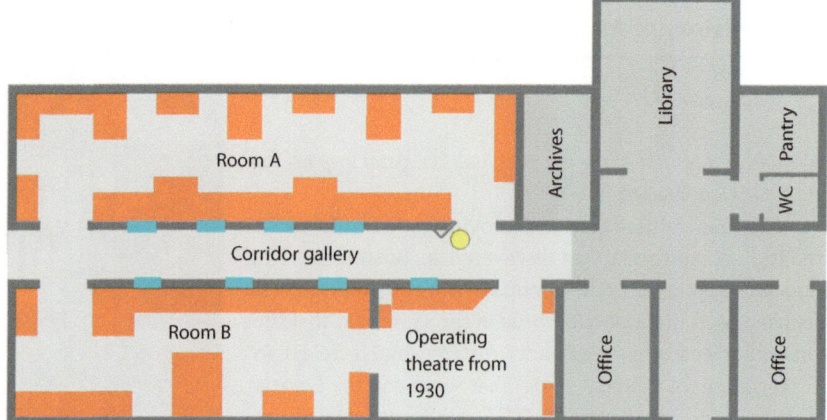

◼ **Fig. 1.59.** Plan of the Horst Stoeckel Museum

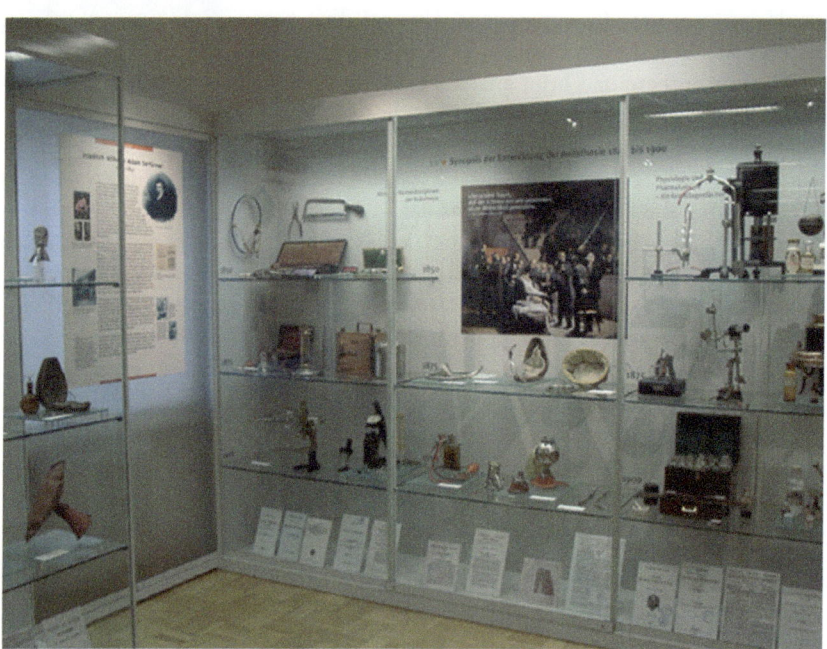

◼ **Fig. 1.60.** View of the exhibits

According to the published comment of a well-known historian of anaesthesia on occasion of its 10th anniversary the museum can be counted amongst the international »big four«.

A vital prerequisite for its success was the committed collaboration of a group of friends and patrons, beginning with the architect, the expert designer, the skilled precision mechanic and the secretary proficient in both multiple modern media and management of the library and the Society of Patrons. Most prominent however is the commitment of the 150 donors and sponsors who ensure continual financial support, in particular the **German Society of Anaesthesiology and Intensive Care Medicine** and the **Professional Association of German Anaesthetists**.

The exhibition is accommodated in the former house for nursing staff transformed by a specially created corporate design. The primary areas of anaesthesia and resuscitation techniques as well as of intensive care medicine are displayed in an instructive manner (◼ Fig. 1.59). A highlight of the 280 m² exhibition area, which particularly impresses visitors, is the complete and authentically equipped operating theatre from 1930. Thirty-six display cases, each devoted to a single main theme, contain more than 850 exhibits. Anaesthesia apparatus – primarily originals – from the nineteenth and early twentieth centuries in Germany is well represented and supported by examples from the UK, the USA, France and other European countries.

The tour begins with a special feature: a large display case containing three horizontal levels, each divided into

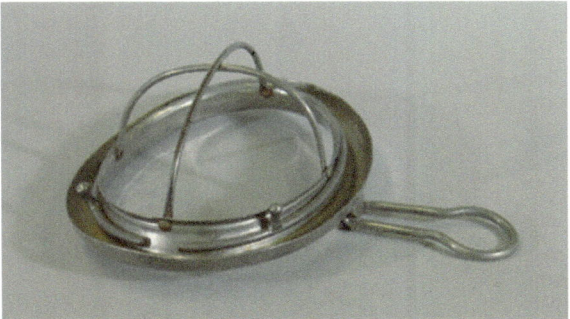

Fig. 1.61. The internationally known mask for ether drip anaesthesia developed in 1890 by Curt Schimmelbusch in Berlin

three vertical sections. Presenting a synopsis of the development of anaesthesia, each horizontal level presents a 25-year period beginning in 1850, 1875 and 1900, respectively. The three vertical sections show the interaction of anaesthesia with its clinical partners and with the basic sciences of pharmacology and physiology (■ Fig. 1.60).

One of the two large rooms is devoted exclusively to the development of inhalation anaesthesia. The variety of exhibits ranges from the first portable anaesthesia glass apparatus from the mid-nineteenth century through the wire mask used for so-called drip anaesthesia, e.g. the internationally known Schimmelbusch mask (■ Fig. 1.61) up to early twentieth century apparatus equipped with advanced dosage controls and compressed oxygen. A prime example of the exhibit is the Roth-Dräger apparatus (■ Fig. 1.62). Another milestone on view is Heinz Oehmig's first anaesthesia work station from 1958, which is the prototype of modern integrated monitoring of the patient's vital parameters.

The second room presents the development of methods for keeping the airways open, for local anaesthesia, rectal and intravenous anaesthesia, muscle relaxation and for respiratory and circulatory resuscitation. The early anaesthetists used cocaine for local anaesthesia until in 1905 the Hoechst Company developed and produced Novocain, the first synthetic local anaesthetic which, unlike cocaine, was not addictive and therefore achieved worldwide use.

A remarkable invention solving the primary problem of keeping the airways open, endotracheal intubation, is represented by F. Trendelenburg's anaesthesia apparatus amongst others. This archetype of intubation still used a tracheostomy cannula, but as early as 1869 included an inflatable cuff. Another important exhibit is F. Kuhn's (Kassel) flexible metal tube (■ Fig. 1.63). He learned the intubation technique using laryngeal cannulas for diphtheria patients in the USA and between 1900 and 1910 was influential in developing the method of oral intubation of the airways.

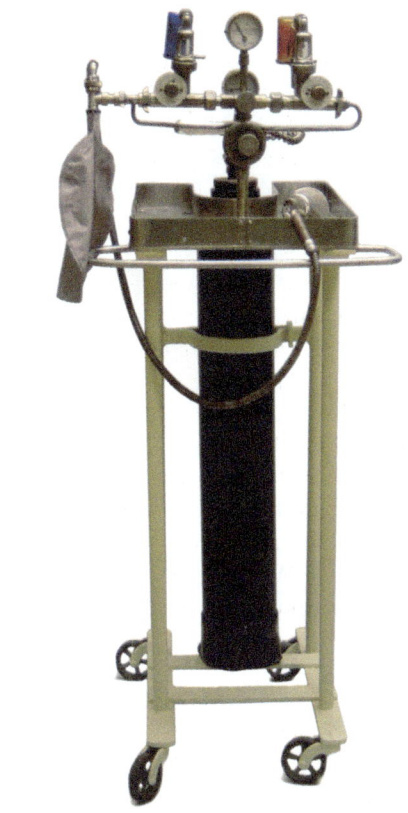

Fig. 1.62. The Roth-Dräger anaesthesia apparatus for ether and chloroform with compressed oxygen and injector dosage system

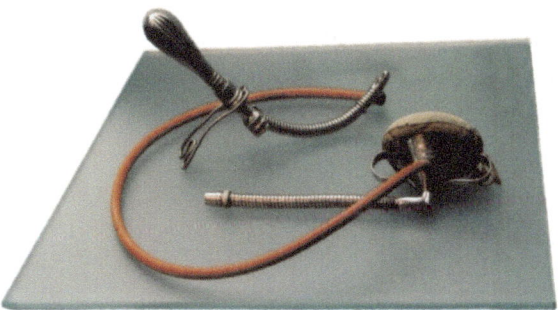

Fig. 1.63. Anaesthetic tube for oral intubation developed in 1900–1910 by F. Kuhn in Kassel

Additionally, the museum contains a fairly extensive collection of intensive care respiratory techniques developed between 1950 and 1990, beginning with its ancestor the so-called iron lung (■ Fig. 1.64), a great attraction for visitors. Development continued with mechanical respiratory apparatus up to the modern electronic high-tech respirators.

One of the most significant technical advances since the Second World War – besides the introduction of synthetic

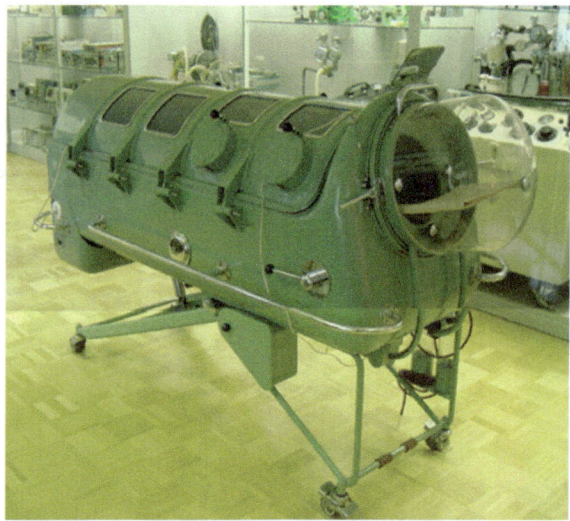

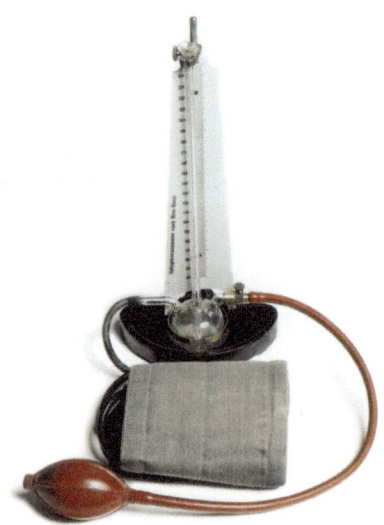

▣ Fig. 1.64. The so-called iron lung manufactured by the Dräger Company in 1952, a forerunner of modern long-term mechanical ventilation used in intensive care medicine

▣ Fig. 1.65. S. Riva-Rocci's original equipment for measuring blood pressure developed in 1900 in Pavia (cuff added)

materials – is the development of apparatus to monitor the patient's vital functions. The development of anaesthesia apparatus and of the anaesthetics themselves has of course also been very important. The exhibits range in scope from Riva-Rocci's device to measure blood pressure from the year 1900 (▣ Fig. 1.65) through the first sphygmographs and the capillary electrometer both from the nineteenth century and culminate in the integrated computer-assisted anaesthesia workstation of the present day.

A remarkable feature is the almost complete collection of anaesthesia drugs. It begins with the first inhalation anaesthetics, laughing gas, ether and chloroform; the first local anaesthetic, cocaine; the first ground-breaking induction anaesthetic Evipan-Natrium (▣ Fig. 1.66). Continuing the collection is the curare preparation Intocostrin first used clinically in 1942 in Canada and circulation medication and analgesics which were used in emergency medicine. The collection also includes the drugs which were then in general use, such as camphor, caffeine and cardiazol, the opium alkaloid morphine or Pantopon and Scophedal (also known as S.E.E. – Scopolamine-Eukodal-Ephetonin).

Banked blood for the Soviet Army has been preserved from the time of the Second World War. The glucose crystals of the stabilizer for blood group A_2 can still be recognized through the glass container. Whilst the US Army contributed to blood substitutes with dried human plasma in a vacuum flask, the Germans already possessed the first blood substitute in a colloid form, Periston from the Bayer Company.

Since the opening of the museum an exhibition of pharmacognosy has been created presenting the three drug groups still essential for modern anaesthesia – opium/mor-

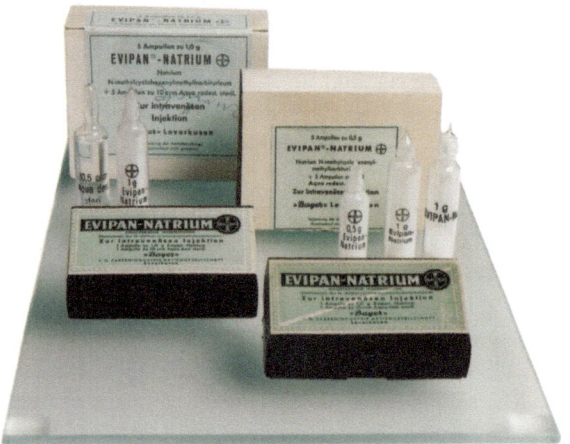

▣ Fig. 1.66. The epoch-making induction anaesthetic Evipan-Natrium, introduced in 1932 by H. Weese, Bayer AG Leverkusen

phine (analgesic, ▣ Fig. 1.67), cocaine (local anaesthetic) and curare (muscle relaxant). Their development can be traced from their early use as drugs or for hunting in Asia and South America through production in pharmacies up to industrial manufacture. The museum pays particular attention to the extensive collection of drugs for all areas of anaesthesia and has so far been able to display 150 drugs (excluding inhalation anaesthetics). Here, as with the equipment, there are still a few gaps which are very difficult to close. This is true especially for the first 100 years of anaesthesia, i.e. the period until the Second World War.

The tour ends with a special highlight, a complete operating theatre from 1930 (▣ Fig. 1.68). The lovely old

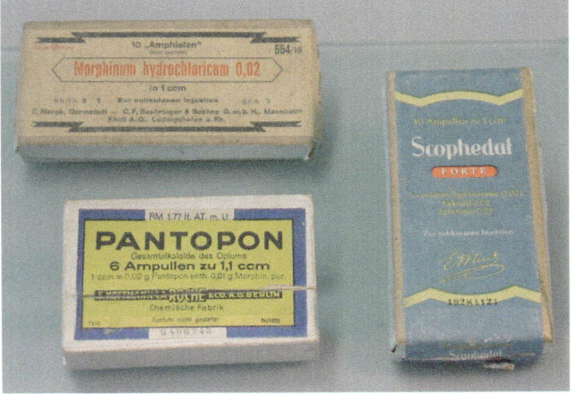

Fig. 1.67. Early opioids: morphine hydrochloride, Pantopon and Scophedal

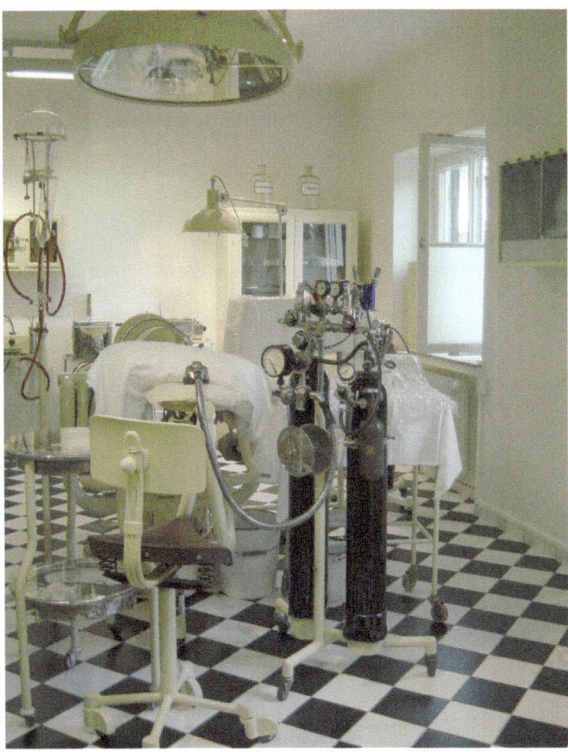

Fig. 1.68. Operating theatre from 1930 with anaesthesia equipment model MÜ from Dräger of Lübeck, infusion and surgical equipment

instrument cabinets are much admired. In this area the two display cases for infusion and transfusion methods are also well worth seeing.

The exhibition is further enriched by the pioneer's gallery. Here the early pioneers – dentists, surgeons, gynaecologists, pharmacologists and physiologists – are presented in large posters with portraits, concise biographies and their pioneering contributions to anaesthesia.

In a corridor gallery the former doorways have been transformed into display cases. On view are the first German-language textbooks, scientific monographs and journals together with photographs and brief biographies of the founding editors. The »explosion-like« spread of ether and chloroform anaesthesia can be traced here.

The museum library with its 12,500 books and the major national and international journals provides the intellectual setting for the intended involvement of young scientists in the evaluation and appraisal of the history of anaesthesia (Fig. 1.69). For this purpose two study rooms with computers and internet connection are available.

What does the museum offer visitors?
The museum is open from 9.00 a.m. to 1.30 p.m. on weekdays. Guided tours for groups of 15–30 are by appointment only and can also be arranged for weekday afternoons and Saturday mornings. The library is available during the museum's opening hours.

The birth of ether anaesthesia in the beginning of modern scientific thought marks one of the first scientific revolutions in the development of modern surgery. The Horst Stoeckel Museum clearly demonstrates how anaesthesia developed in 150 years from a slow beginning into the technically sophisticated, specialized and independent discipline of today. At the same time this example of anaesthesia confirms the theory of Thomas S. Kuhn, who states that the foundation of a science consists of a set of paradigms. Scientific progress consists in the

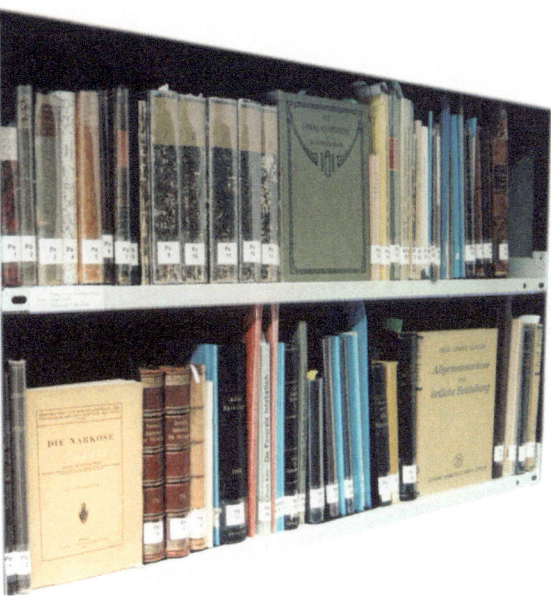

Fig. 1.69. Library with 11,000 books and journals from 1846–2000

gradual accumulation of new information and the subsequent gradual revision of erroneous deductions, until a new revolutionary paradigm arises. Such an event was the discovery of anaesthesia.

On the occasion of the 10th anniversary of the museum a symposium was held in the University Hospital of Bonn on 8th October 2010 [1]. The proceedings of this meeting were published in the following year [2].

References

1. Stoeckel H (2010) 10 Jahre Horst-Stoeckel-Museum für die Geschichte der Anästhesiologie in Bonn. Anästh Intensivmed 51: 376-378
2. Stoeckel H (ed) (2011) Symposium: Deutsche Anästhesie-Pioniere der ersten 100 Jahre – 1847 bis etwa 1950. DCS, Überlingen

For further information:
www.uniklinik-bonn/anaesthesia-museum

The Four Pillars of Anaesthesiology

2.1   Anaesthesia

2.1.1   German Anaesthesia before 1945

J. Schulte am Esch, M. Goerig, K. Agarwal

Surgery has been limited ever since its beginning due to inadequate asepsis as well as insufficient pain management. As the news of the invention of ether as an anaesthetic reached Europe in 1846 it was initially dismissed as »Yankee hogwash« and »typical North American embellishment«. The French physiologist Marie Jean Flourens (1794–1867) issued a warning about its administration by stating: »Ether that kills pain also kills life, and this new substance that will conquer surgery will turn out to be terrific as well as terrifying« [1].

Flourens' judgement was proven right as only a week later the first fatal incident during anaesthesia occurred [2]. Although other various volatile anaesthetics that were considered to be safe were applied during the following decades, fatal adverse events during anaesthesia were observed; hence, patients often would have more reservations about the anaesthesia than the surgical procedure itself or the accompanying pain. As for this apprehension, by the end of the nineteenth century, leading German surgeons, e.g. Johannes von Mikulicz-Radecki in Breslau (1865–1905; ◻ Fig. 2.1), concluded that »anaesthesia is perilous« [3].

At the same time as von Mikulicz-Radecki criticized anaesthesia, knowledge of asepsis well as antisepsis had improved tremendously, and infections of wounds could usually be prevented. Therefore, he would not allow anyone dressed in street clothes to enter the operating theatre, as had still been practised in other hospitals. This was enforced by wearing gloves, face masks and light-coloured, sterilized linen aprons that soon were shown off even outside the operating theatre; hence, surgeons rapidly were nicknamed »demigods attired white«. As opposed to the advances in asepsis during surgery, the evolution of anaesthesia was less stunning. Hardly any significant innovation had been introduced to improve the quality of anaesthesia or reduce its hazards.

Over the decades the belief survived that anaesthetics poisoned the organism; thus, deep stages were to be avoided. Physicians as well as patients were aware of manifold dangers during anaesthesia.

Guidelines for Conducting Anaesthesia in the Year 1922

Even guidelines for conducting anaesthesia in surgery-based training reflected the above-mentioned uncertainties. These had been put into writing by the surgeon Heinrich Braun (1862–1934) of Zwickau who had introduced several

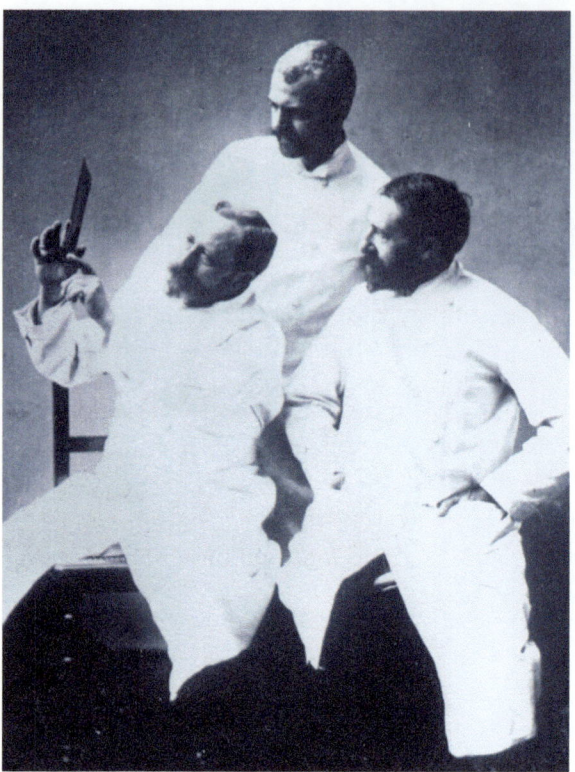

◻ **Fig. 2.1.** The surgeon Johannes von Mikulicz-Radecki of Breslau (centre) studying the first X-ray at the hospital in Breslau; von Mikulicz-Radecki considered anaesthesia to be »the premium category in the art of medicine«

novel techniques in general as well as regional anaesthesia and was reckoned to be an experienced anaesthetist:

> Anaesthesia should not be deeper than necessary. Assuming that a patient is fastened accurately, anaesthesia may be so flat that the corneal reflex is still preserved, no snoring emerges during breathing and the epiglottis does not close [4].

The Airway – a Major Challenge in Anaesthesiology

Many surgeons urged that the anaesthesia not be too deep, as anaesthetic drugs were considered poisonous and upper airway obstruction could be caused when the tongue falls back. Pioneers in ether anaesthesia had already pointed out the »occurrence of suffocation« and deduced that this was related to the incorrect use of the anaesthetic. Their assumption certainly was accurate, though they could not trace the actual cause of this phenomenon [5]. Even John Snow (1813–1858) could not perceive danger in a patient snoring. In 1877 Friedrich Esmarch (1823–1908) of Kiel unveiled several precautions for anaesthesiology in his paperback on surgery at times of war. For patients with inconstant breathing he recommended that »the mouth be opened immediately and the lower jaw pulled with both hands to the front so that the lower row of teeth slips in front of the upper row« [6].

During subsequent years, this simple technique became common knowledge. Threatening dangers of a tongue impeding the airway were described in 1880 by Otto Kappeler (1841–1909) in the first handbook of anaesthesia in German »Anaesthetica«. He also provided a solution for overcoming this hazard by the simple action as described by Esmarch and explained it with the aid of a figure in his book [7].

Simple Techniques and Aids to Keep the Airway Free

During the 1920s, many surgeons described a variety of mechanical aids to keep the airway open. Many of these devices were rather effective but did not become popular once the surgeon Helmut Schmidt of Hamburg (1897–1979) published results on the advantages of the »Mayo tube« in the management of upper airway obstruction caused by the tongue dropping back. Ever since, this simple gadget has become part of an anaesthesiologist's equipment like the endotracheal tube that had already been advocated for decades as an ideal tool for keeping the airway open and reducing the incidence of aspiration [7].

Securing the Airway by Endotracheal Intubation

Endotracheal intubation in anaesthesia was first employed by Friedrich Trendelenburg (1844–1924) in 1869 in Rostock to avoid the aspiration of blood and mucus during intraoral operations. As opposed to modern techniques, Trendelenburg performed tracheotomies the day prior to surgery, inserting the metal tracheal tube immediately before the operation. The anaesthetic agent was then dropped onto a special metal funnel with gauze covering its opening [7].

In 1880, the English surgeon William McEwen (1848–1924) circumvented tracheotomy by orotracheal intubation. His report was overlooked and soon forgotten. Again, by the end of the nineteenth century, surgeons, e.g. Karel Maydl (1853–1903) of Prague or Victor Eisenmenger (1864–1932) of Vienna, described successful tracheal intubation for general anaesthesia. In 1893, Eisenmenger employed a cuffed rubber tube with a pilot balloon [7].

Franz Kuhn's Contribution

In Germany, the surgeon Franz Kuhn (1866–1929; ◘ Fig. 2.2a) of Kassel picked up again the idea of intubation anaesthesia around 1900 and published a large number of articles on his technique (◘ Fig. 2.2b). The tube he had developed was a twistable metal tube of different sizes [8].

At congresses and in articles on this procedure, he recommended the method for resuscitation, in cases of as-

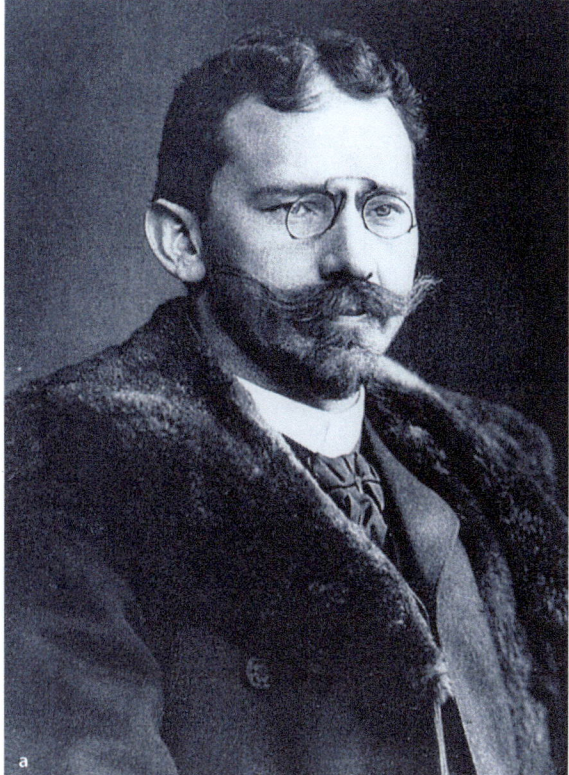

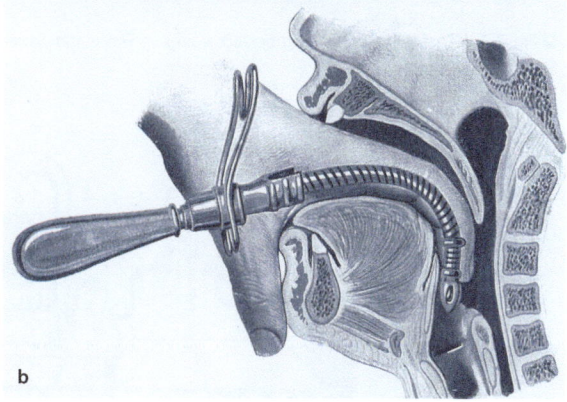

◘ **Fig. 2.2a,b. a** Franz Kuhn, a pioneer in endotracheal intubation. **b** Technique of digital orotracheal intubation as practised by Franz Kuhn: the tongue and the epiglottis are pulled forward with the index finger, as the tube equipped with a mandrin is inserted along the index finger into the larynx

phyxia as well as for chloroform anaesthesia and pointed out the importance of a secure and free airway achieved by means of tracheal »tubage«. The idea of his so-called pulmonary anaesthesia met with incredulity, though, e.g. at the Natural Science Congress in 1902, where he reported his results. Unfortunately, Kuhn did not manage to intubate a patient in deep anaesthesia; hence, opponents of this method felt confirmed, even though advantages were at hand, e.g. unhindered gas exchange via the tube resulting in precisely graded dosing concentrations of volatile anaesthetics as well as improved manipulation of the state of anaesthesia [9].

The Controversy Between Franz Kuhn and Ferdinand Sauerbruch

At about the same time as Kuhn strove to secure the airway by endotracheal intubation and to prevent aspiration, Ferdinand Sauerbruch (1875–1951), who had assisted von Mikulicz-Radecki in Breslau, described the invention

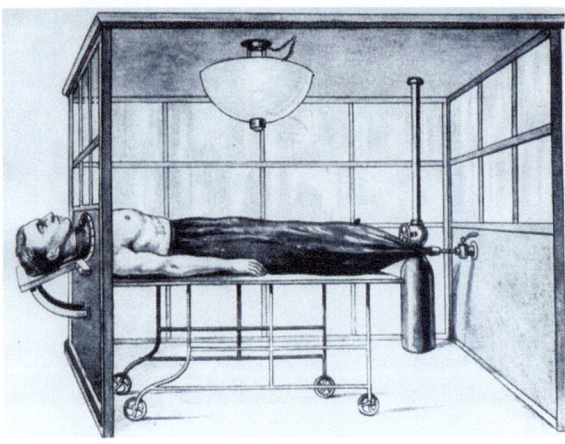

■ **Fig. 2.3.** Negative pressure chamber according to Ferdinand Sauerbruch

of a pressure chamber to perform surgery of the lung in 1904. He employed this method of pressure differences and lowered pressure to avoid pneumothorax, with the chamber surrounding the entire body except the head; thus, a complete collapse of the lung could be prevented [10] (■ Fig. 2.3).

Sauerbruch acquired recognition worldwide by publishing the results of his experiments. He rejected Kuhn's idea of positive pressure ventilation with the aid of an endotracheal tube as not being compatible with human physiology. The suggestion of a positive pressure method by the internist Ludolph Brauer (1865–1951) of Heidelberg, which required the patient to exhale against elevated pressure, utilizing a tight-fitting face mask to prevent the lung from collapsing (■ Fig. 2.4), was also dismissed [11]. Nevertheless, this method was ultimately accepted on the Continent [12]. Respirators like the Tiegel-Henle apparatus and the »Roth-Dräger« high pressure anaesthesia apparatus were commonly used.

In 1913, the surgeon Paul von Bruns (1846–1916) of Tübingen had an amazing idea. He modified an apparatus as follows: instead of the tube for exhalation passing through water to create elevated pressure, he developed a face mask with a valve to adjust pressure [13]. Since Sauerbruch retained enormous influence for decades rejected tracheal intubation for anaesthesia, this method could not become established in Germany or in other European countries for a long time.

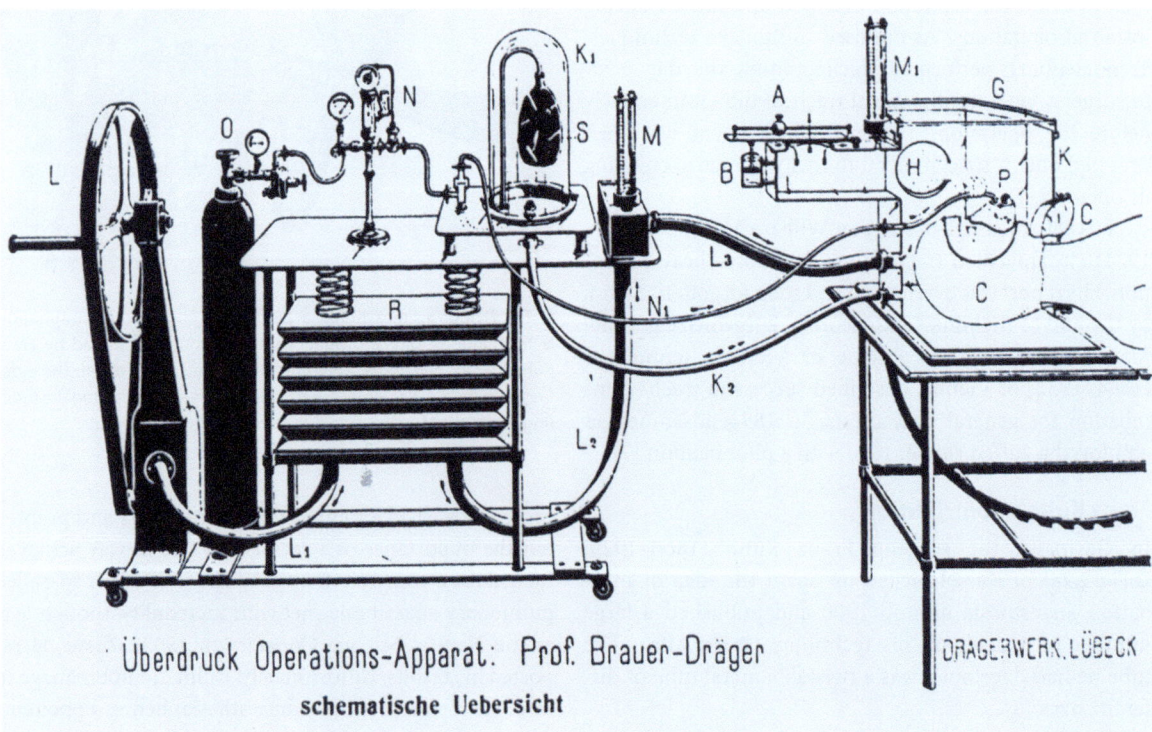

Überdruck Operations-Apparat: Prof. Brauer-Dräger

schematische Uebersicht

DRÄGERWERK.LÜBECK

■ **Fig. 2.4.** The preferred method of preventing pneumothorax in pulmonary surgery according to the internist Ludolph Brauer of Marburg

Insufflation Anaesthesia – Another Technique in Anaesthesiology Rejected by Sauerbruch

Major improvements in thoracic surgery were achieved over the ensuing decades in the United States where the American physiologists Samuel James Meltzer (1851–1922) and John Auer (1875–1948) developed the method of insufflation anaesthesia in 1909 that soon started to spread all over. Sauerbruch rejected this technique of administering a volatile anaesthetic in a mixture of air and oxygen to the pharynx or the trachea via a small catheter. Although the surgeon Charles Elsberg (1871–1948) of New York employed this procedure successfully in surgery of the lungs in the same year and the procedure proved itself a success in thousands of cases, it was refused in Germany due to Sauerbruch's influence [14].

With World War I England was confronted with new challenges as plastic surgery had to be performed on soldiers with facial wounds requiring anaesthesia without the threat of aspiration. The anaesthesiologists Stanley Rowbotham (1890–1985) and Ivan Whiteside Magill (1888–1986), who had worked in London, converted endotracheal intubation for anaesthesia into a routine procedure. Both of them had a superior command of blind endotracheal intubation, without requiring a laryngoscope, which had already been developed in 1895 by the ENT specialist Alfred Kirstein (1863–1922) of Berlin [15].

Paul Moritsch (1896–1966) outlined the lacking popularity of tracheal intubation for anaesthesia after World War II in the German-speaking regions in a figure in his monograph The Management of Pain During Surgical Procedures (Fig. 2.5) [16]. At that point in time, it was regularly used in Anglo-American areas; a detailed description on how it had to be performed with the aid of a laryngoscope was published in popular textbooks. Ether drop anaesthesia utilizing a Schimmelbusch mask as first used in 1890 was still widely employed.

From Ether Drop Anaesthesia and Schimmelbusch Mask to Apparatus-Assisted Anaesthesia

For many years, a mask invented in 1890 by the surgeon Curt Schimmelbusch (1860–1895) of Berlin was prevalent in every operating theatre worldwide [17]. This may not only be attributed to the fact that well-known surgeons with tremendous impact rejected tracheal intubation for anaesthesia, but also to the attitude that only trained and experienced staff could successfully practise a difficult technique like tracheal intubation. As with the advent of intubation, surgeons were reluctant to accept the introduction of apparatus into anaesthesiology.

> Complicated machinery offers no advantage as compared to the air-chloroform/ether mix with our drop technique. Besides, a general practitioner cannot show up with a moving cart to conduct anaesthesia…The apparatus were again relegated to adjacent rooms, and the old mask is back [18].

Apparatus Designed by Ferdinand Junker and Heinrich Braun

Simple blower apparatus were modifications of the model invented in 1867 by Ferdinand Adalbert Junker (1828–1901) [19]. Otto Kappeler's model, patented in 1890, did not become as popular as the one developed by the surgeon Heinrich Braun (1862–1934) of Leipzig [20]. In all these models, a balloon was used to blow air through a bottle filled with chloroform or ether to the patient's face mask (Fig. 2.6). These gadgets could be hung around the physician's neck or onto a stand in order to free the anaesthesiologist's hands: one to hold onto the mask and the other to squeeze the balloon. An overdose of the anaesthetic was likely with the procedure described; nevertheless, this equipment was still being used after World War II [21].

Many complications occurring during anaesthesia could be attributed to hypoxaemia, a fact that surgeons had become conscious of shortly after the invention of the specialty. These were due to obstruction of the upper airway caused when the tongue falls back. This could be managed utilizing the Esmarch manoeuvre. If the desired result could not be obtained, the mouth was opened with the aid of a mouth gag and the tongue was retrieved with a tongue forceps. In cases when this trick also failed, tracheotomy was performed as most of the surgeons were not acquainted with the technique of orotracheal intubation that Franz Kuhn of Kassel had advocated.

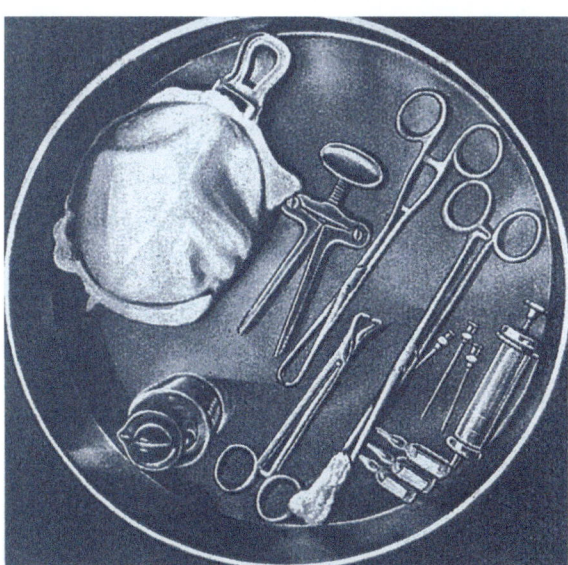

 Fig. 2.5. The anaesthetist's set in the late 1940s

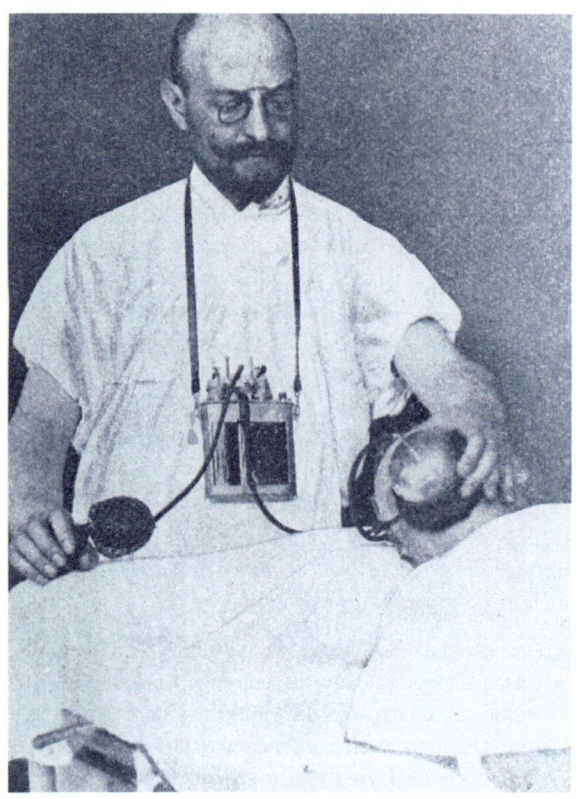

Fig. 2.6. Apparatus developed by Heinrich Braun in 1905. The anaesthetist blew air with the aid of a balloon into the bottle filled with ether or chloroform. The mixture was administered via a tight-fitting face mask

Machines for Anaesthesia with Air-Oxygen Mixtures

As inhalation devices for oxygen therapy had proven to be safe, anaesthesia machines were equipped with air-oxygen cylinders. Various models designed by the Dräger Company in Lübeck had become especially popular, as they were furnished with a patented drip chamber that ensured exact dosage of ether or chloroform for the first time [22] (□ Fig. 2.7).

Respirators for Anaesthesia with Curare

With improved technology that enabled artificial ventilation of patients, it could be expected that surgeons would initiate research on the administration of curare as a muscle relaxant in abdominal surgery; Arthur Läwen (1876–1958) of Leipzig was the first to dare use it [23]. In cooperation with his colleague Roderich Sievers (1878–1943) he developed a respirator that had already been tested in 1910. Tidal volume – as had been emphasized in the original article – could be adapted »observing visible thoracic excursion« so »the thoracic movement during breathing would seem natural« [24].

Again, this might have been influenced by Ferdinand Sauerbruch, who condemned tracheal intubation and positive pressure ventilation as non-physiological. Therefore, use of muscle relaxants was out of the question, as this would have necessitated artificial ventilation. Nevertheless, after World War II the Canadian anaesthesiologists Harold Randall Griffith (1896–1985) and Enid

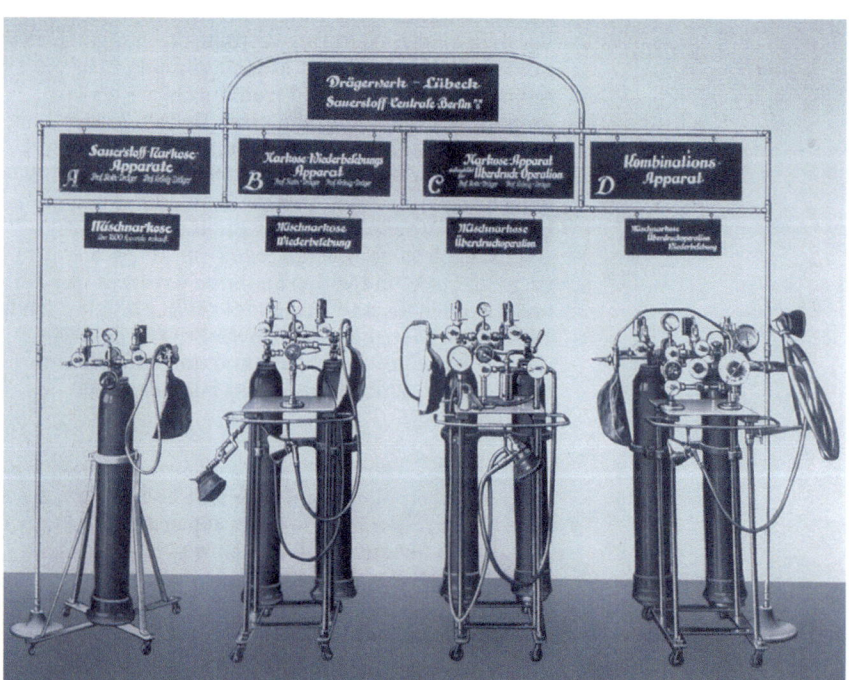

Fig. 2.7. Variety of anaesthesia machines manufactured by the Dräger Company in Lübeck

Johnson (1909–1972) emphasized the advantages of this technique that they had published in 1942; Läwen still lived to see the introduction of curare into the clinical routine in anaesthesiology [25].

The Nitrous Oxide Apparatus Designed by Professor Dr. Sudeck and Dr. Helmut Schmidt – a Modern Anaesthesia Circuit

As nitrous oxide was rather popular among American surgeons and dentists, it also became of major interest to anaesthesiologists in Germany; hence, various efforts were made to introduce an apparatus as well [26]. A machine for the application of nitrous oxide and oxygen was developed in 1910 by the gynaecologist Maximilian Neu (1877–1940) of Heidelberg in cooperation with the Rota-Werke in Aachen. Patented flow meters, the so-called rotameters, permitted exact dosage of both gases; thus, mixtures provoking hypoxaemia could be precluded (◘ Fig. 2.8) [27, 28].

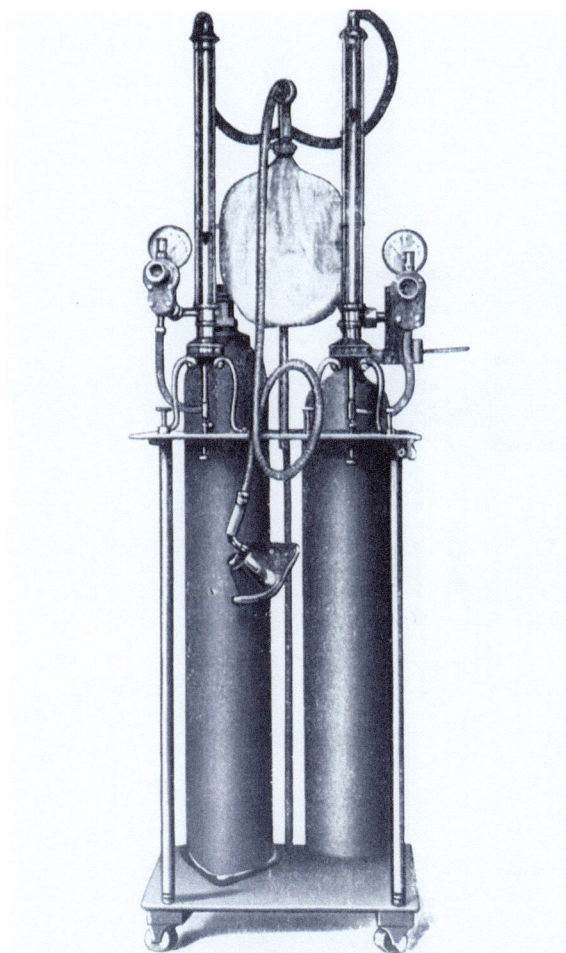

◘ **Fig. 2.8.** The nitrous oxide-oxygen anaesthesia apparatus developed by Maximilian Neu produced at the Rota-Werke in Aachen. Patented rotameters made it possible to avoid hypoxemic gas mixtures

As anaesthesia utilizing nitrous oxide and oxygen did not induce stages deep enough for surgery to be performed, it was primarily employed in gynaecology and obstetrics. This changed when anaesthesia machines were equipped with an additional ether vaporizer. These inventions were associated with famous physicians, i.e. the surgeons Paul Sudeck (1866–1945) and Helmut Schmidt (1895–1979) of Hamburg. In close collaboration with the Dräger Company in Lübeck, the »nitrous oxide apparatus designed by Professor Dr. Sudeck and Dr. Helmut Schmidt« was developed in 1925. Its superior safety and sublime technology comprising separate lines for inhalation and exhalation, low resistance valves, carbon dioxide absorber and bag for manual artificial ventilation contributed to its popularity (◘ Figs. 2.9, b) [29].

The Impact of Narcylene Anaesthesia

The »Model A« introduced by the Dräger Company in 1926 was based technically on a machine developed in 1923 for the administration of the highly volatile anaesthetic narcylene [30].

To reduce the amount required of this expensive agent, a closed circuit was integrated into the device for the first time. This Kreisatmer (rebreathing machine) technique was intended to reduce the extent of evaporating gas and consequently to eradicate the odds of explosions. Nonetheless, explosions still occurred resulting in a temporary ban of narcylene [30]. Investigations of this issue revealed that static charging was the key cause. Thus, several safety guidelines were released that still apply today, significantly reducing the number of explosions. A review published in 1940 on the danger of burns and explosions asserted that »the danger of explosions has nearly vanished« [31].

Anaesthesia Gas Load in Operating Theatres

The load of anaesthesia gases in surgical areas had been discussed in various medical journals as early as 1880 without any effect.

The surgeon Georg Kelling (1866–1945) of Dresden developed a new appliance to redirect volatile anaesthetics outside of the operating theatre as well as a special face mask [32] (◘ Fig. 2.10). In the ensuing years, many surgeons worked out different solutions that seem feasible even from today's point of view. Next to methods both simple and effective like active charcoal filters and the absorption of volatile anaesthetics [33], efficient air-conditioning and ventilation units were installed in hospitals by the 1930s [34].

The effectiveness of these measures could be confirmed by hygiene officials carrying out air analyses at the University Hospital Charité in Berlin as early as 1928: samples were taken before and after a gas draw-out system had been mounted, revealing significantly lower amounts of ether in the air [35].

2

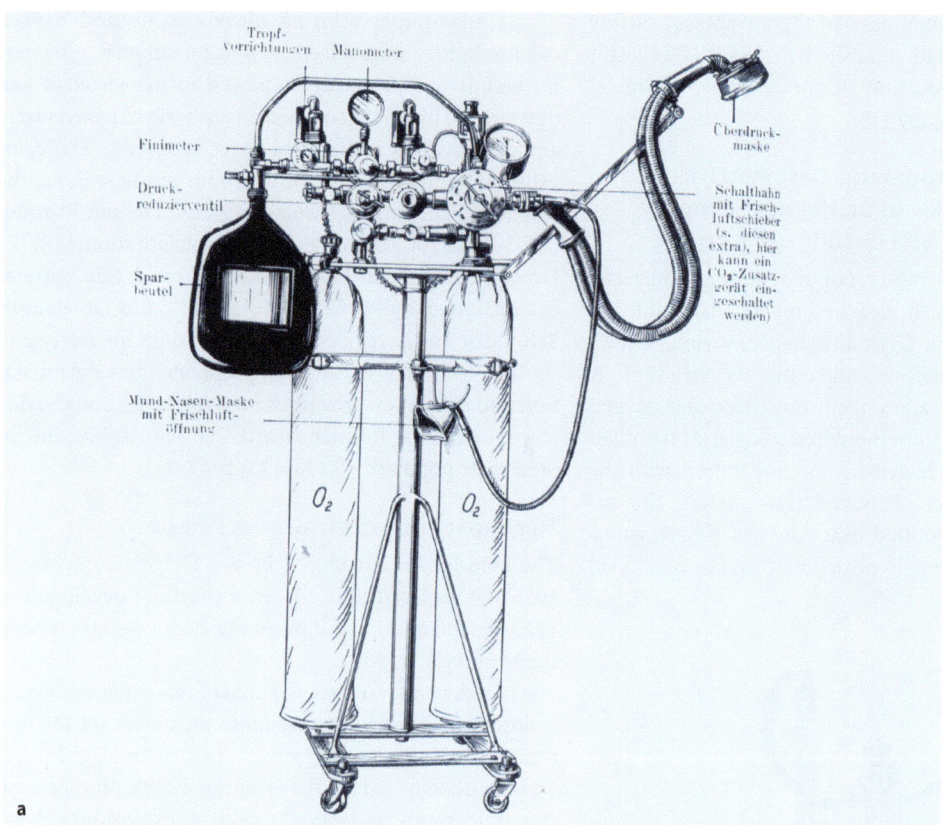

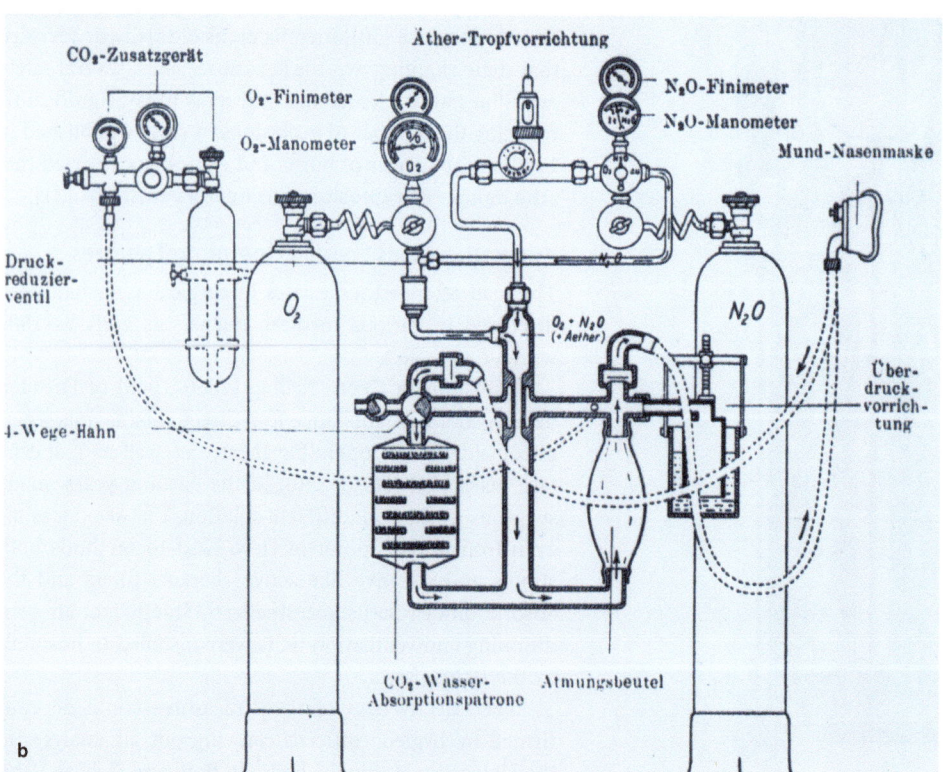

Fig. 2.9a,b. a The »Dräger nitrous oxide-oxygen anaesthesia apparatus according to Professor Dr. Sudeck and Dr. Schmidt, Dr. Ing. Dräger«, »Model A«. It was the first nitrous oxide-oxygen machine to become popular. **b** Technical details of the nitrous oxide-oxygen anaesthetic apparatus manufactured by Dräger, Lübeck, »Model A«, around 1925

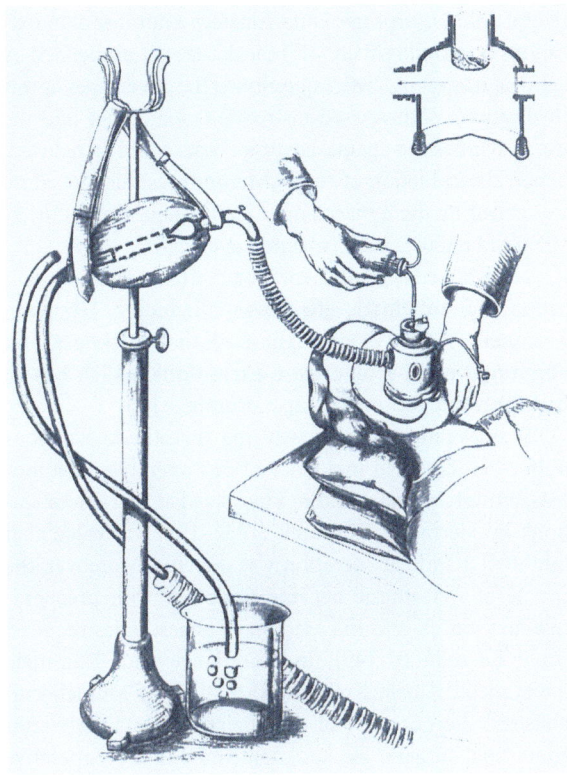

Fig. 2.10. Face mask to dispense volatile anaesthetics according to Georg Kelling

Anaesthetic Techniques for Abdominal Surgery

After the Scottish gynaecologist James Simpson (1811–1870) had ascertained an association between intraoperative aspiration and fatal courses of anaesthesia, preoperative fasting for several hours prior to surgery became common practice. Because physiological time of passage through the stomach was determined to be 6 h, patients were not allowed to eat or drink for this period of time.

Von Mikulicz-Radecki as one of the most important abdominal surgeons at that time was acquainted with the problems of patients who inhaled gastric contents. He rejected »anaesthesia to be carried out according to fixed schemes as it often is so deep that patients become unconscious and reflexes disappear«. He advocated that the so-called half anaesthesia should be practised, a technique that permitted unconsciousness without vanishing reflexes [36]. The anaesthesiologist had to discontinue application of anaesthetics, as soon as aspiration could be anticipated, and keep the patient in trance, so he or she could react to commands and expectorate fluids. Therefore, the technique of half anaesthesia was chosen for abdominal surgery.

Rules to Avoid Complications

Von Mikulicz-Radecki probably was the first surgeon in the German-speaking area to promulgate regulations for avoiding major infringements during anaesthesia in operating theatres and pre-anaesthesia units in his clinic. These included that patients' stomachs had to be drained with the aid of a gastric tube, »if they had not fasted for at least 6 h prior to the operation and if they had any kind of obstruction of the stomach or bowels«, e.g. »stenosis pylori, incarcerated hernias and ileus«.

Technical Aids to Avoid Aspiration During Anaesthesia

Friedrich Trendelenburg was a surgeon who at the end of the nineteenth century had been concerned with how to avoid intraoperative aspiration. As mentioned above, he performed tracheotomy for intraoral surgery in order to insert a special tracheal tube with an inflatable cuff that he had invented. With the aid of an attached funnel even volatile anaesthetics could be dispensed. Nevertheless, aspirations occurred repeatedly due to low-quality material that did not ensure a proper fit [37]. This prompted his colleague Eugen Hahn (1841–1902) to develop a special pressed sponge cannula that was employed until the early 1940s because it was easy to use [38]. Needless to say that »pulmonary anaesthesia« with a tracheal tube – as promoted by Franz Kuhn – offered sufficient protection against aspiration. Nevertheless, this technique did not become prevalent, as it was considered to be intricate, and Ferdinand Sauerbruch refused to admit that it might be advantageous.

Abdominal surgery was rarely successful until asepsis and appropriate anaesthetic procedures were introduced. Surgery of the abdomen along with the chest remained a »noli me tangere area«; thus operations were only performed in hopeless situations as the last choice. Early articles on successful abdominal surgery did not usually mention details on anaesthesia and its course.

At that point in time, anaesthesia was typically performed by applying chloroform that was known to be toxic to parenchymatous organs and depressing cardiovascular function. As the anaesthetic was dropped onto a handkerchief or a simple anaesthesia mask, dosage was difficult to control; thus, intoxications occurred frequently. In view of these risks, patients as well as surgeons hesitated on the decision to perform surgery – abdominal surgery in particular – especially in crucial cases. Until the end of the century, chloroform remained the favourite anaesthetic when it was replaced by ether. This can be attributed to the surgeon Ernst Julius Gurlt (1825–1899) of Berlin, who demonstrated that 1 of 2,907 chloroform anaesthesias was fatal, whereas with ether this number could be reduced to 1 in 14,646 applications. Hence, the scientific quarrel over »ether or chloroform« among

German surgeons came to an end [39]. Due to frequent fatalities in anaesthesia, the surgeon Carl Ludwig Schleich (1859–1922) of Berlin initiated thorough research on techniques to obtain analgesia [40].

After Carl Koller (1857–1944) had determined its analgesic effects cocaine was initially only used to anaesthetize mucous membranes [41]. With topical application, subcutaneous, or intra- and perineural injections of cocaine, new options became available to overcome pain during surgery. With achievements in local anaesthesia as well as the invention of highly effective cocaine derivatives, regional anaesthesia techniques increasingly replaced general anaesthesia in some places. It was preferred in patients who were regarded to be unsuitable for anaesthesia because of their condition, since regional anaesthesia was considered less precarious than general anaesthesia.

Infiltration anaesthesia made it possible to perform minor surgery in outpatients in general practices; in consequence, it became accepted instantly [42]. Surgeons often combined regional anaesthesia with low-dose general anaesthesia or supplemented volatile anaesthetics for painful procedures. Johannes Bakes (1870–1929) employed at the Kaiser-Franz-Joseph Hospital in Vienna named this method »combined anaesthesia« [43].

Other surgeons combined this kind of anaesthesia with morphine injections or induced »twilight sleep« with a mixture of morphine and scopolamine administered subcutaneously [44]. As soon as the desired effect was achieved, regional anaesthesia was supplemented. This procedure became popular quickly. Shortly before his death, the surgeon Ernst von Bergmann (1836–1907) of Berlin, who in 1894 labelled Schleich's invention the »first important surgical endeavour of a German«, underwent abdominal surgery under infiltration anaesthesia according to Schleich's technique [45].

Origins of Premedication

Almost at the same time as orotracheal intubation, ether drop or local anaesthetic techniques were established, by the beginning of the twentieth century preoperative administration of drugs with analgesic, anxiolytic, hypnotic and anti-salivatory effects became en vogue.

In 1900 Eduard Schneiderlin (1875) of the Clinic for Psychiatry in Emmendingen was the first to describe positive effects of a mixture of scopolamine and morphine, a technique he termed »new anaesthesia«. He declared in his original publication that his intention was to relieve the patient and the physician from »the act of anaesthesia…comprising painful sensations« and to »avoid events…that appear to be repulsive to a human being« [46].

The surgeon Bertholt Korff (1859–1918) of Freiburg appreciated the advantages of preoperatively administered scopolamine-morphine. Unfortunately, a number of intoxications occurred initially with the dosage recommended by Schneiderlin; thus, critics questioned the advantages of this medication. With revised instructions for dosage and the use of synthesized agents, adverse events could be reduced; hence, the induction of »twilight sleep«, as this procedure was called by the gynaecologist Carl Joseph Gauß (1875–1957) of Freiburg, soon became popular [47].

Next to sedative and anxiolytic effects of this medication, the antiemetic effect was convincing. Hermann Kümmell (1852–1937) emphasized that »sickness and vomiting« had become »rare exceptions, which has to be highly appreciated in laparotomies« [48].

Besides reduced anxiety during anaesthesia, surgeons noticed a decreased incidence of postoperative pneumonias, a mystery that could not be solved at first. Investigations by Hermann Kümmell (1852–1937) revealed that inhibited glandular secretion was the clue. Moreover, the course of anaesthesia became smoother with preoperative medication and the amount of anaesthetics required could be reduced [49]. In accordance with Kümmell, the surgeon Albert Krecke (1863–1932) of Munich emphasized the necessity of mobilizing patients early after abdominal surgery. He, too, confirmed that preoperative pulmonary exercise was incredibly important and avowed that the patient should take deep breaths 25 times per hour in order to »ventilate alveoli in deeper parts of the lung«. This was to be commenced immediately after anaesthesia under the supervision of an »attendant« [50]. In Hamburg, where Kümmell was in charge, patients inflated rubber cushions.

Arthur Menzel and Ernst Julius Gurlt – Early Protagonists of Securing Quality in Anaesthesiology

As ether and chloroform became widespread for anaesthesia, the incidence of fatal accidents rose; hence, by 1880 several medical committees discussed the adverse effects of different anaesthetics. In the German area, the surgeon Arthur Menzel (1844–1878) of Trieste and a student of Billroth insisted that anaesthesias be systematically recorded and adverse events documented [51]. The surgeon Ernst Julius Gurlt (1825–1899) of Berlin assumed this task and mailed »invitation questionnaires« comprising the following questions:

- *Duration of observation*
- *Information on anaesthetic agents and medications (chloroform-ether, mixtures etc.) administered and how often*
- *Place of purchase*
- *Devices used etc.*
- *Duration of exceptionally extensive (1 h and more) anaesthesias*

- Amount of anaesthetics used per minute, or amount used for extraordinarily prolonged anaesthesias or maximum amount used for outstandingly lengthy anaesthesias
- If and to what extent morphine or other injections have been administered
- Incidents during or after anaesthesias:
  (a) Asphyxia (treatment, e.g. tracheotomy etc.)
  (b) Fatalities (reasons/coroner's report etc.)

These questionnaires were distributed in Germany, Austria, Russia, the Netherlands and the United States and can be categorized as an early contribution to quality control in anaesthesiology. Reports published between 1891 and 1897 as Narkotisierungsstatistik based on completed and returned questionnaires – also known as the »Gurlt Report« – resulted in chloroform, as the favourite anaesthetic, being replaced by ether which was perceived to be less perilous [52]. Nevertheless, anaesthesia still carried significant risks like postoperative nausea and pneumonia.

Local Anaesthesia

The surgeon Carl Ludwig Schleich (1859–1922; ◧ Fig. 2.11) of Berlin developed infiltration anaesthesia during the late nineteenth century, eager to avoid fatal pneumonias after general anaesthesia that were prevalent until then [53].

Infiltration Anaesthesia According to the Surgeon Carl Ludwig Schleich of Berlin

Schleich administered a cooling spray to the area of interest before injecting a highly diluted cocaine solution into the region to be operated on. Circumventing intoxication, he was able to achieve analgesia in almost every operation, even major surgery like laparotomy. Especially in Berlin his virtually safe technique became widespread. Only a few years later, surgeons around the world employed the Schleich method, Anton Freiherr von Eiselsberg (1860–1939) of Vienna being among them. He ascertained »that to argue about infiltration anaesthesia is superfluous« [54].

The Advancement of Local Anaesthesia by Heinrich Braun

The development of local anaesthesia is closely linked to the surgeon Heinrich Braun (1862–1934; ◧ Fig. 2.12) of Leipzig [55]. In 1903 he had already recommended that adrenaline be added to the cocaine solution to decrease the speed of absorption; hence, larger amounts of cocaine could be administered allowing more extensive surgery. The introduction of the synthetically produced Novocain in 1905 can also be attributed to Braun [56]. For many decades it remained the favourite local anaesthetic, although several other high quality drugs were available.

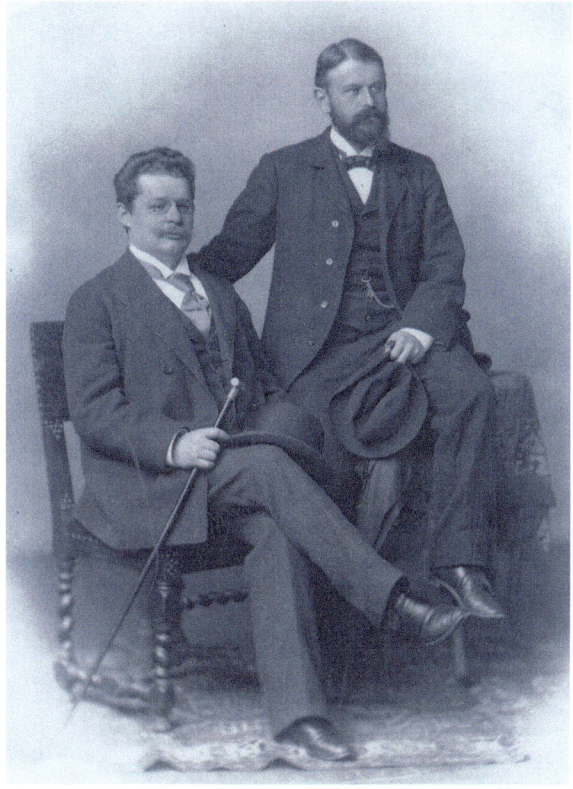

◧ **Fig. 2.11.** The surgeon Carl-Ludwig Schleich (*left*) of Berlin with his friend Karl Briegleb. He made the technique of »infiltration anaesthesia« public. He also was one of the first surgeons to advocate specialized training in anaesthesia. Briegleb acquainted general practitioners with Schleich's infiltrations anaesthesia

Braun contributed to the popularity of local anaesthesia techniques by publishing a Lehrbuch der örtlichen Betäubung (textbook of local analgesia), which first appeared in 1905 and was later released in nine revised editions up until 1951.

August Bier – Father of Spinal and of Intravenous Anaesthesia

When Novocain was introduced, August Bier (1861–1949) (◧ Fig. 2.13a, b) also recommended its application for spinal anaesthesia. Until then, he was obliged to administer the rather toxic cocaine. With spinal anaesthesia, Bier – who first described the procedure in 1899 – attempted to spare patients the nausea accompanying ether anaesthesia that could persist for days [57]. This caused severe discomfort and threatened sutures after abdominal surgery provoking dehiscences and jeopardizing the outcome [58].

After the initial euphoria about the new technique, some fatal incidents occurred; thus, Bier advised against naively employing the method. In addition, the problem

2

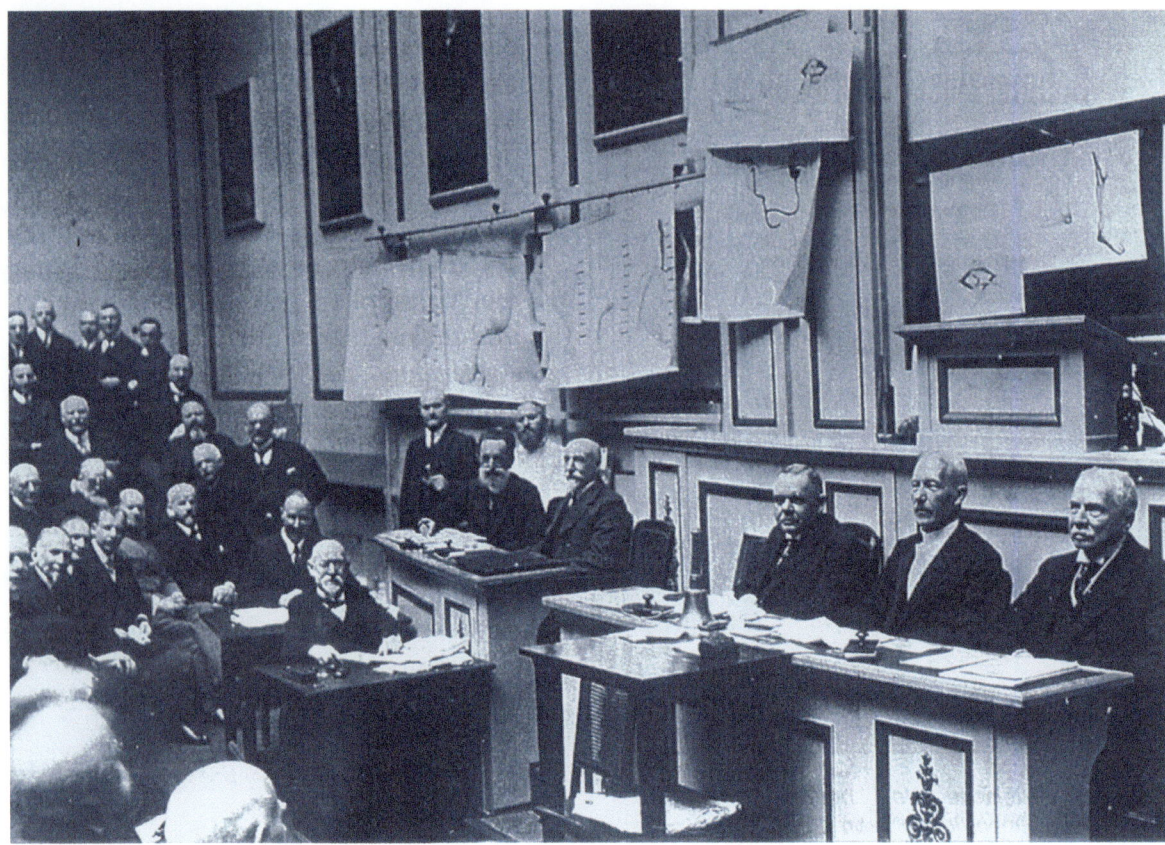

🔹 **Fig. 2.12.** The surgeon Heinrich Braun of Leipzig. He was known as the initiator of scientific research on regional anaesthesia and wrote a text-book on this topic that was published in many editions. The picture shows him (*centre*) at a surgeons' congress in Berlin. To his *left* the surgeon Hermann Kümmell of Hamburg can be seen and to his *right* August Borchard

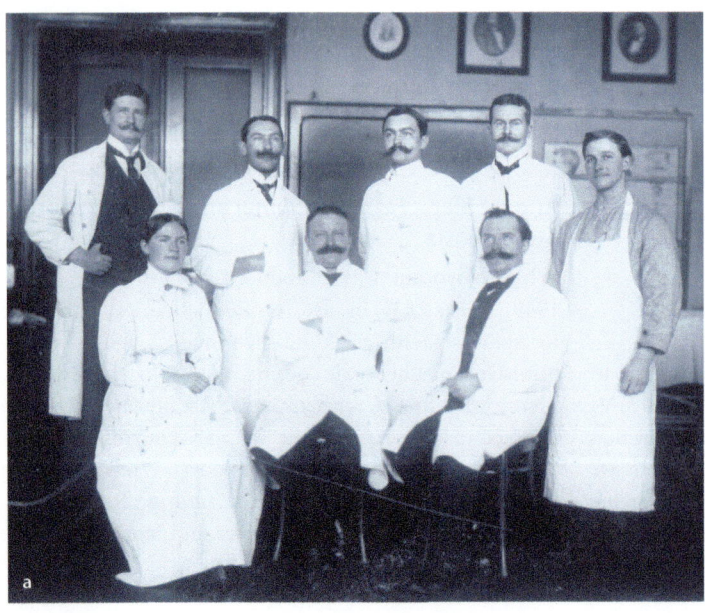

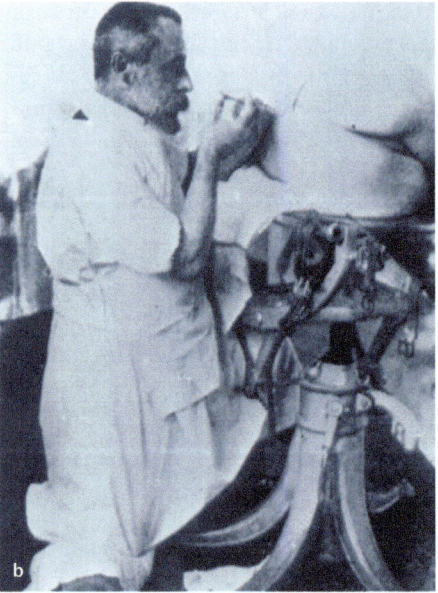

🔹 **Fig. 2.13a,b. a** The surgeon August Bier (*centre*) with his staff at the University Surgical Clinic in Greifswald. **b** Performance of spinal anaesthesia. Notice that the puncture was performed without gloves

of persistent, therapy-resistant headache could not be overcome. Consequently, surgeons performed spinal anaesthesia in special cases only.

Obstetricians, on the other hand, fancied this technique. The gynaecologist Oskar Kreis (1872–1958) of Basel already performed spinal anaesthesia in 1900 for obstetric procedures [59]. With the invention of an axillary block technique to anaesthetize the brachial plexus by Georg Hirschel (1875–1963) and the description of the supraclavicular access by Dietrich Kulenkampff (1880–1963) in 1911, indications for intravenous anaesthesia of the upper extremity diminished [60]. In 1912, Georg Perthes (1869–1927) of Tübingen described the atraumatic electrostimulation for safe localization of peripheral nerves. Perthes' modus operandi was overlooked and finally forgotten, although textbooks of regional anaesthesia referred to it. American authors »re-discovered« it in the early 1960s [61].

Regional anaesthesia experienced a revival in the middle of the 1920s, as blunt, atraumatic spinal cannulae and new local anaesthetics became available. Furthermore, new techniques were invented by the American surgeon George Pitkin (1885–1943) who administered procaine solutions that had been made hypobaric by adding alcohol that he named »Spinocain«. By repositioning his patients, he managed to restrict the spread of the anaesthetic to the required area evading the risk of hypotension [62].

He called attention to the option of restricting anaesthesia to one side by appropriately placing the patient. In order to avoid post-puncture cephalgia, he insisted on employing thin and blunt cannulae with a size of 20-22 gauge (◘ Fig. 2.14) [63]. Pitkin's publications were appreciated in Germany, where they had been spread by Helmut Schmidt of Hamburg by the end of the 1920s [64].

Paravertebral Conduction Anaesthesia

In order to avoid adverse effects of spinal anaesthesia, almost all regional anaesthesia procedures known today were developed during the ensuing years, including the paravertebral and epidural techniques that were applied for pain management after abdominal surgery.

Paravertebral anaesthesia was first described in 1908 by the obstetrician Hugo Sellheim (1871–1936) of Tübingen, although surgeons did not become interested in this technique until Max Kappis (1881–1938) of Hannover published articles on it [65]. Kappis suggested applying it to differentiate indistinct types of abdominal pain, a method that was approved by Arthur Läwen in Leipzig. For toxicological reasons, he already used bicarbonated solutions for regional anaesthesia in 1912, which resulted in improved quality and spread of sensitive and motoric block [66]. Novocain displayed a fast onset as well as an enduring analgesic effect. Läwen approved the extensive performance of paravertebral blocks for postoperative

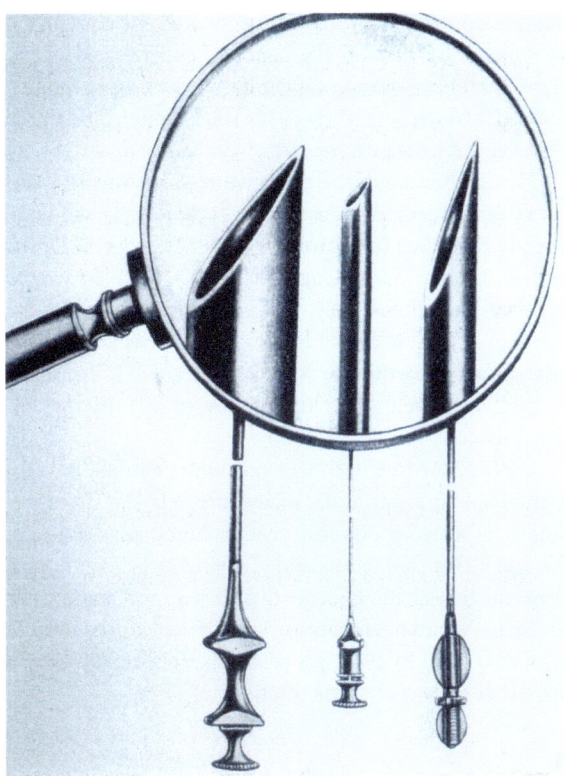

◘ **Fig. 2.14.** The cannulae recommended by Helmut Schmidt for spinal anaesthesia in 1929. Note that he advocated the cannula with the blunt, angled end shown in the *centre* of the picture as it was atraumatic

pain management as he believed this technique exhibited outstanding advantages in patients having undergone cholecystectomies, gastrectomies or nephrectomies. He hoped to decrease the incidence of postoperative pneumonia, as the absence of pain allowed patients to be at ease while breathing.

From Sacral to Epidural Anaesthesia

Läwen also played a role in spreading the use of epidural anaesthesia, which had been developed for pain management in urology and obstetrics. As the needle was inserted via the hiatus sacralis into the epidural space, the technique became known as »sacral anaesthesia«. According to the area covered it was divided into lower and upper sacral anaesthesia. For technical and pharmacological reasons, the quality of conduction anaesthesia was initially inferior; hence, gynaecologists and surgeons rejected it. These doubts did not keep Läwen from improving this technique and developing it into a safe procedure that also permitted operations of the upper abdomen by administering special mixtures of local anaesthetics and appropriately positioning the patient. He already combined epidural and general anaesthesia in 1912. He called attention to the good postoperative »somatic feeling«

that was confirmed by other surgeons. Despite convincing anaesthetic qualities in the hands of experienced physicians, sacral anaesthesia was forgotten and only regained popularity during the early 1930s when spinal anaesthesia experienced its renaissance [67].

Being unaware of the extensive research of the Spanish military surgeon Mirave Pagès (1886–1923), who had already described lumbar epidural puncture in 1920, the Italian Achille Mario Dogliotti (1897–1966) advocated regional anaesthesia [68]. By publishing articles in the German-speaking area his technique – usually called »peridural anaesthesia« – became accepted, especially as Dogliotti gave instructions on how to identify the epidural space.

As for Martin Kirschner's recommendations for segmental spinal anaesthesia, many surgeons, e.g. from Erlangen, reported good results with epidural anaesthesia in the late 1930s [69]. Some added a viscous gel solution to the local anaesthetic in order to affix the local anaesthetic to the nerves to obtain anaesthesia limited to the desired segments [70]. In 1943, gel solutions were replaced by a special viscous »Periston« solution.

Intravenous Techniques
Intravenous Ether Anaesthesia
Looking for alternatives to inhalation and regional anaesthesia, the surgeon Ludwig Burkhardt (1872–1922) of Würzburg invented intravenous chloroform and ether anaesthesia in 1910 that was well accepted for several years. After venesection performed, the patient received a prewarmed 4% ether solution had been inducing anaesthesia within a few minutes. As soon as anaesthesia was deep enough to perform surgery, the infusion was discontinued to be resumed if anaesthesia became too flat [71].

Numerous surgeons, like Hermann Kümmell (1852–1937) of Hamburg, favoured this technique and applied it for oral and facial surgery. Other procedures suitable for this method comprised brain surgery, surgery in patients with hypovolaemic shock, e.g. tubular pregnancy or traumatic rupture of the spleen (◻ Fig. 2.15; [72]). According to Kümmell many anaemic patients survived due to this practice. This seems feasible, since patients received up to 3 l of saline solutions doped with ether.

During World War I, intravenous ether was applied in injured soldiers; hence, the hospital surgeons in Nuremberg felt justified in employing it widely and in 1926 described 1,000 treatments without a single fatality [73].

The discovery of a new »class of sleep-introducing drugs« should also be mentioned: in 1902 Emil Fischer (1852–1919) and Joseph Freiherr von Mering (1849–1909) reported on »diethylbarbituric acid« [74]. »Ve-

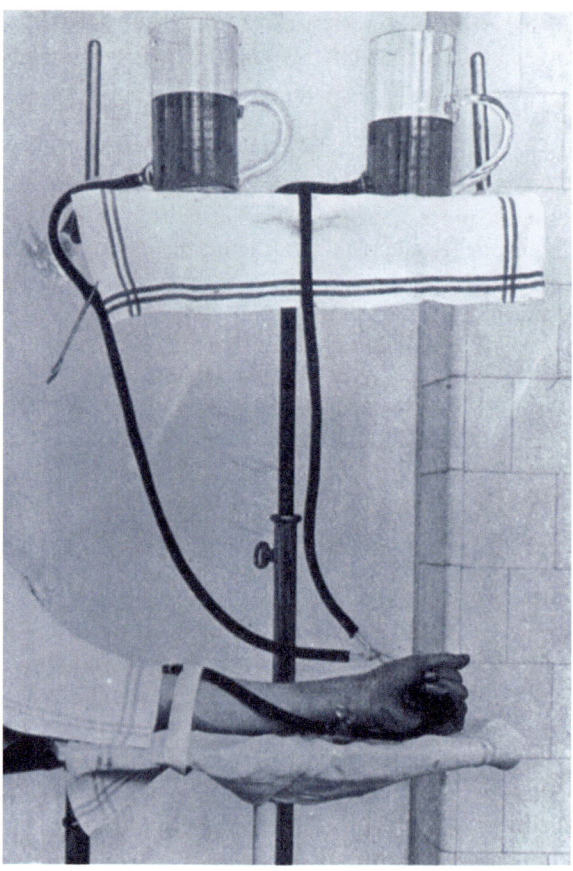

◻ **Fig. 2.15.** Instruments for intravenous ether anaesthesia as used in 1914 at the Eppendorf Hospital in Hamburg

ronal« was the first drug that was used for a long time and became the main substance of this new group of agents. Its pharmacological properties allowed oral application only. With the synthesis of intravenous derivatives of barbiturates in the early 1920s, they could be administered during surgery, too.

Evipan
With the introduction of the derivative Evipan that could be injected intravenously demonstrating a short period of action, Hellmut Weese (1897–1954) (◻ Fig. 2.16a) heralded a new era for anaesthesiology in 1932 [75].

With the »sleep-inducing injection into the arm«, the patients were spared the rather unpleasant sensation experienced during induction with volatile anaesthetics. Within a few months, it was applied countless times, without any documented adverse events. Weese became »the creator of modern, intravenous anaesthesia which triumphed around the world«, as his colleague and friend Hans Killian (1892–1982) declared in 1954 [76]. This was no embellishment: within 10 years, more than 10 million applications could be reported (◻ Fig. 2.16b) [77].

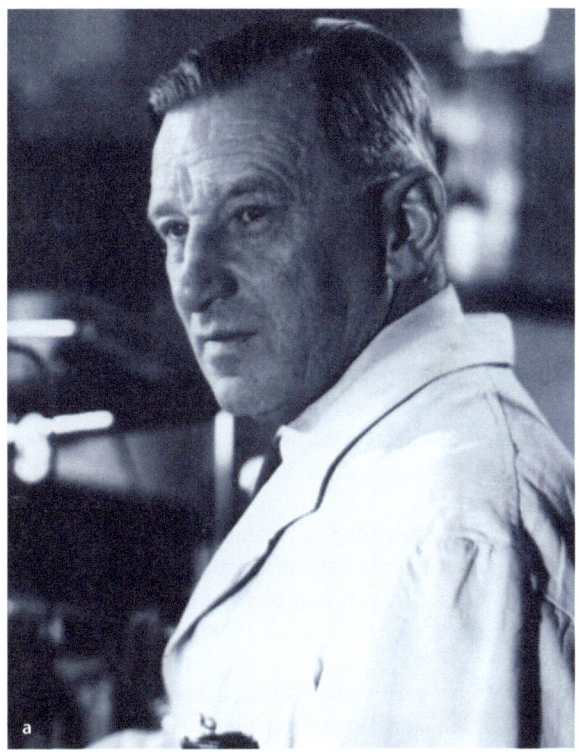

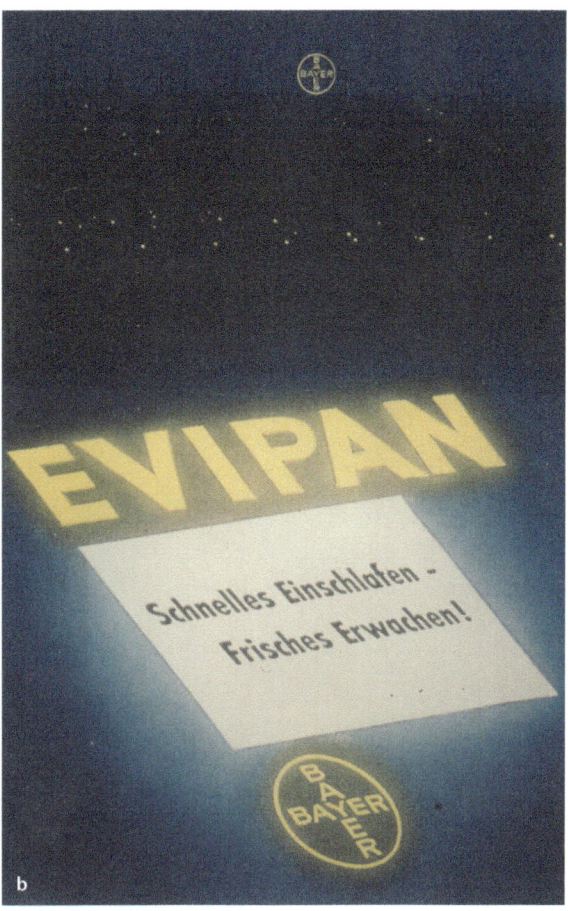

Fig. 2.16a,b. a Helmut Weese (1897–1954). He was involved in the introduction of Evipan in 1932 and also in the development of the blood substitute Periston. After World War II he was influential in the founding of the German Society of Anaesthesia. **b** Advertisement for Evipan

In recognition of his contributions to the introduction of Evipan, Weese was repeatedly honoured, e.g. in 1938, when he became Honorary Member of the International Research Society in New York. Before this, he had assured himself of the high standard of anaesthesia at numerous universities; hence, after World War II he advocated the introduction of anaesthesiology as a specialty in Germany, too.

Rectal Anaesthesia Techniques

With Evipan anaesthesia being accepted by surgeons, other methods were superfluous, especially as they were regarded as controversial right from the beginning: the rectally administered Avertin anaesthesia. The advantages of rectal anaesthesia, such as being convenient, preventing excitation and being accepted by patients, were the main arguments when it was launched in 1927 by the surgeon Otto Butzengeiger (1885–1968; **Fig. 2.17**) of Wuppertal. The action of Avertin was overwhelming as induction of anaesthesia in a quiet environment was smooth and did not show signs of excitation.

Within 4 min, the patient fell asleep, and after 6-8 min, a deep sleep was established; therefore, Avertin was applied in cases where tension, anxiety and restlessness during preparation for anaesthesia and surgery were to be avoided. This technique was chosen for children and those suffering from Basedow's disease. Thus, rectal application of Avertin became a precious tool in anaesthesiology until the middle of the 1960s [78].

Blood Transfusion and Infusion

When the surgeon Rudolph Bumm (1899–1942) of Berlin tried to induce anaesthesia with the aid of the barbiturate Pernocton at the Charité, the transfusion of blood was already known, but not performed regularly, as confirmed by notes from the Department of Surgery at the University of Heidelberg: only 25 blood transfusions were carried out in 1927 [79, 80].

The procedure of transfusing blood became safer when the surgeon Franz Oehlecker (1874–1957; **Fig. 2.18a**) of Hamburg developed a biological test in 1920: the recipient was given a few millilitres of donor blood with a glass

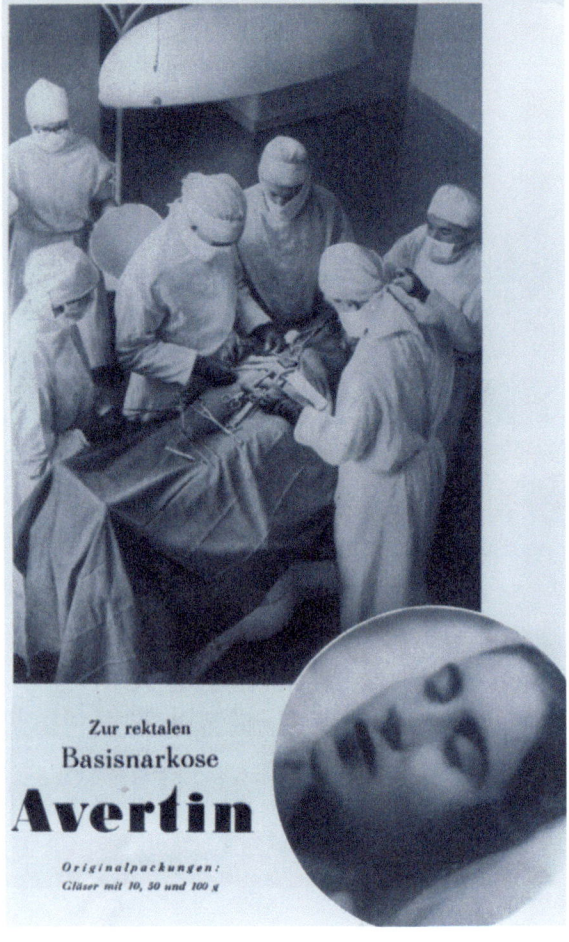

Zur rektalen
Basisnarkose

Avertin

Originalpackungen:
Gläser mit 10, 50 und 100 g

Fig. 2.17. Advertisement for the rectal anaesthetic Avertin

syringe (Fig. 2.18b). If any signs of adverse reactions occurred, like lower back pain or strange sensations in the vein, sweating or tachycardia, the transfusions were stopped. The test was repeated with the blood from another donor [81].

With growing experience and safety of blood transfusions – by the middle of the 1920s kits to determine blood groups had become available – the need for blood grew steadily; therefore, consideration was given to launching »blood donor services«. Institutions within hospitals became known as »institutes for transfusion«, »blood banks« or »blood donation services« and were established in the early 1930s. Usually surgeons were in charge of these organizations, e.g. Paul Clairmont (1875–1942) in Zurich or Ernst Unger (1875–1938) in Berlin [82].

With the increasing acceptance of anaesthesia, subcutaneous and intramuscular injections were introduced. Intravenous techniques were believed to be too dangerous and therefore rejected for a long time; hence, patients with severe hypovolaemia were not supplied with saline solutions. After experiments on animals had been performed by the physiologist Hugo Kronecker (1839–1914) and the gynaecologist Emil Schwarz (1865–1918), predominantly surgeons and obstetricians dared to apply this new technique [83].

Prior to World War I, several solutions for infusion for the management of acute anaemia became available as intravenous administration came into vogue. Their exact configuration, though, was to be discussed for years. »Serum saline solution« developed by the pharmacolo-

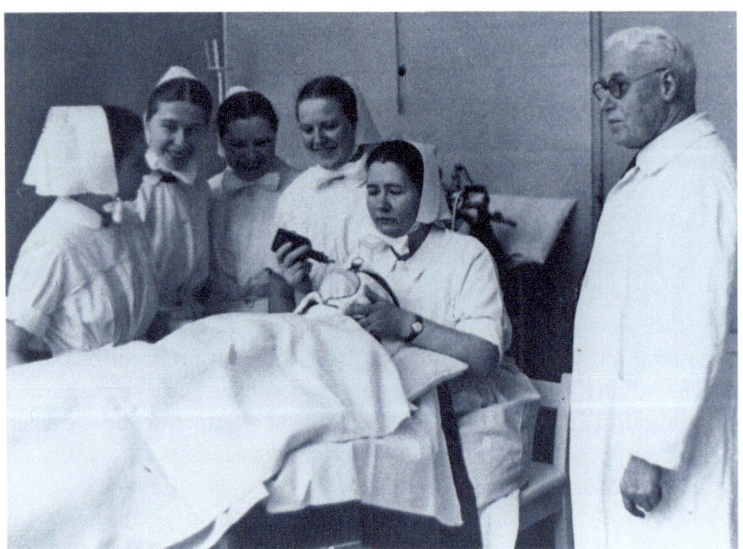

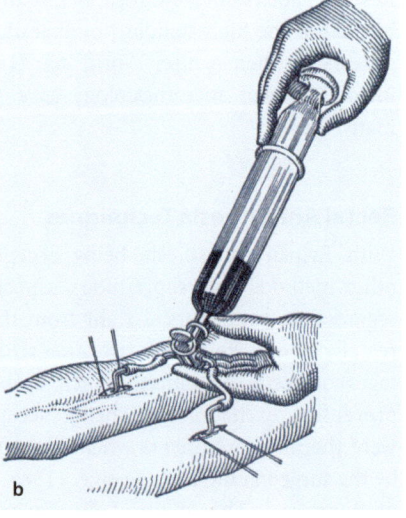

b

Fig. 2.18a,b. a Ether drop anaesthesia around 1940. Nurses usually performed anaesthesia. The picture shows the surgeon Franz Oehlecker of Hamburg, who initiated blood transfusion in Germany. **b** Blood transfusion with a glass syringe as advocated by Oehlecker

gist Walter Straub (1874–1944) became widespread since it could be prepared from hot water and a powder, and »Normosal solution« manufactured at the »Sächsische Serum-Werk« was available in ampoules by the middle of the 1920s [84].

By the end of the 1920s patients suffering from acute anaemia were infused with hypertonic solutions in order to quickly replenish intravascular volume. In a review the surgeon Friedrich Schück (1888–1958) of Berlin pointed out the positive effects on circulation that »usually could be confirmed after 3 min and were definitely present after 5 min« [85].

By the middle of the 1920s, different solutions with various ingredients had become available for infusion, some of them in sterile bottles. During World War II the lack of indifferent and well-tolerated blood volume expanders with an enduring effect became apparent. Hellmut Weese (1897–1954) developed the isotonic colloid solution named »Periston« (◻ Fig. 2.19) to overcome this dilemma. It was administered successfully in severe trauma and cardiocirculatory depression due to infections and burns [86].

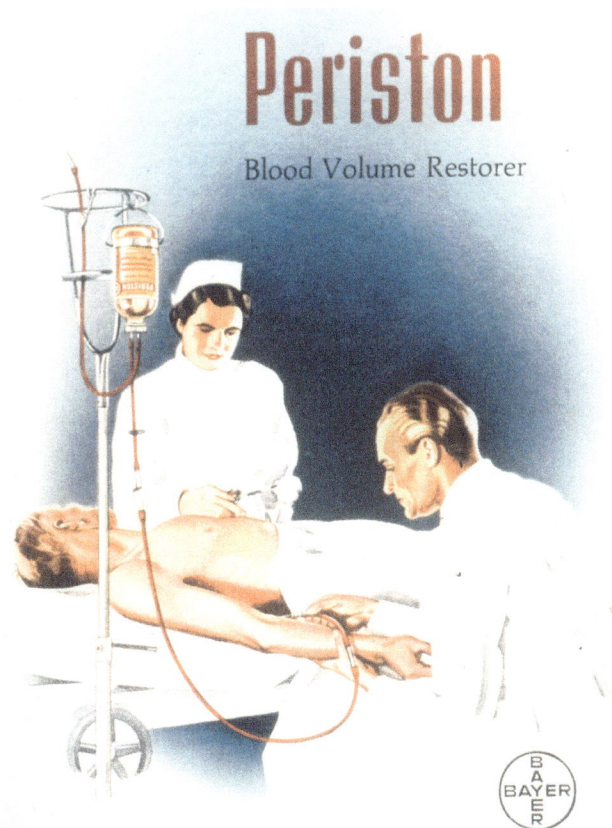

◻ **Fig. 2.19.** Advertisement for the blood volume restorer »Periston«

Monitoring and Documentation of Anaesthetized Patients

Although the surgeon Johann Ferdinand Heyfelder (1798–1868) of Erlangen had already demanded in 1847 that »circulation and respiration be constantly observed during anaesthesia«, no anaesthesia charts were kept [87]. By the turn of the century heart rate, blood pressure and the amount of anaesthetics were noted in »ether charts«, which can be attributed to the efforts of the American surgeon Harvey Cushing (1863–1937). While travelling in Europe, Cushing discovered the sphygmomanometer developed by Scipione Riva-Rocci (1863–1937) and had a similar apparatus built for himself on his return to the United States [88].

In the beginning, his colleagues declined to record blood pressure in anaesthesia charts. In 1903, his recommendation was rejected in an official statement of the Massachusetts General Hospital: »The adoption of blood pressure measurement in surgical patients does not at present appear to be necessary as a routine measure« [89].

Despite this statement, an increasing number of surgeons documented their intraoperative observations, i.e. quality of pulse, blood pressure, breathing as well as amounts of anaesthetics in »anaesthesia protocols«. The introduction of anaesthesia charts into Germany can be attributed to the surgeon Helmut Schmidt (1895–1979) (◻ Fig. 2.20) of Hamburg, who appreciated the advantages of close intraoperative documentation of vital parameters during a trip to the United States at the end of the 1920s. After returning to Germany, he introduced the anaesthesia protocol, which he called »anaesthesia table«, into the Department of Surgery at the Eppendorf Hospital in Hamburg in 1929 (◻ Fig. 2.21). It has been used with minor modifications for many decades. Schmidt was also not supported by his colleagues when introducing this form, which is now a matter of course [90].

Automated Measurement of Blood Pressure

In 1933 the Siemens Company invented the »Autonograph« for continuous measurement of blood pressure that provided a printout of its recordings. It was therefore recommended for »safer anaesthesia«: »...The blood pressure data« can be »consulted at any time as evidence for flawless monitoring of the anaesthesia should any lawsuits arise« [91].

The surgeon Fritz von Schürer-Waldheim (1896–1990) of Vienna was also involved in the development of similar devices and presented the »Kardiotron« at the German Surgeons' Congress in 1937. It allowed the surveillance of cardiocirculatory parameters. Facilitated by the invention of piezoelectronic crystals, the tool recognized even weak levels of the heart rate or blood pressure and transformed this information into acoustic and optical signals to alert the anaesthesiologist [92] (◻ Fig. 2.22). The advantages of

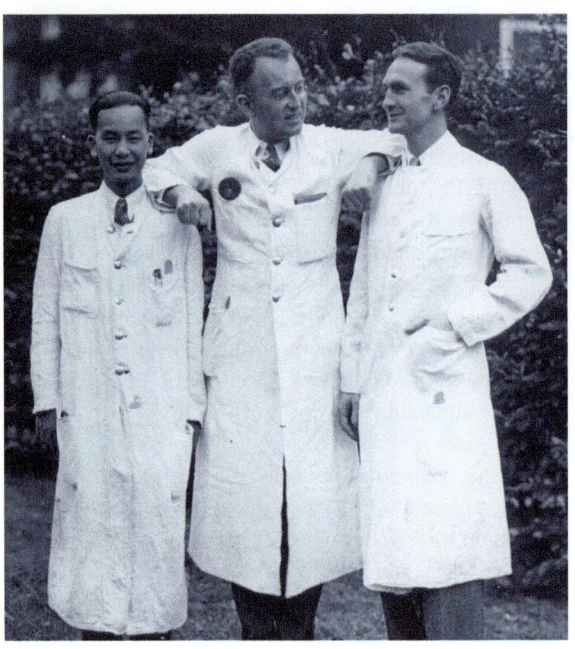

Fig. 2.20. The surgeon Helmut Schmidt (*centre*) of Hamburg with two American guests. Due to his research and publications, nitrous oxide and oxygen anaesthesia could become established in Germany by the beginning of the 1930s

»in somno securitas« were accepted internationally, e.g. by the anaesthesiologist John Silas Lundy (1894–1973) at the Mayo Clinic in Rochester, who had seen such an apparatus at the Karolinska Hospital in Stockholm [93].

Intraoperative Electrocardiogram

Continuous monitoring of electric heart activity was introduced to operating theatres during the 1970s. Initial attempts had already been made at the end of the 1920s, e.g. at the Surgical University Clinic in Freiburg. Using a special arrangement of mirrors, the ECG was projected onto the wall of the operating theatre. However, an analysis was impossible, since artefacts due to the patient's movement as well as surgical or anaesthetic manipulation could not be repressed [94].

Postoperative Monitoring of the Surgical Patient

Early on, surgeons demanded that patients be monitored closely in the intraoperative as well as the postoperative stage; thus, today's standard of recovery rooms or intensive care units cannot be labelled modern achievements. As early as at the turn of the century, surgical units in newly built hospitals were equipped with surveillance rooms. As Walter Kausch (1865–1928) mentioned at the

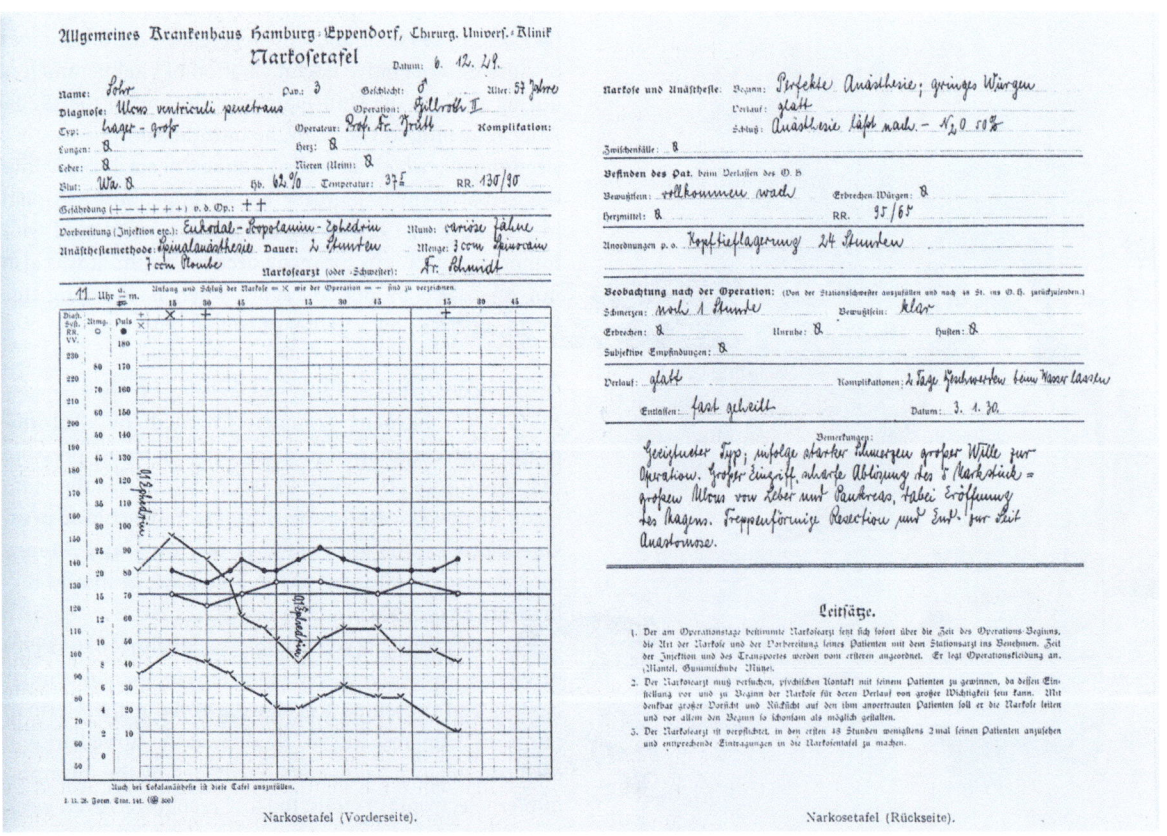

Fig. 2.21. Front and back page of the first anaesthesia chart to be used in Germany introduced in 1928 by the surgeon Helmut Schmidt, who was employed at the Eppendorf Hospital in Hamburg

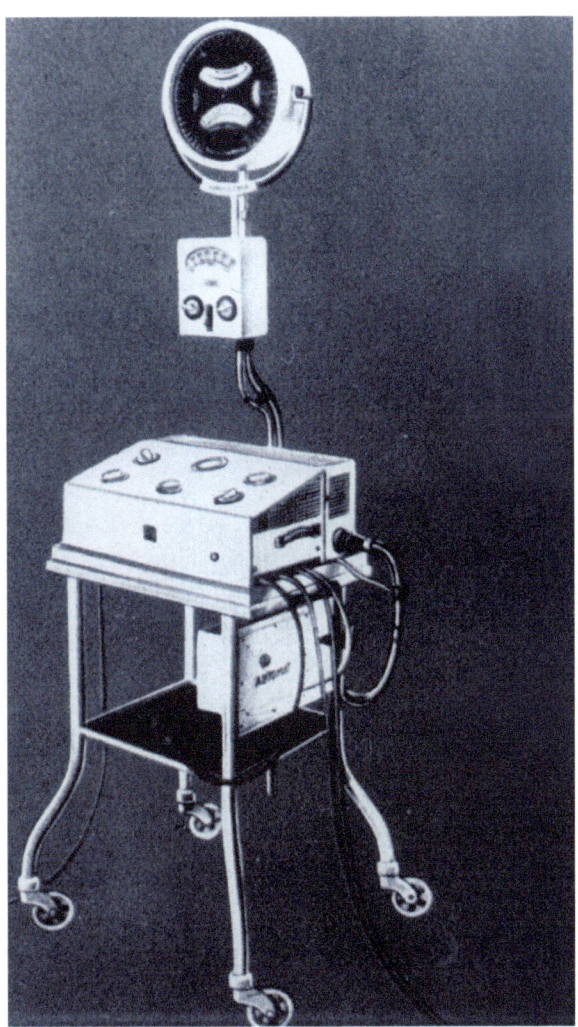

Fig. 2.22. The automatic documentation and printing of recorded parameters of heart rate and blood pressure using the »Kardiotron«, a monitor developed around 1938 by the surgeon Fritz von Schürer of Vienna. The device allowed continuous monitoring of heart rate, blood pressure and respiratory rate. It alerted the anaesthetist with the aid of acoustic or optical signals

inauguration of the new wing at the Urban Auguste-Viktoria Hospital in Berlin: »a recovery room for patients, who require further medical attention« is »an important room that can hardly be found elsewhere« [95].

The surgeon Martin Kirschner (1879–1942) of Tübingen who was open-minded with regard to innovations, appreciated these advantages and insisted that »a department for newly operated and severely ill patients« be built in the wing of the Department of Surgery erected in 1930 where »care during the day and especially at night…provided by trained and experienced personnel« was assured. Next to nurses, this unit was to be staffed with a senior physician, who could make important medical decisions himself. Kirschner also pointed out

the importance of close and trusting collaboration with nurses, as the »impression of a skilful experienced head nurse…would paint a clearer picture than any complicated examination by a physician« [96].

Specialization in Anaesthesiology

Although anaesthesia was conducted by physicians initially, this task soon was conferred to nurses. This was retained through the twentieth century, even though the risks of ether and chloroform were soon disclosed.

Early Suggestion for Specialization in Anaesthesiology

This development should be surprising since Johann Ferdinand Heyfelder (1798–1868) had already demanded in 1847 that

> only lucid and meticulous doctors should be permitted to perform anaesthesia who are able to make distinctions and do not behave tediously by always following the same principle. All lower ranked medical personnel like midwives, barber-surgeons or whatever they are called should not conduct ether inhalation anaesthesia… [87].

Acknowledgement of Well-Performed Anaesthesia

The surgeon Nepomuk Nussbaum (1829–1890) of Munich described in 1878 »the art of anaesthesia« as

> not minor since it requires more knowledge, patience and energy than major surgery. For this reason, there are many more surgeons who can operate beautifully than those who can anaesthetize beautifully with chloroform. This procedure, however, is so important that it is not possible to be too diligent [97].

The Swiss surgeon Otto Kappeler (1841–1909) also acknowledged this improvement and stated in 1890: »Does not the English custom, which transfers responsibility of anaesthesia to an anaesthetetist, and the surgeon therefore leaves the responsibility of anaesthetizing with them, contain significant dangers?« [98].

Despite the obvious connection between a lack of experience and a higher incidence of complications, Kappeler was not able to advocate an independent »chloroformist«, because he, too, was afraid of surgery splintering into separate specialties [99].

Arguments in Favour of Specialization in Anaesthesiology

The requests for specialization continued and elicited statements by several doctors as well as state institutions. The internist Heinrich Quincke (1844–1922) of Kiel encouraged – »if necessary« – state-controlled »development of a specialty«, whereas the Prussian Ministry of

Culture admonished in a publication in 1891 that there was a growing tendency toward specialization that had also taken hold of anaesthesia [100].

This might have contributed to declining requests by the surgeon Carl Ludwig Schleich (1859–1922) of Berlin that anaesthesia be improved by state authorities. He was the first surgeon to condemn the detrimental conditions during anaesthesia and insisted on improved training in anaesthesiology. Schleich was supported in his quest for reorganization of anaesthesiology [101]. His colleague Heinz Wohlgemuth (1863–1936) of Berlin referred to this problem for many years in numerous articles [102].

He was supported by a growing number of renowned surgeons. They pointed out the benefits for their patients and regretted that »professional anaesthetists had not been established here, like for example in England… If this had been the case, voices against general anaesthesia would not be that strong«, as stated by the surgeon Anton Freiherr von Eiselsberg (1860–1939) of Vienna [103].

Hans Kehr (1862–1916) called it »serious nonsense« to leave anaesthesia to just anyone since »skilful anaesthesia is almost more precious than the surgical technique or the most efficient assistance«. Without denying the meticulousness and care of a nurse responsible for anaesthesia, patients in his clinic were anaesthetized by an experienced physician ensuring his slogan: »only a physician should conduct anaesthesia« [104].

According to Benno Wilhelm Müller (1873–1947) working in Hamburg, the deplorable state of affairs in anaesthesia was based on lack of experience and insufficient training of the anaesthesiologists. Nevertheless, he hoped for the future as stated in his textbook of 1908: »It is only a question of time, and even in Germany there will be a change in surgical clinics and we will employ special physicians, who are solely in charge of the anaesthesia« [105].

Opposition Against Specialization in Anaesthesiology Arising

The deplorable state of anaesthesiology must have been severe until the early twentieth century, as Heinrich Braun (1862–1934) states in his biography: »There were very few places in Germany where skilled anaesthesia was conducted and the complaints of von Schleich and Dumont about the insufficient training of medical doctors in anaesthesia and its technique were well justified« [106].

To conclude that Braun supported the establishment of the specialty in anaesthesiology would be embellishing. As opposed to this the surgeon Friedrich Pels-Leusden (1866–1944) of Greifswald argued in a popular textbook: »Fortunately we do not have specialists in anaesthesiology like in the United States and hopefully they will never annoy us« [107].

Pels-Leusden's rigorous rejection has to be judged in the context of requests for reorganization of anaesthesiol-

ogy and establishment of separate specialists that emerged after the end of World War I. This debate culminated in demands for civil servant status of anaesthesiologists that were primarily initiated by military doctors returning from internment or allied detention [108]. They repeatedly stipulated »that the glorious and beneficial institution of the specialty of anaesthesia should soon become established in Germany« [109].

As opposed to the Anglo-American countries, the achievements in anaesthesiology were not appreciated in Germany, and therefore only a few medical doctors were interested in becoming »professional anaesthesiologists« [110]. Max Kappis (1871–1938) argued that this was the main reason for the lack of interest in issues of anaesthesiology:

> I believe that Germany is currently too poor to pay specialists in anaesthesia well enough, which remains the linchpin for anaesthesiologists and trainees. Therefore, surgery in Germany will have to exist without this advantage for years to come, even decades [111].

The Contribution of Ernst von der Porten und Helmut Schmidt of Hamburg

This pessimistic assessment did not prevent physicians from exclusively conducting anaesthesia. Ernst von der Porten (1884–1940; ◻ Fig. 2.23) was among them, as he

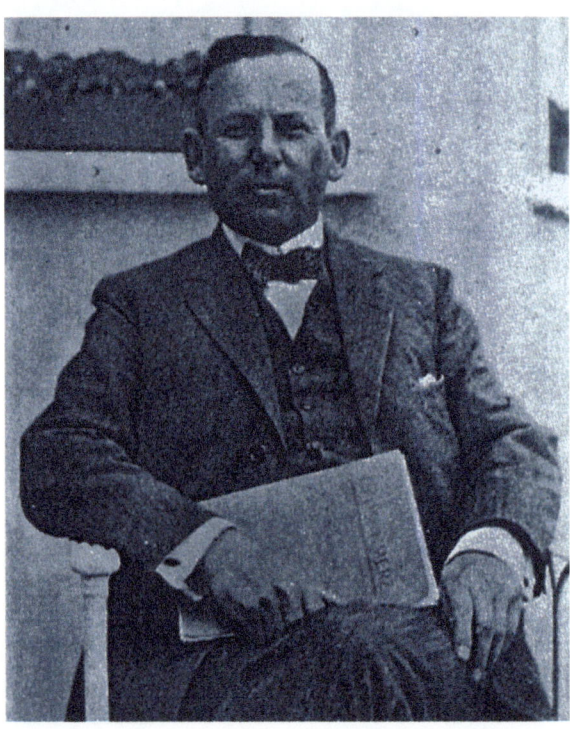

◻ **Fig. 2.23.** Ernst von der Porten, who worked in Hamburg as a specialist in anaesthesia and who advocated establishing anaesthesiology as a specialty

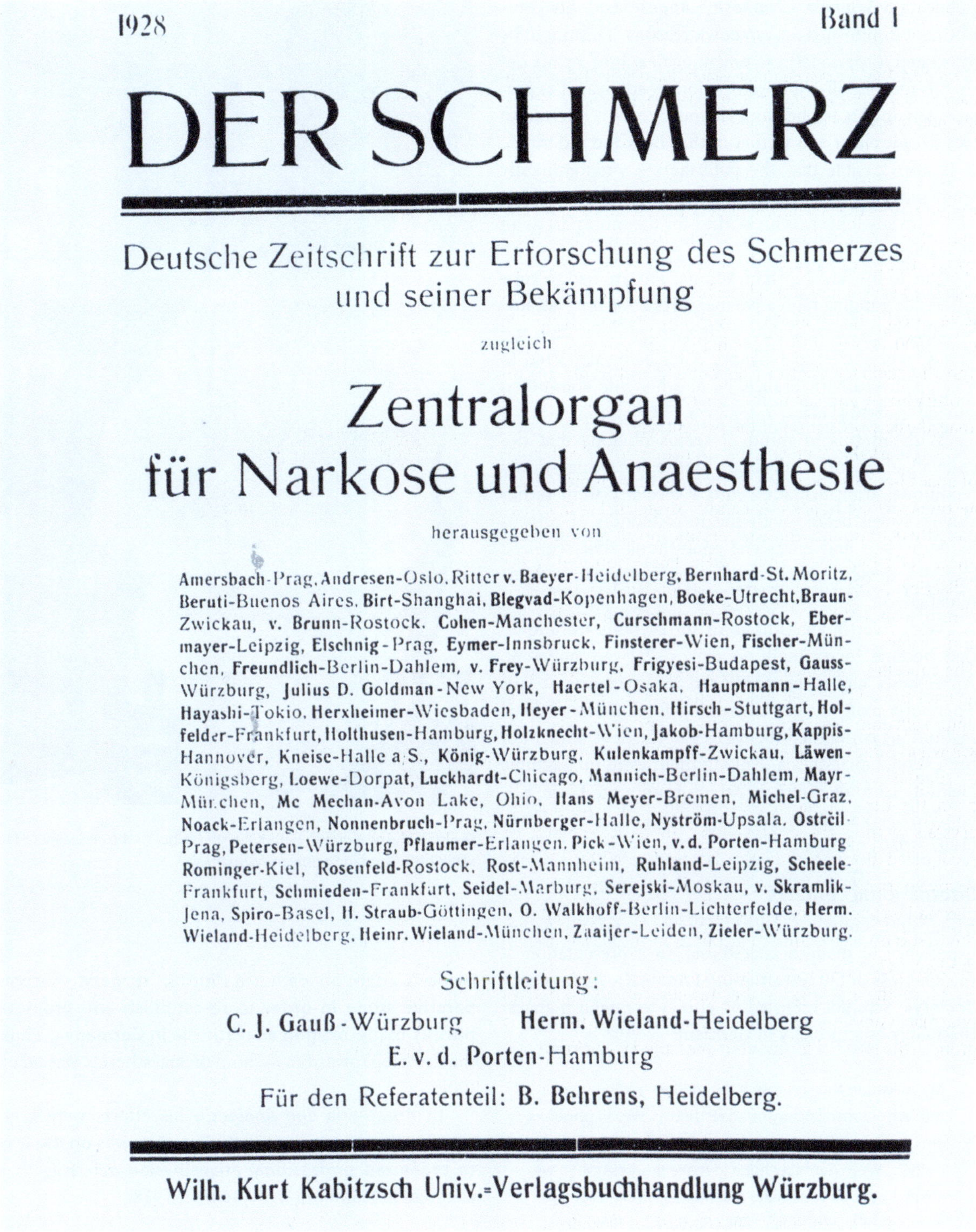

1928   Band 1

DER SCHMERZ

Deutsche Zeitschrift zur Erforschung des Schmerzes
und seiner Bekämpfung

zugleich

Zentralorgan
für Narkose und Anaesthesie

herausgegeben von

Amersbach-Prag, Andresen-Oslo, Ritter v. Baeyer-Heidelberg, Bernhard-St. Moritz,
Beruti-Buenos Aires, Birt-Shanghai, Blegvad-Kopenhagen, Boeke-Utrecht, Braun-
Zwickau, v. Brunn-Rostock, Cohen-Manchester, Curschmann-Rostock, Eber-
mayer-Leipzig, Elschnig-Prag, Eymer-Innsbruck, Finsterer-Wien, Fischer-Mün-
chen, Freundlich-Berlin-Dahlem, v. Frey-Würzburg, Frigyesi-Budapest, Gauss-
Würzburg, Julius D. Goldman-New York, Haertel-Osaka, Hauptmann-Halle,
Hayashi-Tokio, Herxheimer-Wiesbaden, Heyer-München, Hirsch-Stuttgart, Hol-
felder-Frankfurt, Holthusen-Hamburg, Holzknecht-Wien, Jakob-Hamburg, Kappis-
Hannover, Kneise-Halle a. S., König-Würzburg, Kulenkampff-Zwickau, Läwen-
Königsberg, Loewe-Dorpat, Luckhardt-Chicago, Mannich-Berlin-Dahlem, Mayr-
München, Mc Mechan-Avon Lake, Ohio, Hans Meyer-Bremen, Michel-Graz,
Noack-Erlangen, Nonnenbruch-Prag, Nürnberger-Halle, Nyström-Upsala, Ostreil-
Prag, Petersen-Würzburg, Pflaumer-Erlangen, Pick-Wien, v. d. Porten-Hamburg
Rominger-Kiel, Rosenfeld-Rostock, Rost-Mannheim, Ruhland-Leipzig, Scheele-
Frankfurt, Schmieden-Frankfurt, Seidel-Marburg, Serejski-Moskau, v. Skramlik-
Jena, Spiro-Basel, H. Straub-Göttingen, O. Walkhoff-Berlin-Lichterfelde, Herm.
Wieland-Heidelberg, Heinr. Wieland-München, Zaaijer-Leiden, Zieler-Würzburg.

Schriftleitung:

C. J. Gauß-Würzburg   Herm. Wieland-Heidelberg

E. v. d. Porten-Hamburg

Für den Referatenteil: B. Behrens, Heidelberg.

Wilh. Kurt Kabitzsch Univ.=Verlagsbuchhandlung Würzburg.

Fig. 2.24. Cover page of the first German anaesthesia journal *Der Schmerz* in 1928

had assisted Paul Sudeck (1866–1945) – who also was interested in anaesthesia – as an »Anaesthesia Specialist« in Hamburg prior to World War I. Von der Porten advocated improvement of anaesthesiology in Germany and was a founding member of the first German anaesthesia journal *Der Schmerz* in 1928 [112] (Fig. 2.24).

When the journal merged with the competing magazine *Narkose und Anaesthesie* in 1929 to form the new publication *Schmerz – Narkose – Anaesthesie,* his commitment diminished for unknown reasons. This might be attributed to personal resentment against him, as his demands for specialization were no longer advocated as passionately in this publication. Helmut Schmidt referred to this decades later as a victory of the »bearded old men«. It is also feasible that the publishers – predominantly from universities – had not been interested in working with him any longer, as he worked for the most part as an anaesthetist.

Due to his Jewish origin, von der Porten had to cope with wide-ranging repressive measures after the National Socialist Party came to power. He managed to escape and first sought shelter in Belgium. After being deported to a camp in southern France, he and his wife committed suicide in 1940 [112].

With all this in mind, it seems obvious that despite all advances in inhalation and regional anaesthesia techniques transformation into a specialty went rather slowly. Nevertheless, with the introduction of nitrous oxide/oxygen and narcylene anaesthesia that required complex devices, the search for trained personnel intensified.

With Avertin anaesthesia or intravenous techniques that became increasingly popular, risks were apparent. Anaesthesia had to be conducted by specialists at last. Therefore, many surgeons working for university-based institutions committed themselves to the development of professional anaesthesia. Among them were for example Helmut Schmidt (1895–1979) of Hamburg, Hans Killian (1892–1982; ◻ Fig. 2.25) of Freiburg and Fritz Hesse (1897–1980) of Leipzig [113].

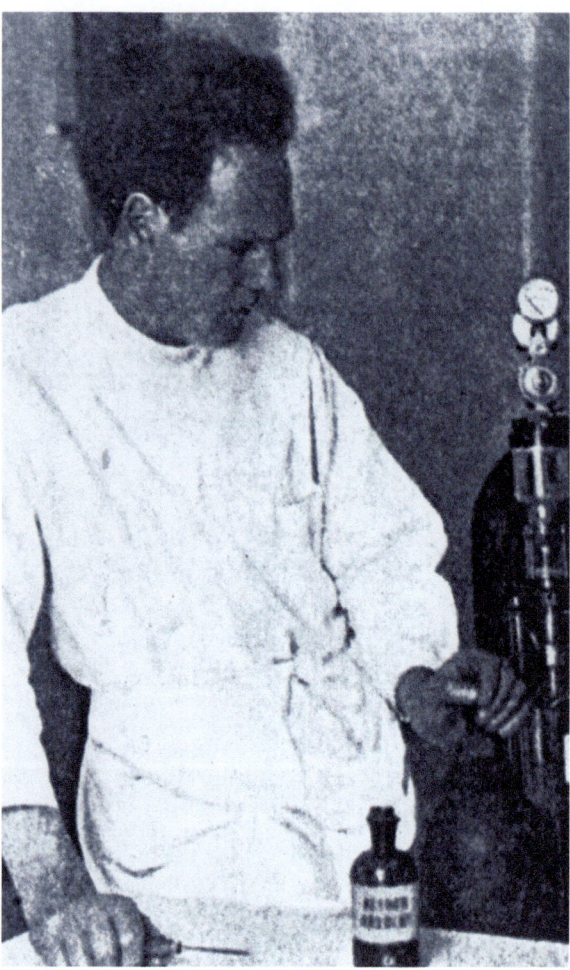

◻ **Fig. 2.25.** The surgeon Hans Killian of Freiburg, who endeavoured to establish a German Society of Anaesthesia

International Contacts

Killian and Schmidt travelled to North America to gather experience in modern anaesthesia. In a presentation at the congress of the »International Anaesthesia Research Society«, Schmidt reported on efforts to establish anaesthesiology as a specialty in Germany:

> My colleague and I represent the modest beginning of a modern German Society of Anaesthetists. We, as surgeons, are convinced of the importance of anaesthesia as a specialty … We in Germany hope to make progress when we are in a position to educate practitioners in the expert methods of anaesthesia … The University of Hamburg is the first in Germany to attempt this and as a lecturer there it will be my special desire to develop the educational aims and progress of this most important branch of medical practice. It is our intention to establish in Hamburg a school of anaesthesia … [114]

In 1928, Schmidt was awarded the title of Professor and published a thesis entitled »The efficiency of nitrous-oxide-oxygen anaesthesia during surgery. A comparative study in order to re-establish and promote nitrous-oxide-oxygen anaesthesia in Germany«. Thus, the first step towards a »school of anaesthesia« was taken [90].

In *Anesthesia and Analgesia* his efforts were honoured with the comment that »Germany was on the way to organized professional anaesthesia«, referring to a congress in Hamburg in September 1928:

> … A congress of physicians and scientists which will take place in Hamburg, Germany, in September of this year and will then be made the basis of a plan for swinging Germany into line for professional anaesthesia and association with the international organization of the specialty.

According to this report everyone was convinced that »when the German medical profession becomes convinced that organized professional anaesthesia is the thing, the specialty will be rapidly developed« [114].

The 90th Meeting of the German Association for the Advancement of Science and Medicine in Hamburg in 1928 – Advertising the Specialty of Anaesthesiology

In September 1928, the 90th Meeting of the German Association for the Advancement of Science and Medicine (Gesellschaft Deutscher Naturforscher und Ärzte) was held in Hamburg. It was a meeting of surgical, pharmacological, obstetrical and gynaecological departments on the subject of »gas anaesthesia and its impact on problems in anaesthesia«, discussing issues in anaesthesiology. After the introduction of the protagonists, a German Society of Anaesthesia was to be founded. In his capacity as General Secretary, Francis Hoeffer McMechan (1879–1939) conveyed greetings from the »International Anesthesia Research Society« and pointed out the significance of the meeting: »When we heard in America that Germany intended to hold a conference on issues in anesthesia for the first time, we spared no efforts to appear at this important meeting« [115].

In a report on the meeting, he again honoured the event: »Thursday, September 20, 1928, will long be remembered as the day on which the specialty of anaesthesia came into its own in Germany« [115]. At that meeting Schmidt as well as Killian had advocated the »specialization of anaesthesiology«. Schmidt especially demanded that the art of anaesthesia be improved, not by employing nurses and occasional anaesthesiologists, but by engaging specialists for »safety first anaesthesia« that could only be achieved when performed by specialists.

The Surgeons' Reactions

Although the problem of separating anaesthesia from surgery was not mentioned in the numerous talks and lectures and there were no further calls for the creation of a German Society of Anaesthesia, one delegate, i.e. the Professor of Surgery Eduard Rehn (1880–1972) of Freiburg, rejected all attempts towards specialization of anaesthesia in his closing speech: »I cannot agree with this suggestion and I believe this is rather too early in view of our circumstances... Likewise, I have to reject the establishment of a lectureship for anaesthesia«. Rehn extended his disapproval, stating that he was not convinced about »the introduction of college-based lessons in anaesthesia on clinical material« [116].

Hans Killian's Suggestions for Reorganization of Anaesthesiology in Germany

The discussions on founding a German Society of Anaesthesia were terminated for the time being. Another

10 years later Hans Killian made another attempt in this direction at the Congress of Surgeons in Berlin in 1939. Since several complaints had been lodged to the *Reichsgesundheitsführer* Leonardo Conti (1900–1945) on deficiencies of the conduction of anaesthesia in German institutions, Killian published his demands – dating back to 1939 – for reorganization of anaesthesia in Germany in the journal *Schmerz – Narkose – Anaesthesie* in 1941, thus making them public [117]. Although this issue was approached at the last Congress of Surgery held during the war in 1943, the turmoil of the war most likely was the reason that prevented further discussions.

Influenced by the advances in the field of anaesthesia in the United States and England during the late 1940s, Germany also started discussions on anaesthesia and the foundation of anaesthesia as its own specialty [118]. Hans Killian as well as Hellmut Weese again belonged to the group favouring the separation of anaesthesiology that finally was to come about in 1953 [119].

Important Developments in Anaesthesia from 1880 to 1950

- 1884 Carl Koller discovers the anaesthetic qualities of cocaine.
- 1888 Maximilian Oberst develops *Oberst'sche Anaesthesie*, which became well-known through an article published by his colleague Ludwig Pernice in 1890.
- 1890 Curt Schimmelbusch presents his anaesthesia mask.
- 1892 Carl Ludwig Schleich advocates the use of »infiltration anaesthesia«.
- 1893 Viktor Eisenmenger develops an endotracheal tube made of rubber equipped with a cuff and a balloon.
- 1895 Julius Ernst Gurlt provides evidence for the advantages of ether over chloroform anaesthesia.
- 1896 Alfred Kirstein publishes his monograph »*Die Autoskopie des Kehlkopfes und der Luftröhre*« (autoscopy of the larynx and the trachea).
- 1898 August Bier conducts the first spinal anaesthesia.
- 1900 Eduard Schneiderlin administers a scopolamine-morphine mixture for analgesia.
- 1901 Hans Horst Meyer and Charles Overton develop the lipoid theory of anaesthesia.
- 1902 The Dräger Company produces anaesthesia machines equipped with cylinders for air-oxygen mixtures containing a patented drip device for chloroform.
- 1903 Emil Fischer and Joseph Freiherr von Mering introduce the first barbiturate »Veronal«.
- 1903 Richard von Steinbüchel asserts the advantages of preoperative application of scopolamine and mor-

phine in obstetrics producing »twilight sleep« according to Carl-Joseph Gauss.

— 1904 Alfred Einhorn synthesizes Novocain.
— 1905 Heinrich Braun administers Novocain to a patient for the first time.
— 1907 The first model of the Pulmotor is presented.
— 1908 August Bier describes intravenous regional anaesthesia.
— 1910 Maximilian Neu presents a nitrous oxide/oxygen anaesthesia apparatus equipped with rotameters for an exact dosage of gases.
— 1911 Franz Kuhn publishes his monograph »*Die perorale Intubation*«.
— 1912 Arthur Läwen applies curare to a human for the first time.
— 1916 Elisabeth Brendenfeld reports on intravenous application of morphine and scopolamine.
— 1918 Georg Kelling points towards hazards of chronic exposure to volatile anaesthetics.
— 1921 Fidel Pagès describes the lumbar access to the epidural space.
— 1922 Anton Hellwig reports on life-saving properties of »Lobelin« during anaesthesia.
— 1923 Carl Joseph Gauß and Hermann Wieland administer narcylene via a closed-circuit anaesthesia device for the first time.
— 1925 invention of the anaesthesia apparatus »Model A« by the Dräger Company for nitrous-oxide/oxygen anaesthesia.
— 1927 Otto Butzengeiger reports on rectal application of the anaesthetic »Avertin«.
— 1927 Werner Forssmann introduces a catheter into his heart.
— 1928 the journals *Der Schmerz* and *Narkose und Anaesthesie* are published in Germany.
— 1929 Hans Berger initiates the observation of the EEG during anaesthesia.
— 1930 Helmut Schmidt proposes the use of anaesthesia charts.
— 1931 Achille Dogliotti again calls attention to the lumbar access for epidural anaesthesia.
— 1932 Hellmut Weese reports on successful application of »Evipan«.
— 1933 devices to automatically measure blood pressure become available.
— 1939 Otto Schaumann and Otto Eisleb manufacture the first artificial opioid »Pethidin«.
— 1940 Norbert Henning proposes intraosseous injections.
— 1942 Carl Joseph Gauss utilizes nitrous-oxide/oxygen analgesia apparatus in obstetrics.
— 1943 Gerhard Hecht and Hellmut Weese publish a report on the blood volume restorer »Periston«.
— 1948 nitrous-oxide/oxygen apparatus equipped with flow meters become available.

— 1949 foundation of a committee by the *Deutsche Gesellschaft für Chirurgie* and the *Deutsche Gesellschaft für Pharmakologie.*

Selected Textbooks of Anaesthesiology That Were Published Between 1880 and 1950 in Germany

— 1880: Kappeler O: *Anaesthetica.* Enke, Stuttgart
— 1881: Tauber E: *Anaesthetica.* August Hirschwald, Berlin
— 1893: Garré C: *Die Aethernarkose.* Laupp'sche Buchhandlungen, Tübingen
— 1897: Czempin A: *Die Technik der Chloroformnarkose für Ärzte und Studierende.* Enslin, Berlin
— 1898: Müller J: *Anaesthetika. Ueber die verschiedenen, gebräuchlichen Anaesthetika, ihre Wirkungsweise und die Gefahren bei ihrer Anwendung.* Mitcher & Röstell, Berlin
— 1898: Hankel E: *Handbuch der Inhalations-Anaesthetica.* Alfred Langkammer, Leipzig
— 1902: Koblanck G: *Die Chloroform- und Äthernarkose in der Praxis.* Bergmann, Wiesbaden
— 1903: Steinbüchel R von: *Schmerzverminderung und Narkose in der Geburtshilfe mit spezieller Berücksichtigung der kombinierten Skopolamin-Morphium-Anästhesie.* Franz Deuticke Verlag, Leipzig Wien
— 1903: Dumont F: *Handbuch der allgemeinen und lokalen Anästhesie.* Urban & Schwarzenberg, Berlin Wien
— 1905: Martin M: *Die Anästhesie in der ärztlichen Praxis.* Lehmanns, München
— 1907: Hirsch M: *Der Ätherrausch.* Franz Deuticke Verlag, Leipzig Wien
— 1908: Müller WB: *Narkologie. Ein Handbuch der Wissenschaft über allgemeine und lokale Schmerzbetäubung (Narkosen und Methoden der lokalen Anästhesie).* Trenkel Verlag, Berlin
— 1913: Brunn M von: *Die Allgemeinnarkose.* Enke, Stuttgart
— 1914: Wein D: Die *Anästhesie in der Zahnheilkunde,* Bergmann, Wiesbaden
— 1919: Winterstein H: *Die Narkose.* Springer, Berlin
— 1921: Kühl W: *Handbuch der Narkose und der Vorbereitung vor Narkosen.* W. Gente, Wissenschaftlicher Verlag, Hamburg
— 1926: Antoine T, Pfab B: *Die Inhalationsnarkose.* Springer, Berlin Wien
— 1934: Killian H: *Narkose zu operativen Zwecken.* Springer, Berlin
— 1934: Hesse F, Lendle L, Schön R: *Allgemeinnarkose und örtliche Betäubung.* Barth, Leipzig
— 1935 Hesse F: *Kleines Narkosebuch – Eine Anleitung zur Allgemeinnarkose für Schwestern und Heilgehilfen.* Barth, Leipzig
— 1936: Härtel F, Jenico H: *Anleitung zur Schmerzbekämpfung.* Steinkopf, Dresden Leipzig

- 1947: Schiffbäumer A: *Grundlagen der Narkose in Theorie und Praxis.* Wissenschaftliche Verlagsgesellschaft, Stuttgart
- 1950: Henley J: *Einführung in die Praxis der modernen Inhalationsnarkose.* De Gruyter, Berlin

Selected Textbooks on Regional Anaesthesia That Were Published in Germany Between 1880 and 1950

- 1887: Viau G: *Die locale Anästhesie bei Zahnextraktionen.* Hirschwald, Berlin
- 1894: Schleich CL: *Schmerzlose Operationen.* Springer, Berlin
- 1897: Hackenbruch P: *Örtliche Schmerzlosigkeit bei Operationen.* Lehmanns, Wiesbaden
- 1905: Braun H: *Die Lokalanästhesie, ihre wissenschaftlichen Grundlagen und praktische Anwendung.* Barth, Leipzig
- 1907: Bosse B: *Die Lumbalanästhesie.* Urban & Schwarzenberg, Berlin Wien
- 1910: Schlesinger A: *Die Praxis der lokalen Anästhesie.* Urban & Schwarzenberg, Berlin Wien
- 1911: Fischer G: *Die lokale Anästhesie in der Zahnheilkunde mit spezieller Berücksichtigung der Schleimhaut- und Leitungsanästhesie.* Meißer, Berlin
- 1913: Hirschel G: *Lehrbuch der Lokalanästhesie für Studierende und Ärzte.* Bergmann, Wiesbaden
- 1913: Homeier F: *Die Anwendungsweise der Lokalanästhesie in der Chirurgie.* Hirschwald, Berlin
- 1916: Härtel F: *Die Lokalanästhesie.* Enke, Stuttgart
- 1922: Brunn M von: *Die Lumbalanästhesie.* Enke, Stuttgart
- 1923: Finsterer H: *Die Methoden der Lokalanästhesie in der Bauchchirurgie und ihre Erfolge.* Urban & Schwarzenberg, Berlin Wien
- 1925: Hirsch C: *Lehrbuch der Lokalanästhesie des Ohres und der oberen Luft- und Speisewege.* Enke, Stuttgart
- 1944: Kirschner M: *Die Hochdrucklokalanästhesie.* Springer, Berlin

References

1. Flourens MJP (1847) Note touchant l'administration de l'éther sur les centres nerveux. C Séances Acad Sci 24:340–344
2. Adams CN (1998) Early reports on deaths under anaesthesia. In: Schulte am Esch J, Goerig M (eds) Proceedings of the Fourth International Symposium on the History of Anaesthesia. Dräger-Druck, Lübeck, pp 157–1563
3. Mikulicz-Radecki J von (1901) Die Methoden der Schmerzbetäubung und ihre gegenseitige Abgrenzung. Arch Klin Chir 64:785–790
4. Braun H (1922) Narkosemethoden. In: Bier–Braun–Kümmell (eds) Chirurgische Operationslehre, vol. I. Barth, Leipzig
5. Wilkinson D (1992) Keeping the airway open. Esmarch's maneuvre or Heiberg's heave? In: Fink BR, Morris LE, Stephen CR (eds) The history of anesthesia. Proceedings of the Third International Symposium, Atlanta 1992. Library-Museum of Anesthesiology, Park Ridge, IL, pp 443–446
6. Esmarch F (1877) Handbuch der kriegschirurgischen Technik. Rumpler, Hannover
7. Goerig M (2001) Geschichte der Sicherung der Atemwege. In: Krier C, Georgi R (eds) Airway Management. Die Sicherung der Atemwege. Thieme, Stuttgart
8. Kuhn F (1911) Die perorale Intubation. Karger, Berlin
9. Kieser F (1964) Die Persönlichkeit und das Wirken von Franz Kuhn. Dissertation, Düsseldorf
10. Sauerbruch F (1904) Zur Pathologie des offenen Pneumothorax und die Grundlage meines Verfahrens zu seiner Ausschaltung. Mitt Grenzgeb Med Chir 13:399–480
11. Brauer L (1903) Die Ausschaltung der Pneumothoraxfolgen mit Hilfe des Ueberdruckverfahrens. Mitt Grenzgeb Med Chir 13:483-500
12. Wiedemann K, Fleischer E (1992) Zur Geschichte der Anästhesie in der Thoraxchirurgie: Pneumothoraxproblem, Intubation, Einlungenventilation. AINS 27:3–10
13. Brunn M von (1913) Die Allgemeinnarkose. Enke, Stuttgart
14. Aiysi K, Goerig M (1992) The merits of Samuel James Meltzer and John Auer for the development of apneic oxygenation. In: Fink BR, Morris LE, Stephen CR (eds) The history of anesthesia. Proceedings of the Third International Symposium. Wood Library-Museum of Anesthesiology 1992, pp 32–40
15. Kirstein A (1895) Autoskopie des Larynx und der Trachea (Besichtigung ohne Spiegel). Berl Klin Wochenschr 22:476–478
16. Moritsch P (1949) Die Schmerzverhütung bei chirurgischen Eingriffen. Maudrich, Vienna
17. Reinhardt M, Eberhardt E (1994) Einführung einer Maske für Chloroform und Äthernarkosen aus ursprünglich aseptischen Überlegungen. AINS 29:30–35
18. Witzel O (1902) Wie sollen wir narkotisieren? Münch Med Wochenschr 48:1993–1998
19. Junker F (1867) Description of a new apparatus for administration of narcotic vapours. Med Times Gaz II: 590
20. Goerig M, Schulte am Esch J (1995) Otto Kappeler – ein Wegbereiter der deutschsprachigen Anästhesie. AINS 30:426–435
21. Weisser Ch (1983) Der Braun'sche Apparat zur Äther-Chloroform-Mischnarkose. Anaesthesist 32:369-373
22. Haupt J (1970) Die Entwicklung der Dräger - Narkoseapparate. In: Dräger - Medizingeräte im Wandel der Zeiten. Drägerwerk Lübeck, Sonderdruck MT 1, Drägerheft 280, 281, 282. Lübeck
23. Läwen A (1912) Ueber die Verbindung der Lokalanästhesie mit der Narkose, über hohe Extraduralanästhesie und epidurale Injektionen anästhesierender Lösungen bei tabischen Magenkrisen. Bruns Beitr Klin Chir 80:168–180
24. Läwen A, Sievers R (1910) Zur praktischen Anwendung der instrumentellen künstlichen Respiration am Menschen. Münch Med Wochenschr 41:2221–2225
25. Griffith HR, Johnson GE (1942) The use of curare in general anesthesia. Anesthesiology 3:418–420
26. Rendell-Baker L (1992) The development of nitrous oxide-oxygen apparatus. Anesthesia History Newsletter, vol 10, no 1: 11–14
27. Neu M (1910) Ein Verfahren zur Stickoxydul-Sauerstoffnarkose. Münch Med Wochenschr 36:1873–1875
28. Goerig M (1994) Historical use of nitrous oxide in Germany. In: Proceedings of the Joint Meeting with the Section of Anaesthetics Royal Society of Medicine, vol. 16. London, 10 December 1994, pp 68-80
29. Wawersik J (1982) Die Geschichte des Narkoseapparates in Grundzügen. Anaesthesist 31:541–548
30. Baum JA (1998) Who introduced the rebreathing systems into clinical practice? In: Schulte am Esch J, Goerig M (eds) Proceedings of the Fourth International Symposium on the History of Anaesthesia. Dräger-Druck, Lübeck, pp 441–449

31. Wilde B (1940) Der heutige Stand der Gasnarkose. Die Narcylen-betäubung. Schmerz Narkose Anästhesie 13:19–32

32. Kelling G (1918) Über die Beseitigung der Narkosedämpfe aus dem Operationssaale. Zentralbl Chir 35:602–606

33. Hölscher F (1925) Zur Beseitigung der ausgeatmeten Narkose-gase. Zentralbl Chir 25:1558–1559

34. Schum H (1935) Die neue Klimaanlage im Operationssaal des Staatskrankenhauses der Landespolizei. Chirurg 7:115–123

35. Hirsch J, Kappus KL (1928) Über die Mengen des Narkoseäthers in der Luft von Operationssälen. Z Hyg Infektionskr 110:391–398

36. Goerig M, Schulte am Esch J (1996) Ursprünge des Nüchternheits-gebotes. AINS 31:245–248

37. Trendelenburg F (1870) Beiträge zu den Operationen an den Luftwegen. Arch Klin Chir 12:112–133

38. Goerig M, Pothmann W (1993) Development of tracheal tubes in anesthesiology. Spring Meeting Anesthesia History Association, Louisville, KY

39. Röse W, Scharff W (1993) Qualitätskontrolle vor 100 Jahren – Die »Narkotisierungsstatistik« von Gurlt aus dem Jahre. AINS 28:254–257

40. Goerig M, Schulte am Esch J (1993) Carl Ludwig Schleich – Weg-bereiter ausschließlich der Lokalanästhesie? AINS 28:113–124

41. Koller C (1884) Vorläufige Mittheilung ueber locale Anästhesie-rung am Auge. Klin Monatsbl Augenheilk 22(Suppl):60–63

42. Hirschel G (1913) Lehrbuch der Lokalanästhesie für Studierende und Ärzte. J F Bergmann, Wiesbaden

43. Bakes J (1905) Zur operativen Therapie des callösen Magenge-schwürs. Arch Klin Chir 76:1129–1150

44. Penkert M (1906) Lumbalanästhesie im Morphium-Skopolamin-Dämmerschlaf. Münch Med Wochenschr 14:646-648

45. Bergmann E von (1894) Über die vor der Sitzung von Herrn Schle-ich demonstrierte Infiltrations-Anästhesie. Verh Dtsch Ges Chir 23:101–102

46. Schneiderlin E (1900) Eine neue Narkose. Aerztl Mitt Baden 10:101–103

47. Gauß CJ (1906) Bericht über das erste Tausend Geburten im Skopolamin-Dämmerschlaf. Münch Med Wochenschr 4:561-562

48. Kümmell H (1905) Diskussionsbemerkung auf dem Deutschen Chirurgenkongress. 1905. Verh Dtsch Ges Chir 34:114–115

49. Kümmell H (1908) Abkürzung des Heilungsverlaufs laparatomier-ter Patienten durch frühzeitiges Aufstehen. In: Verhandlung der Deutschen Gesellschaft für Chirurgie. Hirschwald, Berlin, pp 1–10

50. Krecke A (1910) Ueber Vor- und Nachbehandlung bei Bauchop-erationen, insbesondere über das frühzeitige Aufstehenlassen. Münch Med Wochenschr 39:2037–2041

51. Menzel A (1877) Zur Statistik der Narkose. Ein Vorschlag. Centralbl Chir 4:65–66

52. Röse W (1995) Die »Narkotisierungsstatistik« von Ernst Julius Gurlt aus dem Jahre 1895 – Ein früher Beitrag zur Qualitätskontrolle in der Anästhesie. Anaesthesiol Reanim 20:157–161

53. Sydow FW (1987) Geschichte der Lokal- und Leitungsanästhesie. In: Zinganell K (ed) Anästhesie – historisch gesehen. Springer, Berlin, pp 38–53

54. Eiselsberg F von (1903) Wandlungen in der modernen Chirurgie. Wien Klin Wochenschr 19:563–568

55. Röse W (1982) Heinrich Braun. Anaesthesiol Reanim 20:3–7

56. Braun H (1905) Über einige neue lokale Anaesthetica. (Stovain, Alypin, Novocain). Münch Med Wochenschr 41:1667–1671

57. Bier A (1899) Versuche über Cocainisirung des Rückenmarkes. Dtsch Z Chir 51:361–369

58. Goerig M,Schulte am Esch J (1999) Zur Erinnerung an August Bier (1864–1949). AINS 34:463–474

59. Kreis O (1900) Ueber Medullarnarcose bei Gebärenden. Zentralbl Gynaekol 28:724–729

60. Holmes C (1969) The history and development of intravenous regional anesthesia. Acta Anaesthesiol Scand Suppl 36:11–18

61. Goerig M, Schulte am Esch J (1990) Georg Perthes – Ein Wegberei-ter moderner Regionalanästhesie-Techniken? Anaesth Regionala-naesth 13:1–5

62. Pitkin G (1928) Controllable spinal anesthesia. Am J Surg 5:537–553

63. Schmidt H (1929) Pitkins kontrollierbare Spinalanästhesie mit viskotischen, spezifisch leichteren Novocainlösungen. Arch Klin Chir 157:206–211

64. Schmidt H (1930) Lumbalanästhesie mit spezifisch leichter visko-tischer Novokainlösung (Spinocain) und prophylaktische Stabi-lisierung des Blutdrucks durch Ephedrin. Klin Wochenschr 16:748–756

65. Kappis M (1912) Ueber Leitungsanästhesie an Bauch, Brust, Arm und Hals durch Injektionen am Foramen intervertebrale. Münch Med Wochenschr 12:794–796

66. Läwen A (1910) Ueber die Verwendung des Novokains in Na-triumbikarbonat-Kochsalzlösung zur lokalen Anästhesie. Münch Med Wochenschr 39:2044-2046

67. Läwen A (1913) Die Extraduralanästhesie. Ergeb Chir Orthop 5:38–84

68. Dogliotti AM (1931) Eine neue Methode der regionären Anäs-thesie: Die peridurale segmentäre Anästhesie. Zentralbl Chir 50:3141–3145

69. Weisser C (1992) Martin Kirschner's willkürlich begrenzte und in-dividuell dosierbare gürtelförmige Spinalanästhesie. Grundlagen – Technik – aktuelle Bedeutung. Ein Beitrag zur Geschichte der Regionalanästhesie. Würzb Medizinhist Mitt 10:39–52

70. Göpel H (1943) Die Periduralanaäthesie in der Chirurgie. Chirurg 1:134–145

71. Burkhardt L (1911) Über intravenöse Narkosen. Münch Med Wochenschr 15:778–782

72. Kümmell H (1914) Weitere Erfahrungen über intravenöse Äther-narkose. Bruns Beitr Klin Chir 92:27–36

73. Kreuter E, Streichele E (1926) 1000 Isopral-Äthernarkosen ohne Todesfall. Bruns Beitr Klin Chir 137:455–466

74. Fischer E, Mering J (1903) Ueber eine neue Classe von Schlafmit-teln. Ther Gegenw 5:97–101

75. Goerig M, Schulte am Esch J (1997) Hellmut Weese – Der Ver-such einer Würdigung seiner Bedeutung für die deutschsprachige Anästhesie. AINS 32:678–685

76. Killian H, Weese H (1954) Die Narkose. Thieme, Stuttgart

77. Adams RC (1944) Intravenous anesthesia. Paul B. Höbner, New York

78. Goerig M (1992) The Avertin-story. In: Fink BR, Morris LE, Stephen CR (eds) The history of anesthesia. Proceedings of the Third In-ternational Symposium, Atlanta 1992. Wood Library-Museum of Anesthesiology Park Ridge, IL, pp 223–232

79. Bumm R (1927) Intravenöse Narkosen mit Barbitursäurederivaten. Klin Wochenschr 6:725-726

80. Bauer KH (1958) Eröffnungsansprache zur 75. Tagung der deutschen Gesellschaft für Chirurgie. Langenbecks Arch Klin Chir 289:163–177

81. Öhlecker F (1926) Bluttransfusion. Ergeb Ges Med 9:578–633

82. Schorr M (1956) Zur Geschichte der Bluttransfusion im 19. Jahr-hundert. Benno Schwabe & Co Verlag, Basel

83. Bueß H (1947) Die historischen Grundlagen der intravenösen Injektion. H. R. Sauerländer & Co, Aarau

84. Straub W (1920) Das Problem der physiologischen Salzlösung in Theorie und Praxis. Münch Med Wochenschr 9:249-251

85. Goerig M, Agarwal K (2002) Small-volume resuscitation – histori-cal remarks. In: Diz J et al (eds) The history of anaesthesia. Elsevier, Amsterdam, pp 233–244

86. Hecht H, Weese H (1943) Periston – ein neuer Flüssigkeitsersatz. Münch Med Wochenschr 1:11–15

87. Heyfelder JH (1847) Die Versuche über den Schwefeläther und die daraus gewonnenen Resultate in der chirurgischen Klinik zu Erlangen. Heyder, Erlangen

88. Bause G (1995) History of cardiovascular monitoring. An historical backdrop to cardiovascular monitoring. Bull Anesth Hist 13:6–11

89. Anonymus (1902) Bulletin No 2. Divison of Surgery, Massachusetts General Hospital, p 101

90. Goerig M, Schulte am Esch J (1997) Helmut Schmidt – Ein Protagonist moderner Anästhesie in Deutschland. AINS 31:621–631

91. Anonymus (1932) Werbeprospekt der Firma Siemens-Reiniger für den »Autonograph nach Dr. Lange zum fortlaufenden selbsttätigen Messen und Registrieren des menschlichen Blutdrucks«. Berlin

92. Jaeger F (1937) Die Blutdruck- und Pulskontrolle während der Operation. Schmerz Narkose Anästhesie 1:44–47

93. Lundy (1938) Proceedings of the staff meetings at the Mayo Clinic, vol. 3, 29:449

94. Rehn E, Resinger H (1927) Zur Technik der Projektion und Registrierung von Herzaktionsstromkurven bei Operationen. Klin Wochenschr 1:20–21

95. Kausch W (1909) Das Operationshaus des Auguste Viktoria-Krankenhauses zu Schöneberg. Z Krankenpfl 11:321–327

96. Kirschner M (1930) Zum Neubau der chirurgischen Universitätsklinik in Tübingen. III. Der Behandlungsbau. Chirurg 5:202–215

97. Nussbaum N (1874) Anaesthetica. In: Pitha-Billroth (ed) Handbuch der allgemeinen und speciellen Chirurgie, vol. 1, pt. 2. Enke, Stuttgart

98. Kappeler O (1890) Über die Methoden der Chloroformirung, insbesondere über die Chloroformirung mit messbaren Chloroformluftmischungen. Arch Klin Chir 40:844–868

99. Goerig M, Schulte am Esch J (1995) Otto Kappeler – ein Wegbereiter der deutschsprachigen Anästhesie. AINS 30:426–435

100. Quincke H (1906) Ueber ärztliche Spezialitäten und Spezialärzte. Münch Med Wochenschr 1213–1217, 1260–1264

101. Schleich CL (1894) Schmerzlose Operationen. Springer, Berlin

102. Wohlgemuth H (1908) Bessere Ausbildung in der Narkose und Anästhesie! Dtsch Med Wochenschr 37:1595–1596

103. Eiselsberg F von (1903) Wandlungen in der modernen Chirurgie. Wien Klin Wochenschr 19:563–568

104. Kehr H (1913) Die Chirurgie der Gallenwege. Enke, Stuttgart

105. Müller WB (1908) Narkologie. Trenkel, Berlin

106. Braun H (1925) Heinrich Braun. In: Grote RL (ed) Die Medizin der Gegenwart in Selbstdarstellungen, Vol 5. Felix Meiner, Leipzig, pp 1–34

107. Pels-Leusden F (1925) Chirurgische Operationslehre. Urban & Schwarzenberg, Berlin

108. Busch JP zum (1921) Der Facharzt für Narkose. Dtsch Med Wochenschr 31:900–901

109. Kritzler H (1925) Der Facharzt für Narkose. Dtsch Med Wochenschr 25:719

110. Kausch W (1921) Bemerkung während des Deutschen Chirurgenkongresses. Verh Dtsch Ges Chir 45:139

111. Kappis M (1931) Narkose und Lokalanästhesie. In: Klemperer G, Klemperer F (eds) Neue Deutsche Klinik, vol. 17. Urban & Schwarzenberg, Berlin

112. Tschöp M (1986) Ernst von der Porten. Springer, Berlin

113. Schwarz W, Goerig M (2003) Die Gründungsmitglieder der Deutschen Gesellschaft für Anaesthesie. Anästh Intensivmed 44:461–467

114. Schmidt H (1929) Inhalation or injection narcosis? The development of the specialty of anesthesia in Germany. Curr Res Anesth Analg 8:20–23

115. McMechan FH (1929) Anaesthesia and the Hamburg congress. Curr Res Anesth Analg 8:16–19

116. Rehn E (1929) Schlusswort. In: 90. Versammlung der Gesellschaft Deutscher Naturforscher und Ärzte in Hamburg am 16–22. September 1928. Zentralbl Chir 3:159–174

117. Killian H (1941) Plan zur Neuordnung des Narkosewesens in Deutschland. Schmerz Narkose Anaesthesie 14:73–87

118. Killian H (1950) Gedanken und Vorschläge zur Frage des Narkose Spezialarztes. Dtsch Med Wochenschr 22:739–741

119. Schwarz W (1989) Attemps to establish anaesthesiology as a speciaity in German medicine. In: Atkinson RS, Boulton TB (eds) The history of anaesthesia. International Congress and Symposium Series Number 134. The Parthenon Publishing Group, Carnforth, UK, pp 170–175

2.1.2 Development of Anaesthesia after 1945

J. Schulte am Esch, M. Goerig, K. Agarwal

Introduction

The development of anaesthesia according to Lucien E. Morris is divided into three epochs: the first is the era of »trial and error« with ether and chloroform that lasted until the end of the nineteenth century. This period was marked by limited conceptual possibilities and numerous complications as well as fatalities. The second period until World War II with evolving research was accompanied by important developments in medication and apparatus. This was followed by the third period from the end of World War II until today – the era of anaesthesiologists – with emerging comprehensive perioperative care and pain management, a clear statement regarding further training and education in anaesthesia, with the birth of the specialty of anaesthesiology and the establishment of a specialist society as well as unfolding recognition of the challenges to ensure patient safety [1].

> In the post-war period, we anaesthesiologists were experiencing a new beginning; anaesthesia had its peak moment in time! It was a major discovery in medicine, the anaesthesiologist was the specialist for artificial ventilation, endotracheal intubation, resuscitation, muscle relaxation – preliminary conditions that allowed surgeons to access the thorax including the heart, creating sublime conditions for surgery of the abdomen and inside the skull. The chapter of surgery had to be redefined, which had been impossible before [2].

With these words, Manfred Körner (1923–2012) of Krefeld summarized the situation in a review upon his retirement as Chief of Anaesthesiology in 1983. These conditions along with their challenges which may be present even today, were, at that time, not valued by German surgeons despite the considerable advances in anaesthesiology and surgery in the Anglo-American and Scandinavian world. Techniques hardly differed from those around the turn of the century: anaesthesia was usually performed by young and inexperienced doctors or nurses utilizing Schimmelbusch masks and ether.

German surgeons with vast influence in politics may partly be blamed for this slow development, since disadvantages seemed to be more obvious than advantages in giving birth to a new subspecialty. On top of that during World War II, the international transfer of knowledge that had been initiated in the 1930s became impossible.

Evipan administered intravenously – which was introduced in field hospitals for the induction of anaesthesia – became widespread in numerous hospitals. As opposed to the induction with inhalation of ether, the patient's comfort could be improved since coughing, nausea and the feeling of suffocation were absent. Monosubstance anaesthesia with Evipan became very popular in the 1950s, but required experienced staff to avoid hypotension, depression of the central nervous system leading to apnoea as well as airway obstructions caused when the tongue drops back. At that time, neither artificial ventilation with the aid of an Ambu bag nor a respirator were available. The efficiency of mouth-to-mouth or mouth-to-nose ventilation was rather unknown and only used rarely as opposed to methods invented by Henry Sylvester (1829–1908) and Benjamin Howard (1836–1900) in the previous century.

Analeptics to overcome respiratory or circulatory depression, mouth gags and tongue forceps as well as containers to collect vomit were inevitable for standard procedures in anaesthesia. Concentrated oxygen was rarely added to volatile anaesthetics, since central gas supply had not been introduced at that time. Infusion therapy, even for extensive procedures, was uncommon. If it had to be performed, subcutaneous or rectal as well as in exceptional cases intravenous routes were selected.

Perioperative monitoring comprised frequent palpation of peripheral pulses, less frequent blood pressure control, and respiratory function monitoring by observing rate and quality of unhindered breathing and inspection of the skin. An anaesthetic chart was written in exceptional cases only, although they had already been employed in several German clinics in the 1920s. Due to general conditions in the 1950s the prevalences of perioperative morbidity and mortality under anaesthesia were much higher than today; this limited the scope of patients for whom anaesthesia could be indicated during surgery.

By 2008 the term »unsuitable for anaesthesia« and an age limit hardly existed any longer even for major operations. Thus – as opposed to the post-war period – gastrectomy in a 60-year-old patient may be carried out easily. Blood transfusions were time consuming, recruiting suitable donors was difficult and determination of blood groups was imperfect. Major co-morbidities like insulin-dependent diabetes mellitus, hypertension, renal diseases and/or impaired pulmonary and cardiac performance were classified as contraindications for major surgery, since mortality was increased. These restrictions do not apply anymore, since enthusiastic physicians have refined methods in anaesthesia and therefore facilitated more sophisticated surgical procedures regardless of the uncertain career expectations.

The Establishment of the Specialty since 1945

Since the early 1950s the number of consultants in anaesthesiology has increased continuously resulting in improved care during anaesthetic procedures. As compared to 50 years ago when 1 anaesthesiologist was in charge to 104,000 patients [3], this number is more than 20 times as large today. In 2008, approximately 18,300 physicians are employed in anaesthesia [4]. This increase can be attributed to a growing number of hospitals involved in teaching anaesthesia that were established in the 1960s and 1970s in Germany. These numbers are impressive, but do not depict the multiplicity and extensive conflicts that had to be overcome in operating theatres, which have given rise to the excellent conditions younger colleagues may relish today.

> Today, we have to face the irreversible fact that duties have been split in the operating theatre. The surgeon may completely focus on his operation, while the anaesthesiologist monitors and treats the patient's vital functions. Those who love paradoxes may also express it like this: the anaesthetist is the specialist for non-operative, non-specific objects, more or less for general concerns, as opposed to the surgeon who is the specialist for the operation itself [5].

With this statement, the surgeon Karl-Heinrich Bauer (1890–1978) of Heidelberg had to accept that conducting anaesthesia had become the responsibility of the anaesthesiologist instead of the surgeon. Previous declarations by surgeons – published by the law specialist Karl Engisch (1899–1969) of Munich – that an anaesthesiologist was only an assistant to the surgeon were no longer acceptable [6].

At the request of the Berufsverband Deutscher Anästhesisten (BDA, Professional Association of German Anaesthesists) founded in 1961, the anaesthesiologist Charlotte Lehmann of Munich (*1922) convinced the director at the Bavarian Ministry of Justice, Walther Weißauer (*1921), to publish a report entitled »Division of work and responsibilities between the anaesthesiologist and the surgeon« [7], which reflected the opinion of the community of anaesthesiologists resulting in a clear leverage in favour of anaesthesiologists [8].

This viewpoint also invigorated the newly founded Berufsverband, which also took care of issues concerning labour laws and financial affairs. Establishment of organizations like the BDA and then the DGA (German Society of Anaesthesia) became necessary, since remuneration for anaesthetic procedures by health insurance companies was still not ensured even though anaesthesiology had become a specialty in 1953. These provisions did not exist in the Preußische Gebührenordnung (Prussian Regulation for Charges and Fees for Private Settlement) and in the Allgemeine Deutsche Gebührenordnung (General German Regulations for Charges and Fees). Unsettled questions had to be decided so that young physicians could be offered professional perspectives.

Public discussions on all of the above-mentioned issues in the journal Der Anaesthesist would have jeopardized the non-profit-making reputation of the Deutsche Gesellschaft für Anaesthesie. Hence, it became essential to also establish the Berufsverband Deutscher Anästhesisten [9].

This important standpoint and its impact on anaesthesia, which now had achieved the status of a specialty with equal rights to other specialties, resulted in settling controversies and doubts between anaesthesiologists, surgeons and hospital owners. Contracts between surgeons and anaesthesiologists were arranged: Hermann Krauss (*1899–1972) on behalf of the surgeons and Kurt Wiemers (1920–2004) on behalf of the anaesthetists signed the agreement on »Guidelines on the position of the managerial anaesthetist« in 1964 [10]. This included equal rights of the managerial anaesthetist and the head of the department as well as consultants. At universities separate anaesthesiology departments were established with professors to become chairmen or executive directors. Central anaesthesiology departments were founded in order to cover all kinds of surgery. Consensus was achieved on duties in the recovery room as well as on the intensive or intermediate care unit. Also, an agreement was reached regarding a sufficient number of workplaces for specialty training in anaesthesiology with appropriate working conditions for experienced consultants in larger departments of anaesthesiology.

Ten years prior to this, this rapid evolution in anaesthesiology had been inconceivable. As opposed to many other countries like the USA, the UK, the Scandinavian countries, France and the Benelux countries, in the late 1940s the performance of, and responsibility for, anaesthesia in Germany lay with the surgeons. Furthermore, advances in thoracic surgery for example in the Anglo-American area had to be caught up with in Germany.

Surgeons who were less narrow-minded admitted that these techniques, especially for major abdominal and thoracic surgery, were superior to the traditional techniques. Thus, numerous surgeons favoured and supported a specialty for anaesthesiologists. This was confirmed by demonstrations of visiting foreign anaesthesiologists who presented their repertoire of modern anaesthetic practice, including endotracheal intubation using muscle relaxants.

In this connection, the Swiss thoracic surgeon Karl Eduard Mülly (1909–1986) should be mentioned, who had been working as coworker of the surgeon Alfred Brunner (1890–1972) in Zurich since 1940. He conducted research on relevant issues in anaesthesiology; hence, he contacted English as well as Scandinavian anaesthesiologists. In 1947, while a resident at the clinic for thoracic surgery at the Sabbatsberg Hospital in Stockholm under the expert guidance of Clarence Crafoord, he learned about modern general anaesthesia with endotracheal intubation. Mülly recognized the advantages of intubation for general anaesthesia as opposed to local anaesthesia and introduced it in his department right after his return to Zurich in November 1947, initially for thoracic and major abdominal surgery [11].

Brunner, a former student of Sauerbruch, invited various German surgeons to work in his clinic after the war where they also learned about technical and procedural innovations in modern anaesthesia from Mülly such as endotracheal intubation, closed-circuit anaesthetic systems with carbon dioxide absorption, the use of muscle relaxants and artificial ventilation, shock management as well as anaesthetic charts.

Modern anaesthesia as practised in Zurich epitomized the new anaesthesia specialty, based on scientific facts and requiring professionalism. This gave rise to vast interest in the »new field of anaesthesiology« and many surgeons turned to it.

The female American anaesthesiologist Jean Henley (1910–1994; ◘ Fig. 2.26), who was employed at several university hospitals in the American sector of Germany during the second half of 1949, spread the news of the technique of general anaesthesia and endotracheal intubation [15]. She worked at the Department of Surgery at the University Medical Hospitals in Heidelberg and Giessen for many months. Prior to returning to the USA early in 1950, she completed a short textbook about modern anaesthesia entitled Einführung in die Praxis der modernen Inhalationsnarkose (◘ Fig. 2.27), the first textbook on anaesthesiology published in Germany after World War II [12].

The impact of this book is evidenced by the fact that 15,000 copies were printed. By virtue of her manifold activities and merits, Jean Henley was awarded honorary membership of the German Society of Anaesthesiology and Intensive Care Medicine (DGAI) in 1981.

Significant advances in surgery were facilitated by modern anaesthesia techniques. This was most obvious in thoracic surgery, where surgical treatments for pulmonary tuberculosis and bronchial carcinoma became increasingly important. Hence, institutions specialized in thoracic surgery expected their anaesthesiologists to undergo specific training. Jochen Bark (1918–1963), employed at the Lung Clinic Wehrawald/Todtmoos in the Black Forest, had already been sent to Oxford and to Sir Robert Macintosh in 1949 [13], and Ludwig Zürn (1921–1959) from the University Medical Hospital in Munich acquired specific knowledge in Stockholm [14]. K.H. Bauer was able to send his colleague Rudolf Frey (1917–1981) to Werner Hügin (1918–2001) in Basel, after the latter had worked for the previous 2 years with Henry K. Beecher (1904–1976) in Boston. Trips to Paris or Oxford followed. Many other anaesthesiologists took part in exchange programmes over the subsequent years. Some of them tried to contact foreign universities, while others were sent by Frey who kept in touch with foreign colleagues. Martin Zindler (*1920) was invited to take part in a 3-year training course with

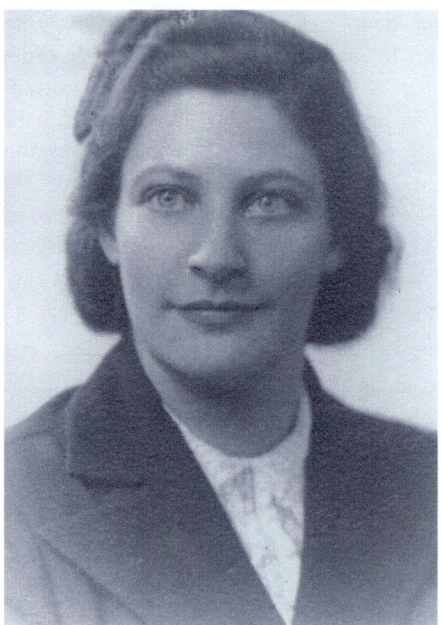

◘ **Fig. 2.26.** Jean Henley

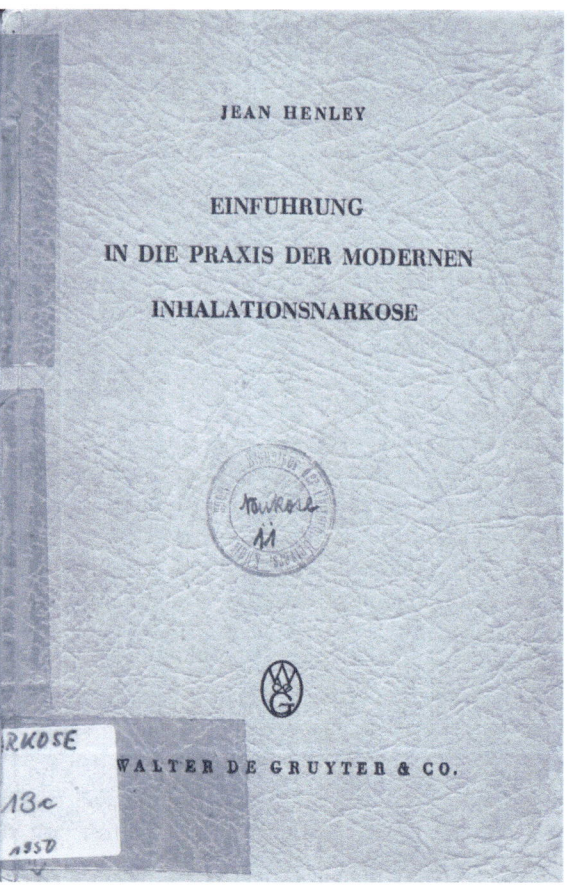

◘ **Fig. 2.27.** The first textbook on anaesthesiology published in Germany after 1945

Robert Dunning Dripps (1911–1972) at the University of Pennsylvania [15]. Among those physicians trained in Europe, especially in England and Sweden, several received the honour of assisting Sir Robert Macintosh (1897–1989) at the University of Oxford. Karl Hutschenreuter (1920–1996) of Jena had had the opportunity to work with Thorsten Gordh (*1920) in Stockholm and Georg Hossli (1907–2010) in Zurich.

At the congress of the German Society of Surgery in Frankfurt in October 1949, where the main issues for the following congress (1950) were selected, protocols on surgical procedures like surgery of the abdomen, endocrine glands and disc prolapse as well as issues in anaesthesia were discussed. To provide participants with information on the current state of the art of anaesthesiology in different European countries, Geoffrey Stephen William Organe (1908–1985), Thorsten Gordh and Sir Robert Macintosh as the most important foreign representatives were invited to speak at a session on »The current state of anaesthesia techniques«. Macintosh clearly voted in favour of anaesthesiology [16].

Surgeons recognized the impact of the development and founded an Anaesthesia Commission in co-operation with the German Society of Pharmacology in 1950 in order to review issues on specialization in anaesthesiology [17, 18]. Legal issues were discussed covering the possibility of training nurses to become anaesthetists »who may be qualified for German circumstances. According to German law, the surgeon is responsible for the whole surgical procedure and the anaesthesiologist is only an aide« [19].

Even though attempts were made towards dismissing the idea of the specialty of anaesthesia, many surgeons like Helmut Schmidt (1895–1979) of Remscheid, who achieved his postdoctoral lecturer qualification in 1928 on an issue in anaesthesiology in Hamburg (❏ Fig. 2.28) and had given lectures on anaesthesiology for many years, could not be discouraged [20].

At the meeting of the Executive Board of the West German Medical Associations in 1952 specialties were endorsed on both sides giving way to general acceptance. The State Chamber of Physicians of the Saarland that was administered by the French government at that time was the first to approve this recommendation [21]. In addition, the Specialist for Narcosis and Anaesthesia was introduced on 31 March 1952, which required 4 years of specialty training as opposed to the 5 years that were recommended by the Specialty Board of the General Council of the West German Medical Associations [22].

The first person to obtain the specialist status accredited by the State Chamber of Physicians of the Saarland was Werner Sauerwein (*1921) who worked in Saarbrücken and had been trained between 1949 and 1953 in Lyon [23].

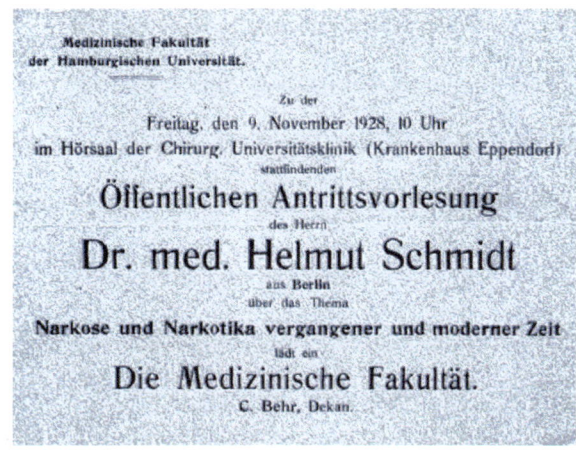

❏ **Fig. 2.28.** Invitation to Helmut Schmidt's inaugural lecture in Hamburg in 1928

Even though anaesthesiologists were appreciated in some parts of the country, they received hardly any support from hospitals and insurance companies since recognition of this speciality as an independent and responsible partner within the system was denied.

Accordingly, many surgeons behaved as if they ruled in their kingdom and became »dictators of the operating theatres«. The surgeon Karl-Heinrich Bauer (1890–1978) of Heidelberg inaugurated the 69th meeting of the German Society of Surgery in Munich in April 1952 with his speech on the topic »Regarding the mental situation of our specialty«, where he also mentioned tendencies within the field of surgery for subspecialization. He was opposed to anaesthesia becoming an independent specialty even though this had happened in the Saarland; he rather wished to see »everything under one roof«.

At the 1st Austrian Congress of Anaesthesia in Salzburg, which took place only weeks later, German delegates founded the German Working Group on Anaesthesiology on 5 September, which later became the German Society [24].

Jochen Bark (1918–1963) was elected Chairman. He had gained experience in intubation anaesthesia for lung surgery at the Thoracic Surgical Clinic in Wehrawald/Todtmoos in the 1940s. With a scholarship from the Swiss »Group to counter tuberculosis in urban areas«, he was educated by Sir Ivan Whiteside Magill (1888–1986) in London between October 1949 and March 1950 and by Sir Robert Macintosh (1897–1989) in Oxford, after having been employed at two Swiss hospitals specialized in pulmonary surgery. At the turn of the year 1952/1953, Bark also invited members of the working group to a scientific meeting at the Surgeon's Congress in Munich. The subjects listed in his letter unmisleading reflected his intention to found the German Society of Anaesthesia:

2

1. Rules of a society and of a medical specialty have been drafted.
2. Contact has been established to the Ärztetag (General Assembly of the German Medical Association): Professor Neuffer, President of the Ärztetag supports the application for specialist status.
3. The Society of Surgery has been contacted: the Chairman, Professor Borchers of Aachen is willing to co-operate. The anaesthesia meeting is scheduled for 11 April.
4. The next business meeting is scheduled for 10 April.
5. The German Society will be founded, the Chairman for the following year has to be elected…

On 10 April 1953, the German Society of Anaesthesia (DGA, ▶ Chap. 1.1) was established at the *Deutsches Museum*. At the end of this meeting the newly elected Chairman Jochen Bark awarded honorary membership to the young society to Hans Killian (1892–1982) and Hellmut Weese (1899–1954) in recognition of their efforts in anaesthesiology. Honorary membership was also granted to the surgeon Helmut Schmidt (1895–1979) of Remscheid [25].

Half a year later at the 56th Meeting of the **Deutscher Ärztetag** (German Medical Assembly) in Lindau, anaesthesiology was chosen to become the 16th area of expertise among recognized medical specialties [26]. Hence, a domain for anaesthesia was established. Professional training time – 2 years had to be carried out in anaesthesia – was set at 5 years. Agreement was reached on transitional regulations for colleagues who had been working as anaesthesiologists for a long time [27].

In 1967, a professional training time of 4 years was proposed in a draft for new rules governing accreditation of the specialty. The specialty expanded over the following years, demanding a revision of the curriculum of professional training including new techniques. A mandatory curriculum was prepared and the guidelines for further professional training were identified. It was designed to be employed in surgery, but since the knowledge of an anaesthesiologist had to cover all areas of surgery, it was initially established merely in anaesthesia-related subjects and consequently defined as follows in the newly decreed rules on accreditation of the specialty:

The specialty of anaesthesia comprises general and regional anaesthesia including pre- and postoperative care; maintaining vital functions during surgery; resuscitation and intensive care in co-operation with the physicians responsible for the patient's overall condition [28].

Unfortunately, the self-confidence and participation of younger physicians did not produce enough trained anaesthesiologists in the 1950s and 1960s. Financial uncertainties, a lack of suitable positions in clinics and training

hospitals as well as personal responsibilities are only some of the reasons to be mentioned. The future development of anaesthesia was uncertain despite official appreciation of the specialty and vivacious interest in the field. Also, influential surgeons were reluctant to grant anaesthesiologists an independent status with the result that physicians turned their backs on the new field and returned to surgery. In comparison to other European countries, only a few Germans specialized in anaesthesiology [29]

In order to overcome this overwhelming lack of personnel, the Executive Committee of the DGA requested broad support. Chairmen of numerous Departments of Anaesthesiology at German Universities had already asserted their demands in February 1959, which later were named the *Göttinger Appell* [30]. Regardless of major advances in the field of anaesthesiology and »outstanding results at surgical centres«, they emphasized that »nearly 95% of all anaesthesias are carried out by non-physicians or by doctors who have not been specially trained for this task«. They pointed out that conditions in England were quite different: more than 2,000 specialists in anaesthesiology were employed in 1959 as compared to about 80 in Germany at the same time. Extrapolations for 1959 revealed that an anaesthesiologist in North Rhine-Westphalia was responsible for 3,500 surgical patients, whereas in Germany as a whole 2,700 patients had to be covered by one anaesthesiologist. In view of these untenable conditions, they demanded that suitable positions be created at hospitals and university clinics.

Since this field lacked sufficient attraction, in 1960 only a small percentage of the 3,604 hospitals in West Germany were staffed with trained anaesthesiologists. There was no adequate relief over the next 10 years with approximately 900 anaesthesiologists at that time. Only 25% of all operations were attended by anaesthesiologists. Often a single doctor was responsible for several patients at the same time in different operating theatres [31]. Severe and fatal incidents repeatedly occurred, resulting in vivid discussions in the lay press as well as in scientific medical publications. The coroner Otto Pribilla (1920–2003) of Kiel stated in his article »Death during anaesthesia« published in 1964 in *Der Anaesthesist* that »Taking a glance at coroners' reports, we have come to the conclusion that the number of cases (fatalities during anaesthesia) has increased in recent years« [32].

As a result of political uproar, physicians from East Germany, some of whom had contributed to founding the DGA in Munich in 1953, were prevented from attending scientific meetings and congresses in West Germany (▶ Chap. 1.4).

This shortage of specialists became obvious in the paper published by the anaesthesiologist Charlotte Lehmann of Munich in *Der Anaesthesist* in 1967: of the 746 members of the then DGAW, 141 were employed in East Germany, only 50 of whom were board-certified anaesthesiologists, as opposed to approximately 400 in West Germany [33].

In the 1960s and 1970s, anaesthesiology experienced enormous scientific and clinical advances. The demand for qualified and well-trained anaesthesiologists in hospitals grew owing to the fact that more sophisticated operative procedures were being undertaken. It became clear that specific training in anaesthesia for thoracic and abdominal surgical procedures had resulted in the neglect of other surgical disciplines. Hence, a new curriculum for anaesthesiology was proposed by the DGAW in 1966 to be approved by the Deutscher Ärztetag in 1968, stipulating specific education on issues of anaesthesia itself: surgery was no longer a part of the specialization in anaesthesiology, 6 months spent in pharmacology, physiology, internal medicine, pulmonary function diagnostics and serology were approved.

It took almost two decades for anaesthesiology to be accepted as a specialty. Various technical and procedural innovations swept over the borders to Germany, many of them originating from the English-speaking area. Anaesthesiology became increasingly integrated, with a solid scientific background especially in physiology and pharmacology.

In 1987 at the 90th meeting of the Deutscher Ärztetag a new curriculum for the board certification in anaesthesiology was passed, again sticking to a 4-year professional training only, even though specialist societies argued that 5 years were necessary [34].

Again in 1992, this discussion was continued and the curriculum was revised at the 95th Deutscher Ärztetag, finally resulting in a 5-year education programme for anaesthesiology.

German anaesthesiology was thus on equal footing with other major European countries. The introduction of pain management as the fourth pillar in anaesthesiology next to anaesthesia for operative procedures, intensive and emergency care medicine was the next major event in the history of anaesthesiology. During the past 10–15 years pain management facilities have been installed at university medical centres as well as at general hospitals with outpatient and walk-in clinics as separate units headed by an anaesthesiologist along the lines of the pain clinic inaugurated by John Bonica (1914–1994) in Washington in 1961, where the »interdisciplinary approach« to pain treatment was born.

With the above-mentioned four components in anaesthesiology, this specialty could be integrated into clinics and hospitals to ensure the patient's health and recovery by providing services ranging from preclinical care and anaesthesia during surgery up to postoperative pain management.

As early as in the 1920s, academic training in anaesthesiology was inaugurated: lectures in this field were held for students and professional training in anaesthesiology was offered to physicians by specialists at university medical centres less reluctant to accept innovative specialties like anaesthesiology [35]. Nevertheless, sophisticated arrangements in anaesthesiology could not be established in Germany until after the end of World War II. Increasing interest in research and improved basic as well as clinical skills created dramatic progress in this field. Some tolerant and open-minded surgeons supported anaesthesiology, partly by employing professionally trained anaesthesiologists at their clinics.

Due to a shortage of board-certified anaesthesiologists at the University of Hamburg, the surgeon Rudolph Nissen (1896–1976) declined the position as chairman in 1950. Right at the beginning of the negotiations, Nissen argued that – based on his experience in the USA – a department of anaesthesiology with consultant and residents was necessary, as »the time has passed…when anaesthesia could be performed by nurses en passant« [36].

Several German university hospitals struggled to create positions for heads of staff in anaesthesiology. By 1960, the surgeon Ludwig Zukschwerdt (1902–1974) was able to establish one for Karl Horatz (1913–1996) at his clinic in Hamburg. In 1960, the first Chairman of Anaesthesiology Rudolf Frey (1917–1981) was employed in Mainz and the second was Martin Zindler (*1920) in Düsseldorf in 1962. In 1966, the position of the head of the department in Hamburg was converted into a Chair of Anaesthesiology with Karl Horatz becoming the first Professor of Anaesthesiology in Germany.

Within 10 years, nearly all German universities had established chairs of anaesthesiology. Physicians with a scientific background became occupied in introducing standard operating procedures in anaesthesiology and intensive care medicine. Clinically relevant issues were examined on a scientific basis; hence, results in basic research were rare. In the 1980s through the late 1990s, research became more structured as a result of an expanding number of departments of anaesthesiology. These reputable scientific results could be published in various respectable journals and presented at numerous congresses.

Regarding the necessity of specific, progressive and qualified scientific research in order to acquire sponsorship for further research and to stay involved in international as well as interdisciplinary investigations, the main focus of this activity had to be revised by the beginning of the twenty-first century (▶ Chap. 2.5).

Starting in the post-war period in 1945, academic teaching in anaesthesiology that had already begun in the 1920s and 1930s was intensified in Germany. At university hospitals obligatory lectures were held on anaesthesia, intensive care medicine and pain management, which had to be attended in order to pass the oral examination of the second part of the medical school final examination.

Academic training in anaesthesiology will remain inevitable in order to get students and physicians interested in this field; hence, superior teaching at universities as well as excellent training for residents is mandatory to secure its status as an academic subject at universities and an important topic for research.

Textbooks and Monographs

For decades, the Lehrbuch der Anaesthesiologie by Rudolf Frey (1917–1981), Werner Hügin (1918–2001) and Otto Mayrhofer (*1920) published in 1955 was the German textbook of anaesthesiology (❒ Fig. 2.29). In contrast to the monograph Die Narkose by Hans Killian and Hellmut Weese published in 1954, this textbook was issued in several editions and also distributed in East Germany. Due to the political upheaval that accompanied the erection of the Berlin Wall, it became increasingly difficult to obtain this book. This was offset by publishing several East German textbooks that were mostly translated from Anglo-American works.

The increasing amount of information and specialization within the specialty of anaesthesiology resulted in a two-volume textbook divided into anaesthesiology and intensive care medicine with the 5th edition of the Frey, Hügin and Mayrhofer textbook. The textbook Anästhesiologie was edited by Alfred Doenicke (*1928), Dietrich Kettler (*1936), Werner List (*1933), Jörg Tarnow (*1940) and Dick Thomson (*1939). The comprehensive book AINS, divided into four volumes (anaesthesiology, intensive care medicine, emergency care medicine and pain management), was published in 2001 by Gunter Hempelmann (*1940), Claude Krier (*1948) and Jochen Schulte am Esch (*1939).

Reflecting the achievements in the field of anaesthesiology accomplished in recent decades, both these textbooks comprise information on more than 1,600 pages each. In comparison, the first textbook of anaesthesiology published in 1950 by the American Jean Henley (1910–1994), Einführung in die Praxis der modernen Inhalationsnarkose, had a total of 120 pages and sold more than 15,000 copies. The description of anaesthesia techniques in the foreword still applies today:

> Advances in agents and techniques in anaesthesiology might be less important than the basic understanding of the anaesthetized patient's physiology as well as the pharmacology of the utilized agents that have become available in recent years because of intensive research. Almost every agent and method can be employed in most cases with the same success rate, if the anaesthesiologist knows what he wishes to accomplish. Current publications are packed with advice on various methods to solve one and the same problem. These are all equally successful in the hands of a person who has acquired the appropriate skills [37].

Fifty years later, the editors of Anästhesiologie issued by AINS included a similar comment in the foreword:

> Major progress in our specialty could be achieved in recent years making it possible to provide patients with individual care tailored to their medical history and peculiarities. Also techniques may be adapted to the specific kind of diagnostic or operative procedure ... Standard operating procedures are issued as precisely as possible based on expert knowledge in physiology and pharmacology ... The editors are aware of the fact that there may be alternative paths to reach the goal [38].

The first edition of Anästhesie published in 1994 by Reinhard Larsen (*1943), who was employed in Göttingen at that time, became very popular; hence, a 9th revised edition has become available meanwhile. In contrast to other available books, »the Larsen« was not a classic textbook, but a book for »further education« to be studied during professional training as reflected by the combination of

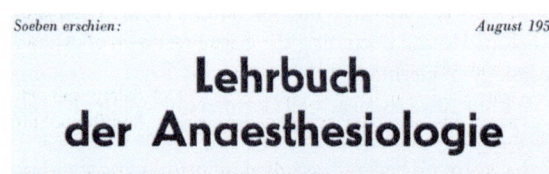

❒ **Fig. 2.29.** Advertisement for the textbook by Frey, Hügin and Mayrhofer in 1955

new didactic and illustrational concepts. A selection of available textbooks is listed below.

Selection of Textbooks of Anaesthesiology Published in West Germany from 1950 to 2001

- 1950 Henley J.: *Einführung in die Praxis der modernen Inhalationsnarkose*. de Gruyter, Berlin
- 1950 Fuchs E.: *Die zentrale Analgesie und Kurznarkose mit Stickoxydul*. Hüllenhagen & Grieh, Hamburg
- 1951 Irmer W., Koss F.H.: *Grundlagen der endotrachealen Narkose mit künstlicher Beatmung in der Thoraxchirurgie*. Barth, Munich
- 1951 Moser H.: *Die Praxis der modernen Narkose*. Maudrich, Vienna
- 1952 Hunter A.R.: *Praktischer Leitfaden der Allgemein- und Spinalanästhesie*. Wiss. Verlagsgesellschaft, Stuttgart
- 1952 Schön F.: *Theorie und Praxis der Allgemeinen Anästhesie*. Hanser, Munich
- 1953 Gillespie N.: *Die Endotrachealnarkose*. Oppermann, Hannover
- 1954 Killian H., Weese H.: *Die Narkose. Ein Lehr- und Handbuch*. Thieme, Stuttgart
- 1954 Wittig G.: *Narkose und Anästhesie*. de Gruyter, Berlin
- 1955 Hügin W., Mayrhofer O., Frey R.: *Lehrbuch der Anaesthesiologie*. Springer, Berlin (2nd edn. 1971; 3rd edn. 1972; 4th edn. 1977)
- 1962 Pflüger H.: *Kurzlehrbuch der modernen Anästhesie*. Schattauer, Stuttgart
- 1973 Herden H.N., Lawin P.: *Anästhesiefibel*. Thieme, Stuttgart
- 1977 Podlesch I.: *Anästhesie und Intensivbehandlung im Säuglings- und Kindesalter*. Thieme, Stuttgart
- 1979 Nemes C., Niemer M., Noack G.: *Datenbuch Anästhesiologie*. Gustav Fischer, Stuttgart
- 1979 Niemer M., Nemes C.: *Datenbuch Intensivmedizin*. Gustav Fischer, Stuttgart
- 1980 Dudziak R.: *Lehrbuch der Anästhesiologie*. Schattauer, Stuttgart
- 1981 Grabow L.: *Hirnfunktion unter dem Einfluss der Allgemeinanästhesie*. Fischer, Stuttgart
- 1982 Doenicke A., Kettler D., List W.F., Tarnow J., Thomson D.: *Lehrbuch der Anästhesiologie und Intensivmedizin*. Springer, Berlin (new edition 1992)
- 1983 Tarnow J.: *Anästhesie und Kardiologie in der Herzchirurgie*. Springer, Berlin
- 1984 Larsen R.: *Anästhesie bei Herz-, Thorax und Gefäßchirurgie. Grundlagen und Praxis. Thoraxanästhesie*. Springer, Berlin
- 1984 Lutz H. et al.: *Anästhesiologische Praxis*. Springer, Berlin
- 1985 Larsen R.: *Anästhesie*. Urban & Schwarzenberg, Munich
- 1985 Kretz F.J.: *Anästhesie im Kindesalter*. Springer, Berlin
- 1987 List W.F., Ostwald P.M.: *Komplikationen in der Anästhesie*. Springer, Berlin
- Osswald, P.M., Hartung H.J.: *Anleitungen zur anästhesiologischen Praxis*. Bergmann, Munich
- 1988 Lipp M. et al.: *Anästhesiologische Aspekte in der Zahnmedizin*. Bibliomed, Melsungen
- 1988 Baum J.: *Die Inhalationsnarkose mit niedrigem Frischgasflow*. Thieme, Stuttgart
- 1989 Kretz F.J., Schäfer J., Eyrich K.: *Anästhesie, Intensivmedizin, Notfallmedizin, Schmerztherapie*. Springer, Berlin
- 1989 Peter K., Frey L., Hobbhahn J.: *Anästhesiologie*. Enke, Stuttgart
- 1992 Jöhr M.: *Kinderanästhesie*. Urban & Schwarzenberg, Munich
- 1995 Georgieff M., Schirmer U.: *Klinische Anästhesiologie*. Springer, Berlin
- 1996 Brandt L., Krauskopf K.H., Somons F.: *Handbuch der Kardioanästhesie*. Wiss. Verlagsgesellschaft, Stuttgart
- 1996 Biro P., Pasch T.: *Anästhesie bei seltenen Erkrankungen*. Springer, Berlin
- 1997 Martin E.: *Facharztlehrbuch Anästhesiologie*. Blackwell, Berlin
- 1998 Heck M., Fresenius M.: *Repetitorium Anästhesiologie*. Springer, Berlin
- 1999 Roewer N., Thiel H.: *Anästhesie Compact*. Thieme, Stuttgart
- 2000 Scherer R.: *Anästhesiologie – Ein handlungsorientiertes Lehrbuch*. Thieme, Stuttgart
- 2000 Jantzen J.P., Löffler W.: *Neuroanästhesie – Grundlagen – Klinik – Neuromonitoring – Intensivmedizin*. Thieme, Stuttgart
- 2000 Schulte am Esch J., Kochs E., Bause H.W.: *Anästhesie und Intensivmedizin*. Thieme, Stuttgart
- 2001 Striebel H.W.: *Die Anästhesie*. Schattauer, Stuttgart
- 2001 Kochs E., Krier C., Buzello W., Adams H.A.: *AINS, Band 1, Anästhesiologie*. Thieme, Stuttgart

The large number of publications reflects the increasing importance of the specialty of anaesthesiology gained within a few years time. In addition to these textbooks, a large number of paperbacks and handbooks have become

2

Moderne Narkose

Theorie und Praxis der Routineverfahren

Von

Lothar Barth

Prof. Dr. med. habil., F.F.A.R.C.S., Facharzt für Anästhesiologie,
Chefarzt der Anästhesieabteilung, Robert-Rössle-Klinik,
Forschungsgemeinschaft der Deutschen Akademie der Wissenschaften
zu Berlin

und

Manfred Meyer

a. o. Dozent Dr. med. habil., Facharzt für Anästhesiologie,
Chefarzt des Laboratoriums für experimentelle Anästhesiologie, Robert-Rössle-Klinik,
Forschungsgemeinschaft der Deutschen Akademie der Wissenschaften
zu Berlin

Zweite, überarbeitete und erweiterte Auflage
Mit 360 zum Teil farbigen Abbildungen im Text und einer Tafel

GUSTAV FISCHER VERLAG · STUTTGART
1965

◻ **Fig. 2.30.** Title page of the first East German textbook by Barth and Meyer

available addressing residents, students and anaesthesia staff, which have become very popular.

Many translations of Anglo-American monographs followed and became prevalent in West Germany, too. Lothar Barth's (1921–1979) textbook **Moderne Narkose** (◻ Fig. 2.30) was first published in 1962. It received considerable attention and a second edition became available in 1966, but because of Barth's emigration to West Germany in 1972, no further editions were published.

Hartwig Ferdinand Poppelbaum (1920–2004), who was considered a pioneer in modern techniques in anaesthesiology in East Germany, translated English textbooks into German for more than 30 years to be published in both parts of Germany, contributing to a transfer of knowledge. Significant translations and monographs are listed below.

Selection of Standard Textbooks by English Authors Translated by Hans Ferdinand Poppelbaum

- 1960 *Grundlagen der Allgemeinnarkose,* VEB Volk und Gesundheit, Berlin
- 1962 *Physik für Anästhesisten.* Hüthig, Heidelberg
- 1962 *Automatische Ventilation der Lungen.* Akademie-Verlag, Berlin
- 1965 *Grundlagen und Praxis der geburtshilflichen Anästhesie.* VEB Volk und Gesundheit, Berlin
- 1967 *Thoraxanästhesie.* VEB Volk und Gesundheit, Berlin
- 1968 *Elektrokardiographie für den Anästhesisten.* VEB Volk und Gesundheit, Berlin
- 1978 *Synopsis der Anästhesie,* 2nd edn. 1985. VEB Volk und Gesundheit, Berlin
- 1982 *Lumbalpunktion, intradurale und extradurale Spinalanalgesie.* VEB Volk und Gesundheit, Berlin
- 1983 *Vorbereitung der Anästhesie.* VEB Volk und Gesundheit, Berlin
- 1985 *Arzneimittelwechselwirkungen in der Anästhesie und Intensivtherapie.* G. Fischer, Stuttgart
- 1990 *Anästhesiologische und internistische Betreuung in der perioperativen Phase.* G. Fischer, Stuttgart

In addition to translated books, several original German monographs were published in East Germany; unfortunately, they were not successfully sold in West Germany.

Selection of Textbooks by East German Authors

- 1962 Barth L., Meyer M.: *Moderne Narkose.* G. Fischer, Jena
- 1975 Schoeppner H., Dietze R., Mielke U.: *Anästhesie und Reanimation in der Kinderneurologie.* Thieme, Leipzig
- 1977 Benad G., Schädlich M.: *Grundriß der Anästhesiologie – Lehrbuch für Studenten,* 4th edn. VEB Volk und Gesundheit, Berlin
- 1980 Langanke D., Warm R.: *Anästhesie und Intensivtherapie in der Geburtshilfe und Neonatologie.* Thieme, Leipzig
- 1983 Meyer M., Schädlich M.: *Allgemeine Anästhesie.* VEB Volk und Gesundheit, Berlin
- 1986 Baust G., Borchert K.: *Interdisziplinäre Intensivtherapie.* VEB Volk und Gesundheit, Berlin
- 1987 Meyer M.: *Physiologische und pharmakologische Grundlagen der Anästhesie.* VEB Volk und Gesundheit, Berlin

Next to German medical journals and the above-mentioned books, several series were published on special issues in anaesthesiology and manifold papers were presented at symposiums or congresses, inducing excellent discussions. A few are mentioned here because of their impact on anaesthesiology:

Anesthesiology and Resuscitation was partly published in English and renamed Anaesthesiologie und Wiederbelebung with the 95th volume. It was first issued by R. Frey, S. Kern and O. Mayrhofer in 1964 and appeared in 226 volumes.

Another series that has to be mentioned here was Klinische Anästhesiologie und Intensivtherapie initiated in 1973 by anaesthetists from Ulm. It was available until 1995, when volume 47 was printed.

Thieme first published a series called Intensivmedizin, Notfallmedizin, Anästhesiologie launched in 1976 by the anaesthesiologists Peter Lawin (1930–2002) and Horst Stoeckel (*1930), the surgeon Georg Rodewald (1921–1991) and the internist Paul Schölmerich (1916–2000). The publication was finished with volume 82 in 1992.

Obviously, publications like these were no longer attractive once online services were inaugurated.

Further Professional Training in Anaesthesiology

»These days, nothing ages quicker than knowledge« (Roman Herzog, 1997)

With the steady and rapid growth of data and knowledge in medicine, education in this subject has to be a lifelong endeavour, as this is the only way to meet future challenges of our specialty. This was accepted early in the history of anaesthesiology; thus, the Deutsche Akademie für Anästhesiologische Fortbildung (DAAF, German Academy of Continuing Education in Anaesthesiology) was established in 1979 by the DGAI and the BDA in order to assure superior education in anaesthesia, intensive and emergency care medicine as well as pain management.

The DAAF adopted some Anglo-American ideas known as »continuing medical education« that will endure in Germany. At the 102nd Deutscher Ärztetag in Cottbus in 1999, it was determined that by 2003 a uniform certificate valid nationwide had to be added or substituted for state credentials. In the future these may be replaced by European diplomas. The Royal College of Surgeons of Ireland and Harvard Medical International designed a concept for further education that spread across Europe and beyond [39].

In addition, training on simulators has become widely accepted in the past 15 years. Adopted from simulation in aviation to eradicate human factors and improve crisis resource management, which might help avoid disastrous crashes, it has become a precious tool in acquiring specific skills in anaesthesiology. Starting in the 1960s, when simulators became available to detect correct endotracheal intubation and positioning [40], major advances could be made ever since inexpensive microchips and suitable software were offered during the early 1980s [41].

Human patient simulators have been installed in different departments of anaesthesiology at university medical hospitals (Aachen, Bonn, Berlin, Düsseldorf, Erlangen, Göttingen, Hamburg, Heidelberg, Mainz, Tübingen and Würzburg), utilizing dummies equipped with software comprising a variety of physiological, pharmacological, respiratory and haemodynamic models. The degree of difficulty can be adapted to the participants' educational levels (◻ Fig. 2.31).

In order to improve performance in critical situations and to convey medical aspects in anaesthesiology, video-assisted debriefing is performed [42]. With the aid of human patient simulators standard situations can be practised in a genuine environment; hence, in some European countries, e.g. Denmark and the Netherlands, board certification in anaesthesiology requires training at the human patient simulator. Various State Chambers of Physicians in Germany validate these courses and issue certificates.

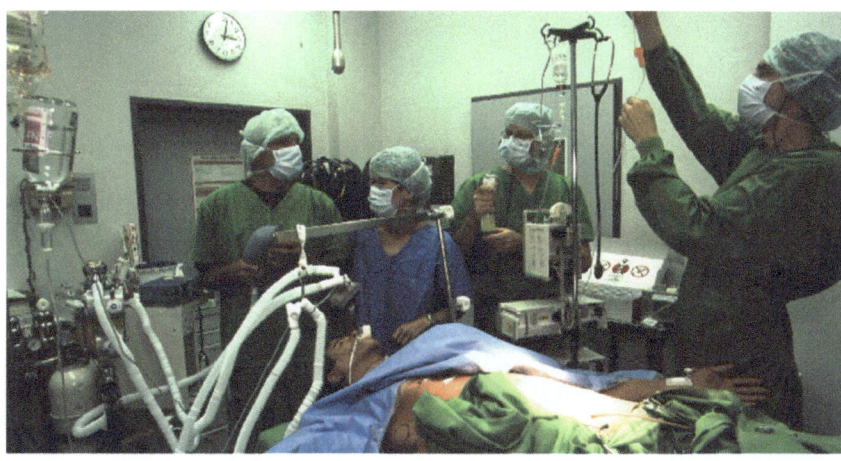

◻ **Fig. 2.31.** Training at the anaesthesia simulator

Leading anaesthesists became increasingly aware of the influence of the quality of undergraduate teaching on the choice of anaesthesiology as a professional career and, therefore, initiated surveys about the knowledge about, and the reputation of, anaesthesiology among medical students [42a]. It was wide-spread experience that courses in advanced life support using full-scale simulators had proven particularly attractive to students if given by anaesthesiologists. This prompted the German Society of Anaesthesiology and Intensive Care Medicine in 2003 to enable 30 university departments to purchase an anaesthesia simulator for the use in undergraduate teaching [42b].

Development of Techniques in Anaesthesiology

Techniques to secure the airway have become essential in anaesthesiology, intensive care medicine and emergency medicine.

With muscle relaxants being available, endotracheal intubation and artificial ventilation for longer surgical procedures became inevitable. Along with the spread of these techniques from the early 1950s, the number of case reports published on incidents and complications grew rapidly. This may be attributed to the fact that traumatizing methods were utilized, e.g. blind nasal intubation of patients with spontaneous breathing, tactile orotracheal intubation according to Kuhn, as well as other blind intubation techniques. Endotracheal intubation became popular in hospitals of various sizes including university medical hospitals. Airway management had to be adapted for a growing number of operative procedures and for distinctive patients with orofacial abnormalities even in neonates, acromegaly, trauma or wounds of the upper airway and the anaesthesiologist had to beware of difficult intubation that could not be handled without specific training.

Various publications on fiberscopes in difficult airway management promoted the utilization of bronchoscopes (❑ Fig. 2.32a, b). First reports by Japanese authors date back to 1967, followed by a paper from Helmut Kronschwitz (*1928) who described findings in Germany in 1969 [43]. By the early 1980s, fiberscopes were available at nearly every large hospital; hence, professional training on handling these fragile devices and techniques was required [44].

Archie Brain's (*1943) invention of the laryngeal mask in 1983 has to be mentioned as another major advance in anaesthesiology [45]. As an alternative to an endotracheal tube or a face mask, it has become an eminent tool in difficult airway management, since terrifying situations like »cannot intubate, cannot ventilate« may be overcome; hence, it is utilized all over the world [46].

With the exclusive usage of disposable materials and the availability of disinfecting solutions, the number of complications caused by sterilization and reuse of tubes as well as the incidence of infections decreased [47].

In the post-war period, nitrous oxide as well as diethyl ether next to cyclopropane, which was introduced by Ralph M. Waters (1883–1979) in the1930s [48], were available in operating theatres. Cyclopropane was a fast-acting powerful gas – and highly explosive when combined with oxygen – so that it was soon banned from operating theatres in contrast to ether, which was also highly explosive in oxygen and was utilized even in the 1960s [49]. Ether mono-anaesthesia was uncomfortable, since it was performed according to the Guedel technique leading to excitation and hypersalivation.

The volatile anaesthetic halothane was developed at ICI, an English company, in 1956 and promptly turned out to be popular. It was introduced by James Raventos (1905–1983) and became available in Germany right after the first clinical trials. It had great advantages compared to other volatile anaesthetics like ether [50].

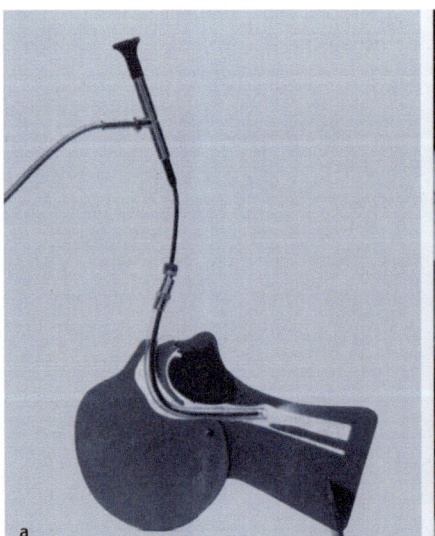
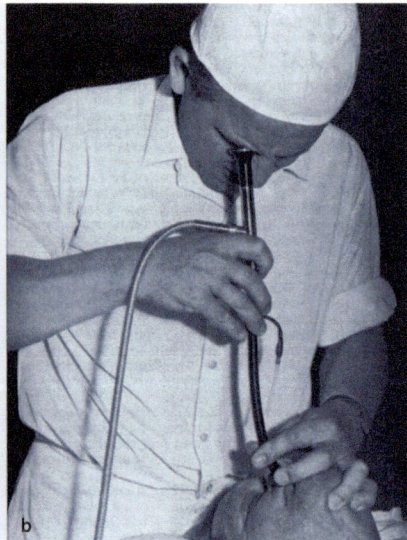

❑ **Fig. 2.32a,b. a** Diagram of fiberoptic intubation. **b** Intubation with a fiberscope (around 1969)

With the introduction of vaporizers in the 1960s, which allowed adjustment of dosage [51], and the invention of devices to measure concentration of gases (»Narkometer«) such as the one developed by Helmut Vonderschmitt (1914–1998) volatile anaesthetics advanced into a growing number of operating theatres [52].

Methoxyflurane, introduced in 1966, a highly potent anaesthetic, became popular very fast and was abandoned as quickly, since 50-70% of the agent were biotransformed to nephrotoxic metabolites [53]. Despite the fact that enflurane, introduced in 1971, was also known to be nephrotoxic and to cause irritations of the CNS in patients with pre-existing CNS maladies – especially epilepsy – it was still utilized. Halothane and enflurane were succeeded by isoflurane with negligible biotransformation and few adverse effects. Two other volatile anaesthetics, i.e. sevoflurane and desflurane, became available in the early 1990s with improved pharmacological characteristics [54]. They exhibited some peculiarities, too, but these did not warrant discontinuation of their use.

Since its introduction in the late 1990s, xenon, which is indicated in patients with cardiocirculatory co-morbidities, has been the subject of research as it seems to be an ideal volatile anaesthetic according to the findings of international clinical studies. Its limited availability and high cost hinder clinical use [55].

In the early 1950s, drugs to be administered intravenously were developed in order to achieve analgesia, hypnosis and muscle relaxation apart from volatile anaesthetics. The American anaesthetist John S. Lundy (1894–1973) named the combination »balanced anaesthesia« in the early 1920s [56]. Walter Henschel (1926–2002) of Bremen promoted the »cocktail lytique« for neuroleptanalgesia (NLA) in Germany [57].

Later, the combination of the neuroleptic agent dehydrobenzperidol with the opioid analgesic fentanyl was termed the »standard NLA technique«; adverse events included postoperative respiratory depression, extrapyramidal symptoms, and states of severe confusion as well as prolonged sedation. Even though large amounts of analgesics were administered, hypertension and tachycardia occurred due to intubation and major surgical stimuli, e.g. sternotomy or manipulation at the peritoneum.

The need for intravenous anaesthetics that could be easily adapted in dosage initiated the search for new hypnotics, analeptics and analgesics in the early 1970s. Pharmacokinetic characteristics like rapid onset and fast elimination of drugs to be administered via precision infusion pumps were new aspects. Numerous tests on pharmacokinetics and pharmacodynamics were performed to identify dosages of agents and the idea of »target

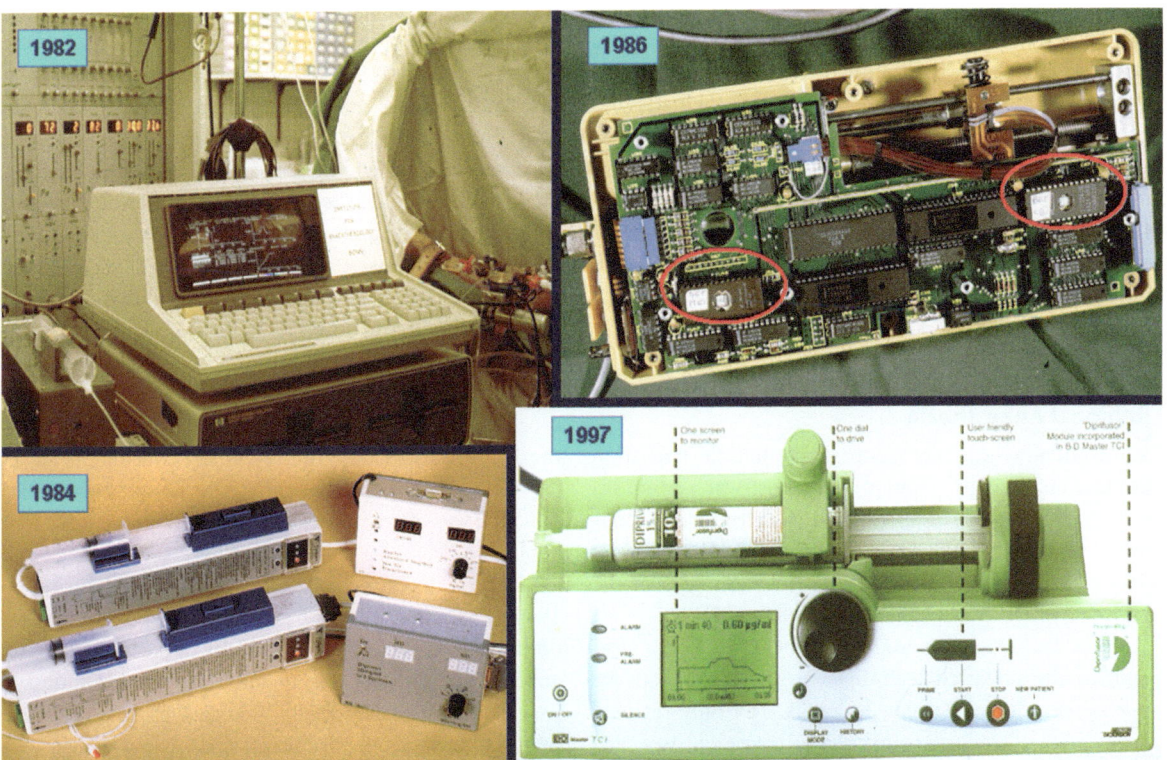

Fig. 2.33. Target-controlled-infusion (TCI): from the first prototype (1982) to the final TCI pump (1997)

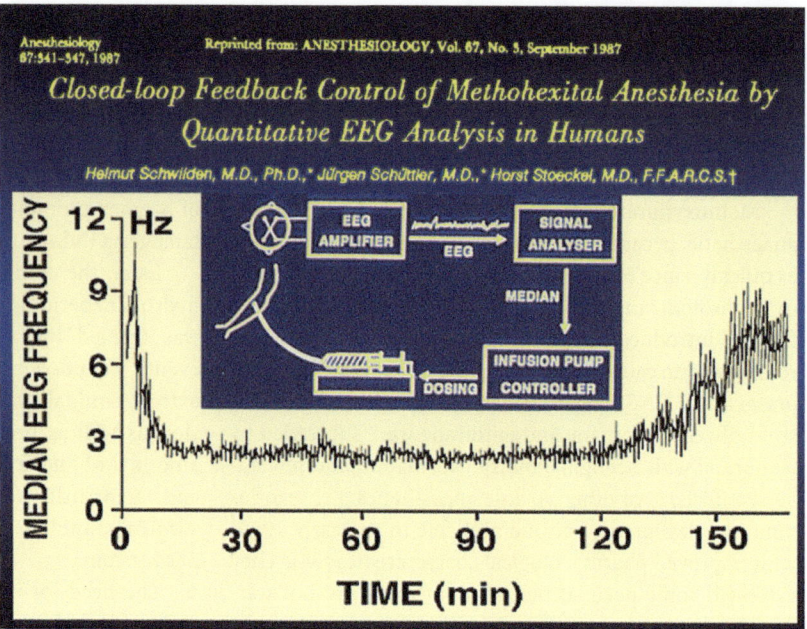

Fig. 2.34. Closed-loop anaesthesia based on the EEG

controlled infusion« (TCI; ▪ Fig. 2.33) was invented with infusion rates and dosage calculated by microprocessors inside the infusion pump [58].

A paper on »closed-loop total intravenous anaesthesia« was published in 1987 by a group of physicians under the expert guidance of Horst Stoeckel (*1930) [59]. As opposed to the open loop in target-controlled infusion systems with no feedback on patients' data, the EEG was the main parameter in estimating pharmacokinetic and pharmacodynamic values in a »closed-loop« technique (▪ Fig. 2.34). These concepts were developed with the findings of the American anaesthesiologists Raymond F. Courtin (1912–2001), Reginald G. Bickford (1913–1998) and Albert Faulconer (1911–1985) in mind, who had tried to adjust dosage of ether according to the patient's EEG signal in the 1950s [60].

Regional Anaesthesia

Since endotracheal intubation under muscle relaxation became increasingly popular in the post-war period, regional anaesthesia was abandoned worldwide: data published in the early 1950s reveal a similar tendency for the Mayo Clinic and for the Department of Surgery of the University Medical Hospital in Heidelberg [61].

After the DGA was founded, general anaesthesia remained the preferred technique in anaesthesiology for several decades at German hospitals. The only regional anaesthesia procedures comprised spinal as well as – even to a lesser extent – epidural anaesthesia; intravenous or plexus anaesthesia were extremely rare. Spinal, epidu-

ral or plexus anaesthesias were mainly performed by surgeons themselves. They had no alternative, as there was a severe lack of professionally trained, experienced anaesthesiologists. With the growing number of departments of anaesthesiology, the use of regional anaesthesia was reduced. This may be explained from today's point of view as follows:

Hans Nolte (1929–1998), who was a pioneer in spreading regional anaesthesia during the early 1970s, argued that regional anaesthesia techniques were neglected because of never-ending discussions with the surgeons on the most suitable technique. Anaesthesiologists preferred general anaesthesia like »balanced anaesthesia« administering muscle relaxants combined with volatile and intravenous anaesthetics as well as modern machines for anaesthesia and respirators that surgeons could not handle.

Hence, the first generation of anaesthesiologists put much more emphasis on general than on regional anaesthesia during specialty training. Many consultants lacked experience in regional anaesthesia techniques so that the outcome was often unsatisfactory if these procedures were applied [62].

Interest in regional anaesthesia rebounded during the 1970s, a fact that was probably influenced by discussions on hepato- as well as nephrotoxicity of particular volatile anaesthetics. In addition, regional anaesthesia found its way into pain management strategies, especially for patients suffering from chronic pain.

As a result a supplement on »Regional Anaesthesia« appeared every 3 months in the journal *Der Anaesthesist* after 1978. It reflected a growing interest in and increasing number of complex regional anaesthesia techniques.

With the growing popularity of regional anaesthesia techniques, an increasing demand for textbooks on regional anaesthesia emerged. The 9th edition of Heinrich Braun's (1862–1934) textbook Die örtliche Betäubung, edited by Arthur Läwen (1876–1958) and published in 1951, no longer met modern standards, but still remained a popular reference book. In 1959, Hans Killian issued the monograph Lokalanästhesie und Lokalanästhetika, which became a precious companion to physicians performing regional anaesthesia [63].

A number of less comprehensive books like the paperback Kompendium der Lokalanästhesie by Hans Georg Auberger (1925–1981) published in 1967 became widespread. In 1982, a considerably more comprehensive 4th edition was published in collaboration with the anaesthesiologist Hans Christoph Niesel (*1936) of Ludwigshafen. In the preface, they proclaimed an interim »renaissance of regional anaesthesia« »since the limits of general anaesthesia« have become obvious and »both techniques can be considered equal« [64].

The Lehrbuch Regionalanästhesie, published in 1981, was just as interesting for anaesthesiologists, since it described different regional anaesthesia techniques for surgery as well as obstetrics. Meanwhile, it has been edited by Hans Christoph Niesel (*1936), Christel Panhans (*1941) and Michael Zenz (*1945).

Hans Nolte published an English as well as a German edition of the monograph Illustrated Manual of Regional Anesthesia with the Indian anaesthesiologist P. Prithvi Raj (*1919) and the American Michael D. Stanton-Hicks (*1937), which was highly recognized for its outstanding academic standard [65]. It was designated »Most Beautiful Book of the Year« in 1988 by the Stiftung Buchkunst of the Börsenverein des Deutschen Buchandels in appreciation of its superior illustrations and sublime didactics (◻ Fig. 2.35).

Local anaesthesia techniques that had been established for many decades were replaced by newer, more invasive procedures during the 1980s; since they carried additional risks, they were the focus of lengthy arguments at congresses and in the scientific literature. Especially thoracic epidural anaesthesia has to be mentioned in this context, since it appears to be a perilous procedure [66].

Epidural analgesia with the aid of implanted catheters has proven successful in pain therapy over extended periods, i.e. weeks and months, e.g. in patients with malignancies or suffering from urologic as well as gynaecological maladies or having undergone abdominal surgery. For the management of trauma patients as well as in orthopaedic surgery, peripheral nerve blocks are gaining further importance in Germany, e.g. various techniques of anaesthesia of the brachial plexus.

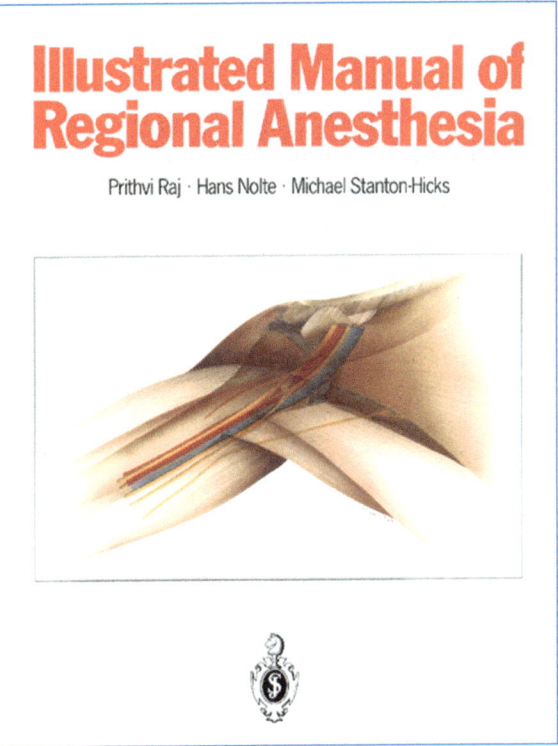

◻ **Fig. 2.35.** Title page of P. Prithvi Raj's, Michael D. Stanton-Hick's and Hans Nolte's textbook, Illustrated Manual of Regional Anesthesia, published in 1988

Artificial Ventilation and Respirators

Growing expertise in endotracheal intubation and muscle relaxation for extensive surgery generated a demand for machines for artificial ventilation. As opposed to this, physicians had favoured manual ventilation for many years, believing that ventilation could be monitored by an »experienced hand« and assuming that this method was more sensible to detect a change in resistance [67].

Their hesitation was prompted by difficulties in handling the respirators as well as their reliability regarding pressure and volume regulation, as the influx of fresh gas influenced the effective respiratory volume. Machines like the Pulmomat manufactured by the Dräger Company, which was developed in 1952 based on the old Pulmotor principle, worked on compressed air or oxygen that could be connected to all Dräger anaesthetic circuits [68]. With the introduction of flowmeters the above-mentioned technical hitches could be overcome [69].

These limitations also applied to many other respirators developed at that time, e.g. a model named after its designer, the Swedish physician Carl-Gunnar Engström (1912–1987) (◻ Fig. 2.36), which delivered a defined volume of gas as opposed to the »Dräger Pulmotor« [70].

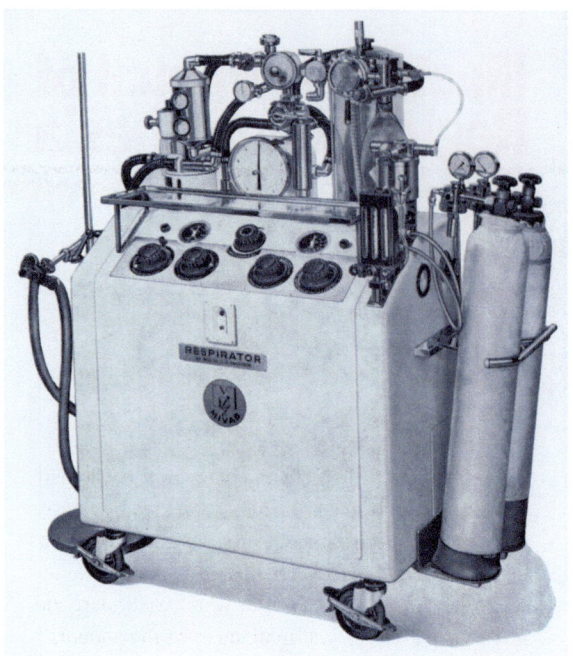

Fig. 2.36. »Engström Respirator 200« (1960)

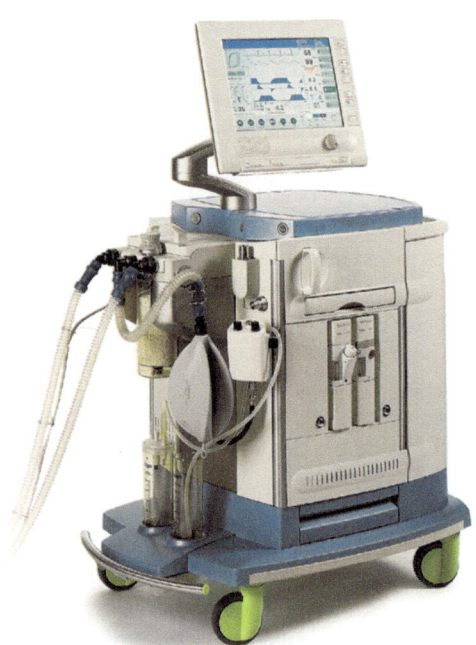

Fig. 2.37. The anaesthetic apparatus of the Dräger Company: the »Zeus« Model (2002)

With the newly elaborated ventilation nomogram, individual patterns for ventilation were accessible [71].

Devices to measure respiratory volume and pressure were introduced in 1960 [72]. Respirators had to be explosion proof, since ether still was en vogue; hence, the »Narkosespiromat 5000« was introduced. It was powered by electricity and offered a large range of respiration patterns [73]: exact selection and adjustment of the respiratory volume between 50 and 1,000 ml, variable frequency of 10–40/min, pressure reserve (+45 mbar) to ensure constant volume even in patients with elevated respiratory resistance as well as choice of inspiration:expiration ratio from 1:1 to 1:2.

For years, vivid discussions were conducted on various ventilation patterns for anaesthesia like alternating pressure or intermittent positive pressure ventilation. Physicians believed the former to interfere less with the patient's cardiac performance. Negative pressure during expiration was supposed to enhance central venous return. Animal models revealed that tension at the alveolar surface was reduced and atelectasis was prominent. Thus, positive pressure respiration prevailed. Further development of electronic devices and evolving monitoring systems for various parameters like inspiratory volume, frequency, peaks and plateaus of pressure as well as inhalation to exhalation ratio facilitated the introduction of distinguished ventilation strategies [74].

Anaesthesia-based ventilators manufactured by the Dräger Company, e.g. »Cicero« and »Cato« as well as »Physioflex« – the latest technological concept as a completely electronically regulated closed-circuit respirator – have to be mentioned in this context next to anaesthesia-based monitoring that was integrated into respirators by the Siemens Company (»Kion«) as well as the Dräger Company (»Zeus«, ▫ Fig. 2.37).

As hospitals were reconstructed or newly built after World War II, central gas reservoirs and supply systems were anticipated. During the early 1960s, the advantages of the American »piping systems« that had already been established in the 1930s were acknowledged. For reasons of economy as well as prevention of possible hazards, gas cylinders made of steel for anaesthesia machines were no longer considered appropriate. The installation of a central gas supply, compressed air and vacuum plants in hospitals permitted the use of many anaesthesia machines, inhalation and insufflation devices, oxygen and climate tents, incubators as well as respirators [75].

Patient Monitoring, Vascular Access and Documentation
Monitoring

»Circulation and respiration should be continuously monitored during anaesthesia« – this statement was made by the surgeon Johann Ferdinand Heyfelder (1798–1869) of Erlangen in his monograph on ether anaesthesia [76]. For decades this was the duty of the so-called *Pulsarius*; later examination of the pupils and

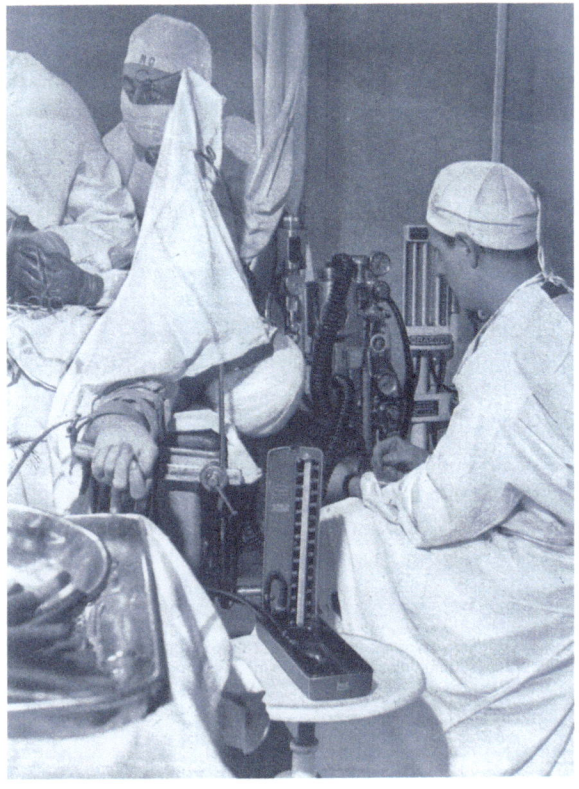

Fig. 2.38. Anaesthesia equipment around 1950

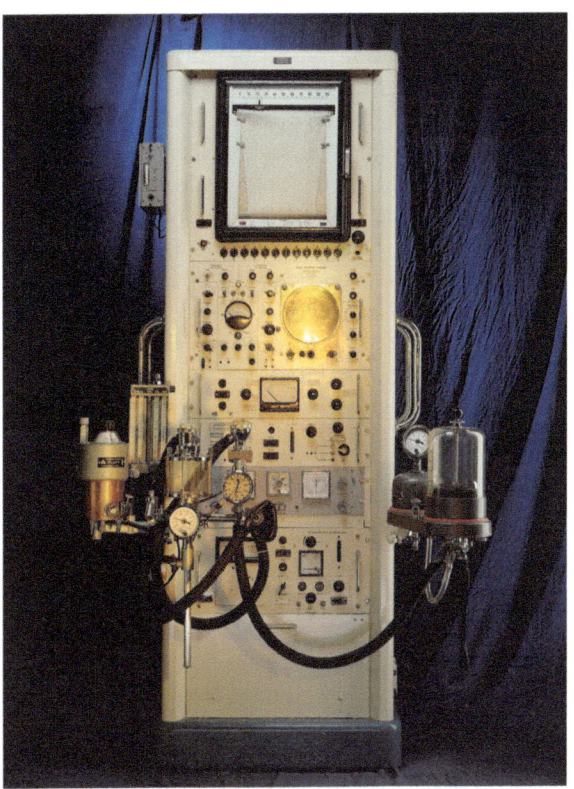

Fig. 2.39. Anaesthesia equipment with integrated monitoring devices developed by Heinz Oehmig (around 1960)

monitoring blood pressure were included, but documentation in an anaesthesia chart as is obligatory today was uncommon.

Monitoring like this was still practiced in the early 1950s in some places, although attempts at continuous automatic recording of vital parameters as well as acoustic and optical visualization had already been made in the 1920s and 1930s in order to detect adverse events early and to avoid complications [77]. War interfered with these efforts and they were not revived until the post-war period (Fig. 2.38).

The German anaesthesiologists Heinz Oehmig (1919–2005) and Helmut Vonderschmitt (1914–1998) recognized the impact of closely monitoring anaesthetised patients according to Galileo Galilei's axiom »Measure everything that can be measured, and make measurable what cannot be measured yet«. During the 1950s, both of them were involved in designing an apparatus to comprehensively monitor physiological parameters in the anaesthetized patient. By the end of the 1950s, Oehmig had invented the »anaesthesia monitoring apparatus with an integrated electronic respirator and anaesthesia machine« (Fig. 2.39), which can be categorized as modern according to today's standard. It allowed continuous assessment and documentation of heart rate and peripheral pulse frequencies, tidal

volume, concentration of end-expiratory and inspiratory carbon dioxide as well as expiratory oxygen.

This device was supplemented by a fast multi-channel recorder for the registration of ECG, EEG, carbon dioxide concentration as well as blood pressure and pulse [78].

The growing demand for monitoring devices for the anaesthetized patient was dismissed as excessive in many places. Some critics were reluctant to accept monitoring systems except for specialized needs, e.g. cardiac surgery or research, »an introduction into operating theatres for general surgery, as has been suggested, seems to be exaggerated« [79]. This reticence is understandable even today because general anaesthesia and endotracheal intubation had not been implemented in many hospitals, and ether anaesthesia with a Schimmelbusch mask was the common technique.

Increasing numbers of general anaesthesia with endotracheal intubation and artificial ventilation and the growing sophistication of surgical techniques made it essential to monitor the anaesthetized patient's vital functions. For unknown reasons devices to detect carbon dioxide in respiratory air, which had been available since the 1950s, only found their way into the theatre much later. The same applies to monitors for saturation of the blood with oxygen that had already been obtainable in the 1940s [80]. The idea of combining oximetry with photoplethysmography to create pulse oximetry can be attributed to Japanese researchers. Nevertheless, in the 1980s, as the microprocessors and light-emitting diodes (LEDs) that were able to constantly emit light of the same quality became available, proper systems for use under clinical conditions could be invented. After that, pulse oximetry spread quickly [81].

The invention of devices for monitoring carbon dioxide concentration in respiratory air was similarly delayed, even though a reliable unit called »URAS« had already become available in the 1950s [82]. These measuring devices were not integrated into the anaesthesia systems until the early 1980s. The DGAI was early to appreciate the value of monitors that measured carbon dioxide and oxygen concentration in the patient's blood and to recommend them in 1989 for all anaesthetic workstations. It took only a few more years until it became compulsory [83] (◘ Fig. 2.40).

Vascular Access

Growing knowledge on the impact of adequate perioperative infusion therapy in patients undergoing surgery by the end of the 1950s raised awareness about it; hence intravenous infusion replaced subcutaneous administration by the 1960s, utilizing a reusable injection needle, butterfly needle or double cannula made of stainless steel. Nevertheless, their tip often perforated the vein resulting in paravascular distribution. The introduction of flexible plastic cannulae, developed by the anaesthesiologist Otto Just (1922–2012) of Heidelberg, produced by the company B. Braun Melsungen AG that were available from 1966 and named Braunüle, eliminated this disadvantage [84].

Having proven successful, infusion therapy for longer periods became popular in the critically ill; thus, thin-walled catheters were placed reaching the intrathoracic vena cava. Since complications occurred, e.g. thrombosis along the catheter or catheter perforation, indications had to be restricted and aseptic insertion was regarded to be inexorable. Because of growing experience with the procedure, improvement of materials used and atraumatic puncture techniques, venesection became unnecessary within a few years time.

Further development of disposable Swan-Ganz catheters with integrated thermistors and stimulation probes allowed determination of cardiac output via temperature dilution techniques, recording of intracardiac ECG and electric stimulation of the right atrium or the right ventricle. German anaesthesiologists commenced to apply them initially for cardiac surgery only; later they were considered advantageous to any critically ill patient. Less invasive percutaneous puncture techniques also diminished any reluctance to use the procedure [85].

Despite all the expertise gained in dealing with invasive devices – especially the Swan-Ganz catheter – complications occurred; hence, controversies that started in the USA reached Germany. This prompted the President's office of the Deutsche Gesellschaft für Anästhesiologie und Intensivmedizin to publish a statement [86].

New Monitoring Procedures

In the search for less invasive diagnostic and monitoring tools, techniques were established in the past two decades based on ultrasound. In anaesthesia, ECG and transcra-

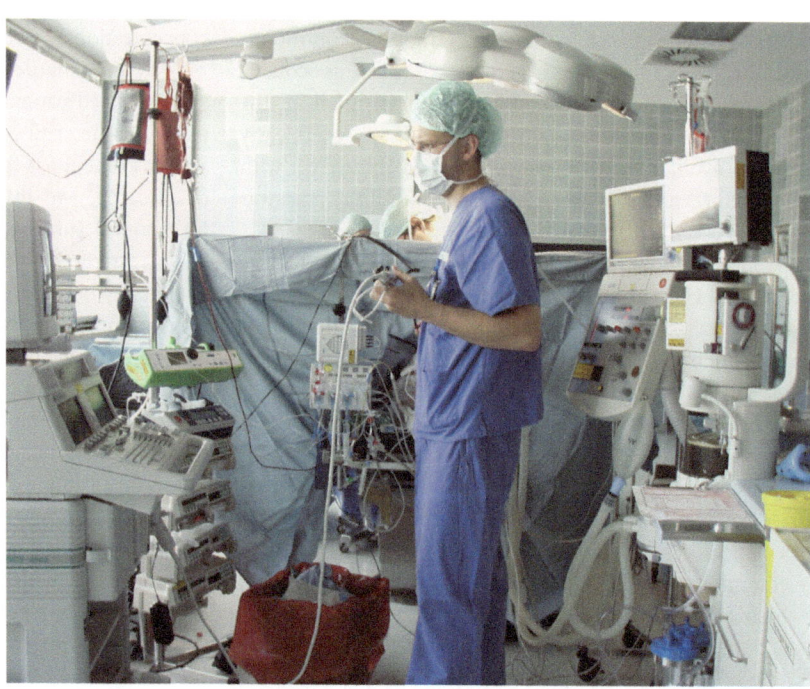

◘ Fig. 2.40. Modern anaesthesia equipment (2002)

nial Doppler were employed [87]. Echocardiography has become part of training guidelines [88] and transcranial Doppler found its way into operating theatres [89].

Continuous ECG monitoring was initially performed with the aid of oscilloscopes. As they were used in the early 1950s in cardiac angiography, they were frequently called »cardioscopes«. However, the quality of the ECG and indicated heart rate was not comparable to today's standard, since artefacts and low-quality signals interfered. For many years needle electrodes or spiral-shaped stylus electrodes poked into the skin were used to obtain the ECG. Artefacts caused by alternating current or the utilization of diathermy could not be suppressed for a long time. Therefore, these devices did not become popular before the 1970s [90].

Devices to monitor respirators in patients receiving artificial ventilation became available by the middle of the 1960s [91]. Next to measuring the concentration of oxygen, airway pressure and tidal volume, alarms signifying disconnection and stenosis were integrated. In addition, appliances for continuous measurement of concentration of volatile anaesthetics were added.

Post-Anaesthesia Recovery Units

As recovery from anaesthesia depends on the type and duration of the anaesthesia as well as surgery, it may take many hours; for this reason, virtually all patients are transferred to a recovery room before being transferred to the ward.

As modern anaesthesia techniques comprising intubation and muscle relaxation were introduced after World War II, and surgical procedures included operations of the abdomen and the chest including the heart in patients of all age groups, special monitoring units became compulsory. As a result, the incidence of adverse events and complications as well as the workload on the wards could be reduced. By the middle of the 1950s recovery units were established in many hospitals [92]. The subject was discussed at anaesthesia congresses, e.g. in 1957 in Vienna, where an English physician gave an account of his 10-year experience with a postoperative recovery unit.

Convinced of the improvement achieved, he recommended taking the following aspects into consideration when establishing recovery units; they still apply today [93]:
1. The unit should be staffed 24 h a day
2. All patients who have received anaesthesia have to go to the unit
3. The staff has to be trained accordingly
4. Not all of the staff should be exchanged at the same time, but one by one
5. Charts have to be recorded properly
6. Recovery units must be located close to the surgical units
7. Emergency doctors have to be available immediately at any time

In 1967, the DGAW published a statement on the organization of recovery rooms, recovery units and intensive care in hospitals [94]. The designations »recovery room«, »recovery unit« and »intensive care« were invented at that time. The recovery room has turned out to be the link between the surgical unit and the wards, being located in the surgical unit and managed by anaesthesiologists.

Reliable Technology, Guidelines and Standards

As explosive volatile anaesthetics like ether and cyclopropane were administered until the middle of the 1960s, various safety problems were encountered. Despite many security measures, explosions occurred because of ignorance regarding safety regulations. Ether-oxygen blends as well as electrostatic anaesthesia machines proved to be especially dangerous [95].

At the same time as efforts were made to improve patient safety during anaesthesia by better training and appropriate monitoring of vital functions, the DGAW created a Standards Committee in the middle of the 1960s: engineers of the German Industrial Standards Committee and members of the specialty were to improve the standardization of anaesthesia equipment. This was a major step on the way to »quality management« [96].

To minimize mixing up of gases, the introduction of a uniform colour code for air, oxygen and nitrous oxide cylinders within Europe was discussed for many years. A new European (EN) standard for connectors for gas was coded [97] by assigning a special geometrical configuration to each connector [98]. Refill systems for vaporizers were designed accordingly [99].

Anaesthesia Protocols and Documentation

At the start of the 1950s the diversity of modern anaesthesia methods with endotracheal intubation, muscle relaxation and artificial ventilation or the combination of regional anaesthesia with general anaesthesia evoked the necessity to introduce charts and protocols for the documentation of procedures applied. This marked the end of the era when a short note was entered into the patient's file. Comprehensive documentation helped avoid complications and charts could be scrutinized for adverse events of the different forms of anaesthesia to be analyzed for statistical purposes (◘ Fig. 2.41).

Devices to electronically process data became increasingly prevalent from the middle of the 1960s, with numerous authors publishing results on their systems. Due to the lack of quality and quantity, results from electronic data processing were seldom accepted, especially with regard to the costs involved in these systems [100].

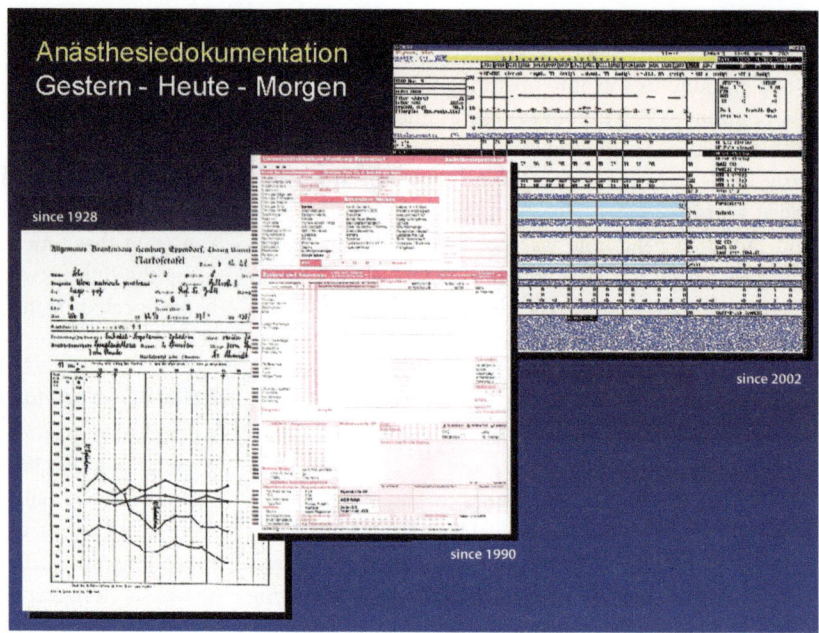

◻ Fig. 2.41. Development of charts in anaesthesiology

Today, regulations require sufficient documentation in anaesthesiology (§11 of the Professional Code of Conduct). To reflect the importance of this requirement, the Society set the standards for minimal documentation in 1989. They were extended to include activity recording and quality management criteria in anaesthesia in 1991–1992. In co-operation with the *German Consulting and Research Society for Hospital Management*, the DGAI added procedure- and quality-related data to medically relevant and patient-related data during the 1990s. These included the listing of adverse events, incidents and complications (*Zwischenfälle, Ereignisse, Komplikationen*, ZEK) during and immediately after procedures, as well as postoperative incidents, malfunctions and complications detected from patient survey or physical examination or analyzing patients' records. In fact, a questionnaire should be included in the postoperative patient survey to estimate patients' satisfaction [101].

Analysis of these results serves to identify when tolerable levels have been exceeded that may require review to determine which quality deficits are responsible. As data are processed for internal and regional use as well as nationwide according to the laws protecting them, a central anaesthesia register could be established to analyze the quality and nature of work in anaesthesiology as well as complications that have occurred.

In addition to securing quality of procedures in anaesthesiology, information on performance can easily be collected in order to estimate the amount of personnel and equipment required as well as to assure the best possible use of work units.

Anaesthesia Techniques in Different Operative Specialities

This section outlines developments in the areas of cardiac surgery, neurosurgery and transplantation surgery as well as gynaecology and obstetrics.

Cardiac Surgery

The importance of cardiac surgery has grown significantly over the past four decades. In 2002, approximately 97,000 patients underwent cardiac surgery in 80 different centres with the aid of extracorporeal circulation of international standard [102].

When Martin Zindler (*1920) anaesthetized the first patient for open heart surgery in surface hypothermia at the University Hospital in Düsseldorf on 9 February 1955 [103], it seemed impossible that the majority of cardiac surgical cases would be performed at non-university hospitals in the future. Important technical advances were part of this quick improvement. Also, it did not appear feasible at that time that patients would be mobilized on the day of cardiac surgery and be healthy enough to be discharged only a few days later. Progress in the field of cardiac surgery may also be attributed to innovations in anaesthesia. Initially, only bubble and rotating disk oxygenators were available, until in the 1980s, screen oxygenators were obtainable. The introduction of heparin-coated circuits was another important step up [104]. Because of the many technical inventions, some problems could be overcome that had accounted for numerous postoperative complications.

Because of superior surgical techniques and new drugs available to the anaesthesiologist, various proce-

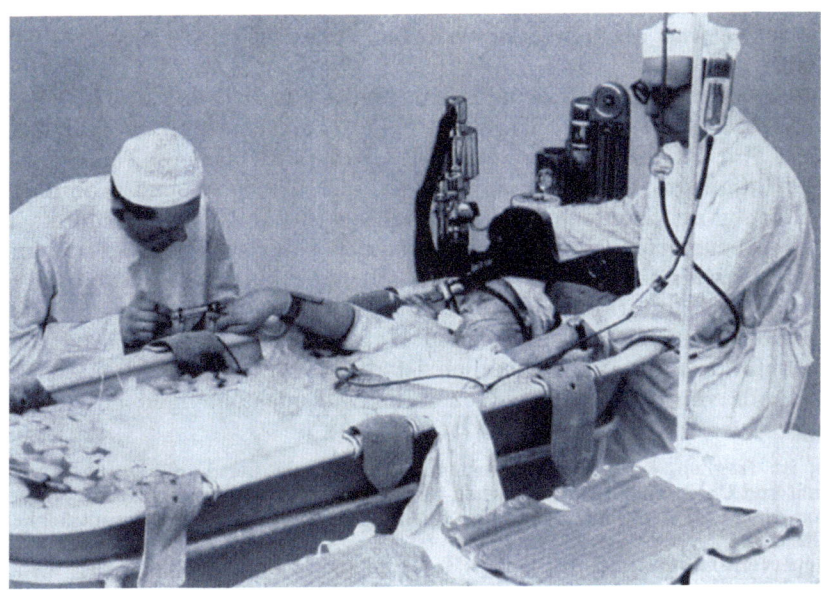

Fig. 2.42. Anaesthetized patient in an ice water bath. Artificial ventilation with ventilation bag (Martin Zindler at the head of the patient)(1955)

dures in cardiac surgery may be performed without the aid of extracorporeal circulation (ECC), i.e. »off-pump coronary artery bypass« [105]), decreasing the incidence of neurological adverse events. Minimally invasive surgery also became popular in cardiac surgery (»minimally invasive direct coronary artery bypass«. Surgery with ECC via alternative access (»port access cardiac surgery«) may be performed with robot assistance. Meanwhile, hypothermia has been omitted in cardiac surgery, only a few patients will experience mild cooling. This technique is called »warm heart surgery«.

Initially, ether anaesthesia and hypothermia in an ice water bath were used (Fig. 2.42). For many years, this technique was continued at the University Medical Hospital in Düsseldorf. The patients' temperature was adjusted by cold water running through mats instead of cooling immersion baths [106]. At this point in time, extracorporeal circulation became available allowing more time for intracardiac procedures. The first effort to utilize this machine proved unsuccessful in Berlin in October 1957, but in 1958 Rudolf Zenker (1903–1979) of Marburg successfully performed surgery on a heart defect with the aid of extracorporeal circulation [107].

Anaesthesia procedures had to be adapted to various demands during surgery. Initially, only volatile anaesthetics were administered. Ether and cyclopropane in nitrous oxide/oxygen were replaced by halothane, enflurane and later isoflurane [108]. Originally methoxyflurane was the favourite anaesthetic in coronary surgery, as it caused less arrhythmias than halothane. By the end of the 1970s »high-dose fentanyl anaesthesia« was chosen the most popular procedure in cardiac surgery and other high-risk surgical interventions [109]. Bal-

anced anaesthesia as well as total intravenous techniques became equally approved methods. Thoracic epidural anaesthesia as a supportive method in cardiac surgery is currently being researched [110]. This is a challenging task because the administration of heparin during the course of the surgical procedure may provoke epidural or spinal haematomas [111].

Efforts to avoid artificial ventilation postoperatively by applying short-acting anaesthetics are based on findings that adverse events can be reduced by early extubation after cardiac surgery named »fast track concepts« [112]. This can only be accomplished if postoperative care comprises the idea of teamwork involving anaesthesiologists, surgeons, intensive care specialists and nurses.

At the same time, more sophisticated monitoring devices became accessible: cathode ray tube monitors were succeeded by high-definition computer-supported systems; displays with an integrated ST segment analysis illustrating trends allow early detection of adverse events. Transoesophageal echocardiography (TEE) provides an inside view of the heart that had seemed to be out of the question 15 years ago. It allows assessment of anatomy and performance as well as comparative estimation of ventricle function before and after the procedure (Fig. 2.43). Intraoperative use of TEE has meanwhile become the »gold standard«, as it permits immediate visualization of function, especially in valve-preserving ventricular reconstruction [113].

Neurosurgery

At the beginning of the twentieth century anaesthetic procedures for neurosurgical cases were restricted to local anaesthesia for trepanation. With the increasing popular-

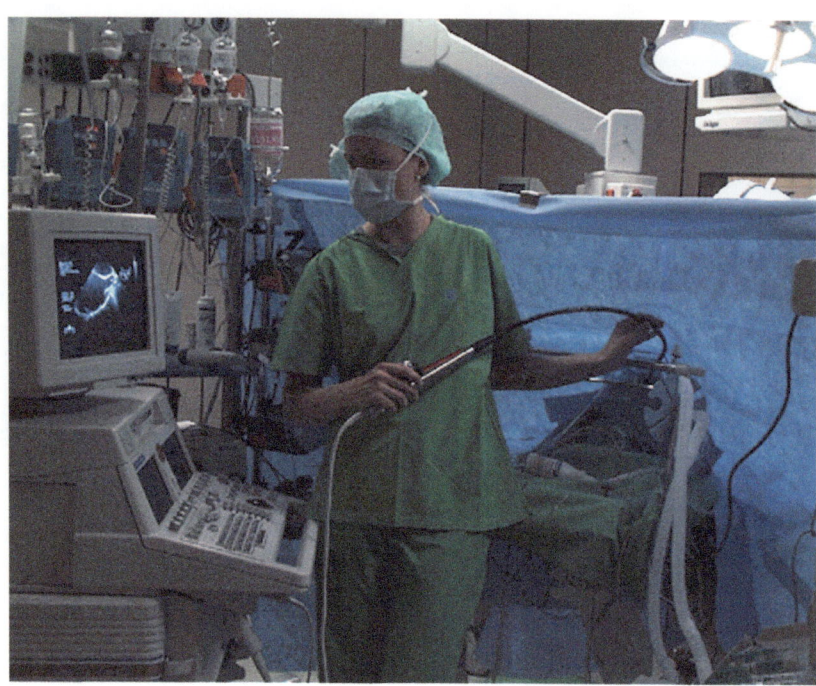

Fig. 2.43. Intraoperative TEE monitoring (2002)

ity of endotracheal intubation in thoracic and abdominal surgery, the majority of neurosurgical operations were performed using endotracheal intubation, muscle relaxation and artificial ventilation in Germany by the 1950s. This seems peculiar since Fedor Krause (1857–1937) had already pointed out the risk of cerebral oedema caused by ether and chloroform in the late nineteenth century.

It was only decades later, in 1942, that the American anaesthesiologist Henry K. Beecher (1904–1976) emphasized that cerebral oedema could be caused by hypoxia and hypercapnia and underlined the importance of an unobstructed airway in neurosurgical patients.

Hypercapnia due to respiratory depression and resulting severe dilation of the cerebral vessels along with cerebral oedema that had been known to occur since the 1940s did not yield artificial ventilation in neurosurgery in every patient. Contemporary textbooks rather advised against artificial ventilation and endotracheal intubation, as this might cause vascular congestion and augment intracranial volume. Up until 1971, in the second revised edition of the **Lehrbuch der Anaesthesiologie** by Frey, Hügin and Mayrhofer, artificial ventilation in anaesthetized patients was not compulsory.

At that time surgery of the posterior cranial cavity was performed without respiratory monitoring of the anaesthetized patient. Even for surgery in the prone position artificial ventilation was not regarded as obligatory, since alterations in spontaneous breathing would reveal impaired brainstem activity that could not be traced during artificial ventilation.

This opinion endured until the middle of the 1960s, even though Seymour S. Kety (1916–2000) and Carl F. Smith (1893–1988) had already been able to prove in 1946 that blood flow and metabolism of the brain were altered by different patterns of ventilation [114].

A leap forward concerning techniques in anaesthesia for neurosurgical procedures could be achieved due to a contribution in the **British Journal of Anaesthesia** by Diana Furness (*1929) of Melbourne in 1957 describing her approach [115]. This included the induction of anaesthesia with thiopental, endotracheal intubation with succinylcholine and local anaesthesia of the trachea as well as sustaining anaesthesia with a nitrous oxide-oxygen mixture, muscle relaxants and artificial ventilation. This model is still valid today, although other drugs are administered.

Controlled hypotension under hypothermia became an important procedure in many German centres for cerebrovascular operations in the late 1950s until the middle of the 1970s. Patients were cooled with the aid of fans and cooling mats to 30°C on the surface to allow pronounced hypotension for a period of 15-20 min for challenging phases of surgery, e.g. surgery of aneurisms or vascular malformations.

Attempts were made to selectively cool the brain by supplying the tissue with blood from the carotid artery, which had been cooled down to approximately 10°C, combined with surface hypothermia of 30°C; additionally, blood flow via the carotid and vertebral arteries was reduced for up to 40 min [116]. Nevertheless, postoperative vasospasms could not be avoided despite the protective effects of hypothermia during ischaemia.

After the introduction of microscopes and calcium antagonists for spasmolysis in the 1970s, a new era commenced for anaesthesia in cerebrovascular neurosurgery [117].

Today, no elementary features have to be added to the notion of Furness from 1957. Anaesthesia for neurosurgical procedures is sustained with volatile anaesthetics and opioids and no specific anaesthetics are required. This may be attributed to less traumatizing neurosurgical techniques.

Clinical and scientific interest has grown along with the development of monitoring devices equipped with available techniques. Next to EEG as well as somatosensory and acoustic evoked potentials, a number of suitable monitoring devices may be employed without interfering signals from within the operating theatre, e.g. the »Cerebral Function Monitor« (1969), deduction of different EEG parameters supported by fast Fourier transformation (1970s and early 1980s) and monitors for trends in bioelectrical brain activities (◻ Figs. 2.44 and 2.45), which anaesthesiologists would not want to miss during several neurosurgical procedures [118].

Gynaecology and Obstetrics

After the War, the gynaecologist Hans Hosemann (1913–1994) of Göttingen introduced an anaesthesia technique in obstetrics that was already popular in England: analgesia with trichloroethylene [119]. The anaesthetic was inhaled with the aid of a special apparatus dangling around the pregnant woman's neck. After 15–30 gasps labour pain would subside for up to 15 min. At the same time drowsiness would set in and the device would slip out of the woman's hand; hence, further uptake of the anaesthetic ceased. Being simple and carrying few hazards, it remained popular in delivery rooms for a long time [120].

A few years later, nitrous oxide-oxygen mixtures were introduced into obstetrics. As suggested by the gynaecologist Carl Joseph Gauß (1875–1957) of Würzburg, the Dräger Company developed an apparatus in the early

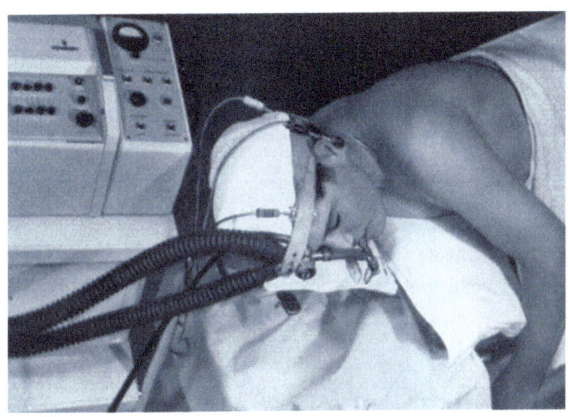

◻ **Fig. 2.44.** Measuring depth of anaesthesia with the aid of an electroencephalogram (1953)

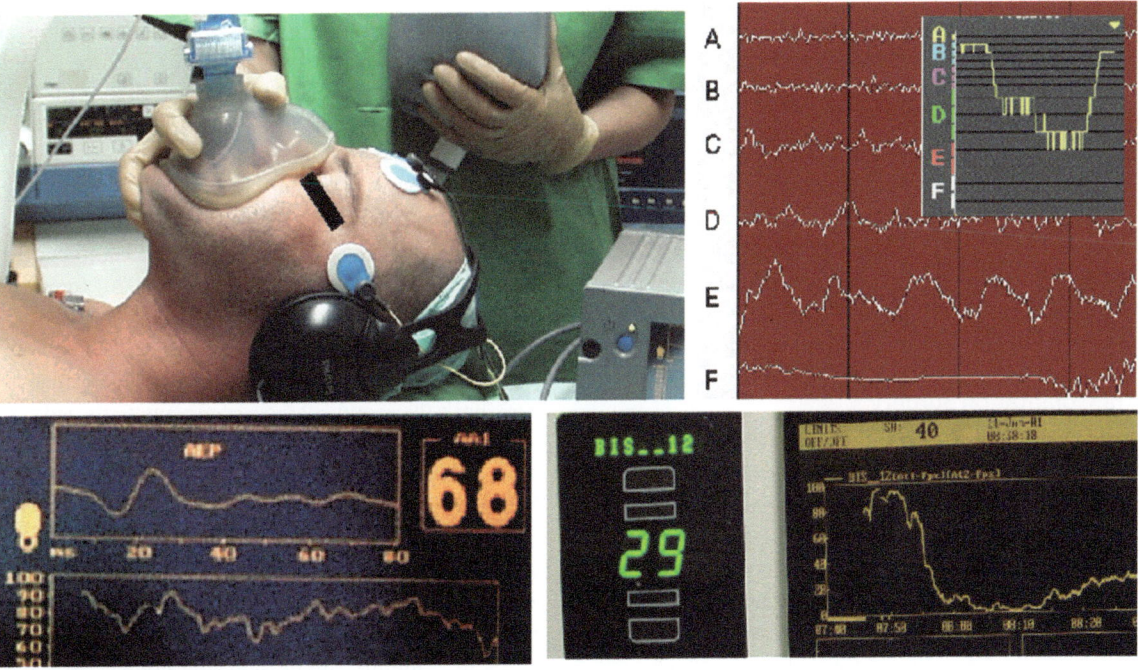

◻ **Fig. 2.45.** EEG monitoring (2002) with contemporary devices such as the bispectral index (*bottom right*), Narcotrend (*top right*) and index of automated analysis of acoustic evoked potentials (*bottom left*)

1940s to be introduced in 1949 as the **Dräger Spezial-Lachgas-Analgesie- und -Narkoseapparat nach Prof. Dr. C.J. Gauss** [121]. After assessment of the nitrous oxide-oxygen concentration by the physician, the woman in labour would inhale the blend via a mask fitted tightly as soon as she felt contractions. As these devices could also be supplemented with an appendage for ether, minor surgical procedures like sutures of the perineum or curettages could be carried out, too [122].

At the same time several regional anaesthesia techniques experienced a renaissance in obstetrics. As lumbar spinal anaesthesia had already been used in the 1920s and 1930s, it was called **»the best technique in anaesthesiology for gynaecology«** [123] and spread widely. From the early 1950s, endovaginal techniques like the paracervical block or the pudendal block supplemented the repertoire of procedures for pain management in obstetrics.

For local anaesthesia, solutions at different concentrations of the newly developed Xylocaine were injected by the obstetricians themselves – which is still common today – in a single-shot injection technique for local, sacral, epidural or spinal anaesthesia. However, during the 1950s first reports on continuous procedures with catheters called **»continuous epidural anaesthesia«** were published. The gynaecologist Hans Karl Wendl (1925–2003) of Hamburg described the advantages of the method that had become common in many places in the USA as early as in 1958 in *Der Anaesthesist*. Wendl ascribed the reluctance to employ this technique to its intricacy and the need for trained anaesthesiologists [124].

By the early 1970s, as a result of increasing experience in regional anaesthesia, continuous analgesia with the aid of epidural catheters during childbirth became customary [125]. It took another 20 years until spinal and epidural anaesthesia could be established for caesarean sections, for general anaesthesia had been the preferred method in Germany in contrast to the Anglo-American area. Thus, mortality due to aspiration or intubation in mothers and neonates could be decreased [126]. Pain relief during childbirth could be achieved with the aid of epidural techniques and the combination of low-dose local anaesthetics and opioids known as **»walking epidurals«** [127].

Transplantation Surgery

Because of advancement in transplantation medicine that will be outlined here with examples of heart, liver and kidney transplantation, anaesthesiologists have to face a rising number of patients with transplanted organs for non-transplant procedures. As a result of this – which had been inconceivable decades ago – chapters in textbooks for anaesthesiology had to be added on special issues of patients with transplanted organs [128].

The first heart transplantation by Christiaan Barnard (1923–2002) in 1967 was a milestone in the history of transplantation medicine. Although the patient did not survive for long, this heightened interest in organ transplantation all over the world. German anaesthesiologists responded in 1970 with an article in *Der Anaesthesist* by the American surgeon William E. Adams (1902–1973) who had performed Lobectomy for lung cancer on Thomas Mann in 1946 [128a]. He did not specify details on the anaesthesiological approach for transplantation, but he did describe problems he had confronted during transplantation of lungs in 1963 and 1964.

Ever since the first orthotopic heart transplantation performed in 1967 with thiopental and halothane [129], various modes of anaesthesia have been applied, e.g. **»balanced anaesthesia«**, **»high-dose opiate anaesthesia«** and total intravenous anaesthesia (TIVA). This emphasizes that the choice of the anaesthetic is less important than the perception of the pathophysiology in terminal myocardial insufficiency. Volatile anaesthetics have been avoided due to their negative inotropic effects causing hypotension. The incidence of hypotension may be reduced when applying intravenous techniques, though co-morbidities like impairment of hepatic and renal function may result in delayed elimination of the agents administered.

Between 1969 and 1977 an average of 30–40 heart transplants were performed annually worldwide; the increased number in the late 1980s and early 1990s can be attributed to sufficient immune suppression with cyclosporine. In 2000, 407 hearts were transplanted in Germany.

Despite decreasing numbers of transplantations, heart transplantations have become a routine procedure at particular centres; advances in immunology, successful treatment of infections and the experience gained with heart transplants led to a decrease in 30-day mortality: it could be reduced from 17% in 1980 to 9% in 1988. At the same time the survival rate increased continuously: in 1990, it was 90% after 1 year, 80% after 5 years and approximately 70% after 10 years [130].

The history of liver transplantation, being one of the most challenging surgical procedures, commences in 1963 when the surgeon Thomas Starzl (*1926) completed it for the first time.

The surgeon Alfred Gütgemann (1907–1985) of Bonn carried out the first liver transplantation in Germany in 1969. Back then, only 39 liver transplantations had been performed worldwide. The patient survived 7 months. Other liver transplantations in Bonn were less successful, though; hence, surgeons refrained from that procedure for some time. Until the early 1980s, liver transplants were only conducted in three centres in Germany: Bonn, Hannover and the Charité in Berlin. The frequency of the procedures was as low as ten per year. With improved means for immune suppression, the number rose from the middle of the 1980s; by 1986 about 100 livers had been transplanted, and this amount increased to 500 in 1991.

The increasing number left an escalating need for organs. As for liver transplantation, this facilitated the invention of new techniques, i.e. transplant reduction, split liver and whole organ grafts [131]. In Germany, the evolution of these sophisticated techniques may be attributed to groups in Hannover and Hamburg [132]. These can be traced by statistics from 2000 when 630 livers were transplanted: 550 patients received whole organ transplants and 80 patients were given split livers in Germany [133].

The techniques described pose challenges to the anaesthesiologist's medical skills and organizational abilities. Basic knowledge in immunology and pathophysiology as well as an interdisciplinary approach are indispensable.

Transplantation of kidneys can be traced back to the early 1950s. The success achieved then paved the way for organ transplantation; hence, an imbalance between the number of patients on the waiting list and organs available for transplantation occurred as early as in the 1980s. As opposed to this, patients with terminal renal insufficiency are in a healthier physical condition before transplantation. Therefore, anaesthesia for these morbid and increasingly elder patients may be performed with predictable risk. Balanced anaesthesia is carried out with opioids and volatile anaesthetics – especially isoflurane because of its low rate of metabolization. Enflurane was abandoned early due to possible nephrotoxic adverse effects of plasma fluorides. In addition to kidneys from brain-dead organ donors, the number of living donors has increased in recent years: in 1981 only 19 kidneys from living donors were transplanted, but in 2000 the number rose to 346.

Academic Meetings of German Anaesthesiologists

Annual meetings with the Austrian and Swiss Anaesthesia Societies had been decided on at the first annual meeting of the DGA in Munich in 1953. Initially, these meetings were held at the same time as the annual meetings of the Deutsche Gesellschaft für Chirurgie (German Society of Surgery).

In the beginning they focussed on special issues and were attended by only a few anaesthesiologists as compared to today's German Anaesthesia Congresses. At the Second Austrian Congress of Anaesthesiology in Velden in 1953, the delegates of the three specialist societies agreed on meeting every 2 years in between the World and European Congresses, at the so-called Zentraleuropäische Anästhesiekongresse (ZAK; Central European Anaesthesia Congresses). After the first two meetings in Austria, the third – held in Munich in 1954 – was named »ZAK« for the first time and turned out to be a successful event during the following 40 years. Conferences on anaesthesiology received international attention. Along

with the meetings of the European Society of Anaesthesiologists (ESA) and events of the European Academy of Anaesthesiology, the 24th ZAK in Vienna in 1995 was to end a well-established tradition. After German reunification, the 23rd ZAK was held in Dresden, chaired by the Congress President Gottfried Benad (*1932) of Rostock (■ Fig. 2.46) [134].

Several German anaesthesiologists participated in the First World Congress of Anaesthesiology in Scheveningen in 1955. With its first President Jochen Bark, the newly founded German Society of Anaesthesia tried to catch up and overcome the lack of experience caused by World War II. International tribute was paid to the DGA by bestowing membership in the European Regional Section of the World Federation of Societies of Anaesthesiologists along with membership in the World Federation as a whole. Twenty-five years later, in 1980, German Anaes-

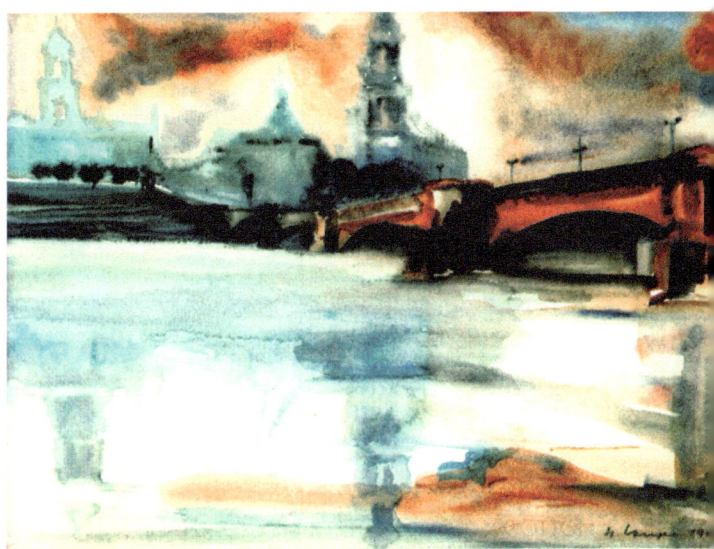

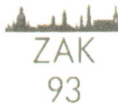

ZENTRALEUROPÄISCHER ANÄSTHESIEKONGRESS

ZAK
93

Vorankündigung

14.–18. SEPTEMBER 1993

Dresden

■ **Fig. 2.46.** Announcement of the *Zentraleuropäischer Anästhesiekongress* (ZAK) in Dresden, 1993

thesiology staged the 7th World Congress in Hamburg under its President Erich Rügheimer (1926–2007) very successfully.

Presidents of the German Society of Anaesthesia arranged annual congresses in their home town or place of work for many years. Nevertheless, it became apparent by the early 1980s that – due to the rising number of delegates and comprehensiveness of the meetings resulting from increasing scientific presentations – it made sense to have professional agencies plan and manage the meetings. For political and tax reasons, a medical congress organization was founded in 1985 by the Berufsverband Deutscher Anästhesisten instead of the charitable scientific association DGAI. Ever since, the Medizinische Congressorganisation Nürnberg (MCN) has been in charge of co-ordinating the annual congress, allowing the President to focus on scientific issues together with the scientific committees.

Since the early 1990s, the importance of regional meetings in anaesthesiology conducted by the DGAI in reunified Germany had increased. The Bavarian section of the DGAI (*Landesverband*) had invited anaesthesiologists for the first time in 1970. These regional events are arranged by the MCN, and the DGAI is trying to achieve that the number of participants in these regional meetings be as high as that at national German Anaesthesia Congresses, i.e. approximately 4,200.

Aspects of Quality

Scientific articles on the hepatotoxicity of halothane have been published since 1959 and on the nephrotoxicity of methoxyflurane since the early 1970s. They sparked discussions on health hazards caused by chronic exposure that were supported by animal trials revealing mutation in liver cells after long-term exposure to subhypnotic doses of halothane. Due to these findings anaesthesia and surgical personnel was considered vulnerable in the early 1970s [135].

Efforts to avoid contamination of personnel with volatile anaesthetics were surprisingly delayed, as the effects of chronic exposure had been understood as early as the 1920s. »We know which security measures radiologists take, but we still lack knowledge on how to protect those who conduct anaesthesias« as stated by the President of the American Society of Anaesthesiologists, Francis Hoeffer McMechan (1875–1939) in 1922 in an obituary for an anaesthesiologist from Chicago who had died of the toxic effects of chronic exposure to ether [136].

McMechan's adage was sustained by the fact that by the 1960s ppm levels (parts per million) of volatile anaesthetics had been identified in operating theatres and recovery rooms representing a potential hazard to the health of the staff. Russian researchers had detected an increased incidence of miscarriages in females employed in operating theatres who had suffered chronic exposure to volatile anaesthetics [137].

The perception that nitrous oxide was inert and the fact that experts of the Deutsche Forschungsgemeinschaft (»German Research Foundation«; DFG) had classified the substance as unproblematic prevented sufficient regulations on maximum levels of the gas in the operating theatre as well as the recovery room. In the early 1980s, this was revised, since pancytopenia as well as megaloblastic proliferation in the bone marrow by inactivation of methionine synthesis occurred after extended exposure to nitrous oxide [138]. With these facts on hand and lacking directives, the Office for Health and Safety in Hamburg set maximum tolerable levels of nitrous oxide at 50 ppm ($\mu l/m^3$) in 1990; nevertheless, a nationwide level for Germany was set at 100 ppm ($\mu l/m^3$) in 1993 [139].

Although no damaging effects had been traced for any other volatile anaesthetic, maximum levels were determined like in other European countries. Already in 1974 the Society demanded that »the provision of powerful exhaust systems should be compulsory for every hospital« [140].

Several trials had shown that the reduction of concentrations of volatile anaesthetics in the air was only viable with the aid of exhaust systems instead of filters. To reduce the risk of leaking gas, especially in induction of anaesthesia in children, an efficient double-mask system became available by the middle of the 1980s [141].

Despite effective exhaust systems and measures to ensure air exchange, in the 1980s evidence surfaced that frequent lifting and replacing of facial masks along with high gas flow and vaporizers set to their maximum induced excessive gas levels in the operating theatre. By applying an optimal technique, official levels for the maximum exposure (MAK levels) do not need to be surpassed. In Germany, MAK levels are determined by a Senate Commission of the DFG that is responsible for estimating hazards caused by different materials.

Quality Assurance and Improvement in Quality

The Society was the first medical specialist society in Germany to improve the safety of apparatus in medicine along with providing recommendations on safety, e.g. education of nurses, introduction of service centres for technical support as well as offering advice on improved security while using machines.

In 1979, the DGAI published a list of recommendations for safely operating technical devices in anaesthesiology, which was revised and extended over the following years. With a number of rules, regulations and directions, technical requirements for conducting anaesthesia were established, partly for national and partly for European use. In Germany, these were summarized in the Medizin-

gerӓteverordnung (MedGV) in 1986. Since 1994, the **Medizinproduktegesetz (MPG)** has been regulating these legal requirements. The latter was completed in 1999 by the **Medizinprodukte-Betreibervorordnung (MPBetreibVO)** with the same objective as before: to protect patients, employees and third parties from hazards deriving from the use of medical products [142]. Currently, the Ministry of Health is compiling an analysis of experience arising from this directive. Equipment at anaesthesia units was described in detail in the **»European Norm 740«** for the first time, focussing on the apparatus at the »standard anaesthesia workstation« as well as the additional equipment of the »extended anaesthesia workstation« with monitoring devices, alarms and safety modules. Guidelines were issued by the **DGAI** and **BDA** in 1989.

As a résumé, these guidelines were extended to different units in detail, e.g. »non-operative workstation«, »general operative medicine« (diagnosis, obstetrics etc.), »paediatric anaesthesia workstation«, »thoracic surgery, or surgery of the major arteries«, »cardiac anaesthesia workstation«, »neurosurgery« as well as »outpatient anaesthesia« [143].

Complications in Anaesthesia

Apart from efforts to ensure safe anaesthesia units and technical devices, complications of various extent and degree may develop. As part of quality assurance in anaesthesiology, these incidents are documented in anaesthesia charts (Fig. 2.47); the term **ZEK** (see above) introduced in 1992 was replaced in 1999 by the name **AVB (Anästhesiologische Verlaufsbeobachtung, monitoring the course of anaesthesia**; Fig. 2.48) [144].

Before 1960, anaesthesia-induced mortality amounted to 4 in 100,000, around 1960, 2 in 100,000, in 1970, 1 in 100,000 and today approximately 0.5 in 100,000. Eighty percent are regarded to be preventable, with severe impact of human factors. Causes comprise difficulties in ventilation due to false intubation (30%), dysfunction of anaesthetic machines (more than 20%) and aspiration (10–20%).

Looking at the 7-day mortality rate as classified by the ASA, patients of category I are unlikely to experience an incident, 0.04% of ASA II patients, 0.06% of ASA III patients and 8% of ASA IV patients will have to cope with adverse events [153]. Mortality may be reduced by: improved training and education, optimal monitoring of the patient, standard operating procedures, minimizing fatigue and sleep deprivation as well as training at the human patient simulator [145].

Legal Issues in Anaesthesiology and Informed Consent

Until the 1960s, adverse events during medical procedures were attributed to fate. Improvement in medical

KOMPLIKATIONEN

Respirations-Tractus

Praeoperativ

Infekt. der ob. Luftwege: Hals .... Nase .... Ohr .... Nebenhöhlen .... Husten.
Singultus .... Obstruktion .... Asthma .... Tracheitis .... Bronchitis ....
Bronchiektasen .... Pneumonie .... Lungenabszeß .... Emphysem ....
Pleuritis .... Empyem .... Tbc: .... aktiv .... stationär .... doppelseitig ...
Vitalkapazität: 33 % .... 33—66 % ....
Andere Komplikationen ....

Postoperativ

Pharyngitis .... Laryngitis .... Husten .... Singultus ....
Obstruktion .... Tracheitis .... Bronchitis .... Aspiration ....
Pneumonie: .... hypostat .... broncho .... lobär .... Atelektase ....
Tbc .... Ödem .... Pleuritis .... Empyem: .... teil .... massiv ....
Andere Komplikationen ....
Kompl. Eintritt: 1.—3. Tag .... 4.—7. Tag .... 2. Wo. .... 3. Wo. ....

Fig. 2.47. Documentation of preoperative and postoperative airway complications in anaesthetized patients according to Jean Henley (1950)

1. AVB-Art

1000 Atmung, nicht näher bezeichnet

1100 Atemwege, nicht näher bezeichnet
1101 Laryngospasmus
1102 Bronchospasmus
1103 Atemwegsverletzung
1104 Stridor (Kehlkopfbereich)
1105 Aspiration
1106 Atemwegsverlegung

1200 Atmungsregulation/Gasaustausch, nicht näher bezeichnet
1201 Hypoxämie
1202 Lungenödem
1203 Hyperventilation
1204 Hypoventilation

1300 Intubation, nicht näher bezeichnet
1301 Unvorhergesehene schwierige Intubation
1302 Sekundär fiberoptische Intubation
1303 Intubation unmöglich
1304 Fehlintubation
1305 Einseitige Intubation
1306 Reintubation
1307 RSI (Crushintubation) mißlungen
1308 Fiberoptische Intubation mißlungen

1400 Tubusprobleme, nicht näher bezeichnet
1401 Dekonnektion
1402 Tubus abgeknickt
1403 Tubus defekt
1404 Akzidentelle Extubation

1900 Sonstiges Atmung, nicht näher bezeichnet
1901 Pneumothorax
1902 Hämatothorax
1903 Pneumonie
1904 Geplante Extubation nicht möglich
1905 Ungeplante (Nach-)Beatmung erforderlich
1999 Sonstige Atmungsstörungen

Fig. 2.48. Codes for adverse respiratory events during anaesthesia (AVB; 2002)

technologies and increasing demand for medical care without adverse events created an escalating amount of medico-legal conflicts as well as civil claims.

Increasing awareness of medico-legal issues due to publication of incidents and the growing number of invasive procedures in anaesthesia, conducted by consultants in anaesthesiology, initiated the generation of questionnaires. A brochure was distributed along with it to inform the patient and to reduce uncertainties before anaesthesia was performed. It facilitates the dialogue between the patient and the physician and ensures that relevant information on patients' medical histories and previous anaesthetic procedures is acquired.

The first form was presented by Ottheinz Schulte-Steinberg (*1920) in the journal *Der Anaesthesist* in 1967, revealing advantages of important information from previous anaesthesias, e.g. difficult endotracheal intubation [146]. It took several years though before a comprehensive form for adults and children was produced by the **BDA** in 1978 [147]. The questionnaire, which was not intended to be a substitute for the necessary physical examination and history taking, was accepted quickly. In close co-operation with the lawyer of the **DGAI** – Walter Weißauer (*1921) – as well as members of the **BDA** and a publishing company, a questionnaire for anaesthesiology compiled for patients was created including a brochure on the procedures and a written informed consent form for anaesthesia [148].

With the printed basic information that was handed to the patient along with the personal communication between the patient and the physician, the requirements of the *Bundesgerichtshof* (Federal Court of Justice) were fulfilled covering different stages of obtaining informed consent [149].

Even before these forms had become available, the relationship between the surgeon and the anaesthetist had been clearly defined in legal terms on the »basis of trust«, which had initially been subject to discussions, and earned appreciation later. It was accepted by doctors as well as scientific specialist societies resulting in the **DGAI** and **BDA** settling arrangements with the surgical societies on co-operating with each other.

Several agreements have been reached since then, confirming that anaesthesiologists perform their duties independently and take sole responsibility. Thus, the kind of procedure for anaesthesia was chosen by the anaesthesiologist, a decision that we take for granted today as opposed to some decades ago.

The central focus of obtaining informed consent and providing the patient with sufficient information on the procedure is to prevent physicians from acting on their own, which is illegal. It is unlawful to treat patients against their wish; thus, written informed consent has to be obtained. The adult patient may take decisions and has to be informed accordingly.

The doctor has to explain the kind, nature, meaning and consequences of the procedure in simple words that even lay people may comprehend and understand what they are agreeing to.

Current legal aspects that have evolved in recent decades comprise the liability for conducted procedures and the approach. The anaesthetic or intensive care procedure that the appropriately informed patient has agreed on is legitimate even if it is unsuccessful. If the patient is harmed due to neglect or lack of diligence on the part of the anaesthesiologist, liability under civil and criminal law will apply. Nevertheless, according to legislation a patient holds a right to receive care at a consultant's standard during and outside of regular working hours. This is implied in order to secure standards of quality, since procedures may be assigned to anaesthesia staff or residents under the expert guidance of a supervising consultant. The specialist standard embraces sufficient amount and training of the required personnel, rooms and machinery at the anaesthesia unit, which are the responsibility of the hospital owner. In addition, the policies of strict division of responsibilities and the basis of trust apply, especially between the surgeon and the anaesthesiologist.

Challenges in Anaesthesiology
Demographic Development, Advances in Medicine and Economic Restrictions

During the past decades, the amount of knowledge and the innovations in technology have increased tremendously in the medical profession as well as in anaesthesiology. Modern concepts of inventive treatment led to further financial expenditures. A growing number of even older patients undergo surgery today. The report of the Enquête Commission »Demographic Changes« published in 2002 calls attention to the rising age in our society: 2.9 million people in Germany are older than 80 years today, and within 20 years this will exceed 5.1 million people. Estimations predict that by 2050 one of ten Germans will be older than 80 years [150]. This development is shown in the table below [151]:

Year	Total population in Germany (millions)	Population aged >65 years (millions)
1950	69.34	6.9
1960	73.15	8.5
1970	78	10.8
1980	78.4	11.5
1990	79.75	11.9
2000	>82	>13.6

Economic constraints and health politics encumber opportunities in medicine significantly due to extreme bureaucracy and restrictions on resources for structural development, which has intensified in the new millennium. Reforms of health care structures in 2000 with a change of paradigms interfered with the financing of medical services: the total budget in hospitals, which had been funded mainly by lump sums for basic care (up to 80%) and to a lesser extent by remuneration (20%), were as from 2004 financed only by case-based lump sums for acute medical treatment, including anaesthesiology. This form of billing, which is based on »diagnosis-related groups« (DRG), posed completely new challenges to hospitals with respect to IT, documentation and controlling. DRGs were developed in the USA to control the use of medical resources and to secure quality assurance in patient care on the wards. In the meantime, similar systems have been implemented internationally, for example in Australia, the UK, France, Scandinavia, Belgium and Ireland, to manage hospital financing, without however noticeably reducing expenses so far. From the medical point of view, such a system is fraught with difficulties as it only reflects the economic category of a case instead of the medical complexity of treatments; hence, the DRG system will not provide sufficient support for securing quality in medicine either.

In order to take the best possible advantage of existing resources, efficient management of surgical procedures is essential; hence, services provided by surgery as well as anaesthesiology have to become part of the complete hospital service package [152]. In this respect, establishing outpatient clinics for preoperative assessment by anaesthesiologists seems feasible. Furthermore, pre- and postoperative care has to be structured and requirements for staff and time have to be adapted accordingly to reduce expensive changing times in order to facilitate more efficient use of operating theatres.

It may be concluded that currently available techniques in anaesthesiology allocate individual procedures for special conditions and specific surgical needs. The increasing number of patients with limiting co-morbidities can be subjected to any surgical procedure required, since anaesthesia may be adapted to prerequisites. Ethical principles underlying the physician's duties have to be kept in mind – especially in anaesthesiology – and have to be re-evaluated constantly to keep pace with the rapid development of medical options in anaesthesiology and economics.

Anaesthesiological procedures have reached a high standard regarding safety and quality. Even though anaesthesiologists have to cope with duties beyond their own specialty and are encumbered by administrative duties, they have to stay in touch with classic clinical anaesthesia, as well as the remaining four pillars of anaesthesiology, i.e. intensive care medicine, emergency care medicine and pain management as well as academic issues.

References

1. Morris E (1998) Pain and analgesia for operative interventions from 1847–1997. In: Schulte am Esch J, Goerig M (eds) The Fourth International Symposium on the History of Anaesthesia – Proceedings. Dräger-Druck, Lübeck, pp 57–72
2. Körner M (1983) Die Entwicklung der Anästhesiologie in Krefeld von 1958–1983. Anästh Intensivmed 11:369–372
3. Lehmann C (1967) Die Deutsche Gesellschaft für Anästhesie und Wiederbelebung. Gründung und Entwicklung. Anaesthesist 9:267–267
4. Sorgatz H (2002) Dipl.-SozW, Geschäftsführer der DGAI/BDA-Geschäftstelle in Nürnberg, Persönliche Mitteilung August 2002
5. Bauer KH (1955) Die Wandlungen der Anästhesie vom Standpunkt des Operateurs. Langenbecks Arch Klin Chir 282:163–176
6. Engisch K (1961) Wie ist rechtlich die Verantwortlichkeit des Chirurgen im Verhältnis zur Verantwortlichkeit des Anästhesisten bei ärztlichen Operationen zu bestimmen und zu begrenzen? Langenbecks Arch Klin Chir 297:236–254
7. Weißauer W (1962) Arbeitsteilung und Abgrenzung der Verantwortung zwischen Anästhesist und Operateur. Anaesthesist 11:239–256
8. Opderbecke HW (2001) Historische Vignette: Als der Berufsverband laufen lernte. In: Landauer B, Sorgatz H (eds) 40 Jahre Berufsverband Deutscher Anästhesisten. Hermann, Nuremberg, pp 16–19
9. Bräutigam HK (1997) Die Entwicklung des Fachgebietes. In: Brandt L (ed) Illustrierte Geschichte der Anästhesie. Wissenschaftliche Verlagsgesellschaft, Stuttgart, pp 176–203
10. Wiemers K, Krauss H (1956) Richtlinien für die Stellung des leitenden Anästhesisten. Anaesthesist 1:31–32
11. Hossli G (1986) Prof. Dr. K. Mülly. Anaesthesist 6:393
12. Zeitlin G, Goerig M (2003) Dr. Jean Henley, an American pioneer of modern German anesthesia. Anesthesiology 99(2):496–502
13. Menzel H (1997) Jochen Bark – a German pioneer of modern anaesthesiology. In: Schulte am Esch J, Goerig M (eds) The Fourth International Symposium on the History of Anaesthesia – Proceedings. Dräger-Druck, Lübeck, pp 117–121
14. Goerig M Schwarz W (2006) Dr. med. Zürn. (Folge 26) Die Gründungsmitglieder der Deutschen Gesellschaft für Anästhesie. Anästh Intensivmed 3:96–98
15. Schwarz W, Goerig M (2005) Prof. Dr. med. Martin Zindler. (Folge 28) Die Gründungsmitglieder der Deutschen Gesellschaft für Anästhesie. Anästh Intensivmed 3:96–98
16. Macintosh R (1951) Aussprachen zu 2–8. Langenbecks Arch Klin Chir 267:59–60
17. Derra (1952) Gedanken zur Neuordnung des Narkosewesens in Deutschland. Das Krankenhaus 44:49–51
18. Hesse F (1951) Aussprache. Langenbecks Arch Klin Chir 267:41
19. Hübner A (1951) Standes- und Berufsfragen. Der Krankenhausarzt 9:92
20. Goerig M, Schulte am Esch J (1996) Helmut Schmidt – Ein Protagonist moderner Anästhesie in Deutschland. AINS 31:621–631
21. Loch F C, Loris W (1997) Der saarländische Sonderweg. Dtsch Ärztebl B 38:1958–1961
22. Anonymus (1953) Fachnachrichten. Ergänzung der Saarländischen Facharztordnung vom 31.3. 52. (Amtsblatt S. 409). Anaesthesist 4:112
23. Fritsche P (1986) Werner Sauerwein zum 65. Geburtstag. Anästh Intensivmed 5:165
24. Bergmann H (1952) Bericht über den Ersten Österreichischen Kongreß für Anaesthesiologie, veranstaltet von der Österreichischen Gesellschaft für Anaesthesiologie, in Salzburg am 5. und 6. September 1952. Anaesthesist 5:150–156

25. Bräutigam KH (1993) 40 Jahre »Facharzt für Anästhesie«. Anästh Intensivmed 34:259–268
26. Killian H (1964) 40 Jahre Narkoseforschung. Verlag der Deutschen Hochschullehrer-Zeitung, Tübingen
27. Anonymus (1953) Stenographische Niederschrift des 56. Deutschen Ärztetages in Lindau vom 19./20. 9. 1953, pp 22–24
28. Ärztekammer Hamburg (1969) Berufsordnung der Hamburger Ärzteschaft vom 20.Mai 1969. In der Fassung vom 19. Januar 1971. Handbuch für das Gesundheitswesen in Hamburg, Ärztekammer Hamburg
29. Anonymus (1959) Mehr Narkoseärzte gefordert. Münch Med Wochenschr 16:820
30. Horatz K, Stoffregen J (1959) Bericht über das Anästhesistentreffen am 1. Februar in Göttingen. Anaesthesist 7:212–213
31. Blüchel K (1976) Die weißen Magier. Fischer, Frankfurt/M
32. Pribilla, O (1964) Tod in Narkose. Anaesthesist 10:340–345
33. Lehmann C (1967) Die Deutsche Gesellschaft für Anaesthesie und Wiederbelebung. Gründung und Entwicklung. Anaesthesist 9:259–268
34. Beschluss des Engeren Präsidiums der DGAI (1984) Empfehlung zur Weiterbildungsdauer in der Anästhesiologie. Anästh Intensivmed 25:441
35. Goerig M, Schhulte am Esch (1998) Helmut Schmidt – an early protagonist of professionalized anaesthesia in Hamburg. In: Schulte am Esch J, Goerig M (eds) The Fourth International Symposium on the History of Anaesthesia – Proceedings. Dräger-Druck, Lübeck, pp 367–378
36. Alnor J (1987) Die Geschichte der Chirurgie im Hamburg-Eppendorf. Medical Dissertation, University of Hamburg
37. Henley J (1950) Einführung in die Praxis der modernen Inhalationsnarkose. de Gruyter, Berlin
38. Kochs E (2001) Vorwort. In: Kochs E, Krier C, Buzello W, Adams HA (eds) Anästhesiologie. Thieme, Stuttgart
39. Van Ackern K, Schwarz W, Striebel JP (2003) 50 Jahre Deutsche Gesellschaft für Anästhesiologie und Intensivmedizin. In: Schüttler J (ed) 50 Jahre Deutsche Gesellschaft für Anästhesiologie und Intensivmedizin. Springer, Berlin, pp 79–119
40. Denson JS, Abrahamson SA (1969) Computer-controlled patient simulator. JAMA 208:504–508
41. Schüttler J, Lussi C (2001) Simulatoren in der Anästhesie. In: Kochs E, Krier C, Buzello W, Adams HA (eds) Anästhesiologie. Thieme, Stuttgart, pp 1601–1606
42. Howard SK Gaba DM, Fish KJ et al (1992) Anesthesia crisis management training: teaching anaesthesiologists to handle critical incidents. Aviat Space Environ Med 63:763–770
42a. Welker A, Baumgart A, Baja J, Schröpl K, Schleppers A. (2010) Das Berufsbild des Anästhesisten. Eine qualitative und quantitative Studierendenbefragung zur Attraktivität unseres Fachs. Anästh Intensivmed 51:318–327
42b. Schüttler J. (2004) DGAI-Projekt zur Optimierung der studentischen Lehre durch Anästhesie- und Notfallsimulatoren erfolgreich angelaufen. Anästh Intensivmed 45:381
43. Kronschwitz H (1969) Die nasotracheale Intubation mit einem Intubations-Fiberskop. Anaesthesist 18:58–59
44. Kleemann P et al (1984) Die Intubation mit dem flexiblen Fiberbronchoskop. Anästh Intensivmed 25:287–295
45. Brain A (1983) The laryngeal mask – a new concept in airway-management. Br J Anaesth 55:801–805
46. Schulte am Esch J (1993) Die Kehlkopfmaske – ein weiteres Konzept zur Atemwegssicherung. AINS 28:133–134
47. Büch H, Neurohr O, Pfleger K et al (1968) Gefährliche Schleimhautschäden durch Endotracheal-Katheter infolge Anreicherung von Phenolen aus einem Desinfektionsmittel. Anaesthesist 17:204–209
48. Waters RM, Schmidt ER (1934) Cyclopropane anesthesia. JAMA 103:975–983
49. Haid B (1953) Die Cyclopropannarkose. Anaesthesist 2:128–131
50. Raventos J (1956) The action of Fluothane – a new volatile agent. Br J Pharmacol 11:394–398
51. Hill DW (1964) Der Dräger-Verdunser »Vapor«. Anaesthesist 13:11–15
52. Vonderschmitt H (1960) Zur Technik der Halothan-Narkose. Anaesthesist 9:112–113
53. Virtue RW, Lund LO, Phelps M et al (1966) Difluoromethyl 1,1,2-trifluoro-2-chloroethlyl ether as an anaesthetic agent: results with dogs, and a preliminary note on observations with man. Can Anaesth Soc J 13:233–241
54. Hobhahn J et al (1997) Der Einfluss von Sevofluran und Desfluran auf die Einleitungs- und Aufwachphase – ein Vergleich mit den herkömmlichen Inhalationsanästhetika und Propofol. Anästh Intensivmed 38:607–615
55. Morris LE (1998) Early encounters with a strange. In: Schulte am Esch J, Goerig M (eds) The Fourth International Symposium on the History of Anaesthesia – Proceedings. Dräger-Druck, Lübeck, pp 359-366
56. Lundy JS (1926) Balanced anesthesia. Minn Med 9:399–404
57. Henschel WF (1990) Standardtechnik auch noch heute? In: Henschel WF (ed) 30 Jahre Neuroleptanalgesie. Urban & Schwarzenberg, Munich, pp 21–29
58. Schüttler J, Schwilden H, Stoeckel H (1983) Pharmacokinetics as applied to total intravenous anaesthesia. Practical implications. Anaesthesia 38(Suppl):53–6
59. Schwilden H, Schüttler J, Stoeckel H (1987) Closed-loop feedback control of methohexital anesthesia by quantitative EEG analysis in humans. Anesthesiology 67:341–347
60. Bickford RG (1950) Automatic electroencencephalographic control of general anesthesia. Electroencephalogr Clin Neurophysiol 2:93–96
61. Frey R, Just O, von Luttichau E et al (1952) Die Schmerzausschaltung an der Chirurgischen Universitätsklinik Heidelberg von 1852–1952. Anaesthesist 1:97–100
62. Nolte H (1993) Die neuere Entwicklung der Regional- und Allgemeinanästhesie in Mitteleuropa. Anästh Intensivmed 34:385–390
63. Killian H (1959) Lokalanästhesie und Lokalanästhetika. Thieme, Stuttgart
64. Niesel HC, Auberger HG (1982) Regionalanästhesie, Lokalanästhesie, Regionale Schmerztherapie. Thieme, Stuttgart
65. Nolte H, Stanton-Hicks MD, P. Raj (1998) Illustrated manual of regional anesthesia. Springer, Berlin
66. Weis KH (1994) Cave: Thorakale Katheter-Epiduralanästhesie zur postoperativen Schmerztherapie. Kasuistik zweier Patienten mit irreversibler Querschnittslähmung. Anästh Intensivmed 35:202–203
67. Herden HN, Lawin P (1973) Anästhesiefibel. Thieme, Stuttgart
68. Fürniss H (1984) Vom Dräger Poliomaten zum Spiromaten. In: Lawin P, Peter K, Scherer R (eds) Maschinelle Beatmung gestern – heute – morgen. Thieme, Stuttgart, pp 28–43
69. Fürniss H (1959) Narkose, Narkosebeatmung und Beatmung in der Ersten Hilfe. Lübeck
70. Resse G (1956) Zur automatischen Narkosebeatmung. Chirurg 4:186–190
71. Radford EP, Ferris BG, Kriete BC (1954) Clinical use of a nomogram to estimate proper ventilation during artificial respiration. N Engl J Med 251:877–882
72. Haupt J (2001) Ehemaliger leitender Ingenieur der Dräger-Werke, Lübeck. Correspondence of Juli 2001, p 113
73. Haupt J (1970) Die Entwicklung der Dräger-Narkoseapparate. Dräger-Werke, Lübeck
74. Rügheimer E (1984) Bilanz der Beatmung. In: Lawin P, Peter K, Scherer R (eds) Maschinelle Beatmung gestern – heute – morgen. Thieme, Stuttgart, pp 75–89

75. Wilke HJ (1970) Die Dräger Zentralversorgungsanlagen für in der Medizin verwendete Gase und Vakuum im Krankenhaus. Dräger-Sonderdruck MT 1 aus dem Drägerheft Nr.280–282, Lübeck, pp 40–52

76. Heyfelder JF (1847) Die Versuche mit dem Schwefeläther und die daraus gewonnenen Resultate in der chirurgischen Klinik zu Erlangen. Heyder, Erlangen

77. Schürer F von (1937) Das Kardiotron, ein Apparat zur objektiven Messung der Pulsfrequenz, des Blutdruckes und der Atmung während der Operation. Arch Klin Chir 189:388–392

78. Oehmig H (1972) Intraoperative Patienten-Überwachung. Anästh Inf 13:68–73

79. Kern ER (1964) Gegensätzliche Strömungen der heutigen Anästhesiologie. Anaesthesist 13:277–279

80. Ritsema CR et al (1955) Über Oximetrie und Carboxymetrie während der Narkose. Anaesthesist 3:250–259

81. Severinghaus W, Astrup P (1998) History of blood gas analysis. In: Schulte am Esch J, Goerig M (eds) The Fourth International Symposium on the History of Anaesthesia – Proceedings. Dräger-Druck, Lübeck, pp 591–596

82. Göpfert H, Frey R (1954) Ein schnellanzeigendes Messgerät für die Kohlensäure in der Ausatemluft. Langenbecks Arch Klin Chir 279:804–809

83. Beschluss des Engeren Präsidiums der DGAI (1989) Qualitätssicherung in der Anästhesiologie. Anästh Intensivmed 30:307–314

84. Just OH, Dietzel W (1966) Die historische Entwicklung der intravenösen Injektionstechnik und die heutige Verwendung der Plastikkanüle (Braunüle). Schwester 12:30–34

85. Opderbecke HW (1999) Zur Entwicklung der intravenösen Infusionstechnik – ein persönlicher Erfahrungsbericht. Anaesthesist 48:919–923

86. Beschluss des Engeren Präsidiums der DGAI (1997) Rechtsherzkatheter (Swan-Ganz-Katheter). Anästh Intensivmed 38:246–247

87. Margreiter J et al (2000) Einsatzmöglichkeiten der transösophagealen Echokardiographie in der perioperativen Überwachung. Anaesthesist 49:74–91

88. Loick M et al (1999) Richtlinien zur Weiterbildung in der transoesophagealen Echokardiographie für Anästhesisten: Indikationen – Ausbildung – Zertifizierung – »TEE in der Anästhesiologie«. Anästh Intensivmed 40:67–71

89. Schregel W (1997) Stellenwert der transkraniellen Doppler-Sonographie bei erhöhtem intrakraniellem Druck. Zentralbl Neurochir 58:43–46

90. Janssens U, Hanrath P (1999) Medizinisch-methodische Entwicklung und Monitoring. Anaesthesist 48:733–743

91. Rentsch HP (1967) Der »Ventitrol« – ein neues Gerät zur direkten und kontinuierlichen Messung des Atemzeitvolumens. Anaesthesist 16:113–115

92. Schwarz W (2002) Vom Aufwachraum zur Aufwachstation. Abstractband DAK 2002. Diomed, Ebelsbach, p 77

93. Davies RM (1957) Die postoperative Wachstation. Anaesthesist 6:335

94. Beschluss des Engeren Präsidiums der DGAI (1967) Stellungnahme der DGAW zur Organisation von Aufwachraum, Wachstation und der Intensivbehandlung am Krankenhaus. Anaesthesist 16:282–284

95. Forgacs J, Voszka R, Orban I (1960) Über Explosionen im Operationssaal. Anaesthesist 9:357–362

96. Horatz K, Frey R (1967) Bericht über das Symposium zur Standardisierung von Anästhesiegeräten. Anaesthesist 16:290–291

97. DIN (1997) Umstellung der Gaskennfarben an Anästhesiearbeitsplätzen. Der Übergang von der nationalen Norm DIN 13252 auf die europäische Norm EN 740. Anästh Intensivmed 38:268–269

98. Beuster H (1998) Normen erfüllen. Neue Europäische Normen für Rohrleitungssysteme für medizinische Gase und Versorgungseinheiten. Medizin-Technik aktuell. Dräger-Druck, Lübeck, pp 10–11

99. Zelk M (1998) Farbe bekennen. Medizin-Technik aktuell. Dräger-Druck, Lübeck, pp 8–9

100. Lejhanec J, Lempert J, Mayrhofer O et al (1972) Erfahrungen und Probleme mit einer computergerechten Datenerfassung. Anaesthesist 21:496–505

101. Kersting T (1991) Qualitätssicherung und Qualitätskontrolle in der Anästhesie. Anästh Intensivmed 32:308

102. Anonymus (2002) Herzchirurgie. Nach wie vor Spitzenplatz. Dtsch Ärztebl 36:1948

103. Zindler M (2000) Hypothermie für Herzoperationen mit Kreislaufstillstand – Beginn der offenen Herzchirurgie in Deutschland. AINS 35:340–345

104. Böttcher W (1999) Die historische Entwicklung der extrakorporalen Zirkulation. In: Lauterbach G (ed) Handbuch der Kardiotechnik. Urban & Fischer, Munich, pp 1–22

105. Arom KV, Flavin TF, Emery RW et al (2000) Safety and efficacy of off-pump coronary artery bypass graft. Ann Thorac Surg 69(3):704–710

106. Zindler M (1987) Geschichte der Thorax- und Kardioanästhesie. In: Zinganell K (ed) Anästhesie – historisch gesehen. Springer, Berlin, pp 54–70

107. Zenker R, Heberer G, Gehl H et al (1958) Zur Aufrechterhaltung der Organfunktionen und des Stoffwechsels im extrakorporalen Kreislauf. Langenbecks Arch Klin Chir 289:294–302

108. Tarnow J et al (1975) Die Wirkung von Ethrane auf die Hämodynamik und die Sauerstoffversorgung des Myocards im Vergleich zu Halothane. In: Bergmann H, Blauhut B (eds) Respiration Zirkulation Herzchirurgie. Springer, Berlin, pp 127–133

109. Spencer FC, Benson DW, Liu WC et al (1959) Use of a mechanical respirator in the management of respiratory or pulmonary disease. J Thorac Cardiovasc Surg 38:758–770

110. Ganapathy S, Dobkowski WB, Murkin JM et al (1999) Thoracic epidural analgesia (TEA) increases graft flow and reduces cortisol release in minimally invasive coronary bypass surgery (MIDCAB). Anesthesiology 91:A3–A130

111. Kessler P, Neidhart G, Lischke V et al (2002) Koronare Bypass-Operation mit kompletter medianer Sternotomie am wachen Patienten in hoher thorakaler Periduralanästhesie. Anaesthesist 51:533–538

112. Silbert BS, Santamaria JD, O'Brien JL et al (1998) Early extubation following coronary artery bypass surgery: a prospective randomized controlled trial. The Fast Track Cardiac Care Team. Chest 113:1481–1488

113. Pasch T, Spahn DR (2001) Herzkreislauffunktion. In: Kochs E, Krier C, Buzello W, Adams HA (eds) Anästhesiologie. Thieme, Stuttgart, pp 480–488

114. Kety SS, Smith CF (1946) The effect of active and passive hyperventilation on cerebral blood flow, cerebral oxygen consumption, cardiac output, and blood pressure of normal young men. J Clin Invest 25:107–119

115. Furness D (1957) Controlled respiration in neurosurgery. Br J Anaesth 29:415–418

116. Gött U (1966) Selektive Hirnkühlung. Anaesthesist 15:372–375

117. Meyer SA (1995) Intensive care management of subarachnoid hemorrhage. Curr Opin Anesth 8:139–144

118. Maynard D, Prior PF, Scott DF (1969) Device for continuous monitoring of cerebral activity in resuscitated patients. Br Med J 4:545–546

119. Hosemann H (1951) Die Schmerzlinderung unter der Geburt. Med Klin 46:70–74

120. Ahrens P, Braun U (1998) The Göttinger model – a trichchlorethylene- vaporizer. In: Schulte am Esch J, Goerig M (eds). Proceedings of the Fourth International Symposium on the History of Anaesthesia. Dräger-Druck, Lübeck, pp 549–551

121. Fauvet E (1951) Schmerzlinderung unter der Geburt. Z Geburtsh Gynäkol 135:149–169

122. Imholz G (1949) Wehennarkose mit einem neuen lungenautoma-tisch gesteuerten Lachgasnarkosegerät. Dtsch Med Wochenschr 42:1277–1278

123. Jaschke T von (1930) Die Lumbalanästhesie – das beste Anästh-esieverfahren in der Gynäkologie. Schmerz Narkose Anaesthesie 4:3–7

124. Wendl KH (1958) Die epiduralen Leitungsanästhesien zur Schmerzausschaltung in der Geburtshilfe. (Bericht über 1000 Fälle). Anaesthesist 7:301–303

125. Strasser K (1980) Lumbale Periduralanästhesie in der Geburts-hilfe. Urban & Schwarzenberg, Munich

126. Hawkins JL, Koonin LM, Palmer SK et al (1997) Anesthesia-related deaths during obstetric delivery in the United States, 1979–1990. Anesthesiology 86:277–284

127. Morgan BM (1995) »Walking« epidurals in labour. Anaesthesia 50:839–840

128. Bornscheuer A et al (2001) Transplantierte Patienten. In: Kochs E, Krier C, Buzello W, Adams HA (eds) Anästhesiologie. Thieme, Stuttgart

128a.Adams WE (1970) Probleme der Organtransplantation. Anaesthe-sist 19:57–60

129. Ozinsky J (1967) Cardiac transplantation – the anaesthetists view. A case report. S Afr Med J 41:1268–1270

130. Schmidt ER, Toric M (1990) Anästhesiologische Probleme bei Herztransplantation. Ther Umschau 472:122–128

131. Broelsch CE, Burdelski M, Rogiers X et al (1994) Living donor for liver transplantation. Hepatology 20:49S–55S

132. Pichlmayr R, Ringe B, Gubernatis G et al (1988) Transplantation einer Spenderleber auf zwei Empfänger – eine neue Methode in der Weiterentwicklung der Lebersegmenttransplanatation. Lan-genbecks Arch Klin Chir 373:127–130

133. Persijn GG, Cohen B (2000) Eurotransplant International Founda-tion. Annual Report 2000

134. Pasch T (2000) Anästhesiologie. In: Regierungsrat des Kantons Zürich (ed) Zürcher Spitalgeschichte, vol. 3. pp 623–638

135. Dudziak R (1981) Nebenwirkungen von flüchtigen Anästhetika auf das Anästhesiepersonal unter besonderer Berücksichtigung des Mutterschutzgesetzes. Anästh Intensivmed 4:81–92

136. McMechan FH (1922) Obituary. Curr Res Anesth Analg 1:18

137. Vaisman AI (1967) Work in surgical theatres and its influence on the health of anesthesiologists. Eksp Khir Anaestheziol 3:430–437

138. Nunn JF (1987) Clinical aspects of interaction between nitrous oxide and vitamin B12. Br J Anaesth 59:3–13

139. Amt für Arbeitsschutz Freie und Hansestadt Hamburg (1996) Merkblatt für den Umgang mit Narkosegasen

140. Henschel WF, Lehmann C (1975) Schädigung des Anästhesie-Personals durch Narkose-Gase und -Dämpfe. Springer, Berlin

141. Derting F, Bovenkamp U (1981) Studie zur Verbesserung der Sicherheit von Beatmungs- und Narkosengeräte. Idis, Bielefeld

142. Prüssner P (1999/2000) Medizinprodukterecht. Referat g2/AS 205 Medizinprodukte

143. Beschluss des Engeren Präsidiums der DGAI (1989) Qualitätssi-cherung in der Anästhesiologie. Anästh Intensivmed 30:307–314

144. Beschluss des Engeren Präsidiums der DGAI (1999) Modifikation des Kerndatensatzes Anästhesie. Anästh Intensivmed 40:649–658

145. Böhrer H (2001) Komplikationen und Sicherheitsaspekte: Allge-meine Aspekte und Definitionen. In: Kochs E, Krier C, Buzello W, Ad-ams HA (eds) Anästhesiologie. Thieme, Stuttgart, pp 1430–1432

146. Schulte-Steinberg O (1967) Ein Patientenfragebogen für den Anästhesisten. Anaesthesist 16:109–111

147. Weißauer W (1978) Das Konzept des Aufklärungs- und Anam-nesebogens aus rechtlicher Sicht. Anästh Inf 19:245–246

148. Weißauer W (1981) Zur Neufassung des Aufklärungs- und Anam-nesebogens. Anästh Intensivmed 2:52–52

149. Weißauer W (1994) Neue Aufklärungs- und Anamnesebögen – Anpassung an die medizinische und forensische Entwicklung. Anästh Intensivmed 35:253–255

150. Clade H (2002) Pflegeversicherung: Handlungsbedarf. Dtsch Ärztebl 99:A-1325

151. Statistisches Bundesamt (2002) Persönliche Mitteilung, Corre-spondence of April 2002

152. Alon E, Schüpfer G (1999) Operationssaal-Management. Anaes-thesist 48:689–697

153. Heck M, Fresenius M (1999) Repetitorium Anästhesiologie. Springer, Berlin, pp 571–572

2.2   Intensive Care Medicine

2.2.1   The Development of Intensive Care Medicine in the Framework of Anaesthesiology in the Federal Republic of Germany[1]

P. Lawin (†), H.W. Opderbecke, H. Van Aken

Introduction

Hardly any field of clinical medicine has had a stronger influence on modern medicine in recent decades than intensive therapy. With the development of intensive medical treatment procedures to restore and maintain disturbed vital functions, the resources of surgical medical care in particular expanded to a tremendous extent. In addition, new ethical and legal issues arose, such as determining the time of death, the limits of the medical duty to treat and, linked to this, medico-legal questions on problems of euthanasia. Finally, intensive care medicine, with its interdisciplinary character, has led to the development of new organizational forms in hospitals, with interdisciplinary bed units. Last but not least, the qualification requirements for intensive care staff provided the initial stimulus for the development of further in-service specialist training for nursing staff, analogous to the additional training available for doctors.

In this process, developments in the Federal Republic of Germany to some extent took a different direction in comparison with the international situation. In Germany, due to the special characteristics of the regulations for the medical profession, a separate discipline of »intensive care medicine« did not develop, and neither the title »physician specializing in intensive care medicine« nor a »German Society of Intensive Care Medicine« exist that are comparable to the scientific and medical specialist societies representing other disciplines. Instead, at an early stage there was already a structuring into three separate areas of internal medicine intensive care, surgical and anaesthesiological intensive care, and paediatric and neonatal intensive care. The effect of this was that intensive care medicine did not lose its connection to the associated specialist fields. One expression of this structure was the foundation of the German Interdisciplinary Association of Critical Care and Emergency Medicine (Deutsche Interdisziplinäre Ver-

einigung für Intensiv- und Notfallmedizin, DIVI), which only had corporate membership by the specialist societies and professional associations in the neighbouring fields and which for over 20 years now has been characterized by effective and harmonious interdisciplinary collaboration.

The course of the developments leading to the current situation, which we believe should be regarded as a favourable one, now covers a period of around 50 years. It has been shaped to a decisive extent by the German Society of Anaesthesiology and Intensive Care Medicine (Deutsche Gesellschaft für Anästhesiologie und Intensivmedizin, DGAI).

Initial Development Trends

At the end of the Second World War, German medicine, which had once led the world, had, due to its many years of isolation, substantially fallen behind in comparison with the international standard and the Anglo-American standard in particular. Surgery in particular was affected by this. One of the reasons for this was the anachronistic level of anaesthetic technology available. As had been customary for decades, anaesthesia in German hospitals was usually passed over to nursing staff or young, inexperienced resident physicians. The main technique used was still ether drop anaesthesia, although various modifications of the induction method were used. Compared to the anaesthetic technique, monitoring and maintenance of vital functions during the procedure were grossly neglected. These serious shortcomings became particularly noticeable when it came to catching up with deficiencies in the field of chest surgery. This now required the introduction of tracheal intubation that had long since been customary in the Anglo-American countries, so as to allow open chest surgery to be carried out without time pressure. The fact that it was actually a German physician, the surgeon Franz Kuhn in Kassel, who first recognized the importance of the intubation technique and used it for anaesthetic purposes, can be described in retrospect as tragic [48–50]. As is well known, the procedure he developed was unable to hold its own against Sauerbruch's differential pressure procedure [90, 91].

In order to catch up with international developments at the end of the war, therefore, German surgery had to cast off its old habits and promote the introduction of these modern anaesthetic procedures, whether it wanted to or not. But this necessarily implied the specialization of an independent discipline of physician anaesthetists. The difficult and sometimes controversial negotiations on this issue between the German Society of Surgery and the German Society of Anaesthesia (Deutsche Gesellschaft für Anaesthesie, DGA), conducted in the spring of 1953, have been described by Bräutigam in a detailed article on medical history [19].

---

[1] Based on articles written by the authors Lawin and Opderbecke for the series »*The historical development of intensive care medicine in Germany*«, published in the annual volumes of the journal *Der Anaesthetist* in 1998–2000 and in book form under the title *Die Intensivmedizin in Deutschland* (Springer, Berlin, 2001).

The emergence of physician anaesthetists with their own independent authority meant that, unlike the earlier anaesthesia nurses, they were not responsible only for anaesthesia and the elimination of pain but also relieved the surgeon of the need to look after monitoring and maintaining vital functions. As the surgical procedures became more extensive and cumbersome – not least as a result of the new methods of intubation anaesthesia – the task of monitoring and maintaining vital functions became all the more important in comparison with the actual anaesthetic procedure.

Postoperative patient care thus also grew in importance simultaneously – particularly continuous monitoring and adequate fluid substitution. It soon became clear that, in view of limited staffing and equipment resources, this type of care could only be provided optimally by placing patients who had undergone serious operations in special centralized bed units. It was recalled that even before the Second World War, the surgeons Kirschner [44] and Sauerbruch had established »supervision wards« of this type in their hospitals for the same purpose.

Another model was provided by the internal medicine ventilation wards that developed at the end of the 1940s and in the early 1950s, particularly in Scandinavia and Germany, for artificial ventilation of poliomyelitis patients with respiratory insufficiency. This initial developmental stage, which ultimately led to the creation of conservative medical intensive care units analogous to surgical intensive care units, is closely linked with the name of the Hamburg internists Aschenbrenner and Dönhardt, who carried out magnificent pioneering work with what were then extremely limited means [12, 13, 26].

In the surgical field, the first bed units of this type developed in the form of department-related surgical »supervision wards«. With regard to medical care, it seemed an obvious step to assign responsibility for monitoring and maintaining vital functions to the anaesthetist, as he was already carrying out this task intraoperatively. The natural result was thus that interdisciplinary collaboration in the operating room continued without interruption into the supervision ward. To begin with, there were hardly any conflicts of responsibility, since although the anaesthetist was broadly independent in specialist terms during the initial stages of these developments, within the hospital hierarchy he still did not yet have a position of equality and independence. His position was more that of an assistant medical director with a special function, and he was at best entitled to call himself »head of the division of anaesthesia in the surgical department«.

The equipment available in these first supervision wards that were set up in individual hospitals during the 1950s was modest, and even almost primitive from today's point of view. ECG monitors in the modern sense were not yet available; in the absence of a central gas supply, oxygen bottles stood at the bedside and had to be constantly exchanged; suction drains were kept operating by water jet pumps and the only circulatory monitoring available consisted of frequent manual blood pressure measurements. However, these blood pressure checks were the first step towards introducing timed daily charts instead of the usual »temperature curve«. It need hardly be mentioned that there were initially no single-use infusion sets and hardly any differentiated infusion solutions.

Virtually nothing was known about the perioperative pathophysiology of surgical procedures. Fatal courses after serious operations were simply regarded as unavoidable. The treatment provided for what the French surgeon Leriche [64] described in 1953 as a »secondary disease« – *maladie postopératoire anatomique* with disturbance of the *milieu intérieur* – was scarcely capable of having a »targeted« effect in comparison with today's standard postoperative therapies.

In the 1950s, there was still a lack of almost everything that would be regarded today as necessary for the postoperative phase after large abdominal operations. I can describe from my own memory a course observed in 1958:

> A medical invigilator was assigned to monitor a patient after total colectomy due to ulcerative colitis. But what could the – usually extremely young – doctor do?
> To maintain blood pressure, an adrenaline drip was placed in this patient, in addition to an infusion with so-called physiological saline. It was essential to check the blood pressure and »titrate« the adrenaline drip accordingly. The patient's urinary discharge ceased during the course of the night and the patient died the following morning.

For a long period, infusion solutions adjusted to catabolism and energy turnover, such as glucose, amino acids or fat emulsions, were not available.

Older doctors may still recall the way in which, after the introduction of systemic infusion therapy, the Strauss winged cannula was replaced by plastic cannulas such as the Braun cannula and AbboCath, and how frequently thrombophlebitis developed due to the infusion of higher percentage solutions. This problem, which seems banal today but was then a serious one, was only solved using the caval vein catheter technique, initially via the basilic vein and later via the subclavian or jugular vein [78].

In the same context, at the beginning of 1960, central venous pressure became an important monitoring parameter for fluid balance and assessing filling pressure in the right heart [21]. The laborious hunt for the last air bubble under the dome of the Statham element for intra-arterial blood pressure measurement became a mere legend once simple pressure transmission systems were introduced.

Since the introduction of the Swan-Ganz catheter, pulmonary arterial occlusion pressure – known as wedge pressure – has also allowed assessment of the functional condition of the left heart, as well as parameter-guided titration of positive inotropic substances.

These initially serious deficiencies were relieved by the explosive development of new treatment approaches and a flood of publications on topics such as parenteral nutrition [2], the treatment of disturbances of the acid-base balance and electrolyte substitution [55, 58], to mention only three examples here. These topics were a rich field of research for many people at the time. The results led to clear progress and today form part of the clinical routine. It was mainly anaesthetists who introduced the new discoveries into clinical work and thereby created the conditions in which surgeons were able to carry out expanded and new methods of surgery.

This was the period in which shock was defined as a pathophysiological condition [1] and it was discovered that different damaging factors lead to various forms of shock and various courses, but all resulting in failure of the microcirculation [68]. Allgöwer and Burri introduced a »practicable« shock index [10]. Renal function became a criterion for the extent of shock, with the parameter of »urinary output« being defined. The concepts »kidney in shock« and »shock kidney« made it possible to distinguish between still reversible and irreversible conditions [93, 96].

Medical Developments: the Examples of Long-Term Ventilation and Parenteral Nutrition

Long-Term Ventilation

Despite this, treatment of shock and compensating for metabolic disturbances were not able to save all of the patients. Increasingly often, patients who had survived an initial shock state or the initial postoperative phase were now dying of respiratory insufficiency.

Forty years ago, pneumonia was the most frequent and dangerous postoperative complication. In these cases our medical reports closed with the words »Postoperatively, the patient developed pulmonary inflammation and unfortunately died of its effects«.

The patients concerned had a peaceful death. At this time, at the end of the 1950s, no one had yet thought of ventilation.

As mentioned in the introduction, as »wards for freshly operated patients«, the first surgical supervision wards were initially more like intensive monitoring units in character. However, these wards were soon increasingly accepting non-surgical patients with respiratory insufficiency of various causes. These particularly involved patients with severe tetanus conditions, patients with neurological deficits and also poisoning. Up to this time, internists had used tank respirators (iron lungs) for artificial ventilation, particularly in cases of respiratory paralysis due to poliomyelitis. For the conditions of the time, this was a very successful form of treatment, which in Germany was particularly associated with the names of the Hamburg internists Aschenbrenner and Dönhardt [13, 26].

Following the introduction of endotracheal intubation and positive pressure ventilation into anaesthetic technique, it was soon found that this procedure was suitable for long-term ventilation of patients with respiratory insufficiency and that it was far superior to treatment with the iron lung. As this was primarily an anaesthesiological technique, the anaesthetist thereby acquired direct competence for the intensive treatment of non-surgical cases. The equipment initially available consisted of the Scandinavian Engström respirator, as well as the Poliomat and the Pulmomat manufactured by Dräger. These devices were later largely replaced by Bird and Bennett respirators and other pressure-controlled constructions from the USA.

Although this represented the beginnings of ventilation treatment, it was still a considerable time before the relationship between the oxygen supply and demand and haemodynamics was capable of being incorporated into the treatment approach.

The indication for controlled long-term ventilation gradually extended to include primary pulmonary-related forms of respiratory insufficiency [57, 60, 62]. However, adult respiratory distress syndrome (ARDS) required more sophisticated and individually variable ventilation techniques – positive end-expiratory pressure (PEEP), intermittent mandatory ventilation (IMV), high-frequency ventilation (HFV), etc. These requirements were met by newly developed respirators with electronic control elements. Devices that may be mentioned include the Servoventilator 900 (Siemens) and the UV 1 and UV 2 (Drägerwerk) [98]. Further progress was provided by devices for technically simplified blood gas analysis, which allowed tight control of ventilation therapy. The first device of this type was the Analysator (Radiometer, Copenhagen), developed by Astrup.

As ventilation quite often lasted for several weeks, the question soon arose of whether tracheotomy or long-term intubation was preferable. To begin with, tracheotomy was considered preferable even after several days of ventilation, particularly after a special flexible spiral tube developed by Rügheimer became available for this purpose. Later, prolonged intubation using »low-pressure, high-volume« cuff tubes became increasingly predominant, in order to avoid cicatricial tracheal stenoses as a late complication of long-term respirator therapy [88, 89].

Today, the procedure of controlled or assisted long-term ventilation for pulmonary or extrapulmonary respiratory insufficiency can be described as having been largely technically perfected. It has remained a field for the anaesthetist, although internists and paediatricians also used it successfully. Not all of the details of the development of this complex form of treatment can be presented in the brevity required for this cursory survey. A more detailed description is available in the article by Hachenberg and Pfeiffer published as part 15 of the series »The historical development of intensive care medicine in Germany« [37].

Infusion Therapy and Parenteral Nutrition

With the development of long-term intensive treatment of severely ill patients with respiratory insufficiency, balanced intravenous infusion therapy and parenteral nutrition also increased in importance. The problems involved are extremely varied, and the various issues involved can only be touched on in keywords here: the selection of sugar and sugar substitutes such as glucose, fructose, sorbitol, xylitol, intravenous administration of alcohol and fat emulsions as calorie vectors, and finally the use of protein hydrolysates and amino acid mixtures and the optimal combination of them. Here again it was anaesthetists who were decisively involved in the relevant discussions [2, 5, 9, 16, 17, 27, 28, 51, 97].

An overview of the historical development of parenteral nutrition by C. Puchstein was published as part 11 of the series »The historical development of intensive care medicine in Germany« [86].

With the development of long-term infusion therapy, particularly with the administration of hyperosmolar solutions, the problem of infusion-related thrombophlebitis as a limiting factor also had to be solved. This was achieved by developing strict administration criteria, which reduced the complication rate of central venous catheterization (caval catheter) to an acceptable level and thus created the conditions for widespread use of this infusion technique [22, 36, 77, 78].

In the present context, only these two aspects of intensive therapy can be highlighted here as examples, since the topics of ventilation, infusion therapy, and parenteral nutrition were researched and advanced by German anaesthetists in particular. There are of course other procedures in intensive care medicine that are equally important, such as ECG monitoring, renal substitution treatment, specialized intensive care methods in neonatology, etc. Mention should also be made of the complex topics of shock and sepsis, scientific research on which has always been a common interdisciplinary task for everyone involved in intensive care – including surgeons as well.

Publications

The first reports of experience in intensive care medicine published in the German-language literature after the Second World War were by the Department of Surgery at the University of Vienna, associated with the names of P. Fuchsig, R. Kucher, O. Mayrhofer and K. Steinbereithner

[33, 33, 46, 65]. In 1959, H. Franke and H.W. Opderbecke of Nuremberg described their surgical and anaesthesiological collaboration on a surgical supervision ward [31]. P. Lawin of Hamburg reported in 1964 on the »reorganization of an anaesthesia department with a supervision ward in an old hospital« – the first anaesthesia department in Germany that officially had an interdisciplinary ward attached to it [52]. Articles on other topics by anaesthetists and surgeons followed [11, 30, 41, 47, 53, 66, 79, 83, 92, 104]. Valuable encouragement for an approach using centralized postoperative care was provided by Scandinavian authors, since at that time these countries were the leaders in this field [14, 42, 100]. With their publications and lectures in Germany, the Scandinavian anaesthetists M. Holmdahl of Uppsala and H. Poulsen of Aarhus [39, 84, 85] can take special credit for this. Retrospective accounts of this initial phase of development have been published by P. Lawin [56] and K. Wiemers [105].

In the literature, this initial phase of development was concluded in many respects with the publication in 1968 of the textbook edited by P. Lawin, **Praxis der Intensivbehandlung** (The practice of intensive treatment). A chapter by Lawin and Opderbecke on »The organization of intensive treatment« was included in the second edition of the book in 1971 and continued to be revised up to the sixth edition in 1994 [59].

In parallel with these publications on organizational structures, architecture, equipment and operational procedures in intensive care units, numerous medical and scientific publications on issues in intensive treatment were also appearing. The extent of the literature is now almost unmanageable. We can only list here the most important books, publication series and journals published in the German-speaking countries and dealing with intensive care topics from an anaesthesiological point of view:

Books (arranged chronologically)

1. Wiemers K, Kern E (1957) 1st edn. Wiemers K, Kern E, Günther M, Burchardi H (1969) *Postoperative Frühkomplikationen*, 2nd edn. Thieme, Stuttgart
2. Lawin P (ed) (1st edn. 1968) (6th edn. 1994) *Praxis der Intensivbehandlung*. Italian and Spanish editions. Thieme, Stuttgart
3. Satter P, Dudziak R (1971) *Frischoperiertenstation und Intensivpflege*. Barth, Heidelberg
4. Kucher H, Steinbereithner K (eds) (1st edn. 1972) *Intensivstation, -pflege, -therapie*. Steinbereithner K, Bergmann H (eds) (2nd edn. 1984) Thieme, Stuttgart
5. Frey R, Hügin W, Mayrhofer O (eds) (3rd edn. 1972) *Lehrbuch der Anästhesiologie, Reanimation und Intensivtherapie*. Springer, Berlin. Benzer H, Burchardi H, Larsen R, Suter PM (eds) (7th edn. 1995), title changed to: *Lehrbuch der Anästhesiologie und Intensivmedizin*. Springer, Berlin
6. Glatz G (ed) (1st edn. 1977) *Anästhesie und Intensivmedizin*. Bibliomed, Medizinische Verlagsgesellschaft. Scherer R, Schöngart C (eds) (3rd edn. 1989) *Anästhesie und Intensivmedizin*. Bibliomed, Med. Verlagsgesellschaft

7. List WF, Osswald PM (eds) (1st edn. 1989, 2nd edn. 1992) *Intensiv-medizinische Praxis*. Springer, Berlin
8. Neander KD, Meyer G, Friesacher H (1993) *Handbuch der Intensiv-pflege*. Ecomed, Landsberg/Lech

Publication series

1. Anaesthesiologie und Wiederbelebung. Frey R, Kern F, Mayrhofer O (founding editors; founded 1965) Renamed: Anaesthesiologie und Intensivmedizin. Springer, Berlin
2. INA-Intensivmedizin-Notfallmedizin-Anästhesiologie, Lawin P, Loewenich V v, Schuster HP, Stoeckel H, Zumtobel V (founding editors; founded 1977). Thieme, Stuttgart
3. Klinische Anästhesiologie und Intensivtherapie, Ahnefeld FW, Burri C, Dick W, Halmágyi M (founding editors; founded 1974). Springer, Berlin

Journals (arranged chronologically)

1. *Der Anaesthesist*
    Founded 1951. Founding editors: Frey R, Hügin W, Mayrhofer O.; editor 1969–1997: Doenicke A.; editor since 1997: Peter K. Springer, Berlin
2. *Informationen*
    Issued by the *Deutsche Gesellschaft für Anästhesie* and *Berufsverband Deutscher Anästhesisten* by its own publishing house. Editor: Lehmann C; renamed 1970 as *Anästhesiologische Informationen*. Eds: *Deutsche Gesellschaft für Anästhesie und Wiederbelebung* (DGAW) and *Berufsverband Deutscher Anästhesisten* (BDA). Demeter, Gräfelfing/Munich. Editor: Opderbecke HW until 1994, renamed 1978 as *Anästhesiologie u. Intensivmedizin*. Eds: DGAI and BDA. Perimed, Erlangen. Editor since 1994 Landauer B., since 1996 Blackwell, Berlin. From 2002 DIOmed, Nuremberg. Editor: Taeger K.
3. *Zeitschrift für Praktische Anästhesie und Wiederbelebung*
    Founded 1965. Founding editor: Just OH, Thieme, Stuttgart; renamed 1974 as *Praktische Anästhesie, Wiederbelebung und Intensivtherapie*. Ed: Just OH; renamed 1991 as *AINS Anästhesiologie-Intensivmedizin-Notfallmedizin-Schmerztherapie*. Eds: until 1994 Lawin P, Stoeckel H; eds: from 1995 Hempelmann G, Schulte am Esch J, Krier C
4. *European Journal of Intensive Care Medicine*
    Founded 1975. Founding editors: Lutz H, Kachaner J, Peter K, Tinker J, Wolff G; renamed from vol. 3, 1997 as *Intensive Care Medicine*. Springer, Berlin

Approaches to Organization and Incorporation into Hospital Structures

The advantages of centralized care for newly operated patients were in the meantime so clear that other surgical disciplines now also claimed the right to a share in these facilities. While initially it was only individual patients with a particularly high risk of complications who were admitted to the supervision wards in addition to surgical patients, this soon raised the question of which physicians had jurisdiction and responsibility for these »guest patients«, leading in turn to the question of who the medical heads of centralized units of this type should be.

To meet the growing demands of intensive care medicine, it was usually possible in university hospitals to establish additional specialty-related bed units when needed – particularly since at that time, as mentioned above, the costs and effort required for the technical equipment were comparatively small. By contrast, in most hospitals the costs and effort, and staffing requirements in particular, appeared to be too great for a separate supervision ward – or, as it soon came to be called, intensive care ward – to be assigned to each surgical specialist department and to the internist as well. This resulted in the need to establish interdisciplinary bed units and to give consideration to what their organizational structure should be and which physicians should head them.

The journal of Germany's senior hospital doctors, *Der Krankenhausarzt*, devoted two special issues in 1967 to the development of anaesthesiology. Both issues have a preface by M. Zindler of Düsseldorf. The preface to the first special issue states:

> It has proved to be a particular blessing for the most seriously ill patients that the work of the anaesthetist has extended beyond the operating room to supervision wards, wards for newly operated patients and intensive treatment wards. Many patients who would otherwise have been lost have been saved thanks to constant monitoring and care, as well as mechanical long-term ventilation when necessary.

In addition to other articles more on questions of principle, the issue also includes articles on »Duties and experience of an anaesthesia department in a 340-bed hospital« (G. Weise of Hüttental-Weidenau) [101], »Duties and work of the anaesthesia departments in a medium-sized hospital« (H.A. Berkel of Lüdenscheid) [15] and »The anaesthesia department in a 1000-bed hospital« (M. Körner of Krefeld) [45]. All three authors describe anaesthetists' duties and working conditions not only in the operating room but also in surgical intensive care medicine.

The second special issue of the journal *Der Krankenhausarzt* (issue 5, 1967) is devoted exclusively to the organization of surgical intensive care medicine. In the preface to this issue, Zindler draws clear distinctions between the various duties in the recovery room, supervision ward and intensive treatment unit on the basis of a resolution then being prepared by the German Society of Anaesthesia and Resuscitation (Deutsche Gesellschaft für Anaesthesie und Wiederbelebung, DGAW), and he discusses medical responsibilities with particular attention to the role of the anaesthetist.

The first article in this second special issue, by P. Lawin of Hamburg, deals with »Intensive care treatment in large hospitals«. In addition to considerations of principle on the organization of intensive care medicine, he describes his experience in intensive care medicine in the old hospital in the Altona district of Hamburg; he also assesses the prospects for the planned intensive care ward in the new

Hamburg-Altona General Hospital in Othmarschen [54]. His remarks are supplemented by an article by C. Lehmann of Munich on organizational and clinical experience in an intensive treatment ward in the Rechts der Isar Hospital (which at that time was a municipal hospital) [61]. M.H. Holmdahl and W. Duvernoy of Uppsala then report on 15 years' experience in surgical intensive care medicine in Sweden [39]. The authors distinguish between intensive treatment and intensive observation, and provide information on the principles of organization, depending on the number of acute beds in the hospital, on staffing requirements and on bed requirements in intensive care for the individual specialties. Finally, the authors explain that the accepted practice in Sweden is to transfer the administrative management of interdisciplinary intensive care units to the anaesthetist, who shares medical responsibility with the referring physician.

The series of articles in these special issues is concluded by W. Vogel and K. Wiemers of Freiburg on »Duties and functioning of a department of anaesthesiology« [99]; K.H. Bräutigam of Stuttgart, »Staffing plan for an anaesthesia department« [18]; B. Haid of Innsbruck, »Planning a department of anaesthesiology at a university« [38]; and H. Nolte and F.W. Ahnefeld of Mainz, »The organizational, staffing and material requirements for modern hospital resuscitation facilities« [71].

In these articles as well, intensive care medicine is regarded as an integral component of specialist duties in anaesthesiology.

On 1 July 1967, the German Hospital Institute (Deutsches Krankenhausinstitut, DKI) in Düsseldorf and the German Association of Senior Hospital Physicians held a seminar in Düsseldorf on »Intensive care and intensive treatment«. Three of the papers presented at the meeting were also published in the journal Der Krankenhausarzt [69, 106]. Under the title »The organization of intensive treatment, intensive monitoring and intensive care«, S. Eichhorn, a member of the Executive Committee of the German Hospital Institute, for the first time discussed the set of problems involved from an economic and administrative point of view [29]. He compares the nursing and medical services in German hospitals, traditionally divided into specialist departments, with the Anglo-American structures, which are primarily divided – in accordance with the level of intensive care needed – into intensive care units, intermediate care units and self-care units. The development of intensive care medicine, he states, makes it necessary at least in this field to adopt the practice of arranging the facilities in accordance with the intensity of care in German hospitals as well and to provide interdisciplinary bed units for this purpose. The previously widely varying data on bed and staffing requirements led Eichhorn as well to draw a distinction between intensive monitoring and intensive treatment. In

addition, he mentions postoperative observation in the recovery room as an additional functional category.

The author goes into detail on the issue of medical jurisdiction and responsibility. His remarks include the following statements:

1. The jurisdiction and thus the primary responsibility for intensive treatment remain with the individual physicians in the individual specialist disciplines.

2. The jurisdiction and thus the primary responsibility for intensive treatment pass to a specialist physician responsible for this. At the same time, this raises the question of whether this then represents a new medical specialist discipline, or whether at least in this area the classical division according to specialist disciplines is to be abandoned. On the part of doctors, intensive monitoring also usually requires collaboration between several specialists. Usually, however, the responsibility here remains with the specialist discipline concerned, while the other specialists only join in with assistance. In the field of surgical monitoring, there will be a smooth transition between the anaesthetist's responsibility for the recovery phase and the surgeon's responsibility for further treatment.

   The necessity to clearly regulate the issue of medical jurisdiction thus primarily arises in the field of intensive treatment and less so in the field of intensive monitoring – provided at least that there is no dissolution of the specialist departments as is the case in the USA, for example, when the idea of progressive care is pursued to its logical conclusion. It will be the task of the specialist medical organizations to reach clear decisions on all of these questions as soon as possible.

Eichhorn's article includes additional remarks on the organizational structure relative to the size of the hospital, on requirements for medical and nursing staff and notes on the architecture, furnishing and equipping of intensive care units. From today's point of view, this comprehensive presentation can be regarded as the first fundamental publication on this topic in the German-language specialist literature, setting the standard for further developments.

Further Developments as Exemplified by Hamburg's Municipal Hospitals

The situation in the 1960s in Hamburg can be regarded as a typical example for the period.

In 1956, L. Zukschwerdt, then Chairman of the Department of Surgery of the University Hospital in Eppendorf, Hamburg, transferred the management of the supervision ward with 27 beds to a surgeon and anaesthetist, K. Horatz, as Senior Physician. All trainee surgeons and anaesthetists had to work there for 1 year. Hardly anyone at the time suspected how fruitful the pioneering spirit that predominated there was to be for the later development of intensive care medicine.

When P. Lawin was appointed as Head of the newly founded Department of Anaesthesia at the General Hospital in Altona in Hamburg in 1962, he also wanted to have a supervision ward available as a counterpart to the already existing internal medicine ventilation unit, in the same way as at the University Hospital in Eppendorf, Hamburg. Dr. H. Nachtrab, Departmental Head of the Medical and Hospital Service of the Health Authorities in the Free and Hanseatic City of Hamburg, found this approach convincing, approved a new type of organizational form termed »anaesthesia department with supervision ward« and provided the necessary funding. On 2 January 1963, the Anaesthesia Department originally founded on 1 December 1962 was able to put the ward into operation. It was one of the first interdisciplinary surgical intensive care wards in Germany to have an independent Anaesthesia Department attached to it.

The Heads of the Anaesthesia Departments in Hamburg's other general hospitals now understandably had similar wishes, but at the same time there was increasing resistance to the idea on the part of the surgeons. It was then hardly conceivable that anaesthetists should have beds at their own disposal, when in the eyes of the surgeons the patients were »theirs«.

It was probably 1964 when Nachtrab therefore invited the Heads of the Surgery Departments, Diebold from St. Georg General Hospital and Lichtenauer from Harburg General Hospital, as well as the Heads of the Anaesthesia Departments Bermann from St. Georg and Nüssgen from Harburg, as well as Lawin from Altona General Hospital, to a discussion at the Hamburg Health Department in order to reach a mutually acceptable joint approach. It was a difficult task, since Diebold's emotionally presented objections for a long time got in the way of an objective discussion. Finally, thanks to Lichtenauer's open-minded and friendly style, agreement was successfully reached: the approach developed by Nachtrab, who had become an enthusiastic advocate of the anaesthesiologists' ideas, was accepted by the group.

Later, in 1968, Nachtrab published an article in the *Zeitschrift für Praktische Anästhesie und Wiederbelebung* stating his views and the experience that had been gained in the meantime [70]. He summed up as follows:

> In smaller and medium-sized hospitals, only one ward of this type will be present, and it will be appropriate for the anaesthetist to be in medical and administrative charge of it. In large hospitals with around 1,000 beds, there will inevitably be one surgical and one conservative intensive care treatment area; it will then be appropriate for the latter to be managed by an internist. Patient care in these wards will take place on a team basis – i.e. the personal doctor-patient relationship will be maintained. Patients who have undergone surgery, for example, will continue to be the patients of the surgeon, who will be responsible for everything needed in postoperative treatment. He will use the medical staff of this department in the context of his responsibilities.
>
> The anaesthetist who carries out special treatment measures such as ventilation etc. is responsible in the context of the measures lying within his field. In the context of current care, he is also responsible for immediate action to fight acute, life-threatening complications. Intensive treatment wards of this type therefore require a specialized standby team of doctors who can be available immediately within minutes to fight life-threatening conditions effectively.
>
> This type of organization would be inconceivable without having a leading medical figure with responsibility for it. It is therefore appropriate to assign the medical and administrative management of wards of this type to the anaesthetist in the surgical field or to an internist in the conservative field. In Hamburg, this approach has been practised in all intensive treatment wards so far established and it has proved its value.

This model became the obligatory form of organization in Hamburg, the largest hospital local authority in Germany with its 15,000 beds, and it was also pioneering because it was recommended as an exemplary approach by Germany's »Standing Conference of Senior Medical Officers of the Federal States«.

Initial Activities of the DGA

In the early 1960s, continuing developments and resulting issues led the DGA to address the problem as well. It could hardly have been expected at the time that the problems would continue to be debated right down to the present day. At the time, in negotiations then being conducted by the German Society of Surgery's specially formed »Anaesthesia Committee«, the primary concern was with the recognition of anaesthesiology as an independent specialty, delimitation of medical responsibilities in the operating room and the representation of the new specialty in teaching and research. In addition, there now arose the problem that – expressed in a polemical and rather pointed way – led to the question: »Whom does intensive care medicine belong to?« In particular, developments in the hospitals were leading to intensive care medicine having an interdisciplinary character, with the anaesthetist holding a key position. By contrast, the German Society of Surgery even until very recently never tired of postulating the existence of »surgical intensive care medicine«.

When one reads the minutes of the Executive Committee meetings of the DGA of these years, it appears that detailed discussion on the functions and definitions of terms for postoperative units first took place at the meeting in Mainz on 29 October 1964, chaired by the then DGA President, K. Wiemers of Freiburg. In a letter of 26 October 1964, Wiemers had previously written to the then Chairman of the Association of the Scientific Medical Societies in Germany (Arbeitsgemeinschaft Wissenschaftlicher Medizinischer Fachgesellschaften, AWMF), a surgeon named Junghanns in Oldenburg, stating the following observations:

> The recovery rooms in which the patients remain after the operation until they are transferred to the ward are the responsibility of the head anaesthetist. The supervision ward (ward for newly operated patients and acute patients) is usually headed by the surgeon in close collaboration with the anaesthetist. If there is a central intensive care unit in which patients from various disciplines are cared for, it can be recommended that the organizational management of it should be transferred to the anaesthetist.

The letter also counters an objection on the part of the surgeons – that the anaesthetist cannot take responsibility for a surgical supervision ward simply because his postgraduate training would not include any compulsory surgical periods – by saying that his work in the operating room would provide the anaesthetist with sufficient insight into surgical work.

It was during Wiemer's Presidency, in November 1964, that the long years of negotiations with the German Society of Surgery were finally concluded and an initial agreement »Guidelines on the position of the managerial anaesthetist« was reached [107].

With regard to postoperative patient care, point 6 in these guidelines states:

> The recovery rooms in which the patients remain after the operation until they are transferred to the ward are the responsibility of the head anaesthetist. The supervision ward (ward for newly operated patients and acute patients) is usually headed by the surgeon in close collaboration with the anaesthetist. If purely resuscitation tasks also have to be carried out in the supervision ward (e.g. ventilated patients), it can be recommended that the anaesthetist should take over this part. It has proved valuable to assign anaesthesia nurses to support these duties.

The ideas Wiemers had previously developed were thus taken over almost verbatim into the agreement.

The DGA's subsequent efforts focused on making surgical intensive care medicine to a firm component of the specialty without staking any claim to exclusivity. In the same way as in politics in general, the motto in our professional politics at that time was to sacrifice what was impossible in order to achieve what was possible. Any claim to exclusivity would have set all of the other disciplines against us and in addition would have contradicted the stipulations of the Postgraduate Training Regulations (*Weiterbildungsordnung*) requiring specialist physicians to restrict themselves to their own specialty.

A first step in this direction was the renaming of the DGA as the German Society of Anaesthesia and Resuscitation (Deutsche Gesellschaft für Anaesthesie und Wiederbelebung, DGAW). This move was prepared at the request of M. Zindler of Düsseldorf and K. Horatz of Hamburg, K. Wiemer's successor as President, at the meeting of the Executive Committee in Munich on 21 April 1965, and was adopted at the Society's general assembly in Zurich in September 1965. This established the specialist jurisdiction of the anaesthetist for emergency medicine, but here again with no claim to exclusivity.

Initial Contacts with the DKG

A further step involved efforts by the DGAW to make contact with the German Hospitals Federation (Deutsche Krankenhausgesellschaft, DKG). These resulted in initial talks held in Düsseldorf on 31 March 1967.

The representatives of the DKG participating in the talks were: Prelate Mühlenbrock (President), District Chief Administrative Officer Adam (General Secretary) and Wirtzbach (Secretary); on the anaesthesiology side, the participants were Henschel (President of the BDA), Lehmann (Secretary of the DGAW/BDA), Opderbecke (President of the DGAW) and Weißauer (DGAW/BDA Legal Advisor).

The atmosphere of the talks, thanks to Mühlenbrock, was surprisingly friendly and accommodating. Basically, three main topics were discussed: first, the position of the head anaesthetist in the hospital; second, the anaesthetist's duties in the recovery room, in the supervision ward and in the intensive care unit; and third, issues of staffing requirements.

The German Association of Cities *(Städtetag)*

At almost the same time, German Association of Cities declared, in a reply dated 2 March 1967, to a letter of 27 February 1967 from Opderbecke (K. Horatz's successor as DGAW President), that it was willing to listen to representatives of the DGAW on issues involving the way in which intensive care medicine was organized in municipal hospitals.

The hearing was held on 29 June 1967, in Munich's City Hall. Those present included the members of the Health Committee of the German Association of Cities and its »municipal hospital« working group. The DGAW was represented by Lehmann and Opderbecke. After a presentation by Opderbecke, the discussion was initially marked by the fact that the advisory doctors belonging to the committees were mainly surgeons and internists, the majority of whom expressed reservations regarding anaesthetists having capacities of responsibility in intensive care units. Objections to this view were stated in particular by Nachtrab, Chief Medical Director of the Hamburg Health Authorities, who described Hamburg's municipal hospitals [70], and by Matussek, the Mayor of Stuttgart. The latter reported his favourable impressions of a visit to the intensive treatment centre at the University of Vienna, headed by the anaesthetists Kucher and Steinbereithner.

The hearing by the relevant committees of the German Association of Cities was reflected in a »Recommendation to establish and operate intensive care wards« that was adopted by the Committee of the German Association of Cities on 20 December 1972 [119].

First DGAW Resolution

At the latest, these contacts with the DKG and the German Association of Cities showed the need to express in concrete terms the existing ideas regarding the organizational structures for intensive care facilities that had in the meantime been established – consisting of the recovery room, supervision ward and intensive treatment unit – and to define the individual terms relative to the nature of the duties involved, so that a clear and consistent approach could be defended in the future. At the DGAW's Executive Committee meeting on 30 March 1967, it was decided to develop an approach of this type, and the result was conclusively discussed and agreed at the DGAW Executive Committee meeting held in Salzburg on 20 September 1967 in the form of a »Position statement on the organization of the recovery room, supervision ward and intensive treatment in hospitals« and published the same year [108]. This finally brought some order into the variety of terms previously used, such as »newly operated patients' ward«, »monitoring ward«, »supervision ward«, »intensive care ward«, »ventilation centre« etc. The approach, inaugurated by Opderbecke, designates »intensive care medicine« as the generic term, subdivided into »intensive treatment« and »intensive monitoring«. The term »intensive care« was only used to refer to the nursing aspects of intensive medicine.

The Nuremberg Symposium

A symposium initiated by Opderbecke at the conclusion of his period of office as President of the DGAW and held in Nuremberg on 15–16 November 1968, entitled »Planning, organization and furnishing of hospital intensive treatment units« (◘ Fig. 2.49), represented a decisive turning-point. The meeting was co-organized by the DGAW together with the German Hospital Institute (Deutsches Krankenhausinstitut, DKI), based in Düsseldorf, and the Institute of Hospital Architecture of the Technical University of Berlin, giving the occasion an interdisciplinary character.

The number of speakers participating matched the variety of the topics dealt with. In addition to numerous German anaesthetists (F.W. Ahnefeld and M. Halmágyi of Mainz, H.A. Berkel of Lüdenscheid, P. Lawin of Hamburg, C. Lehmann of Munich, E. Rügheimer of Erlangen and K. Wiemers of Freiburg), the Vienna research group was represented by R. Kucher, O. Mayrhofer and K. Steinbereithner, and Scandinavian anaesthetists by M. Holmdahl of Uppsala and H. Poulsen of Aarhus.

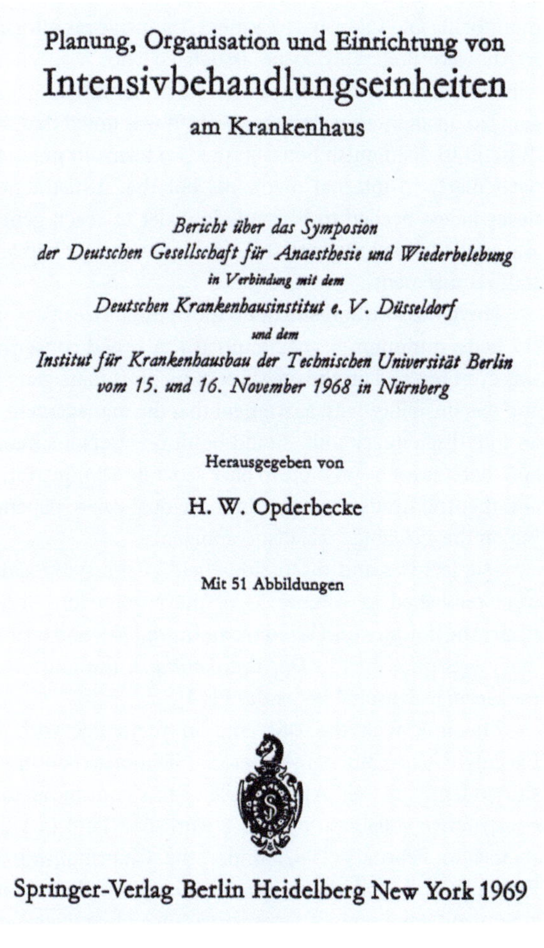

Planung, Organisation und Einrichtung von
Intensivbehandlungseinheiten
am Krankenhaus

*Bericht über das Symposion
der Deutschen Gesellschaft für Anaesthesie und Wiederbelebung
in Verbindung mit dem
Deutschen Krankenhausinstitut e. V. Düsseldorf
und dem
Institut für Krankenhausbau der Technischen Universität Berlin
vom 15. und 16. November 1968 in Nürnberg*

Herausgegeben von

H. W. Opderbecke

Mit 51 Abbildungen

Springer-Verlag Berlin Heidelberg New York 1969

◘ **Fig. 2.49.** Cover of the report on the symposium of the German Society of Anaesthesia and Resuscitation held in Nuremberg, 15–16 November 1968

Surgery was represented by P. Fuchsig of Vienna and paediatric medicine by D. Berg and V. von Loewenich of Frankfurt, as well as B.K. Jüngst and U. Köttgen of Mainz. Internal medicine was represented by U. Gessler of Nuremberg, K. Ibe of Berlin and P. Schölmerich of Mainz. Issues of hygiene were addressed by E. Kanz of Munich and legal issues by W. Weißauer of Munich. The situation of intensive care nurses was presented by the anaesthesia–nurse manager T. Valerius of Mainz. Representing the DKI, S. Eichhorn spoke about economic and management considerations; P. Poelzig spoke about architecture and equipment as a representative of the Institute of Hospital Architecture at the Technical University of Berlin; and W. Jung as Chairman of the Specialist Association of Administrative Managers of German Hospitals discussed questions of economic viability.

In the concluding discussion, in which H. Nachtrab of Hamburg took part as a representative of the hospital funding bodies, there was consensus on the necessity for all hospitals, independent of their size, to establish intensive care wards; particularly in larger hospitals, a distinction in principle needed to be made between intensive monitoring and intensive treatment. Intensive monitoring wards were preferably to be associated with a specialty, while intensive treatment wards were preferably to be organized on an interdisciplinary basis. It was noted that it is difficult to distinguish between the two terms in practice, particularly in internal medicine, but that a distinction nevertheless needed to be made in order to reach generally applicable solutions to still-open questions of bed and staff requirements.

There was also agreement on the optimal size of a ward (12 beds; minimum 8, maximum 16). A broad consensus was even reached on the question of medical management and responsibility, with agreement that the management of an interdisciplinary unit should be in one person's hands and that it must be possible to have separate administrative and medical heads of a ward in individual cases, depending on the available specialist competence.

The lectures and discussions held at the symposium were published as volume 33 of the publications series Anaesthesiologie und Wiederbelebung [73], and a summary was published in Das Krankenhaus, the journal of the German Hospital Federation [74].

The link with the DKI, and in particular with its Executive Committee member S. Eichhorn, continued subsequently as well. An example of this continuing and constructive collaboration was a workshop held in Düsseldorf in February 1982, under the Chairmanship of Eichhorn and Opderbecke, on »Principles of the organization and equipping of recovery rooms in hospitals«, the results of which were published as a resolution with the same title [131]. The workshop had been preceded by a symposium arranged by E. Rügheimer in the fall of 1981,

held in Merano, on »Recovery room – recovery phase: an anaesthesiological task« [87].

In September 1992, the DGAI awarded S. Eichhorn the Franz Kuhn Medal in recognition of his services to the status of anaesthesiology in German hospitals.

The Working Group on Internal Medical Intensive Care

The response to the Nuremberg meeting was unexpectedly strong. In particular, internists suspected that anaesthetists were wanting to assert a claim to exclusivity with the topic and were wanting in the future to treat patients with internal diseases in intensive care units that would be managed by anaesthetists on their own independent responsibility.

The German Society of Internal Medicine and the Professional Association of Internists reacted to these fears by founding a »Working Group on Internal Medicine Intensive Care« at the 72nd meeting of the Northwest German Association of Internal Medicine held in Hamburg on 30 January 30–1 February 1969, on the basis of a report on the Nuremberg meeting presented by W. Nachtwey of Hamburg.

The foundation of this group led to a joint Executive Committee meeting being held by the DGAW and BDA in Munich on 22 February 1969, under the Chairmanship of DGAW President K. Hutschenreuter of Homburg/Saar, who had been elected for the 1969–1970 period of office. After a detailed discussion, it was decided that as a countermeasure, a joint »Committee on Issues of Intensive Therapy« should be founded within the DGAW and BDA, with Horatz, Lawin, Opderbecke (Chair) and Wiemers as its members. The tasks of this group were described as follows:

> The task of the Committee is to pursue further political development of the specialty in the sector of intensive therapy. For this purpose, conciliatory and mediating discussions between the Committee, the President of the DGAW, the Chair of the Professional Association and specialist societies and professional bodies with an interest in this topic (surgery, gynaecology, internal medicine, neurosurgery) are necessary. The aim of the negotiations will be to develop a unified view regarding the way in which intensive treatment should be organized in hospitals. The composition of the participants from our side will be decided by Opderbecke on a case-by-case basis.

Agreement with the Internists

The situation was exacerbated when the Working Group on Internal Medicine Intensive Care (Arbeitsgemeinschaft für Internistische Intensivmedizin, AGII) sent a circular dated 5 August 1969 to all West German hospital funding bodies and heads of medical departments in which internal medicine stated its claim to intensive care medicine.

In reaction, the DGAW and BDA wrote a joint letter dated 6 September 1969 to the DKG and its members, clarifying the position of both associations. Signed by Hutschenreuter and Henschel, the letter stated in part:

> The circular [by the internists – ed.] of 5 August 1969 must be emphatically contradicted to the extent that it insinuates that a claim to exclusivity has been made by our specialty that has in fact never been raised. Our specialty is attempting neither to establish a monopoly on intensive therapy nor a claim to the management of intensive treatment units; however, it also expects the same approach to be taken by other specialties. Modern intensive therapy makes such complex demands on medical treatment that it can never be the domain of only a single discipline and instead requires, in our view, close collaboration between all disciplines at the bedside.

This tense atmosphere was finally defused through the willingness of both sides to negotiate. An initial discussion between the AGII and the DGAW and BDA's Committee on Issues of Intensive Therapy was held in Hamburg as early as 3 October 1969. The participating internists were: Broglie, Dönhardt, Gerok, Gessler, Gross (Spokesman), Haan, Nachtwey, Schölmerich and Spang, along with Pril as legal advisor; the anaesthetists were Henschel, Lawin, Lehmann, Opderbecke (Spokesman) and Wiemers, along with Weißauer as legal advisor.

After a statement from the anaesthesiology side clarifying that there was no intention of making an exclusive claim to the whole field of intensive care medicine, it was possible to reach consensus on the principles of an agreement surprisingly quickly.

The draft produced was agreed at a joint meeting of the Executive Committees of the DGAW and BDA in Munich on 4 April 1970. Agreement from the decision-making bodies in internal medicine followed at the annual meeting of the German Society of Internal Medicine held in Wiesbaden in 1970.

The »Joint recommendation on the organization of intensive care medicine in hospitals« [112] is based on the following principles:

1. **University hospitals and large hospitals.** Specialty-linked intensive care units should be planned for intensive monitoring and for special tasks in intensive treatment. In addition, university hospitals and large hospitals require both an interdisciplinary surgical unit and a conservative medical intensive treatment unit.

2. **Large and medium-sized hospitals.** In large and medium-sized hospitals with more than 300 beds, two separate units should usually be established for intensive care medicine: an interdisciplinary surgical unit and a conservative medical unit. The former should be managed by an anaesthetist and the latter by an internist. This does not affect the option of establishing specialty-linked surgical supervision wards in addition.

3. **Small hospitals.** If it is possible for financial or other reasons to establish an intensive care unit in hospitals with fewer than 300 beds, a participating head of department familiar with the principles of intensive care medicine should take charge of it.

The fourth and fifth points should be quoted here verbatim, as they led to renewed debate between the two specialties later on:

4. **Duties of the director of interdisciplinary units.** The organization of an interdisciplinary unit must lie in one person's hands. In close collaboration with the representatives of other specialties, the director must ensure monitoring, maintenance and restoration of vital functions in accordance with regulations. He is responsible for timely consultation with the treating and co-treating specialist physicians and must co-ordinate their work. The director of the unit must assign the required general and specialist instructions to the subordinate physicians and medical ancillary staff working in the unit and must monitor their work. He is responsible for the correct maintenance of the unit's medical and technical equipment.

5. **Treatment of the primary disease, collaboration.** In an interdisciplinary intensive care unit, the diagnosis and treatment of the primary disease remain the domain of the representative of the specialty responsible for it, who carries out diagnosis and therapy in close collaboration with the other physicians working in the unit. In this form of medical teamwork, each of those involved has responsibility for his or her aspect of diagnosis and therapy.

In retrospect, one can hardly overestimate the importance of this agreement with the internists, as it was to serve later as a model for subsequent agreements with the surgical specialties and in addition had a decisive influence on the DKG's »Guidelines for the organization of intensive care medicine in hospitals«.

Agreements with Other Specialties

Following the Nuremberg meeting in 1968, surgeons were initially hesitant about entering into negotiations regarding the allocation of responsibilities in intensive care medicine, apparently because they initially wished to await the results of the controversy between anaesthetists and internists. When the surprisingly speedy agreement between the two specialties was announced, the surgeons also declared their willingness to enter into discussions.

The seminal joint meeting between the German Society of Surgery and the Professional Association of German Surgeons, on the one hand, and the DGAW and BDA on the other, was held in Frankfurt on 28 November 1969. On the surgeons' side, the participants were von Brandis, Major, Müller-Osten and Rathke, and the anaesthetists included Henschel, Hutschenreuter, Lehmann and Opderbecke. Weißauer, who in the meantime had also started working for the Professional Association of German Surgeons as legal advisor, chaired the meeting as a neutral moderator. The list of principles for the assignment of duties and collaboration that had been agreed with the internists served as the basis for the negotiations. However, the discussions proved to be more difficult since in this case it was not only a question of drawing boundaries between duties in intensive care units, but also of establishing regulations for the indispensable collaboration needed in specialty-related surgical supervision wards and interdisciplinary centralized intensive treatment units. Despite these difficulties, it was possible to conclude the negotiations within a few months. At the Executive Committee meeting of the DGAW and BDA held in Munich on 2 April 1970, the draft that had been drawn up was adopted and, when agreement from the negotiating partners on the surgical side was forthcoming, it was published as the »Agreement between the specialties of surgery and anaesthesia regarding the delimitation of duties and collaboration in intensive care medicine«, along with a commentary by Weißauer [102, 113].

In the meantime, Wiemers had established contacts with the German Society of Neurosurgery. An initial discussion between representatives of the two specialist societies was held in Giessen during the annual meeting of the German Society of Neurosurgery on 5 July 1969. The participants on the neurosurgical side were: Jenssen of Kiel, Kuhlendahl of Düsseldorf, Pia of Giessen and Schürmann of Mainz. The anaesthetists were L'Allemand, Hutschenreuter, Opderbecke and Wiemers. Once the outlines of agreement on the most important points had been established, Jenssen and Wiemers continued negotiations sometimes through personal meetings and sometimes by letter. The »Recommendations for the organization of anaesthesia in the context of neurosurgery« were finally signed by the two Presidents, Hutschenreuter and Kuhlendahl, in October 1970 and were subsequently published [114].

In the section on »Collaboration in preoperative and postoperative care«, definitions and functional descriptions of the terms »recovery room«, »supervision ward« and »intensive treatment unit« were taken over verbatim from the DGAW statement of 1967, and it was established that the recovery room would be under the control of the anaesthetists and the specialty-related supervision ward

under the control of the neurosurgeon. An interdisciplinary surgical intensive treatment unit would usually be managed by the anaesthetist. The same regulations were listed for medical collaboration in the unit as had previously been agreed between anaesthetists and internists.

Analogous agreements were made between the Professional Association of German Urologists and the BDA in 1972 [121], between the specialist societies and professional associations on collaboration in ENT medicine in 1976 [125], between the professional associations on collaboration in the orthopaedic field in 1984 [132] and between the specialist societies and professional associations on collaboration in gynaecology and obstetrics in 1988 [134]. The last agreement was with the German Ophthalmological Society in 1998 [138]. All of these agreements basically include the same statements on collaboration in intensive care medicine as those agreed with the neurosurgeons.

Regulations had thus been agreed with nearly every surgical specialty field regarding the distribution of duties and collaboration in intensive care medicine, and these largely corresponded to the views held by the DGAW and BDA.

These agreements have been published, along with other resolutions and recommendations, in an anthology compiled and edited by H.W. Opderbecke and W. Weißauer [81]. Updated editions have regularly been published, the most recent one in 2011 [40].

Renegotiations with the Internists

In the »Joint agreement« between the two specialties of anaesthesiology and internal medicine, it was assumed that two separate intensive care units – one surgical and the other conservative – would be established in hospitals with more than 300 beds. In fact, however, many hospitals set the limit higher for economic reasons, so that joint surgical and conservative bed units were created more frequently than had originally been planned. This led to difficulties in implementing the agreed principles for the distribution of medical duties, as the boundaries between treatment of the primary disease on the one hand and maintenance of vital functions on the other are more fluid in internal medicine disease patterns than in surgical cases. When the unit was directed by anaesthetists, internists in these mixed units often felt excluded from care for their patients, as the competence boundaries were unclear, and they requested that the agreement should be modified.

Both sides made efforts to solve the problem, so as not to harm the good relations that had in the meantime been established between the specialties. After preparations for the meeting by letter, negotiations took place in Sprendlingen on 4–5 May 1979. The internists were represented by: U. Gessler of Nuremberg, K.D. Grosser of Krefeld, W. Nachtwey of Hamburg and L. Pippig of Gütersloh; Opderbecke, Rügheimer, Weis and Weißauer represented the anaesthesiology side. Consensus was achieved on modifying the »Joint agreement« and in particular on rewriting the section on »Medical competence and responsibility«. The following text was agreed:

> For collaboration between the internist and the anaesthetist, the following principle applies: the assignment of patients to each area of medical care is guided in hospitals of all sizes by the primary disease. The internist is responsible for diagnosis and therapy in patients in whom the primary disease is mainly medical, including life-threatening courses and complications; the anaesthetist, along with the representative of the relevant surgical specialty, is responsible for the diagnosis and treatment of patients in whom the primary disease is mainly surgical, including life-threatening courses and complications. Helpful and considerate collaboration between the anaesthetist and internist is indispensable. The principles of medical consultancy work apply.
> In joint conservative and surgical intensive care units, the medical and non-medical staff are subject to specialist instructions from the representative of the specialty responsible for the patient's treatment. The two representatives of the specialties concerned shall agree on joint guidelines for intensive care. Without giving consideration to who has the organizational responsibility for the conservative-surgical intensive care unit, the two representatives of the specialties shall agree on the main organizational issues.

The text of the new agreement was approved by the Executive Committees of the DGAI and BDA at their meetings in Saarbrücken on 22 November 1979, and subsequently published [130].

With the resolution of the controversy, the assignment of medical roles in intensive care medicine was largely concluded. Subsequent activities in professional politics were thereafter mainly initiated by the German Interdisciplinary Association of Critical Care Medicine (Deutsche Interdisziplinäre Vereinigung für Intensivmedizin, DIVI).

The DKG's Recommendations

Due to the Nuremberg meeting and discussions in the German Association of Cities, the DKG now considered it appropriate to take up the group of topics involving the »organization of intensive care medicine«. It therefore organized a hearing in Düsseldorf on 12 November 1969, chaired by G. Hopf of Hamburg, who in his capacity as President of the German Association of Senior Hospital Physicians was a member of the DKG's Organization Committee. Other medical participants were Major of Solingen, representing the German Society of Surgery; Schölmerich of Mainz, representing the German Society of Internal Medicine; and Dönhardt and Haan of Hamburg, representing the AGII. Anaesthesiology was represented by Henschel, Hutschenreuter and Opderbecke.

The fact that consensus had been reached between internists and anaesthetists shortly beforehand on the basic structural issues proved to be an inestimable advantage during the discussion. The medical ideas offered by the DKG's representatives were convincingly presented.

As a result of this discussion, the DKG in 1970 drafted an initial »Recommendation on the organization of intensive care medicine in hospitals« [111] – 2 years before the publication of the recommendations of the German Associations of Cities. As the DKG's recommendations were aimed at its member associations and thus at all West German hospital funding bodies, together with the subsequent statements by the DGK they had a decisive influence on the subsequent structural development of intensive care medicine in the hospitals.

For larger general hospitals with more than about 650 beds upwards, the statement recommends the establishment of one intensive care unit for the surgical field and one for the conservative field. In addition, specialty-related units with special tasks may be necessary. For hospitals with 300–350 beds or more, one intensive care unit is suggested. Here it is stated: »So far as this is divided into a surgical and a conservative department, the two departments should form a single unit both in terms of the rooms occupied and organizationally«. Finally, for smaller hospitals with basic care, a »group for intensive care medicine« is envisaged. The following statement is made regarding its medical management:

> The management and organization of the intensive care unit should be transferred to a physician with special training in intensive care medicine. He has responsibility for the routine care of patients.
> In close collaboration with the representatives of other specialties, the director of the interdisciplinary intensive care unit must ensure monitoring, maintenance and if necessary restoration of vital functions of patients in accordance with regulations. He is responsible for timely consultation with treating and co-treating specialist physicians who remain responsible for the treatment of the primary disease for each patient; he must co-ordinate their work. As the person responsible for the organization, the director of the intensive care unit can give the necessary general and specialized instructions to the medical, medical-technical and other members of staff in the intensive care unit; he must also monitor their work in this respect. He is responsible for proper maintenance of the medical and technical equipment in the intensive care unit.

The following details on staffing requirements are based on the »Reference figures for staffing of hospitals with nursing staff« published by the DKG on 19 September 1969:

(a) In intensive monitoring units (supervision wards) from 1:1.9 to 1:1.0 (proportion of nursing staff members to average occupied beds)

(b) In intensive treatment units, from 1:0.7 to 1:0.5 (proportion of nursing staff members to average occupied beds)

For staffing requirements in the medical service it is stated:

(a) Intensive treatment requires the uninterrupted 24-h presence of a physician. The total number of physicians necessary is based on the number of patients requiring intensive treatment and the type and severity of their diseases.

(b) Intensive monitoring requires the constant standby presence of a physician, with the type and extent of medical work being based on the patients' disease pictures.

Finally, with regard to bed requirements, it is stated:

»At present, the requirement for beds in intensive care medicine is 3–5% of hospital beds«.

The DKG recommendation had thus adopted in principle the general structural conceptions of the anaesthetists and internists, but departed from them on the issue of the size of hospital in which two separate intensive care units, one surgical and one conservative, were necessary so that the recommendation met with reservations from internists in particular.

The DKG itself apparently also found its recommendations unsatisfactory, although for quite different reasons. In any case, as early as 1972 it surprisingly, and without having previously contacted any representatives of the medical specialties again, published a revised version that deviated from the relatively precise details on staffing requirements and severely watered down the DKG's guidance figures [118]. The question of staffing requirements in intensive care medicine was subsequently to become a persistently contentious issue between the DKG and the physicians' associations [67, 75, 80, 110, 129].

Two years later, the DGK published a third version of its »Guidelines on the organization of intensive care medicine in hospitals«, dated 9 September 1974 [123]. On this occasion, it had previously set up a preparatory committee, with members including Haan as an internist and Opderbecke as an anaesthetist. This final recommendation now also adopted without reservations the physicians' ideas regarding the structure of intensive care medicine relative to hospital size and its still applies today.

Renaming of the Society

In the early 1970s, societies of intensive care medicine were established in several countries – in the USA, the Society of Critical Care Medicine, in the UK the Intensive Care Society and in Switzerland the Swiss Society of Intensive Care Medicine. The British and American groups jointly organized the »First World Congress on Intensive Care« in London on 24–27 June 1974. The German participants included R. Frey of Mainz and K. Hutschenreuter of Homburg/Saar. It was decided in London that a second World Congress would be held in Paris in September 1977 and that in the meantime preparations would be made to found a World Federation of Societies of Intensive and Critical Care Medicine.

At the meeting of the DGAW's Extended Executive Committee held in Erlangen on 2 October 1974, under the Chairmanship of E. Rügheimer of Erlangen who was DGAW President for 1973–1974, Frey and Hutschenreuter reported on their impressions of the London meeting. During the discussion, the question was raised of which society would in the future represent German intensive care medicine at the international level; the potential consequences of the foundation of a society of intensive care medicine in Germany were also pointed out. There was broad agreement that the foundation of such a society would be a first step in the direction of intensive care medicine becoming a separate specialty and that it might imply the introduction of a qualification as »specialist in intensive care medicine« into the medical postgraduate training regulations in Germany. Since Germany's postgraduate training regulations, as part of the regulations for the medical profession, not only define the contents of the specialties but also their boundaries, which the specialist has to observe as a matter of principle in his work, the logical consequence of a development of this type would have been that the parent surgical and conservative specialties would lose their responsibility for the intensive treatment of their patients, which would pass to a specialist in intensive care medicine. A loss of this type would have had particularly severe consequences for anaesthesiology.

Against this background P. Lawin in a letter of 22 July 1975 to the acting DGAW President, W. Henschel of Bremen, officially applied to found a »Working Group on Intensive Care Medicine« within the DGAW, or alternatively to rename the DGAW as the »German Society of Anaesthesiology, Resuscitation and Intensive Care Medicine«. The text of the letter was as follows:

Dear Mr. President,
I would courteously request you to place the following item on the agenda for the next meeting of the Executive Committee:

It is proposed that a Working Group on Intensive Care Medicine should be founded within the German Society of Anaesthesia and Resuscitation.

The task of this working group will be to better represent the interests of intensive care medicine matters in the scientific field and through contacts with other societies of intensive care medicine that already exist abroad.

In addition, it is requested that the meeting of the Executive Committee should consider whether, as an alternative to the above, the German Society of Anaesthesia and Resuscitation should be renamed and have the term »intensive care medicine« added to its name.

(signed) P. Lawin.

This proposal was discussed several times in subsequent DGAW Executive Committee meetings. At the meeting in Saarbrücken on 20 November 1975, Lawin was able to present detailed reasons for his proposal. In view of international developments, he considered that it was urgently necessary to give the close connection between anaesthesiology and intensive care medicine clearer expression in relation to external bodies as well.

In preparation for the DGAW general meeting in Saarbrücken in September 1977, a previously prepared official resolution was submitted to the meeting of the Extended Executive Committee held in Erlangen on 7 May 1977, chaired by K.-H. Weis of Würzburg, who was President for 1977–1988. The resolution was to rename the DGAW as the German Society of Anaesthesiology and Intensive Care Medicine (Deutsche Gesellschaft für Anästhesiologie und Intensivmedizin, DGAI). The required changes to the statutes involved also envisaged a corresponding extension of the Society's goals. Paragraph 2 of the statutes received the following wording:

The purpose of the Society is to unite physicians in common work on improving and advancing anaesthesiology, intensive care medicine and emergency medicine and to ensure the best possible provision of care to the population in these fields.

The Executive Committee's proposal to change the statutes was approved with the required two-thirds majority at the DGAW general meeting held in Saarbrücken on 19 November 1977, and the new name came into force legally on being entered into the official register of associations, societies and clubs in Heidelberg.

Foundation of the DIVI

Despite the justified reservations on the part of the DGAW with regard to the formation of a German Society of Intensive Care Medicine, the idea was initially pursued further

by several colleagues in the specialty who were motivated by international developments. For example, at an interdisciplinary symposium on dopamine held in Mainz on 2 October 1976, R. Frey of Mainz invited the participants to a meeting with the aim of founding a »German Society of Intensive Care Medicine«. Henschel and Opderbecke took part in the meeting in order to represent the DGAW's interests. Initially, Frey as an anaesthetist and H.-G. Lasch of Giessen as an internist spoke in favour of the foundation of an association of this type; other participants warned against hasty decisions. In a statement made in the name of the DGAW, Opderbecke categorically spoke against the efforts to found an independent society of intensive care medicine. The meeting was finally adjourned without any resolutions being passed.

Even before Frey's initiative, Opderbecke had contacted W. Nachtwey in Hamburg, the new General Secretary of the AGII, which had in the meantime been renamed the German Society of Internal Medicine Intensive Care (Deutsche Gesellschaft für Internistische Intensivmedizin, DGII). There was quick agreement that the two specialties shared the same interests on this issue. To counter trends that were recognizable on both sides, an alternative approach needed to be developed, preferably with an interdisciplinary »Working Group on Intensive Care Medicine« serving as an umbrella organization.

Under the influence of this development, a resolution of principle was made at the meeting of the DGAW's Extended Executive Committee held in Lübeck-Travemünde on 7 October 1976, chaired by W. Henschel, President for 1975–1976, to open official negotiations with the DGII with the goal of founding a joint interdisciplinary »Working Group on Intensive Care Medicine«, for which only corporate membership by scientific and medical specialist societies and professional associations of specialist physicians involved in intensive care medicine would be envisaged. W. Weißauer was requested to develop appropriate draft statutes for the group.

An initial discussion with representatives of the DGII and – new on the scene – the Working Group on Neonatology and Paediatric Intensive Care Medicine was held in Frankfurt on 4 December 1976. The participants from the anaesthesiology side were Henschel, Lawin, Opderbecke, Weis and Weißauer.

On the basis of previous contacts between Nachtwey and Opderbecke, consensus on principles was quickly reached and at a second meeting on 10 January 1977, the foundation of a German Interdisciplinary Association of Critical Care Medicine (Deutsche Interdisziplinäre Vereinigung für Intensivmedizin, DIVI) was decided. The resolution was based on the draft statutes prepared by Weißauer, who had succeeded in solving the difficult legal issues involved in the planned structure of the association.

The founding meeting of the DIVI, chaired by Opderbecke, was held in the Sheraton Hotel at Frankfurt Airport on 29 January 1977. Those present were the anaesthetists P. Lawin of Münster, H.W. Opderbecke of Nuremberg and K.-H. Weis of Würzburg; the internists H.-G. Lasch of Giessen, W. Nachtwey of Hamburg, K.D. Scheppokat of Gehrden and H.P. Schuster of Mainz as well as the paediatricians P. Emmrich of Mainz, P. Lemburg of Düsseldorf and V. von Loewenich of Frankfurt. The Executive Committee that was elected consisted of Lasch (President), Emmrich (Vice-President), Lawin (General Secretary), Opderbecke (Secretary) and Schuster (Treasurer) (◘ Figs. 2.50 and 2.51). The association's foundation was then announced as follows:

> Representatives of the German Society of Anaesthesia and Resuscitation, the German Society of Internal Medicine Intensive Care, the Working Group on Neonatology and Paediatric Intensive Care Medicine and the Professional Association of German Anaesthetists founded a German Interdisciplinary Association of Critical Care Medicine (DIVI) in Frankfurt on 29 January 1977.
> The Association will serve to promote the science and practice of intensive care medicine. It envisages as its main tasks:
> - Strengthening the collaboration between the scientific societies and associations involved in issues of intensive care medicine
> - Representing the common interests of intensive care medicine to government bodies, medical professional associations and third parties
> - Communicating with foreign scientific associations concerned with the science and practice of intensive care medicine
> - Participating in international conferences in the field of intensive care medicine and representing the interests of intensive care medicine at the international level
>
> The medical and scientific societies and professional associations of medical specialists that have joined in this Association will send representatives who as regular members of the Association will carry out tasks in accordance with its statutes in the interests of their specialist societies and professional associations. The Association is open to all other medical and scientific specialist societies and professional associations of medical specialists involved in issues of intensive care medicine in accordance with its statutes.

The first societies to join the DIVI were the German Society of Surgery and the Professional Association of German Surgeons in spring of 1978. They were shortly afterwards followed by the German Society of Gynaecology and Obstetrics and the German Society of Neurosurgery. Finally, the German Society of Neurology joined in 1987.

```
Am 29. Januar 1977 fanden sich im Sheraton-Hotel am
Flughafen Frankfurt ein:

     Professor Dr. med.  P. Emmrich
     Professor Dr. med. Hans-Gotthard Lasch
     Professor Dr. med. Peter Lawin
     Priv.-Doz. Dr. med. Peter Lemburg
     Professor Dr. med. Volker v. Loewenich
     Priv.-Doz. Dr. med. W. Nachtwey
     Dr. med. H.W. Opderbecke
     Professor Dr. med. K.D. Scheppokat
     Professor Dr. med. Hans-Peter Schuster
     Professor Dr. med. Karl-Heinz Weis

Herr Dr. Opderbecke eröffnete um 10.⁰⁰ h die Versammlung. Er
begrüßte die Erschienenen und erklärte, daß die Zusammenkunft
erfolgt sei, um die "Deutsche interdisziplinäre Vereinigung
für Intensivmedizin" in der Form eines rechtsfähigen Vereins
zu gründen.

Her Dr. Opderbecke gab den Wortlaut der für den zu gründenden
Verein ausgearbeiteten Satzung bekannt und stellte sie zur
Diskussion.

Von den Anwesenden wurde einstimmig beschlossen, die
"Deutsche interdisziplinäre Vereinigung für Intensivmedizin"
als Verein zu errichten, ihm die dieser Niederschrift als An-
lage beigefügte Satzung zu geben und ihm als Gründungsmit-
glieder anzugehören.

Die Anwesenden übertrugen sodann einstimmig Herrn Dr. Nachtwey
die Leitung der Wahl des 1. Vorstandes und sprachen sich ein-
stimmig für Wahl durch Akklamation aus. Vorgeschlagen und bei
Enthaltung des jeweiligen Bewerbers wurden einstimmig gewählt

                                                          -2-
```

◘ **Fig. 2.50.** First page of the minutes of the founding meeting of the DIVI

In the meantime, the German Society of Paediatric Surgery, the German Society for Thoracic and Cardiovascular Surgery and the Professional Association of German Neurosurgeons have also joined the DIVI.

In accordance with the goals stated in its statutes, the DIVI has in the course of its now 30 years of existence formulated numerous resolutions on topical problems in intensive care and emergency medicine and represented them to state bodies, the DKG, the German Medical Association (Bundesärztekammer, BÄK), the Association of the Scientific Medical Societies (AWMF) and others [43].

In connection with the foundation of the European Society of Intensive Care Medicine in Geneva on 13 March 1982, the DIVI general meeting held in Düsseldorf on 19 November 1982 decided to apply to organize the Third European Congress on Intensive Care Medicine. Not least through the influence of H.-P. Schuster of Hildesheim, as a member of the Executive Committee of the European Society, the DIVI succeeded in having its application accepted. The date of the conference was set for 11–14 July 1986 and the location as Hamburg.

This conference was the first scientific meeting in which the DIVI presented itself to an international public. It was also the first interdisciplinary meeting in Germany

DEUTSCHE INTERDISZIPLINÄRE VEREINIGUNG FÜR INTENSIVMEDIZIN
GERMAN INTERDISCIPLINARY SOCIETY OF CRITICAL CARE MEDICINE

PRÄSIDENT
Professor Dr. H.-G. Lasch
Direktor der medizinischen Klinik und
Poliklinik der Universität Gießen
Klinikstraße 32 b
6300 Gießen

VIZEPRÄSIDENT
Professor Dr. P. Emmrich
Universitäts-Kinderklinik Mainz
Langenbeckstraße 1
6500 Mainz 31

GENERALSEKRETÄR
Professor Dr. P. Lawin
Direktor der Klinik für Anästhesiologie
und operative Intensivmedizin der
Universität Münster
Jungeblodtplatz 1
4400 Münster/Westf.

SCHRIFTFÜHRER
Priv.-Doz. Dr. H. W. Opderbecke
Vorstand der Anästhesie-Abteilung der
Städt. Krankenanstalten Nürnberg
Flurstraße 17
8500 Nürnberg

KASSENFÜHRER
Professor Dr. H.-P. Schuster
II. Med. Univ.-Klinik und Poliklinik Mainz
Langenbeckstraße 1
6500 Mainz 31

Sehr geehrte Damen und Herren !

Wir dürfen Sie davon in Kenntnis setzen, daß sich die Deutsche Gesellschaft für Anästhesiologie und Intensivmedizin,
die Deutsche Gesellschaft für internistische Intensivmedizin
und die Arbeitsgemeinschaft für Neonatologie und pädiatri-
sche Intensivmedizin sowie die Berufsverbände Deutscher Internisten und Deutscher Anästhesisten zu einer

DEUTSCHEN INTERDISZIPLINÄREN VEREINIGUNG
FÜR INTENSIVMEDIZIN

zusammengeschlossen haben. Die Vereinigung steht auch anderen wissenschaftlichen Fachgesellschaften und ärztlichen Be-
rufsverbänden offen, die an der Intensivmedizin interessiert
sind.

Die Vereinigung will der Förderung der Intensivmedizin in
Wissenschaft und Praxis dienen. Sie befaßt sich mit allen, die
Intensivmedizin berührenden, fachübergreifenden Fragestellun-
gen und steht zu diesem Themenkreis als Gesprächspartner und
für Stellungnahmen zur Verfügung.

Mit vorzüglicher Hochachtung

Prof. Dr. H.G. Lasch
Präsident

Priv.-Doz. Dr. H.W. Opderbecke
Schriftführer

◻ **Fig. 2.51.** Official announcement
of the foundation of the DIVI

that brought German intensive care physicians together in a European forum.

The success of the conference led P. Lawin, successor to Lasch as President of the DIVI, to advocate with great decisiveness and persuasiveness the creation of a standing German Interdisciplinary Congress for Intensive Care Medicine. Despite reservations on the part of several members, his proposal was approved by a majority; the first German Interdisciplinary Congress for Intensive Care Medicine was held in Hamburg on 27–30 November 1991, presided over by P. Lawin. With over 3,000 partici-pants (including physicians and nurses), the response by far exceeded that for the European Congress and showed that there was a strong demand among German intensive care physicians in every specialty for an interdisciplinary forum of this type in addition to the annual meetings of the individual specialist societies.

Since then, the DIVI has held a regular German Inter-disciplinary Congress for Intensive Care Medicine every 2 years, with each meeting having approximately 5,000 participants.

The DIVI has thus established a tradition in which the individual conference participants and the partici-pating scientific and medical specialist societies can see for themselves the shared interests they have and prob-lems they face, as well as the advances that have been made in the field of intensive care medicine. In addition to the so far exclusively existing corporate membership the DIVI created two personal membership categories in 2008 (▶ Chap. 2.2.2).

The Foundation of the World Federation

As one of the first activities undertaken by the DIVI, Lasch and Lawin took part as the official German del-egates in the Second World Congress for Intensive Care Medicine, held in Paris on 19–23 September 1978. The foundation of a World Federation of Societies of Inten-

sive and Critical Care Medicine, previously announced at the London congress, took place at this meeting. Lawin was able to have a decisive influence on the difficult and sometimes controversial discussions concerning the statutes that accompanied the foundation of the World Federation. The discussion in particular concerned the problem of which of the various national societies would be entitled to be a member and thus national representative to the World Federation. In the case of intensive care medicine in Germany, this issue was solved by the foundation of the DIVI. A. Gilston (President), S. Bursztein (General Secretary) and P. Lawin (Treasurer) were elected to the three-member Executive Committee for a period of 4 years.

Additional Training of Nurses in Intensive Care

The DGAI can claim to be the first organization ever to have developed concrete ideas for additional training in nursing care and to have implemented them in the anaesthesia and intensive care sector. The development of intensive care medicine was associated with a substantial expansion of the duties expected of nursing staff in this field. Not only did continuous monitoring of vital functions become a component of basic care, but treatment was also expanded with numerous components such as monitoring and technical performance of infusion therapy, operating and monitoring of respirators, and bronchial lavage for intubated patients and those with tracheotomies, etc. In addition, to manage incidents the nursing staff also had to familiarize themselves with the principles and techniques of modern resuscitation procedures, particularly since in the initial period the constant presence of a physician in the intensive care unit was more of an exception than a rule. Since this specialized information did not form part of the training for general nursing care, individual hospitals started to establish supplementary training courses of various lengths and with varying content.

To prevent chaotic developments, the DGAW Executive Committee took up this topic in the spring of 1967 and set up a committee with the aim of developing recommendations for uniform »additional training«.

After initial contacts with the **Working Group of German Nursing Associations** and the **Agnes Karll Association**, the committee – consisting of C. Lehmann of Munich, K. Horatz and P. Lawin of Hamburg and K. Wiemers of Freiburg (Chair) – developed a draft resolution that was adopted at a DGAW Executive Committee meeting held in Munich on 18 April 1968 [109].

Publication proceeded despite the fact that it had not yet been possible to establish a consensus with the nursing associations regarding the general principles of additional nursing training. While the **DGAW** favoured an additional training system analogous to the postgraduate training provided for physicians, the nursing associations advocated full-time courses with more college-like characteristics.

The first DGAW resolution recommends practical work for at least 1 year in an anaesthesia department with theoretical instruction consisting of a total of 100 teaching hours, based on a detailed curricular catalogue.

This initial resolution was already based on the following principles, which continued to be influential on all subsequent drafts initiated by the physicians' side:
1. The further training should consist of in-service training in the same way as for physicians.
2. There should be a balanced relationship between theory and practice.
3. Anaesthesia and intensive care should be linked.

Although the framework and content of the statement may seem inadequate from today's point of view, its importance at that time can scarcely be overestimated. With this announcement, the **DGAW** for the first time developed principles for in-service additional training for the nursing professions on analogy with additional training for physicians, and thus provided the stimulus for a wide variety of initiatives participated in, in one way or another, by other associations of physicians and nurses, the **DKG**, the Public Services and Transport Workers' Union (ÖTV) and not least also the German states' Working Group of Senior Medical Officers and a number of the ministries responsible in the various states. In addition, the **DGAW** proposals also led to models for further nursing training being developed in other fields such as the surgical service and psychiatry.

The immediate effect of this first recommendation for further training was two discoveries:
1. It soon emerged that a 1-year course with only 100 teaching hours was too short and that a 2-year in-service further training course with an expanded curriculum appeared to be necessary.
2. Further developments also showed that a recommendation from only one medical specialist society had far too little authority and scope to prevent the feared »chaotic growth« of numerous different course approaches and that instead it was necessary to achieve as broad a consensus as possible with other associations and state authorities.

For these reasons, the **DGAW** considered it necessary – as early as at the Executive Committee meeting held in Saarbrücken on 2 September 1969 – to address the topic again. A new committee was set up (consisting of F.W. Ahnefeld of Ulm as Chair, C. Lehmann of Munich, H. Pflüger of Frankfurt and K. Wiemers of Freiburg) with the task of further developing the 1968 resolution to produce a general framework recommendation. The goal was that this would make it easier to achieve recognition for the courses at the level of the federal states.

At the following Executive Committee meeting held in Munich on 2 April 1970, Ahnefeld was already able to report that it had been possible to reach basic agreement on a common approach to additional training with the AGII's representative, W. Nachtwey of Hamburg. Ahnefeld also reported on successful negotiations with the ÖTV, with the aim of achieving a higher salary rate for specialist nursing staff [6].

At the Executive Committee meeting in Nuremberg on 11 November 1970, Ahnefeld presented the draft »Recommendations for an additional training qualification for specialist nurses in anaesthesia and intensive care« for discussion. The recommendations were to be approved at a subsequent general meeting. Publication was initially postponed so as not to anticipate the planned negotiations with the federal states' Working Group of Senior Medical Officers and with the DKG. Ahnefeld had already contacted both of these organizations.

In this situation, the DKG surprisingly and without any prior contacts published recommendations, »Additional training for qualification as specialist nurse/specialist paediatric nurse« in issue 6 for 1971 of its journal, *Das Krankenhaus*, dated 25 May 1971 [115].

These recommendations envisaged three further training courses:
(a) For qualification as a nurse in the surgical service
(b) For qualification as a nurse in the anaesthesia service and in intensive care
(c) For qualification as a psychiatric nurse

An additional training period of 1 year was set for all of these fields. For additional training in anaesthesia and intensive care, 44 weeks of practical work and a total of 320 h of theoretical instruction in accordance with a structured curriculum were envisaged.

It was obvious that with the overloading of the theoretical part, both in terms of time and content, this approach could not be carried out in the form of in-service training and that its implementation would give rise to almost insuperable staffing and financial difficulties [116].

The DGAW then decided to publish the recommendations that had been adopted in November 1970 [117] and at the same time to initiate talks with the DKG.

After several reminders pointing out the urgency of the matter, and in particular after a joint and detailed letter sent to the DKG's General Secretary, H.W. Müller, by Ahnefeld on behalf of the DGAW and by Nachwey on behalf of the AGII, the long-awaited negotiations finally began in Düsseldorf on 19 February 1976, chaired by the DKG Secretary, Lauterbacher. The participants consisted of the DGAW (represented by Ahnefeld and Dick), the AGII, the German Society of Social Paediatrics (later renamed as the German Society of Neonatology and Paediatric Intensive Care Medicine), the German Society of Specialist Nursing (founded in 1975) and a representative of the State of Lower Saxony's Ministry for Social Affairs. The further training guidelines prepared jointly by the DGAW and AGII and the DGAW working group's planned curriculum, which had in the meantime been published [7], served as the basis for the negotiations.

Thanks to the preliminary work that had been done, the negotiations were already successfully completed on 24 June 1976, with consensus on a draft recommendation, »Model for a state-law regulation on the additional training and examination of nurses and paediatric nurses in intensive care«.

A final meeting was held on 20 October 1976, including the nursing associations. While approving the goal of state recognition for the courses and further training establishments, the nursing associations were resolutely opposed to state recognition for the final diploma and to the planned term »specialist nurse«. In their view, both of these would lead to discrimination of nurses who did not have additional training. The DKG declared its willingness to dispense with the term »specialist nurse« but declined to make further concessions.

The recommendation was approved by the Executive Committee of the DKG with the agreed wording and with the limitation mentioned on 16 November 1976 and was published the same year [124].

A reprint of the DKG recommendation in the journal *Anästhesiologische Informationen* followed in the second issue for 1977, together with comments by W. Dick and F.W. Ahnefeld [25].

After adopting and publishing the recommendation, the DKG set up an additional training committee with the task of developing principles for the recognition of additional training establishments and advising the DKG regarding their recognition. Dick took part in this committee's work on behalf of the DGAW [23, 24, 126].

In 1989, G. Golombek, the DKG's Secretary responsible for the issue, published a 10-year report [35]. The report initially provides a survey of the development in the federal states in which state regulation of additional training in intensive care had in the meantime taken place. For the other federal states, the DKG had also received and processed during the report period 1,000 applications from hospitals to obtain recognition as training establishments. A total of 638 training establishments had been recognized, 380 of which were focused on anaesthesia and intensive care medicine, 192 on internal medicine and intensive care medicine and 66 on paediatrics and intensive care medicine. Golombek estimated that at that time more than 5,000 members of the nursing staff had successfully completed a 2-year further training course at one of these recognized additional training establishments.

Unfortunately, this extremely fruitful work was questioned in the early 1990s when the individual federal states – which are legislatively responsible for additional professional training – took up the matter and passed outline legislation for additional training in nursing care. This legislation permitted the state ministries concerned to enact special additional training regulations by decree, including regulations for intensive care. This started an unfavourable trend to the extent that it meant abandoning the principle of uniformity at federal level and largely removing additional training in intensive care nursing from the influence of physicians.

Lemburg (representing the German Society of Neonatology and Paediatric Intensive Care Medicine) and Opderbecke (representing the DGAI) reported on this situation using the example of the State of North Rhine-Westphalia (NRW) [63]. Difficulties were already faced in obtaining any access at all as medical representatives to the working group set up by the NRW Ministry of Labour. The attempt to exert influence as physicians on the consultations, to provide support for practically oriented, patient-related additional training, failed to a large extent due to the fact that the Ministry and the nursing associations represented in the working group had quite different goals and regarded the additional training regulations more as a tool of professional and educational politics. According to their views, a successfully completed additional training course was to serve among other things as an admission requirement for a study course at an additional education college.

The curricula were also designed in accordance with these goals and envisaged stronger weight being given in terms of time and content to the theoretical instruction, inevitably at the cost of the practical aspect of additional training. When the representatives of the physicians found that no further influence on the consultations was to be granted to them in relation to these fundamental questions, they ultimately relinquished further participation in the working group in order to avoid being later identified with the results of the consultation process.

Similar developments took place in the states of Bremen, Hamburg, Lower Saxony, Schleswig-Holstein and the Saarland.

Evidently in order to adapt its 1976 recommendations to the developments just described, the DKG in September and October 1998 published a new Recommendation for additional training for nursing staff in intensive care [137]. The recommendation is prefaced by the following preamble:

> On 11 May 1998, at the 196th meeting of its Executive Committee, the DKG adopted the following »Model for federal-state legal regulation of additional training and examination of nurses and paediatric nurses

in intensive care« in the form of a recommendation. It decided at the same time that – for as long as any one federal state does not have in place a state legal regulation for additional education as foreseen in the recommendation – the DKG will carry out recognition of additional training establishments according to the standards stated in the recommendation. The recommendation will take effect on, and the start of the transitional period in Paragraph 23 of the recommendation shall be, 1 October 1998. If necessary, the DKG will hear expert advice regarding applications for recognition.

With this modified DKG recommendation for additional training, only one distinction will in the future be made between the fields of »intensive care and anaesthesia« and »paediatric intensive care«. The previous field of »internal medicine and intensive care medicine« will lapse, as the earlier division of further training into separate specialties within the context of intensive care (anaesthesia and intensive care medicine and internal medicine and intensive care medicine, respectively) no longer corresponds to today's requirements for interdisciplinary care for the most seriously ill intensive care patients and their complex clinical pictures. This is particularly evident in the fact that the majority of intensive care units in hospitals have interdisciplinary structures and that no clear distinction is made any longer between surgical and conservative intensive care. For the reasons stated above, the contents presented below have therefore been developed for the teaching subjects and exercise fields concerned.

Following the trend of the time, the medical specialist associations affected by this had not previously been informed by the DKG regarding its intention to amend its 1976 recommendation, nor were they consulted regarding it.

From the physicians' side, it is regrettable that with this new recommendation, the DKG abruptly ended its many years of constructive collaboration with the specialist societies representing physicians in the field of intensive care medicine. This was particularly disappointing for those physicians who in the past had devoted themselves with tremendous commitment to developing and promoting additional training in the field of intensive care nursing. These include F.W. Ahnefeld and W. Dick in Ulm, as well as M. Halmágyi in Mainz. Together with the senior anaesthesia nurse Therese Valerius in Mainz, this research group had edited a publication series on additional training and education for nurses, published by Springer [8], and had given numerous additional training courses in anaesthesia and intensive care in collaboration with H. Bergmann of Linz and H. Nolte of Minden. The regular Aachen conferences organized by G. Kalff and his senior anaesthesia nurse F.-G. Müller should also be mentioned.

The DKG's 1998 recommendation for additional training represents a decisive break. It abandons the original approach of organizing additional nursing training on analogy with postgraduate training for doctors in favour of courses arranged on a college basis.

Postgraduate Training of Physicians

The structural development of intensive care medicine in Germany is also reflected in the various stages of development of the regulations for qualification as a specialist physician and for postgraduate training of physicians. These stages are marked by the increasing specialization of medicine, due to the continuing advances being made, and simultaneous efforts to maintain the unity of the profession of physician despite this. In the course of these developments, the postgraduate training regulations ultimately became a regulatory tool serving not only to regulate the postgraduate training of physicians but also to establish boundaries between specialties preventing specialist physicians from normally working outside of these boundaries.

This principle represents the root cause of the joint efforts made by the affected disciplines, despite certain conflicts of interest, to prevent the formation of an independent specialty of intensive care medicine and instead to integrate the contents of postgraduate training in intensive care medicine into postgraduate training in the individual disciplines and thereby maintain the connection between a specialty-related form of intensive care medicine and its parent disciplines.

The first regulations for specialist physicians were adopted by the German Medical Assembly held in Bremen in 1924. At that time, the term »intensive care medicine« was of course completely unknown. The risks of specialization within the medical profession had already been recognized at the time and thoroughly discussed. This »Bremen Guideline« already includes the principle that the specialist physician should restrict himself to his specialist field and that holding double qualifications should only be permitted in exceptional cases [95].

In the early years after the war, there were initially no substantial changes with regard to postgraduate training. The fields listed in the 1937 regulations for professional and specialist physicians were initially maintained: ophthalmology, surgery, gynaecology and obstetrics, ENT diseases, skin diseases and venereal diseases, internal medicine, paediatrics, urinary tract diseases, lung diseases, neurology and psychiatry, orthopaedics, roentgenology and radiotherapy and dental, oral and maxillary diseases. In 1949, the additional terms »spa doctor« and

»psychotherapist« were included. The specialist physician of anaesthesia was introduced in 1953 and the specialist physician in neurosurgery and specialist physician in laboratory medicine in 1956.

Up to this time, the typical procedure was that the regulations for specialist physicians only specified minimum training periods for the individual fields. Until then, definitions of the fields and details of the contents of postgraduate training involved had been absent. For example, for the specialist physician in anaesthesia, the regulations stated:

- Postgraduate training period: 4 years
- 1 year's work in the field of surgery
- 2 years' work in the field of anaesthesia
- 6 months' work in the field of pharmacology or physiology
- 6 months' work in the field of internal diseases

This simple system was fundamentally altered when H.J. Sewering of Munich in 1957 became Chairman of the »Conference of Specialist Physicians' Committee Chairmen of the State Chambers of Physicians«, which later became the »Standing Conference on Postgraduate Medical Training« of the German Medical Association (BÄK). In his own dynamic style, he carried through a fundamental expansion of the Postgraduate Training Regulations (Weiterbildungsordnung, WO), as they were from then on known. This new approach, adopted in 1968 at the 71st German Medical Assembly in Wiesbaden, now included not only minimum periods for postgraduate training but also definitions of the fields and summaries of the contents of the postgraduate training. In an appendix, »Guidelines on the content of postgraduate training«, the contents were listed in detail. This established the prerequisites for the new regulations not only to regulate postgraduate training but also to set the boundaries between specialties [94]. This now allowed rigorous implementation of the demand that physicians should not outstep the boundaries of their own specialty.

Services that were not listed in the »Guidelines on the content of postgraduate training« were now regarded as alien to the specialty and could not be charged for by physicians in private practice, for example. It was consequently disputed by the BÄK, with reference to the WO, for example, that anaesthetists were entitled to carry out an anaesthetic preoperative examination – leading to extensive controversies [82, 103].

A competitive situation of this type would undoubtedly have also arisen in intensive care medicine if it had been included as an independent field in the WO. Instead, parallel in time with the developments described here, the specialist scientific and medical societies and professional medical associations with interests in intensive care medicine had broadly agreed on the principles of collaboration and division of duties in the field of intensive care medicine [136]. As a result, no significant rivalries developed between the disciplines concerned with regard to the contents of postgraduate training courses in intensive care medicine. The DIVI, as a body amalgamating the medical specialist societies and professional associations representing intensive care medicine, also subsequently played a conciliatory role in this context.

The term »intensive therapy« first appears in the 1968 WO, in the definition of the specialty of anaesthesia, as it was then still termed. The definition was worded as follows:

> The specialty of anaesthesia covers general and local anaesthesia, including pretreatment and post-treatment, maintenance of vital functions during surgical procedures, resuscitation and intensive therapy in collaboration with the specialist physicians responsible for the primary disease.

This wording was the result of an extensive correspondence between the then President of the DGAW, Opderbecke, and the Chairman of the BÄK's Standing Conference on Postgraduate Medical Training, Sewering – ultimately leading to this compromise formulation that satisfied everyone involved [72]. The qualifying addition, »in collaboration with the specialist physicians responsible for the primary disease«, was intended to express the fact that the anaesthetist's responsibilities in intensive care medicine only lay within the boundaries of his specialty.

The guidelines on the content of postgraduate training in the 1968 WO also use the term »intensive treatment« for the first time. The text on the contents of postgraduate training in anaesthesia states, for example:

1. Conveying and acquiring detailed knowledge and experience…
1.5 In long-term ventilation with mechanical respirators, including analysis of blood gases and the acid-base balance and associated problems of intensive treatment…

The entire duration of postgraduate training was still 4 years.

The DGAI subsequently attempted, in a »Recommendation on the granting of authorization to provide postgraduate training« to introduce time guidelines for the required intensive care medical activity in the framework of postgraduate training in anaesthesiology. In 1979, the BÄK for the first time published »Guidelines on authorization to provide postgraduate training« [127]. For bed-using areas, »guideline bed numbers« were given in the form of minimum requirements.

This led the DGAI to update an earlier »Recommendation on the granting of authorization to provide postgraduate training« [128]. The new version includes the statement in relation to intensive care medicine:

Authorization to provide postgraduate training can be given to…

4. For 4 years the head physician in a central anaesthesia division in a hospital, who in addition to a general surgical division provides anaesthesiological services in more than two additional surgical fields (as defined by the postgraduate training regulations) working as independent specialist divisions authorized to offer postgraduate training with a total of at least 300 surgical beds and in addition a surgical intensive care unit with at least six beds or an interdisciplinary conservative-surgical intensive care unit with at least eight beds.

It must be ensured here…

2. That a physician receiving postgraduate training works under instruction and supervision for at least 6 months – with at least 3 months of these being full-time – in an intensive care unit as specified in sections 3 and 4.

The formulation »…6 months – with at least 3 months of these being full-time« indicates the difficulty of incorporating 6 months of full-time intensive care medical work into the framework of a postgraduate training period consisting of a total of only 4 years.

To overcome this bottleneck with regard to time, the DGAW had already applied to the BÄK in a letter of 11 October 1974 for an extension of the postgraduate training duration from 4 to 5 years. The application was justified as follows:

> The state of knowledge in this specialty has expanded in such a way that the knowledge and experience required can no longer be fully conveyed in a period of only 4 years. The expansion affects above all the fields of emergency medicine and intensive therapy. With advancing developments in the ambulance service and the interdisciplinary organization of intensive care medicine in hospitals, the anaesthetist has acquired, in addition to his work in the operating room, two additional comprehensive areas of responsibility that go well beyond purely anaesthetic work. In the future, therefore, greater weight needs to be given in specialist postgraduate training courses to conveying knowledge and experience in the field of emergency medicine and intensive care medicine.

In response to this, the DGAW received a letter from the BÄK dated 3 December 1975, giving a negative decision without any reasons being stated.

In the following years as well, the DGAI on several occasions repeated its application to have the postgraduate training period extended to 5 years in view of the complex requirements of intensive care medicine, without receiving a favourable response from the BÄK or the Standing Conference on Postgraduate Medical Training. The extension was finally only achieved through the postgraduate training regulations (WO) adopted by the German Medical Assembly held in Cologne in 1992.

The impossibility of ensuring at least 6 months of full-time intensive care work within a 4-year postgraduate training period led the DGAI in 1984 to publish a »Recommendation on the period of postgraduate training in anaesthesiology« [133]. This states among other things that:

> The Executive Committee of the DGAI takes this development as an occasion to point out to those anaesthetists who are authorized to provide postgraduate training, in accordance with the letter from the Chairman of the Standing Conference on Postgraduate Medical Training, that the 4-year postgraduate training period envisaged in the postgraduate training regulations is a minimum period that must not be shortened but may be exceeded if required. The Executive Committee recommends anaesthetists who are authorized to offer postgraduate training to check whether, when their special conditions are taken into account, the goal of postgraduate training can be achieved in 4 years in their postgraduate training establishment. In view of the enhanced requirements that must be made, this will usually no longer be possible. In this case, the Executive Committee would hereby suggest to anaesthetists who are authorized to offer postgraduate training that they should base their postgraduate training courses on a 5-year time frame from the very outset. However, this presupposes that colleagues newly starting their postgraduate training should be informed that existing conditions require that the minimum period should be exceeded by 1 year.

Despite the futile attempts to obtain an extension of the minimum postgraduate training duration, the DGAI President for 1987–1988, K. Peter of Munich, applied in a letter of 8 January 1987 to have the passage »...and a 6-month period of work in an intensive care unit« added to the time requirements for postgraduate training in anaesthesiology.

This suggestion was fortunately taken up at the 90th German Medical Assembly held in Karlsruhe. In the version adopted, the postgraduate training duration for anaesthesiology was now defined as follows:

- Four years in a postgraduate training establishment in accordance with Paragraph 6, Section 1
- At least 3 years in the surgical field and 6 months in intensive care medicine

The advances in intensive care medicine that had in the meantime taken place led in the specialties affected by it to a recognition that although basic knowledge and experience could be conveyed and acquired even within a 6-month period, qualifications sufficient for independent work in an intensive treatment ward or for serving as head physician in such a ward could not. In addition, not all of the physicians undergoing postgraduate training were interested in obtaining deeper knowledge and experience in intensive care medicine – particularly those whose professional goal was to establish a private practice. However, the postgraduate training system implied in the WO did not allow any differentiation capable of taking this into account. The only way of intensifying the postgraduate training offered would have been to classify intensive care medicine as a »branch«. However, this route could not be considered, since according to Paragraph 18, Section 1 of the WO, a physician holding a title of qualification for a branch may »... generally only work within that branch«. This regulation would thus have cut him off from the parent discipline.

Efforts to solve this problem led to consideration by the scientific and medical specialist societies of the introduction of what was termed a »voluntary qualification certificate« outside the framework of the WO. The internists went furthest down this path. In 1989, the German Society of Internal Medicine Intensive Care presented a model »Qualification certificate for medical intensive care« [135]. The basis for this qualification was to be 2 years of work in intensive care medicine (1 year during postgraduate training in internal medicine and an additional year after successfully completing postgraduate training) and a final examination by a committee established by the Society.

This development naturally led to similar considerations by the DGAI and DIVI. Talks were consequently held between the DGAI and the German Society of Surgery with the aim of co-ordinating ideas for a voluntary qualification certificate in the field of surgical intensive care medicine.

In parallel with this, with the agreement of the DIVI, the DGAI in a letter of 27 September 1990 to the Chairman of the BÄK's Standing Conference on Postgraduate Medical Training applied for the introduction into the WO of a 2-year »supplementary postgraduate training course in anaesthesiological intensive care medicine«. The application was accompanied by detailed arguments and a detailed list of the planned contents of the postgraduate training course.

This led to two hearings being held in Munich on 18 October and 19 December 1990 by the Standing Conference on Postgraduate Medical Training, chaired by H.J. Sewering. The participants were representatives of the specialist societies amalgamated in the DIVI and professional associations, including the anaesthetists K. Fischer, H.W. Opderbecke, K. Peter and K. Zinganell. The representatives of the DIVI unanimously spoke in favour of introducing a »supplementary postgraduate training course in specialist intensive care medicine«. The various specialties within the DIVI had previously developed catalogues listing the contents of the postgraduate training course and had co-ordinated these with each other [136].

In the final session held on 21 December 1990, Sewering expressed his definitively negative attitude to the introduction of a »supplementary postgraduate training course«. He referred to the alternative option of a »voluntary qualification certificate« awarded by the specialist societies or the DIVI, although a certificate of this type could not be regarded as obligatory in any way by the Chambers of Physicians in their legal capacity as public corporations.

As a result of a restructuring of the Executive Committee of the BÄK, its committee on »postgraduate medical training« also underwent personnel changes and was reconstituted on 19 June 1991 under the Chairmanship of J.D. Hoppe. With this grouping, which represented a change of generations, new stimuli also developed with regard to intensive care medicine and the introduction of a »supplementary postgraduate training course«.

The aim of this new committee's work was, in addition to harmonizing postgraduate medical training between the old West German states and the new federal states in East Germany, to undertake a fundamental revision of the 1987 version of the WO. This was to be on the agenda of the 95th German Medical Assembly in Cologne.

During the preparatory negotiations, the committee's Chairman Hoppe and the BÄK's General Secretary P. Knuth ensured the greatest possible transparency and established close contacts with the specialist societies and professional associations involved [40, 76].

The WO adopted by the 95th German Medical Assembly in May 1992 contained a number of new elements including the »optional postgraduate training course in specialist intensive care medicine«.

According to Paragraph 3 of the WO, this is open to the following disciplines: anaesthesiology, surgery, cardiac surgery, internal medicine, paediatric surgery, paediatrics, neurosurgery, neurology and plastic surgery.

For anaesthesiology, the new WO also features an addition to the definition of the specialty and an extension of the postgraduate training period to 5 years – finally meeting a demand that the specialty had been pursuing since 1974.

The detailed contents of the optional postgraduate training course in »specialized intensive care medicine« in the individual fields are based on a »basic catalogue« developed by the DIVI under the Chairmanship of H. Burchardi of Göttingen [20].

With the 1992 WO, the position of intensive care medicine has been definitively established within the spectrum of independent fields. In spite of its basically interdisciplinary character and its largely standardized methodology, it now has an established departmental assignment to each of its parent disciplines. Opinions may differ on

whether the terms introduced in the new WO are well chosen. Terms such as specialized anaesthesiology and surgical, cardiac-surgical and neurosurgical intensive care medicine sound at the very least unusual; however, they correspond to the basic system used in the WO, which not only establishes specialty-related contents but also thereby determines the boundaries between disciplines. For this reason, the differentiation that developed for structural reasons between surgical and conservative intensive care medicine could not be reflected in the WO.

More important than this semantic issue is the clarification of medical responsibility and competence resulting from the departmental assignment. Since the optional postgraduate training course in »specialist intensive care medicine« is defined in a strictly field-related way, each specialist physician also has to observe the boundaries of his field in this area as well. Only the anaesthetist is able to work comprehensively within the framework of specialist anaesthesiological intensive care medicine, although still with the previously applying restriction »...in collaboration with the physicians responsible for the primary disease«.

For the time being, the 1992 WO represents the conclusion of the structural development of intensive care medicine in Germany. To this extent, it supplements the interdisciplinary agreements and recommendations on the division of duties and collaboration in the field of intensive care medicine and on organizational structures in hospitals and university hospitals. In addition, it provides the physician working in intensive care medicine with a framework for acquiring the necessary knowledge and experience and provides a means of formally certifying that this qualification has been obtained.

New standard regulations for postgraduate training were adopted at the 106th German Medical Assembly held in Cologne in 2003 [139].

Section A, Paragraph 2.2 specifies that the definition of the field also determines the limitations on the specialist medical work that a physician is entitled to carry out. In other words, the standard regulations for postgraduate training are synonymous with a regulation restricting professional practice in medicine. The new standard Postgraduate Training Regulations also continue to define intensive care medicine as an additional descriptive term. This qualification can be added to the relevant specialist term, i.e. anaesthesiological, surgical, internist, paediatric, neurosurgical and neurological intensive care medicine.

The prerequisite for acquiring this qualification is recognition as a specialist in the fields of anaesthesia, surgery, internal medicine, general medicine, paediatric medicine, neurosurgery or neurology.

The period of postgraduate training is 24 months. Of this, 6 months can be served during the postgraduate training period needed to qualify as a specialist. However, for the field of anaesthesia, 12 months can be recognized during the postgraduate training period needed to qualify as a specialist, since 12 months of intensive care medicine are a requirement for postgraduate training in anaesthesia. Six months can also be served in intensive care medicine in another field.

The contents of additional training courses in intensive care medicine for anaesthesia are as follows:

- Perioperative intensive medical treatment
- Intensive observation and treatment after trauma
- Differentiated diagnosis and treatment for cardiac and pulmonary diseases
- Treatment of intensive care disease patterns in collaboration with physicians treating the primary disease

The postgraduate training regulations have fully confirmed the basic structure of the agreements that have existed for decades between anaesthesiology and the surgical specialties, as well as internal medicine, in the regulations on additional postgraduate training in »anaesthesiological intensive care medicine« [112, 113, 114, 118, 121, 130, 139].

The anaesthetist therefore has authority to provide interdisciplinary intensive care medical treatment for patients in all specialties. Intensive care medical treatment directed by and on the responsibility of the anaesthetist thus corresponds both to the practical requirements of rational management and also to all legal requirements for the organization and quality of intensive care treatment.

Conclusion

Fifty-five years of the DGAI: this also means nearly 55 years of intensive care medicine in Germany. From the time when the Executive Committee of the DGA in October 1964 for the first time addressed the topic, to the Nuremberg Symposium in November 1968, the subsequent agreements with other specialities, the founding of the DIVI in January 1977, the efforts to achieve adequate postgraduate training in intensive care, right down to the anchoring of intensive care medicine in the postgraduate training regulations for physicians – all of this has been the result of consistent professional policy work on the part of the DGAI with the aim of making intensive care medicine into a firm and indispensable component of our specialty [34].

The increased demands that surgical medicine places on the anaesthetist today make it absolutely necessary for anaesthetists to have detailed knowledge and experience in intensive care medicine as well. To this extent, the developments described here have not only decisively influenced the specialty's position of importance today and its status within modern medicine, but have also determined the high level of quality that has been achieved in Germany in the anaesthesiological care of patients.

References

1. Ahnefeld FW (1962) Der Schock. Dtsch Med Wochenschr 87:425
2. Ahnefeld FW, Frey R, Halmágyi M, Kreuscher H (1964) Infusionstherapie und parenterale Ernährung bei chirurgischen Kranken. Dtsch Med Wochenschr 89:1871
3. Ahnefeld FW (1976) Das Problem der Schwesternweiterbildung. Anästh Inf 17:107
4. Ahnefeld FW, Burri C, Dick W, Halmágyi M (ed.) (1975) Infusionstherapie I. Klin Anästhesiol Intensivther, vol. 6. Springer, Berlin
5. Ahnefeld FW, Burri C, Dick W, Halmágyi M (ed.) (1975) Infusionstherapie II: Parenterale Ernährung. Klin Anästhesiol Intensivther, vol. 7. Springer, Berlin
6. Ahnefeld FW, Dick W (1972) Das Berufsbild von Anästhesie- und Intensivtherapie-Schwestern bzw. -Pflegern. Anästh Infm 13:201
7. Ahnefeld FW, Dick W, Halmágyi M (1975) Zur Entwicklung einer Weiterbildungsordnung zur Fachschwester/zum Fachpfleger für Anästhesie und Intensivmedizin – Lehrplan für den theoretischen Unterricht Narkose und Leitungsanästhesie – Lehrplan für den theoretischen Unterricht Intensivmedizin und Wiederbelebung. Anästhesiol Intensivmed 16:60
8. Ahnefeld FW, Dick W, Halmágyi M, Valerius Th (eds) (1975) Weiterbildung I – Richtlinien, Lehrplan, Organisation.Springer, Berlin
9. Ahnefeld FW, Frey R, Halmágyi M, Kreuscher H (1964) Infusionstherapie und parenterale Ernährung bei chirurgischen Kranken. Dtsch Med Wochenschr 89:1871
10. Allgöwer M, Burri CW (1967) Schockindex. Dtsch Med Wochenschr 92:1947
11. Alter H (1969) Intensivpflegestationen im mittleren Krankenhäusern. Münch Med Wochenschr 111:954
12. Aschenbrenner R (1968) Intensivpflege im modernen Krankenhaus – warum und wie? Münch Med Wochenschr 110:984
13. Aschenbrenner R, Dönhardt A (1953) Künstliche Dauerbeatmung in der eisernen Lunge. Erfahrungsbericht über 105 atemgelähmte Poliomyelitis-Patienten der Jahre 1947 – 1952. Münch Med Wochenschr 95:748, 770
14. Bauer Ä (1968) Fünfzehn Jahre postoperative Überwachung und Intensivbehandlung. Anaesthesist 17:65
15. Berkel HA (1967) Aufgaben und Tätigkeit der Anästhesie-Abteilung an einem mittleren Krankenhaus. Krankenhausarzt 40:74
16. Bock E (1984) Grundzüge des Aminosäurestoffwechsels. Anästhesiol Intensivmed 25:223
17. Bock E (1986) Totale parenterale Ernährung beim posttraumatischen Nierenversagen. Anästhesiol Intensivmed 27:45
18. Bräutigam KH (1967) Stellenplan einer Anästhesie-Abteilung. Krankenhausarzt 40:138
19. Bräutigam KH (1993) 40 Jahre »Facharzt für Anästhesie«. Die Entwicklung 1945 – 1953. Anästhesiol Intensivmed 34:259
20. Burchardi H (1994) Die neue Weiterbildungsordnung stimuliert die interdisziplinäre Kooperation. Anästhesiol Intensivmed 35:357
21. Burri CW, Müller W, Kuner E, Allgöwer M (1966) Methodik der Venendruckmessung. Schweiz Med Wochenschr 96:624
22. Burri CW, Gasser D (1971) Der Vena-Cava-Katheter. Anaesthesiol Wiederbeleb, vol. 54. Springer, Berlin
23. Dick W (1978) Gemeinsame Weiterbildung der Disziplinen mit intensivmedizinischen Versorgungsaufgaben – Schwerpunkt Anästhesie und Intensivmedizin. Anästhesiol Intensivmed 19:194
24. Dick W (1983) Weiterbildung Fachkrankenpflege Anästhesie und operative Intensivmedizin. Anästhesiol Intensivmed 24:110
25. Dick W, Ahnefeld FW (1977) Kommentar zur Weiterbildungsempfehlung der DKG. Anästhesiol Intensivmed 18:89
26. Dönhardt A (1955) Künstliche Dauerbeatmung. Springer, Berlin
27. Eckart J, Kleinberger G, Lochs H (1980) Klinische Ernährung – Grundlagen und Praxis der Ernährungstherapie. Zuckschwerdt, Munich

28. Eckart J, Tempel G, Kaul A, Schürnbrand P (1973) Untersuchungen zur Utilisation parenteral verabfolgter Triglyceride nach Operationen und Traumen. Infusionstherapie 1:138

29. Eichhorn S (1967) Organisation von Intensivbehandlung, Intensivüberwachung und Intensivpflege. Krankenhausarzt 40: 321

30. Eigler FW, Schildberg FW (1969) Einrichtung und Organisation einer chirurgischen Wachstation. Chirurg 40:162

31. Franke H, Opderbecke HW (1959) Die Bedeutung einer »Wachstation« in der Überwachung und Behandlung Frischoperierter. Chirurg 30:487

32. Fuchsig P, Brücke P, Kucher R, Steinbereithner K (1966) Intensivbehandlungs-Station. Münch Med Wochenschr 108:2473

33. Fuchsig P, Mayrhofer O (1965) Die Intensivpflegestation – ein modernes Forum interdisziplinärer Zusammenarbeit. Wien Klin Wochenschr 49:961

34. Götz E, Hack G, Sorgatz H, van Eimeren W, Wulff A (1995) Umfrage zur Situation der Anästhesiologie in Deutschland. Anästhesiol Intensivmed 36:218

35. Golombek G (1989) Seit 10 Jahren einheitliche Fachweiterbildung Intensivpflege. Anästhesiol Intensivmed 30:231

36. Gülke Ch, Kipke EH, Opderbecke HW (1972) Der Kava-Katheter – Ein zehnjähriger Erfahrungsbericht. Münch Med Wochenschr 114:1503

37. Hachenberg T, Pfeiffer B (2000) Beatmung, Tracheotomie und prolongierte Intubation. Anaesthesist 49:434

38. Haid B (1967) Planung eines Institutes für Anästhesiologie an einer Universität. Krankenhausarzt 40:140

39. Holmdahl MH, Duvernoy W (1967) Intensivbehandlung in Schweden. Krankenhausarzt 40:131

40. Hoppe JD (1991) Leitlinien einer Reform der ärztlichen Weiterbildung. Dtsch Ärztebl 88:C-2138

41. Horatz K (1969) Einrichtung und Betrieb einer Anästhesieabteilung mit Wachstation und Intensivpflegeeinheit. Krankenhausumschau 38:630

42. Ibsen B (1968) Organisation einer Intensivtherapieabteilung in Kopenhagen. Rückblick und Ausblick. Anaesthesist 17:272

43. Karimi A (ed.) (1991) Deutsche Interdisziplinäre Vereinigung für Intensiv- und Notfallmedizin (DIVI): Stellungnahmen, Empfehlungen zu Problemen der Intensiv- und Notfallmedizin, 1st edn. Karimi A, Dick W (eds) (1995) 3rd edn. Eigenverlag

44. Kirschner M (1930) Zum Neubau der Chirurgischen Universitätsklinik Tübingen II. Der Krankenhausbau. Chirurg 2:30

45. Körner M (1967) Die Anästhesie-Abteilung in einem 1000-Betten-Krankenhaus. Krankenhausarzt 40:77

46. Kucher R (1965) Funktion und Einrichtung einer Intensivbehandlungsstation – Krankengut und Ergebnisse. Wien Klin Wochenschr 49:969

47. Kügler J, Horatz K (1967) Zwei Jahre Intensivbehandlung an der Anästhesieabteilung. Anästh Praxis 2–53

48. Kuhn F (1901) Die perorale Intubation. Zentralbl Chir 28:1281

49. Kuhn F (1905) Perorale Intubation mit Überdrucknarkose. Dtsch Z Chir 76:148

50. Kuhn F (1906) Die perorale Intubation mit und ohne Druck. III. Apparat zur Lieferung des Drucks für die Überdrucknarkose. Dtsch Z Chir 81:63

51. Lang K, Frey R, Halmágyi M (ed.) (1966) Infusionstherapie. Anaesthesiol Wiederbeleb, vol. 13. Springer, Berlin

52. Lawin P (1964) Neu-Organisation einer Anaesthesie-Abteilung mit Wachstation in einem alten Krankenhaus. Krankenhausarzt 37:32

53. Lawin P (1966) Organisationsformen der Intensivpflege im Krankenhaus. Medizinalmarkt 14:412

54. Lawin P (1967) Intensivbehandlung im Grosskrankenhaus. Krankenhausarzt 40:116

55. Lawin P (1968) Störungen des Säure-Basen-Haushaltes – Differentialdiagnose und Therapie. Dtsch Med Wochenschr 93:1664

56. Lawin P (1978) Die Entwicklung der Intensivmedizin. Anästhesiol Intensivmed 19:418

57. Lawin P (ed) 1987 Aktuelle Aspekte und Trends der respiratorischen Therapie. Springer, Berlin

58. Lawin P, Burchardi H (1965) Erkennung und Behandlung von Störungen des Säure-Basen-Haushaltes. Münch Med Wochenschr 107:107

59. Lawin P, Opderbecke HW (1971, 1975, 1981, 1989, 1994) Die Organisation der Intensivbehandlung. In: Lawin P (ed) Praxis der Intensivbehandlung, 2nd–6th edn. Thieme, Stuttgart

60. Lawin P, Peter K, Scherer R (eds) (1980) Maschinelle Beatmung gestern – heute – morgen. Intensivmed Notfallmed Anästhes, vol. 48. Thieme, Stuttgart

61. Lehmann Ch (1967) Die Intensivbehandlungs-Einheit: Ausstattung, Organisation und Erfahrungen. Krankenhausarzt 40:124

62. Lehmann Ch (ed) (1968) Langzeitbeatmung. Anaesthesiologie und Wiederbelebung, vol. 29 Springer, Berlin

63. Lemburg P, Opderbecke HW (1994) Die Weiterbildung von Pflegekräften in der Intensivmedizin – Rückblick und Ausblick. Anästhesiol Intensivmed 35:40

64. Leriche R (1953) De la maladie post-opératoire anatomique. La Presse medicale 41:61

65. Mayrhofer O (1971) Definition, Funktion und Bedeutung der Intensivmedizin. In: Frey R, Hügin W, Mayrhofer O (eds) Lehrbuch der Anästhesiologie und Wiederbelebung. Springer, Berlin

66. Meisner H, Struck E, Sebening F (1966) Sechsjährige Erfahrungen auf einer Intensivbehandlungs-Station. Münch Med Wochenschr 108:2479

67. Menzel H (ed) (1982) Personalbedarfsermittlung für Intensivbehandlungsstationen. Perimed, Erlangen

68. Messmer K (1971) Pathophysiologische Aspekte des hypovolämischen, kardiogenen und bakteriotoxischen Schocks. Med Welt 22 (N.F.):1159

69. Mürtz R (1967) Intensivbehandlung und Reanimation aus der Sicht des Internisten. Krankenhausarzt 40:334

70. Nachtrab H (1968) Anästhesiedienst und Stellung des Anästhesisten in Hamburg. Z Prakt Anästh 3:353

71. Nolte H, Ahnefeld FW (1967) Die organisatorischen, personellen und materiellen Voraussetzungen zur modernen Wiederbelebung im Krankenhaus. Krankenhausarzt 40:144

72. Opderbecke HW (1968) Zur neuen Weiterbildungsordnung. Informationen DGAW/BDA No. 4:15

73. Opderbecke HW (ed) (1969) Planung, Organisation und Einrichtung von Intensivbehandlungseinheiten am Krankenhaus. Anaesthesiologie und Wiederbelebung, vol. 33. Springer, Berlin

74. Opderbecke HW (1969) Die Organisation der Intensivmedizin im Krankenhaus. Krankenhaus 61:304

75. Opderbecke HW (1976) Die Anhaltszahlen der DKG. Anästh Inf 17:424

76. Opderbecke HW (1992) Die neue Weiterbildungsordnung. Anästhesiol Intensivmed 33:364

77. Opderbecke HW (1999) Zur Entwicklung der intravenösen Infusionstechnik. Anaesthesist 48:919

78. Opderbecke HW, Bardachzi E (1961) Die Verwendung eines »Kava-Katheters« bei langdauernder Infusionsbehandlung. Dtsch Med Wochenschr 86:203

79. Opderbecke HW, Pohl O (1961) Planung und Gestaltung einer »Wachstation« für Frischoperierte. Krankenhaus 53:70

80. Opderbecke HW, Sorgatz H (1993) Leistungseinschränkung in der Intensivmedizin als gesundheitspolitisches Konzept. Anästhesiol Intensivmed 34:285

81. Opderbecke HW, Weißauer W (eds) (1983) Entschliessungen – Empfehlungen – Vereinbarungen. Perimed, Erlangen

82. Opderbecke HW, Weißauer W (1987) Die Pflicht des Anästhesisten zur Voruntersuchung und die Fachgebietsgrenzen. Anästhesiol Intensivmed 28:382

83. Pichlmaier H, Jabour A, Besirsky Hw, Kanz E, Linke K, Altmeyer E, Edel HH, Müller R (1968) Intensivbehandlung nach Organverpflanzung unter aseptischen Bedingungen. Bruns' Beitr Klein Chir 216:122

84. Poulsen H (1965) Abteilung für intensive Therapie-Aufgaben. Einrichtung und Funktion. Anaesthesist 14:19

85. Poulsen H (1967) Allgemeine Problematik der Intensivbehandlung. In: Just OH, Stoeckel H (eds) Die Ateminsuffizienz und ihre klinische Behandlung. Thieme, Stuttgart

86. Puchstein C (1999) Die Entwicklung der parenteralen Ernährung. Anaesthesist 48:827

87. Rügheimer E (ed) (1982) Aufwachraum – Aufwachphase. Eine anästhesiologische Aufgabe. Klinische Anästhesiologie und Intensivtherapie, vol. 24. Springe, Berlin

88. Rügheimer E (1982) Die Tracheotomie. In: Benzer H, Frey R, Hügin W, Mayrhofer O (eds) Anaesthesiologie, Intensivmedizin und Reanimatologie. Springer, Berlin

89. Rügheimer E (ed) (1983) Intubation, Tracheotomie und bronchopulmonale Infektion. Springer, Berlin

90. Sauerbruch F (1904) Zur Pathologie des offenen Pneumothorax und die Grundlagen meines Verfahrens zu seiner Ausschaltung. Mitt Grenzgeb Med Chir 8:399

91. Sauerbruch F (1920) Das Druckdifferenzverfahren. Springer, Berlin

92. Schülke K, Ungeheuer E, Pflüger H (1968) Intensivpflege in der chirurgischen Klinik. Fortschr Med 86:338

93. Seybold D, Gessler U (1984) Die Niere im Schock und Schockniere – Nosologie, Pathophysiologie, Klinik und Therapie. In: Rieker G (ed) Schock. Springer, Berlin

94. Sewering HJ (1968) Die Weiterbildungsordnung. Dtsch Ärztebl 65:1445

95. Sewering HJ (1987) Von der »Bremer Richtlinie« zur Weiterbildungsordnung. Dtsch Ärztebl 84:B-1595

96. Sieberth HG (1979) Akutes Nierenversagen. Thieme, Stuttgart

97. Striebel JP, Peter K, Rabold M, Schaub P, Schmidt R, Schmitz ER (1976) Das Verhalten der freien Plasmaaminosäuren und einiger Stoffwechselparameter während parenteraler Ernährung in der postoperativen-posttraumatischen Phase. Infusionstherapie 3:162

98. Suter PM (1989) Beatmungsgeräte. In: Lawin P (ed) Praxis der Intensivbehandlung, 5th edn. Thieme, Stuttgart

99. Vogel W, Wiemers K (1967) Aufgabe und Funktion eines Institutes für Anästhesiologie mit Beatmungszentrale und Betreuung einer chirurgischen Wachstation. Krankenhausarzt 40:134

100. Wählin Ä, Westermark L, van der Vliet A (1972) Intensivpflege und Intensivtherapie. Neuhaus GA (ed) Springer, Berlin

101. Weise G (1967) Aufgaben und Erfahrungen einer Anästhesie-Abteilung an einem 340-Betten-Krankenhaus. Krankenhausarzt 40:70

102. Weißauer W (1970) Zu den Vereinbarungen zwischen den Fachgebieten Chirurgie und Anästhesie über die Aufgabenabgrenzung und die Zusammenarbeit in der Intensivmedizin. Anästh Inf 11:168

103. Weißauer W (1988) Fachgebietsgrenzen der Anästhesiologie bei Laborleistungen. Anästhesiol Intensivmed 29:257

104. Wiemers K (1966) Allgemeine Gesichtspunkte, Organisation und Aufbau von Intensivbehandlungsstationen. In: Horatz K, Frey R (eds) Probleme der Intensivbehandlung. Anaesthesiologie und Wiederbelebung, vol. 17 Springer, Berlin

105. Wiemers K (1986) Anästhesist und Intensivtherapie. Anästhesiol Intensivmed 27:166

106. Zindler M (1967) Intensivbehandlungseinheit, Wachstation und Aufwachraum. Krankenhausarzt 40:330

Recommendations, position papers, agreements (in chronological sequence)

107. Deutsche Gesellschaft für Anästhesie und Deutsche Gesellschaft für Chirurgie (1965) Richtlinien für die Stellung des leitenden Anaesthesisten. Anaesthesist 14:31

108. Deutsche Gesellschaft für Anästhesie und Wiederbelebung (1967) Stellungnahme zur Organisation von Aufwachraum, Wachstation und Intensivbehandlung am Krankenhaus. Anaesthesist 16:282

109. Deutsche Gesellschaft für Anästhesie und Wiederbelebung (1969) Stellungnahme zur Ausbildung von Schwestern und Pflegern für den Anaesthesiedienst und die Intensivpflege. Anaesthesist 18:229

110. Deutsche Krankenhausgesellschaft (1969) Anhaltszahlen für die Besetzung der Krankenhäuser mit Pflegekräften. Krankenhaus 61:420

111. Deutsche Krankenhausgesellschaft (1970) Empfehlung zur Organisation der Intensivmedizin in Krankenhäusern. Anästh Inf 12:3

112. Deutsche Gesellschaft für Anästhesie und Wiederbelebung, Deutsche Gesellschaft für Innere Medizin, Arbeitsgemeinschaft für internistische Intensivmedizin, Berufsverband Deutscher Anästhesisten, Berufsverband Deutscher Internisten (1970) Gemeinsame Empfehlung zur Organisation der Intensivmedizin am Krankenhaus. Anaesthesist 19:265, Krankenhausumschau 39:696

113. Deutsche Gesellschaft für Chirurgie, Deutsche Gesellschaft für Anästhesie und Wiederbelebung, Berufsverband der Deutschen Chirurgen, Berufsverband Deutscher Anästhesisten (1970) Vereinbarungen zwischen den Fachgebieten Chirurgie und Anästhesie über die Aufgabenabgrenzung und die Zusammenarbeit in der Intensivmedizin. Anästh Inf 11:167

114. Deutsche Gesellschaft für Neurochirurgie, Deutsche Gesellschaft für Anästhesie und Wiederbelebung (1971) Empfehlungen zur Organisation der Anästhesie im Rahmen der Neurochirurgie. Anästh Inf 12:34

115. Deutsche Krankenhausgesellschaft (1971) Weiterbildung zu Fachkrankenschwestern/Fachkrankenpflegern/Fachkinderkrankenschwestern. Krankenhaus 63:269

116. Bundesanstalt für Arbeit (1971) Anordnung über die induviduelle Förderung der beruflichen Fortbildung und Umschulung vom 9. September 1971. Amtl. Nachrichten der Bundesanstalt für Arbeit 19:No. 11

117. Deutsche Gesellschaft für Anästhesie und Wiederbelebung (1971) Empfehlungen für die Weiterbildung zur Fachschwester oder zum Fachpfleger für Anästhesie und Intensivpflege. Anästh Inf 12:251

118. Deutsche Krankenhausgesellschaft (1972) Empfehlung zur Organisation der Intensivmedizin in den Krankenhäusern. Krankenhaus 64:339, Anästh Inf 13:223

119. Deutscher Städtetag (1972) Empfehlungen für die Einrichtung und den Betrieb von Intensivstationen. Anästh Inf 14:285

120. Arbeitsgemeinschaft für internistische Intensivmedizin und Deutsche Gesellschaft für Anästhesie und Wiederbelebung (1972) Definition und Bedingungen von Intensivbehandlungseinheiten am Krankenhaus. Anästh Inf 13:305, Anaesthesist 22:546

121. Berufsverband der Deutschen Urologen, Berufsverband Deutscher Anästhesisten (1972) Vereinbarung zwischen den Fachgebieten Urologie und Anästhesie über die Aufgabenabgrenzung und die Zusammenarbeit im operativen Bereich und in der Intensivmedizin. Anästh Inf 13:219

122. Deutsche Gesellschaft für Anästhesie und Wiederbelebung (1973) Entschliessung über die Weiterbildung von Fachschwestern und Fachpflegern. Anästh Inf 14:28

123. Deutsche Krankenhausgesellschaft (1974) Richtlinien für die Organisation der Intensivmedizin in den Krankenhäusern. Krankenhaus 66:457, Anästh Inf 16:29

124. Deutsche Krankenhausgesellschaft (1976) Muster für eine landesrechtliche Ordnung der Weiterbildung und Prüfung zu Krankenschwestern, Krankenpflegern und Kinderkrankenschwestern in der Intensivpflege. Krankenhaus 68:439; Anästh Inf 18:96

125. Deutsche Gesellschaft für Anästhesie und Wiederbelebung, Deutsche Gesellschaft für Hals-, Nasen-, Ohrenheilkunde, Kopf- und Halschirurgie, Berufsverband Deutscher Anästhesisten, Berufsverband Deutscher Hals-, Nasen-, Ohrenärzte (1976) Vereinbarung über die Zusammenarbeit in der HNO-Heilkunde. Anästh Inf 17:354

126. Deutsche Krankenhausgesellschaft (1978) Grundsätze und Verfahren zur Durchführung der Empfehlung der Deutschen Krankenhausgesellschaft vom 16. November 1976. Anästh Inf 19:205

127. Bundesärztekamm (1979) Richtlinien über die Ermächtigung zur Weiterbildung. Dtsch Ärztebl 76:113

128. Deutsche Gesellschaft für Anästhesiologie und Intensivmedizin (1979) Empfehlungen zur Erteilung einer Weiterbildungsermächtigung. Anästhesiol Intensivmed 20:XXIX

129. Deutsche Interdisziplinäre Vereinigung für Intensivmedizin (1979) Stellungnahme zur Besetzung von Intensiveinheiten mit Pflegepersonal. Anaesthesist 28:416

130. Deutsche Gesellschaft für Anästhesiologie und Intensivmedizin, Deutsche Gesellschaft für Innere Medizin, Deutsche Gesellschaft für internistische Intensivmedizin, Berufsverband Deutscher Anästhesisten, Berufsverband Deutscher Internisten (1980) Gemeinsame Empfehlung für die Fachgebiete Anästhesiologie und Innere Medizin zur Organisation der Intensivmedizin am Krankenhaus. Anaesthesist 29:395, Anästhesiol Intensivmed 21:166

131. Deutsches Krankenhausinstitut Düsseldorf, Institut für Krankenhausbau der Techn. Universität Berlin, Deutsche Gesellschaft für Anästhesiologie und Intensivmedizin (1982) Grundsätze für die Organisation und Einrichtung von Aufwacheinheiten in Krankenhäusern. Anaesthesist 31:632, Anästhesiol Intensivmed 23:373

132. Berufsverband Deutscher Anästhesisten, Berufsverband der Ärzte für Orthopädie (1984) Vereinbarung über die Zusammenarbeit bei der operativen Patientenversorgung. Anästhesiol Intensivmed 25:464

133. Deutsche Gesellschaft für Anästhesiologie und Intensivmedizin (1984) Empfehlung zur Weiterbildungsdauer in der Anästhesiologie. Anästhesiol Intensivmed 25:441

134. Deutsche Gesellschaft für Anästhesiologie und Intensivmedizin, Berufsverband Deutscher Anästhesisten, Deutsche Gesellschaft für Gynäkologie und Geburtshilfe, Berufsverband der Frauenärzte (1988) Vereinbarung über die Zusammenarbeit in der operativen Gynäkologie und in der Geburtshilfe. Anästhesiol Intensivmed 29:143

135. Deutsche Gesellschaft für Internistische Intensivmedizin (1989) Qualifikationsnachweis für Internistische Intensivmedizin. Intensivmed 26:334, 27:499

136. Deutsche Interdisziplinäre Vereinigung für Intensivmedizin (1989) Empfehlungen zum Inhalt der Weiterbildung in der Intensivmedizin im Rahmen der Gebiets- und Teilgebiets-Weiterbildung. Anästhesiol Intensivmed 29:224

137. Deutsche Krankenhausgesellschaft (1998) DKG-Empfehlung zur Weiterbildung für Krankenpflegepersonen in der Intensivpflege. Krankenhaus 90:537, 608

138. Deutsche Gesellschaft für Anästhesiologie und Deutsche Ophthalmologische Gesellschaft (1998) Gemeinsame Empfehlung über die Zusammenarbeit in der operativen Ophthalmologie. Anästhesiol Intensivmed 39:309

139. Neue (Muster-)Weiterbildungsordnung http://www.bundesaerztekammer.de/30/Weiterbildung/03MWBO/index.html

140. Deutsche Gesellschaft für Anästhesiologie und Intensivmedizin, Berufsverband Deutscher Anästhesisten (2011) Entschließungen, Empfehlungen, Vereinbarungen, 5th ed. Aktiv & Verlag, Ebelsbach

2.2.2 German Society of Anaesthesiology and Intensive Care Medicine and German Interdisciplinary Association of Critical Care Medicine (DIVI)

W.F. Dick

Introduction
Founding of the DIVI

On 29 January 1977, representatives of three scientific societies and two professional organisations founded the German Interdisciplinary Association of Critical Care Medicine (DIVI) in Frankfurt/Main: The German Society of Anaesthesia and Resuscitation and the German Professional Association of Anaesthetists, represented by P. Lawin and H. W. Opderbecke, the German Society of Internal Medicine Intensive Care and the German Professional Association of Internists, represented by H.G. Lasch and H.P. Schuster, as well as the Working Group on Neonatology and Paediatric Intensive Care Medicine, represented by P. Emmrich.

This association, which is now 25 years old, serves to co-ordinate intensive care medicine in Germany.

Essential Tasks and Goals

- To further intensive care medicine in science and practice and to deepen the cooperation between the scientific societies and associations dealing with issues of intensive care medicine
- To represent the joint interests of intensive care medicine vis-à-vis the authorities, medical associations and third parties
- To communicate with scientific associations abroad, which deal with intensive care medicine in science and practice
- To participate in international congresses in the field of intensive care medicine
- To represent the interests of intensive care medicine at an international level

Further Developments up to the Present Structure

In the years following the foundation of the DIVI, other scientific societies and professional organizations joined DIVI, including:
- German Society of Surgery
- German Society of Gynaecology and Obstetrics
- German Society of Internal Medicine
- German Society of Neurosurgery
- German Society of Neurology
- German Society of Paediatrics
- German Society of Paediatric Surgery
- German Society for Thoracic and Cardiovascular Surgery
- Association of German Surgeons
- Association of German Neurosurgeons
- Association of German Paediatricians

The member societies and associations are represented by a specific number (at present 34) of individuals. According to the Standing Rules, the Board and the Executive Committee are equally represented; the position of the President is reserved for members of the founding societies. (H.G. Lasch and D.L. Heene, internal medicine, P. Lawin, and W.F. Dick, anaesthesiology, A. Enke and F.W. Schildberg, surgery).

In 2008, the DIVI created, by approving new Statues, two personal membership categories in addition to the corporate membership exclusively in force up to this time. From now on, the DIVI consisted of 3 divisions: A, Division of scientific societies and professional organizations; B, Division of individual medical specialists with or in training in intensive care medicine; C, Division of non-medical members active in intensive care medicine.

Sections of the DIVI

The goals and objectives of the DIVI were initially focussed on intensive care medicine only. Subsequently, aspects of emergency medicine, scientific research and other fields of interest to intensive care medicine were added, which led to the foundation of different sections. Ordinary members of these sections are nominated by the member societies, and supporting members are selected by the respective organizations. Ordinary members shall represent the entire spectrum of the DIVI.

The Section of Emergency and Disaster Medicine

The section of emergency medicine was founded initially (14 March1980), to be followed a few years later (27 November 1988) by the section of disaster medicine. The two sections merged on 26 October 1990 into the section of emergency and disaster medicine. This led to the integration of the goals and objectives of emergency and disaster medicine into those of the DIVI. The following members chaired and guided the section from its inception: H. Hochrein, P. Sefrin, H.U. Lehmann, A. Karimi and E. Martens.

The section has exerted a considerable influence on the development of accredited training programmes in emergency medicine. Consequently, the DIVI enlarged its name into German Interdisciplinary Association of Critical Care and Emergency Medicine in 1989. Uniform qualitative criteria of training have become prerequisites of emergency physicians' activities in the field .The concepts of training programmes such as »Medical EMS Director«, »Chief Emergency Physician« and »Total Quality Management« have been influenced considerably by the section. Unfortunately, the realization of these concepts continues to be hindered by a small number of professional organizations.

The Section of Science and Research

On 25 November 1997, the section of science and research was created. Together with its interdisciplinary working groups, the goal of the section is to promote the scientific interests and activities of basic and clinical research in intensive care and emergency medicine. The section was formally founded on 24 November 2000. The following interdisciplinary working groups were established: multiorgan failure, total quality management, multitrauma, coma, cardiovascular risk factors, artificial ventilation, acute pancreatitis, shock and artificial organs.

The section has an identical number of regular members of the DIVI and appointed members of the working groups.

Other working groups are to be established in the near future. The section is presently chaired by H.P. Schuster, Hildesheim, to be followed by E. Klar, Heidelberg.

Congresses and Meetings
DIVI Congress

In the early years of its existence, the DIVI concentrated almost exclusively on the co-ordination and support of different medical activities of its member societies and on assisting in solving different interdisciplinary problems. It was, however, due to the initiative of P. Lawin that the board decided – against considerable opposition – to hold a regular interdisciplinary meeting. In 1991, the first DIVI Congress was held with great success in Hamburg. From that time on, regular meetings have convened in Hamburg every second year and annually since 2010.

- 1993: 2nd DIVI Congress, Congress President A. Encke, Frankfurt (surgery)
- 1995:3rd DIVI Congress, Congress President H.P. Schuster, Hildesheim (internal medicine)
- 1997: 4th DIVI Congress, Congress President W.F. Dick, Mainz (anaesthesiology)
- 2000: 5th DIVI Congress, Congress President F.W. Schildberg, Munich (surgery)
- 2002: 6th DIVI Congress, Congress President W. Seeger, Giessen (internal medicine)
- 2004: 7th DIVI Congress, Congress President K. Reinhart (anaesthesiology)
- 2006: 8th DIVI Conress, Congress President K.W. Jauch (surgery)
- 2008: 9th DIVI Concress, Congress President G.W. Synbrecht (internal medicine)

DIVI Congresses today represent the most comprehensive meetings on intensive care medicine and emergency medicine in the German-speaking countries.

Meetings of the Section of Emergency and Disaster Medicine

These meetings have been held regularly since 1982 under the Chairmanship of the following clinicians:

- 1982/1983   H. Hochrein
- 1984   E. Ungeheuer
- 1985   H. Gillmann
- 1986   J.G. Schöber, R. Strigl
- 1987   A. Karimi

- 1988   H.U. Lehmann
- 1989   G. Hierholzer
- 1990   H.N. Herden
- 1991   F.W. Ahnefeld
- 1992   M. Harloff
- 1994   P. Sefrin

Since 1995, meetings of this section have been organized in the form of satellite meetings of DIVI Congresses.

Meetings of the Section on Science and Research

Sessions of this section represent an integral part of DIVI Congresses.

Further Activities of the DIVI – Recommendations, Guidelines, Journals
Statements and Recommendations

The DIVI has thus far issued a considerable number of statements and recommendations on intensive care and emergency medicine [partly in cooperation with the German Medical Association, the National Association of Emergency Physicians (BAND) and the standing conference on emergency medicine, etc.]. These statements and recommendations are regularly published in the »Pink Book« in English and German. The most recent German edition dates back to 2005. The statements and recommendations serve as a basis for decision making by the authorities.

The most important statements and recommendations are as follows:

- Emergency medicine by hospital physicians
- Qualification of emergency physicians
- Undergraduate, postgraduate and specialist training in emergency medicine
- Qualification of chief emergency physicians in mass casualty situations
- The national emergency medical services protocol
- The national emergency physician protocol
- The intensive care transport protocol
- Qualification of physicians in the transport of intensive care patients
- Delegation of emergency measures in the emergency medical service
- The Emergency Medical Services Director
- Quality management in emergency medicine
- Supraspecialty status in emergency medicine
- Prehospital thrombolysis in patients with AMI
- Prehospital treatment of patients with cerebral and multiple trauma

The following statements and recommendations are considered milestone statements in intensive care medicine:

- Training of physicians and nurses in intensive care medicine
- Personnel requirements of physicians and nursing staff in intensive care medicine

- Humane aspects of design and equipment of intensive care units
- Physical design and equipment of intensive care units
- Equipment and apparatus for patient care in intensive care units
- A new concept for the training of nurse specialists in intensive care medicine
- Scope of activities of nurses in intensive care medicine
- Catalogue of postgraduate training requirements for physicians in intensive care medicine
- Common core curriculum for optional specialist training in intensive care medicine
- Accreditation of training institutions for specialist training in intensive care medicine

Guidelines

DIVI guidelines have been issued on topics such as acute respiratory failure, acute renal failure, central venous catheter insertion, care and monitoring, mechanical ventilation modes and settings, graduated plan for the treatment of increased intracranial pressure in severe head injury, etc.

An interdisciplinary working group guaranties that the guidelines are both evidence based and co-ordinated between the various specialties represented in the DIVI.

Journals

The DIVI agreed not to publish its own journal. Instead, statements, recommendations, guidelines, etc. issued by the DIVI are published in journals of the member societies, including: *Anästhesiologie & Intensivmedizin, Der Anaesthesist, Notfallmedizin, Der Notarzt, Intensivmedizin und Notfallmedizin, Informationen des Berufsverbandes Deutscher Chirurgen, Zentralblatt für Chirurgie, Der Unfallchirurg, Aktuelle Chirurgie, Zeitschrift für Kardiologie, Medizinische Klinik, Monatschrift für Kinderheilkunde, Der Kinderarzt, Aktuelle Neurologie, Kardiochirurgie, Neurochirurgia and Zentralblatt für Neurochirurgie.* Later this policy was changed and the first issue of the journal »DIVI« was sent to the members in March 2010.

Structure of Intensive Care Medicine in Germany

Thanks to the persistent efforts and continuous discussions of the DIVI, intensive care medicine (comparable to emergency medicine) is not a separate specialty in Germany today, but has been defined as a supraspecialty. In order to achieve special competence in intensive care medicine, base specialty training has to be successfully completed in a first step. In addition to base specialty-related knowledge and skills, the syllabus of a supplemental specialist training programme in intensive care medicine has to provide for the acquisition of relevant

skills. This additional programme is designed to enable the achievement of supraspecialty status in intensive care medicine, anaesthesiology, surgery, cardiac surgery, internal medicine, neurology, neurosurgery or paediatrics, respectively. A common core (common trunk) curriculum of 6–12 months provides knowledge and skills in basic intensive care medicine. An additional 12–18 months are dedicated to training in special intensive care medicine.

The above-mentioned 6–12 months training in basic intensive care medicine is integrated into the base specialty training programme, enrolment in the additional 12–18-month course is possible only on successful completion of base specialty training.

Topics of basic training programmes include cardiopulmonary resuscitation, post-resuscitation care, pathophysiology, diagnosis and treatment of organ dysfunctions, shock, multiorgan failure, sepsis, chest pain and injuries, intoxication, infectious diseases, etc. In addition, special knowledge, practical skills and experience have to be obtained in a number of intensive care procedures such as artificial organ replacement procedures. Further topics included in the programme deal with hygienic, administrative, organizational, ethical and medico-legal aspects.

The following recommended number of procedures should be documented: 75 documented completed cases with complicated intensive medical clinical courses, including 50 patients receiving long-term ventilation, specified minimum numbers of endotracheal intubations, bronchoscopies, haemofiltrations, haemodialyses, central venous and pulmonary artery catheters, chest drains, etc. The described requirements have been developed by working groups and subsequently agreed upon by the member societies, as well as by the Federal and State Medical Associations.

This concept has further facilitated the discussion process on the achievement of uniform training structures and programmes in Europe, which serve as a basis for standardized quality of care by all specialties involved in intensive care medicine, including internal medicine, paediatrics, surgery, anaesthesiology, etc.

Postgraduate Training of Nurse Specialists

Due to the sustained efforts, especially of anaesthesiology (H.W. Opderbecke), internal medicine (H.P. Schuster) and paediatrics (P. Emmrich, P. Lemburg), a uniform, standard qualification of nurse participants in courses in intensive care medicine has been ensured. The course programme was further designed to include special aspects pertaining to the different specialities such as the special requirements of anaesthesiology in the operating theatres, or ICUs, respectively. More self-serving considerations, not only of professional associations of nurses, but also of different ministries, were responsible for the abandonment of these uniform training concepts. Consecutive projects only required 12 weeks of training in anaesthesia, which was too much for those not interested in anaesthesia and too little for those particularly interested in anaesthesia in the OR.

The consequences are already acutely felt today. Qualified anaesthesia nurses are insufficiently trained, and new training programmes for nurses interested in anaesthesia in the OR have to be developed and organized.

Executive Committees and Presidents of the DIVI

The initial Executive Committee (H.-G. Lasch, P. Emmrich, P. Lawin, H.W. Opderbecke, H.P. Schuster) was continuously active from 1977 to 1982. A Second Vice President, A. Encke, Frankfurt, and a Second Treasurer, A. Karimi, Cologne, were elected in 1982 and served until 1988. From 1989 on, the President was elected regularly every 2nd or 3rd year, starting with President P. Lawin, Münster, Vice President A. Sturm, Herne, and General Secretary A. Enke, Frankfurt. H.W. Opderbecke and A. Karimi continued in office for several years as Honorary Secretary and First Treasurer, respectively. D. Heene, Mannheim, started his term of office as Second Treasurer in 1988. From 1990 to 1992, P. Lemburg, Düsseldorf, and W. Dick, Mainz, were elected Second Vice President and Honorary Secretary, respectively. From 1994 to 1998, D. Heene served as President, F.W. Schildberg, Munich, as General Secretary, and R.W.C. Janzen, Frankfurt, as Second Treasurer.

From 1998 to 2000, W.F. Dick acted as President, and W. Bock, Düsseldorf, as Honorary Secretary. From 2001 to 2002, F. W. Schildberg served as President, and H. Burchardi, Göttingen, was elected General Secretary. From 2003 to 2004 W. Hacke, Heidelberg, was elected to the office of President. From 2004 to 2006, E. Martin, Heidelberg, served as President and G. Kreymann, Hamburg, as General Secretary, and from 2006 to 2008, A. Markewitz, Koblenz, acted as President and G. Jorch, Magdeburg, as General Secretary.

Honorary Members

The DIVI may elect those members to honorary membership who have made an outstanding contribution to the development of the DIVI. This illustrious group includes Prof. Dr. med. Dr. vet. h.c. Dr. med. h.c. H.G. Lasch (internal medicine), Prof. Dr. med. H.W. Opderbecke (anaesthesiology), Prof. Dr. med. Dr. med. h.c. P.Lawin (anaesthesiology), Prof. Dr. med. A. Encke (surgery), Prof. Dr. med. Dr. med. h.c. F.W. Ahnefeld (anaesthesiology), Prof. Dr. med. Dr. med. h.c. mult. H. Gillmann (internal medicine), Prof. Dr. med. D.L. Heene (internal medicine), Prof. Dr. med. A. Karimi (neurosurgery), Prof. Dr. med. Dr. med. h.c. W.F. Dick (anaesthesiology), Prof. Dr. med. Dr. med. h.c. F.W. Schildberg (surgery) and Prof. Dr. med. H. Burchardi (anaesthesiology).

Support of Young Researchers

Highly regarded scholarships and awards bestowed by the DIVI serve to promote and support young researchers and clinicians such as the Traveller Scholarship (3–4× 5,000 €/year) and the Else Kröner Memorial scholarship (25,000 €/year).

Future Aspects

Over the past 25 years the DIVI has repeatedly demonstrated justification for its existence as an interdisciplinary organization for intensive care and emergency medicine.

The DIVI faced its greatest challenge in 2000 when the Federal Medical Council had to be convinced of the validity of the interdisciplinary common trunk concept of training in intensive care medicine and emergency medicine. On approval by the Council, the concept of a supraspecialty in intensive care and emergency medicine could be realized. It was thus this very concept which prevented the DIVI from becoming defunct.

In 2001 the DIVI restated that the different specialties involved in intensive care medicine and emergency medicine agreed on their commitment to train nurses and physicians, and to practise intensive care medicine according to a common trunk concept. As demonstrated in the past, special requirements of the individual disciplines may be met from 25 to 50% by a common trunk part and from 50 to 75% by an additional part providing specialist training.

The DIVI Foundation

For a more extensive support of scientific activities, especially of young researchers, a foundation was established by the DIVI (Executive Committee: W.F. Dick, A. Karimi, D.L. Heene). The initial funding was in the amount of 400,000 DM or 200,000 €, respectively. It is hoped that this amount will increase rapidly in the future to enable the support of research projects with substantial grants.

Intensive Care Medicine and Health Authorities

DRGs were introduced into the German health care system as from 2004. Unfortunately, the German health care authorities have failed to give adequate consideration to the importance of intensive care medicine and the respective required procedures. Working groups and experts from the DIVI have recently made substantial contributions to an adequate representation of the requirements of the different specialties. This has raised greater awareness on the part of the Ministry of Health and the Federal Council of Experts of Health Care Systems of the importance of intensive care and emergency medicine. Hopefully this will lead to an even better mutual understanding of the thoughts and perspectives of all parties involved.

2.2.3 The History of Intensive Care Medicine in Europe

H. Burchardi

Structures and conditions of education and training in intensive care medicine vary fundamentally in European countries. They have been developed on the historical background and reflect the balance of power in the professional competition between the various medical specialties.

Already in the 1970s special societies of intensive care medicine had been founded abroad, such as the »Society of Critical Care Medicine (SCCM)« in the USA, the »Intensive Care Society« in the UK and the »Schweizerische Gesellschaft für Intensivmedizin (SGI)« in Switzerland. In 1977 the »World Federation of Societies of Intensive and Critical Care Medicine« was established.

In contrast to the national societies a supranational »European Society of Intensive Care Medicine (ESICM)« was founded in 1982 which was a society of individuals devoted to intensive care medicine and which did not lay claim to national representation.

All these societies articulated the increasing self-confidence of those who were dedicated to intensive care medicine, but they also reflected the necessity to care for the special matters of intensive care medicine without the constraints of the traditional specialties' interest.

Previous Development in Europe

A survey of the ESICM demonstrates the situation of 1996 [3]. It is shown that the multidisciplinary approach to intensive care medicine has been realized in many European countries (in 10 of 19), however with considerable variations. On the other hand, in 8 countries, such as in Scandinavia, Italy and the East European countries, intensive care medicine is exclusively linked to anaesthesiology – as was the case in the former German Democratic Republic.

The ESICM firmly promotes the multidisciplinary approach, because this ensures a broad basis of competence in medical care as well as in research.

In this spectrum of educational structures the situation in Spain is a unique exception: Since 1978 the Spanish system of medical education has been centralized. Based on the ranking list from the final, government-controlled medical examination, the young physician can choose his specialization, with the consequence that those with lower ranking numbers have to be content with what is left. As there are no subspecialties, this is a decision for a lifetime. In this context intensive care medicine is a specialty by its own with a training time of 5 years. This special Spanish way has produced much unease in other European countries as it blocks the multidisciplinary

approach to intensive care medicine and contradicts the general European trend.

Switzerland also found its own way very early. In 1985 the SGI created a certificate of special competence in intensive care medicine, based on a definied curriculum at an accredited ICU and an examination [15]. Five years later, this certificate was made an official additional qualification by the Swiss Medical Association (FMH) obtainable by anaesthetists, surgeons, internists and paediatricians. This qualification with 2 years of training introduced a concept of education for intensive care medicine which in 1988 has been taken over quite similarly as a qualifying certification by the German Society of Internal Medicine Intensive Care (Deutsche Gesellschaft für Internistische Intensivmedizin, DGII) [16]. Later on, the German Interdisciplinary Association of Critical Care and Emergency Medicine (Deutsche Interdisziplinäre Vereinigung für Intensiv- und Notfallmedizin, DIVI) proposed this concept as the model for the official structure of education and training in intensive care medicine (*fakultative Weiterbildung Spezielle Intensivmedizin*) which has been introduced in Germany by the Federal Medical Association (Bundesärztekammer) (see below).

As an important modification, the FMH established the specialization for intensive care medicine in 1997. This, however, can be obtained as a »secondary specialty«, open for physicians with basic specialties such as internal medicine, surgery, anaesthesiology and paediatrics/neonatology. Thus, the multidisciplinary approach is still maintained, but in Switzerland, intensive care medicine is now a specialty by its own (details can be found under www. fmh.ch/). The duration of training and education is 6 years (3 years for non-specific education + 3 years for specific intensive care education). It must be done at specially certified ICUs, finished by an examination [21].

I am convinced that the multidisciplinary concept for intensive care medicine is a good, comprehensible solution [6]. However, the future of intensive care medicine will depend on how much freedom will be offered to that innovative specialty. If the perspectives to develop intensive care remain too restricted by the basic specialties, then a specialty by its own will sooner or later become attractive. The recent development in Switzerland clearly indicates this direction. In any case, the decisions in other European countries will certainly influence the structural development in Germany as well.

Examinations and Diplomas in Intensive Care Medicine

In the context of this multidisciplinary concept the ESICM established in 1989 a European Diploma in Intensive Care (EDIC) which is open to physicians who have completed their basic specialties in anaesthesiology, internal medicine, surgery or paediatrics. The multi-disciplinary diploma consists of a written examination (multiple choice questions in English) and an interview at the bedside. The certification of the European Diploma requires in addition to the successful examination 2 years of full-time practice in intensive care. The Diploma does not compete with existing official national certifications. In some countries (such as in Scandinavia and The Netherlands) the EDIC has already been accepted as the official diploma by the national societies or has been incorporated into their existing diploma.

On the level of a European diploma an unpleasant competition happened between the ESICM and the European Academy of Anaesthesiology (EAA) in the early 1990s: the EAA had established in 1984 a »European Diploma in Anaesthesiology« which became very successful over the years. After the ESICM was going to establish its own diploma for intensive care medicine in 1988, the EAA changed the name of their diploma to »European Diploma in Anaesthesiology and Intensive Care«. Mediating interventions to co-ordinate both diplomas failed. Ultimately all the problems were solved when the ESICM in 1998 became recognized by the »European Union of Medical Specialists« (UEMS) as the official European body representing intensive care medicine. In this context the ESICM received the mandate for defining the aims of education and training in intensive care medicine in Europe (see below).

Today the European Community is progressively becoming a reality. The free migration of working persons within the European Community requires that national professional regulations are adapted to the conditions valid in other European countries. This is particularly true also for medicine.

Harmonization of Professional Education in Europe

In 1957, the Treaty of Rome promoted the free movement of people between the European Member States, but primarily it did not guarantee migrating doctors the right to exercise their medical profession in other Member States. Several Medical Directives from 1975 to 2006 (75/362/EEC, 75/363/EEC, 93/16/EC, 2005/26/EC, and 2006/100/EC) provided a legal basis for mutual recognition of basic medical qualifications and postgraduate training. All Member States were thus obliged to harmonize their medical training systems in order to comply with the European minimum requirements [9].

For this purpose the »European Union of Medical Specialists« (UEMS) was created in 1958 with the aim of harmonizing the medical professional structures and improving the quality of medical care in the European Economic Community (EEC). The UEMS develops guidelines, recommendations and statements concerning general problems of professional structures, medical qualification and education as well as other general questions. Among others such general guidelines have been defined in (for details see the UEMS website: www.uems.net):

- The Charter on Training of Medical Specialists (1993)
- The Charter on Continuing Medical Education (1994)
- The Charter on Quality Assurance (1996)
- The Charter on Visitation of Training Centres (1997)
- The Charter on Continuing Professional Development (2001)
- The Policy Statement on Assessments during Postgraduate Medical Training (2006)

The guidelines of the UEMS can only be regarded as recommendations. The final decision on the national level is made by the national authorities. In the different Member States this is organized in different ways: In some countries the Ministries of Health Care are authorized, in other countries this task has been assigned to the medical societies. In Germany this competence is given to the State Chambers of Physicians (Landesärztekammern). As a result, a long period of time usually elapses before all regulations are realized in all Member States. Nevertheless, such recommendations will finally point the way to go for the European countries. The general recommendation of the UEMS always defines minimal requirements, so that all Member States will be able to follow. It remains possible for countries to define advanced regulations and requirements on their own national level.

The ambitious aim to harmonize the European professional structures initially appeared to be inaccessible. The pressure to come to a compromise and a vision of common pathways was probably missing. During a long period of time the chances for a common future were not perceived. This may also have been the reason why the German Society of Anaesthesiology and Intensive Care Medicine (DGAI) over a period of 13 years abstained from any representation in the UEMS.

According to the statutes of the UEMS Germany is officially represented through the Union of Professional Organisations of Medical Specialists (Gemeinschaft Fachärztlicher Berufsverbände, GFB). As the corresponding representation of the German anaesthesiologists the Professional Association of German Anaesthetists (Berufsverband Deutscher Anästhesisten, BDA) was a member of the GFB until the early 1980s, the BDA could send its delegates to the UEMS. However, in 1983 the BDA left the GFB, because membership in the GFB did not seem to be beneficial compared to the inappropriately high financial burden (calculated from the large number of members). Consequently, the German anaesthesiologists were only accepted in the UEMS as observers without any voting power. Thus during a long period of time, one of the largest national societies of anaesthesiologists in Europe was not present in the official European institution responsible for harmonization of professional education!

Meanwhile it became apparent that membership in the GFB could become increasingly important for German anaesthesiologists, mainly for problems involved in setting up private practice. As it became more and more important to contribute to the general discussion on professional education in Europe, the BDA decided in 1996 to join the GFB again. Since then, German anaesthesiologists have again been present in the UEMS as delegates with full voting rights.

As already mentioned, only the officially recognized specialties are represented by sections in the UEMS. This means that until recently intensive care medicine was not represented at the UEMS. Since about 1990 the UEMS Section of Anaesthesiology has taken care of intensive care matters through a special subcommittee, but this in no way reflected the multidisciplinary concept of intensive care medicine which is now predominant in Europe.

By a joint effort of the ESICM (H. Burchardi) and the UEMS Section of Anaesthesiology (S. de Lange and H. van Aken) a UEMS »Multidisciplinary Joint Committee of Intensive Care Medicine« (MJCICM) was established in 1998. This committee is composed of UEMS delegates from the various specialties involved in intensive care medicine, such as anaesthesiology, internal medicine, pneumology, surgery, neurosurgery and paediatrics as well as by a »Standing Advisory Board« where delegates of the ESICM and the European Society of Paediatric and Neonatal Intensive Care (ESPNIC) are present [10]. This committee, which was a completely new structure within the UEMS, was adapted from the concept of the DIVI, the German Interdisciplinary Association of Critical Care and Emergency Medicine – an indication of how convincing the multidisciplinary concept of the DIVI appears to others. Meanwhile the UEMS has created similar committees also for other multidisciplinary fields such as emergency medicine, pain medicine, etc.

By virtue of this committee, intensive care medicine was for the first time officially represented within the UEMS. Simultaneously the ESICM received the mandate to officially participate in the process of harmonizing professional structures and educational recommendations in Europe. In this connection some of the already existing ESICM recommendations have been officially adopted by the UEMS.

This committee, which is so important for intensive care medicine in Europe, has presented initial activities undertaken so far (for details see the UEMS-MJCICM website: www.uems.net):

Definition of Intensive Care Medicine

Intensive care medicine combines physicians, nurses and allied health professionals in the co-ordinated and collaborative management of patients with life-threatening single or multiple organ system failure, including stabilization after major surgical interventions. It is continuous (i.e. 24 h) management including monitoring, diagnostics, support of failing vital functions and treatment of the underlying diseases.

Guidelines for Education and Training in Intensive Care Medicine

Special competence in intensive care medicine can be acquired by physicians who already have their certification in an appropriate primary speciality such as anaesthesiology, internal medicine, paediatrics, pneumology and surgery, etc. This requires 2 years of additional full-time education and training in intensive care medicine at an officially accredited ICU; 6–12 months of the training period in intensive care can be accepted as part of the primary speciality. A catalogue of special knowledge and skills in intensive care medicine (»core curriculum«) must be fulfilled by all physicians independent of their primary specialty. The acquirement of sufficient knowledge and skills should be certified by a specialty-specific training logbook. For accreditation of training centres certain minimal requirements have to be fulfilled: continuous (24-h) presence of physicians in the ICU, a minimum of six beds, vital organ support (such as mechanical ventilation, renal replacement therapies) on at least 40% of the intensive care days. Consultant services (such as laboratories, radiology, blood bank) in the hospital or affiliated to the hospital must be available at any time.

It is obvious that these recommendations resemble those defined by the DIVI [12]. The multidisciplinary concept and recommendations of the DIVI have demonstrated their convincing effect on the European level. Thus, the DIVI played the pioneering role for such recommendations.

Intensive Care Accreditation Visiting Programme

Based on the UEMS Charter on Visitation of Training Centres (1997) some specialties (e.g. anaesthesiology, neurosurgery) have already established an external auditing programme by which hospitals on an optional basis and after an auditing visit can be certified as an official European training centre. As these external audits have been well accepted and valued, the MJCICM established an Intensive Care Units Accreditation Visiting Programme (ICUAVP) for external qualification of training ICUs. The external visit can be requested by the hospital at its own expense.

The visiting commission is composed of experts delegated by the UEMS-MJCICM and the ESICM, including a national representative. The certification (**Approved European Centre for Training and Education of Intensive Care Medicine**) is valid for 5 years and is granted jointly by the UEMS and ESICM.

Future Development of Education and Training in Intensive Care Medicine

According to European regulations the professional diploma and the specialty qualifications have been recognized by the different Member States since 1975. The logical consequence of that harmonization would be the mutual recognition of the various concepts of professional education and training; but there is still a long way to go before that point is reached.

In January 2000 the UEMS created the »**European Accreditation Council for Continuing Medical Education**« (**EACCME**) which on a supranational level will reward successful participation at meetings for professional education by CME qualification points (www.uems.net). The aim of this institution is to harmonize professional further education in Europe and to improve its quality.

However, the problem is that the national institutions authorized for CME certification are not always willing to hand over their power of control to a supranational European authority and to abandon their (supposed) higher standard of quality. The introduction of a Europe-wide continuous professional education would be so important – particularly for intensive care medicine which progresses so fast.

To keep or even to improve the high professional standard for intensive care medicine requires first of all long-term practice in this field. Experience and expertise can only be gained by continuous and long-term practical activity in intensive care medicine. Today, intensive care medicine cannot be done casually if quality is the aim!

This is where a special dilemma arises: in Germany, positions which require long-term and exclusive practice of intensive care medicine are still rare (recently such a development seems to making some progress).

However, even if a few long-term careers for intensive care medicine can be created, the number of experts exclusively devoted to intensive care medicine remains small. For physicians it has become evident that they should not be involved in intensive care medicine for too long a period of time, because at present attractive professional careers in that field are missing.

The German specialists' society DGAI should strive for better structures of long-term careers for intensivists. From the professional view the position of anaesthesiologists in intensive care medicine is still regarded as very strong. Only if the field of anaesthesiology continues to maintain a high level of quality and professional education in the future can it retain this leading role in intensive care medicine. In the multidisciplinary competition anaesthesiology is able to claim high levels of educational quality. It would be wrong to decrease the quality standards.

Research in Intensive Care Medicine

Intensive care medicine in Europe has a good reputation. Very early research groups were established in which special clinical problems of intensive care were studied. They were created by some prominent experts who over a long period of time and on an international level were able to explore intensive care problems continuously and thoroughly.

It may be audacious to acknowledge some of them and run the risk of omitting other important names. Only a few European intensivists shall be mentioned who on an international level and over a long time have been identified with specific intensive care topics. Some names that can be mentioned include L. Gattinoni (Milan) and P. Suter (Geneva) for the topic of mechanical ventilation, G. Hedenstierna (Uppsala) and C. Roussos (Athens) for physiology of mechanical ventilation, J.-L. Vincent (Brussels) for cardiovascular functions, C. Ronco (Vicenza) for renal replacement therapies, C. Brun-Buisson (Paris) and K. Reinhart (Jena) for infection and sepsis, L. Thijs (Amsterdam) and M. Lamy (Liège) for inflammatory mediators, A. Artigas (Barcelona) for epidemiologic questions and J.-R. LeGall (Paris) for development of severity-of-illness scores.

Large international conferences have contributed considerably to the international opinion of the high quality of intensive care medicine in Europe. Since 1980 the **European Society of Intensive Care Medicine (ESICM)** has annually organized a large conference where intensivists from all over the world convene and exchange their scientific results and clinical experiences. In addition, a large international symposium with high-level professional education has been organized by J.-L. Vincent in Brussels every year since 1980.

There are good reasons why intensivists from North America are frequent guests and speakers at these conferences. They appreciate these excellent meetings and notice how much the quality of European intensive care medicine profits from its multidisciplinary concept. Likewise European intensivists participate regularly at the corresponding conferences in the USA and Canada, as invited speakers and even sometimes as members of the Organizing Committee. In the USA intensivists who have been trained by PACT, the educational programme of the ESICM, are accredited with adequate CME points. It follows that the intercontinental contacts between Europe and North America are particularly close – a transatlantic partnership for intensive care medicine.

In the context of this transatlantic partnership large international consensus conferences have been taking place regularly since 1992, in joint co-operation between the **European Society of Intensive Care Medicine (ESICM)**, the American Thoracic Society (ATS) and the Societée de Réanimation de Langue Française (SRLF), recently also joined by the US Society of Critical Care Medicine (SCCM). These international consensus conferences are organized according to a strict and very ambitious structure, a concept previously developed by the SRLF [7]. The topics of these international consensus conferences were up to now (1) selective decontamination of the digestive tract [23], (2) predicting outcome in ICU patients [22], (3) tissue hypoxia [16], (4) ARDS, parts 1 and 2 [1, 2], (5) mechanical ventilation, parts 1 and 2 [19, 20], (6) non-invasive positive pressure ventilation in acute respiratory failure [13], (7) ICU-acquired pneumonia [14], (8) challenges in end-of-life care in the ICU [8] and necrotizing pancreatitis [to be published].

In the active international competition of research in intensive care medicine, Germany plays a relatively minor role. At international conferences on intensive care medicine, by the frequency of scientific publications and in respect to international research activities, Germany is represented only to a modest degree [4, 5, 18] – and this despite the fact that for many years now Germany since has had the highest number of members in the ESICM. In my opinion, there are structural reasons for such inefficiency. There are no structures offering an attractive professional and scientific long-term perspective for those who really want to be active in intensive care medicine. Directors responsible for long-term research concepts require a certain independent, autonomous position with personal responsibility for their scientific activities and their own financial budget. Scientists require a long-term perspective and clinical research in intensive care medicine needs a lot of staying power.

In the past this problem has not been sufficiently recognized in Germany. The German Society of Anaesthesiology and Intensive Care Medicine, but also the societies of internal medicine and surgery, were mostly concerned with not losing control over intensive care medicine; they were extremely frightened by the idea of an independent intensive care medicine. Presumably important chances have been missed. Now economic priorities also dictate activities in the teaching hospitals. Official grants and other financial support clearly privilege basic research. It is true that clinical practice always appeals to evidence-based medicine, and the German research community has called for improvements in clinical research [11], but the sufficient financial support is lacking. Governmental as well as industrial support is scarce.

Anaesthesiology as a clinical specialty may particularly suffer from such restrictive development. Now economic efficiency dictates the new directions. Misinterpretation of the scientific importance of intensive care medicine could lead to great disappointment for anaesthesiology – the independence of intensive care medicine may be the consequence.

Perspectives

The free movement of professionals within the European Community requires harmonization of regulations. Even before such harmonization has been realized, physicians are already seeking better working conditions within Europe, a fact we are currently experiencing in Germany. Therefore, it is urgent that the preconditions and quality criteria for professional employment in Europe are defined and harmonized on an international level.

Presumably the future development of intensive care medicine in Europe will still be dominated by the national preconditions, the professional structures and regulations, as it has been the case in the past. Thus, the national authorities for professional affairs in Germany, the Medical Associations, will probably also in future determine the speed of development in Europe. However, in the long term they will not be able to act against the general evolution in Europe. The German Medical Association has already demonstrated its readiness to respect European aspects.

References

1. Artigas A, Bernard G, Carlet J et al, and the Consensus Committee (1998) The American-European Consensus Conference on ARDS, Part 2. Am J Respir Crit Care Med 157:1332–1347
2. Bernard G, Artigas A, Brigham K et al, and the Consensus Committee (1994) Report of the American-European consensus conference on ARDS: definitions, mechanisms, relevant outcomes and clinical trial coordination. Intensive Care Med 20:225–232
3. Bion J, Ramsay G, Roussos C, Burchardi H, on behalf of the Task Force on Educational Issues of the European Society of Intensive Care Medicine (1998) Intensive care training and speciality status in Europe: international comparisons. Intensive Care Med 24:372–377
4. Boldt J, Maleck W (1999) Intensivmedizinische Forschung in Deutschland – eine Analyse von Beiträgen in wichtigen internationalen Journalen. Anasthesiol Intensivmed Notfallmed Schmerzther 34:542–548
5. Boldt J, Maleck W (2001) From which countries do chairpersons and invited speakers at important anaesthesia and intensive care meetings come? Eur J Anaesthesiol 18:194–196
6. Burchardi H (2001) Specialty status for intensive care medicine? (editorial). Eur J Anaesthesiol 18:67–69
7. Carlet J, Artigas A, Bihari D et al (1992) The first European Consensus Conference in Intensive Care Medicine: introductory remarks. Intensive Care Med 18:180–181
8. Carlet J, Thijs LG, Antonelli M et al. (2004) Challenges in end-of-life care in the ICU. Statement of the 5th International Consensus Conference in Critical Care: Brussels, Belgium, April 2003. Intensive Care Med 30:770–784
9. De Lange S (2001) The European Union of Medical Specialists and speciality training. Eur J Anaesthesiol 18:561–562
10. De Lange S, Van Aken H, Burchardi H (2002) Intensive care medicine in Europe: structure, organisation and training guidelines of the Multidisciplinary Joint Committee of Intensive Care Medicine (MJCICM) of the European Union of Medical Specialists (UEMS). ESICM Statement. Intensive Care Med 28:1505–1511
11. Deutsche Forschungsgemeinschaft (1999) Klinische Forschung. Denkschrift. Wiley-VCH, Weinheim

12. Deutsche Interdisziplinäre Vereinigung für Intensiv- und Notfall-medizin (DIVI) (2004) Stellungnahmen, Empfehlungen zu Proble-men der Intensiv- und Notfallmedizin, 5th edn. DIVI: Karimi A, Burchardi H

13. Evans TW (2001) International Consensus Conferences in Intensive Care Medicine: non-invasive positive pressure ventilation in acute respiratory failure. Organised jointly by the American Thoracic Society, the European Respiratory Society, the European Society of Intensive Care Medicine, and the Societé de Réanimation de Langue Française, and approved by the ATS Board of Directors, December 2000. Intensive Care Med 27:166–178

14. Hubmayr RD, Burchardi H, Elliot M et al (2002) Statement of the 4th International Consensus Conference in Critical Care on ICU-Acquired Pneumonia (Chicago, IL, May 2002). Intensive Care Med 28:1521–1536

15. Mitteilungen der Deutschen und der Österreichischen Gesell-schaft für Internistische Intensivmedizin (1986) Ausbildung von Ärzten in Intensivmedizin. Fähigkeitsausweis in Intensivmedizin der Schweizerischen Gesellschaft für Intensivmedizin. Inten-sivmed 23:1–4

16. Mitteilungen der Deutschen und der Österreichischen Gesellschaft für Internistische Intensivmedizin (1989) Qualifikationsnachweis für internistische Intensivmedizin der DGII. Intensivmed 26:334–337

17. Richard C (1996) Tissue hypoxia. How to detect, how to correct, how to prevent? Intensive Care Med 22:1250–1257

18. Shahla M, Verhaeghe V, Hedeshi AR, Friedman G, Vincent JL (1995) European participation in major intensive care journals. Intensive Care Med 21:7–10

19. Slutsky AS (1994) Consensus conference on mechanical ventila-tion – January 28–30, 1993 at Northbrook, Illinois, USA. Part I. Intensive Care Med 20:64–79

20. Slutsky AS (1994) Consensus conference on mechanical ventila-tion – January 28–30, 1993 at Northbrook, Illinois, USA. Part II. Intensive Care Med 20:150–162

21. Stocker R, Frutiger A, Berner M (2002) Facharzttitel »Intensivme-dizin« in der Schweiz. Intensivmed 39:131–141

22. Suter P, Armaganidis A, Beaufils F et al (1994): Predicting outcome in ICU patients. 2nd European Consensus Conference in Intensive Care Medicine. Intensive Care Med 20:390–397

23. The First European Consensus Conference in Intensive Care Medi-cine (1992) Selective decontamination of the digestive tract in intensive care unit patients. The European Society of Intensive Care Medicine; The Societé Réanimation de Langue Française. Infect Control Hosp Epidemiol 13:609–611

2.3   Emergency Medicine

W.F. Dick and J. Schüttler

2.3.1   Historical Notes

Emergency medicine in Germany looks back on a long tradition, despite having often been neglected, ignored or forgotten in favour of the history of Anglo-American emergency medicine. While the article by Pantridge [41] published in the early 1960s is regarded as the first description and start of prehospital defibrillation in the USA and the UK, this measure had also been described in German-speaking countries and was carried out there at that time, e.g. at the Mobile Life Support Units (MLSU) in Cologne, Mainz, Heidelberg, etc.

The name of one of the most famous German-speaking physicians, Paracelsus [12], who worked in 1527 as City Physician and Professor of Physics and Surgery in Basel (Switzerland), for centuries has been associated with emergency medicine. He might even be regarded as a historical representative of evidence-based medicine. Paracelsus refined the ancient techniques (Galen) of mouth-to-mouth ventilation by introducing a ventilation bag whose nipple was inserted directly into the nostrils of apnoeic patients in order to ventilate them properly. Another eminent name associated with emergency medicine in the nineteenth/twentieth century was F. Trendelenburg (1844–1924: Halle, Leipzig, Jena, Göttingen, Berlin and Rostock [20]). He rediscovered what was known in the Middle Ages as the head-down position – originally used for surgical procedures – and is today referred to as the Trendelenburg position. In addition, his name is connected to the first description of the Trendelenburg operation for the surgical therapy of fulminant pulmonary embolism, a procedure which was, however, first carried out by Kirschner in 1924. Furthermore, Trendelenburg used tracheotomy and artificial ventilation for the treatment of respiratory complications due to chloroform anaesthesia.

Another name of great importance for the history of emergency and disaster medicine in Germany is that of the surgeon J.F.A. von Esmarch [6]. It was his firm conviction that the efficient organization of medical resources and medical personnel (including ambulances, mobile pharmacies and field kitchens) decisively influences both the quality and the outcome of medical care. He further postulated that different parts of equipment needed to be designed so that the different parts would fit together. As early as 1875 he predicted that disasters would expand in proportion to technological advances and that the development of concepts and strategies to ensure availability of adequate equipment at all times was essential. The introduction of mobile hospitals and hospital trains

were additional innovations which were realized on his initiative. One of the first trains carrying injured soldiers back from the battlefields in France to Berlin (1870) was launched on his initiative, although it was sponsored by private individuals instead of by the German army. Furthermore, he was the driving force behind the ruling that all soldiers had to carry first aid kits as of 1873. Von Esmarch was thus one of the first physicians to recognize the importance of first aid by laypersons, a concept he supported actively. His name is, however, most closely associated with the Esmarch manoeuvre, i.e. a simple to perform measure which ensures upper airway patency.

Equally important for the development of emergency medicine is the name of F. Kuhn (1866–1929 [48]). Although Kuhn was a surgeon, his special focus of interest was the advancement of anaesthesia and emergency medicine. He developed various techniques of endotracheal intubation and different types of endotracheal tubes. He recommended the performance of endotracheal intubation in asphyxial patients, because this provided more adequate ventilation in this patient population. Additional points of emphasis in his work were the application of positive pressure ventilation in chest operations, the administration of oxygen, the infusion of pre-warmed fluids, as well as cardiac compression by intermittent chest compression. His scientific career was at times overshadowed by controversies with F. Sauerbruch, who strongly favoured the application of negative pressure ventilation (negative pressure chambers) over positive pressure ventilation in thoracic surgery, and did everything possible to thwart the »Kuhn concept«.

2.3.2   Development of Modern Emergency Medicine in Germany

The development of emergency medicine in German-speaking countries in the twentieth century was decisively influenced by the surgeon M. Kirschner; he initiated prehospital emergency medicine by postulating at the 62nd national congress of the German Society of Surgery in 1938 that: »The doctor should go out to see the injured at the scene, instead of the injured being brought to the hospital to see the doctor«. K.H. Bauer [5], a surgeon working in Heidelberg, introduced the first MLSU in Germany on 5 February 1957 – the Clinomobil (◘ Fig. 2.52). This unit was initially used as a mobile operating unit, intended primarily for the treatment of trauma patients.

Only a few months later, Friedhoff introduced an emergency ambulance in Cologne; its principal aim was to stabilize the patient's vital functions during transport and may thus be regarded as the first compact emergency ambulance system (◘ Fig. 2.53)

Anaesthetists contributing to the development of mobile life support unit (MLSU) systems in the following years

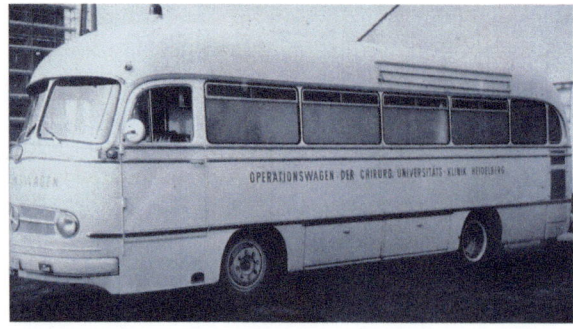

Fig. 2.52. Clinomobile of the Surgical University Hospital Heidelberg

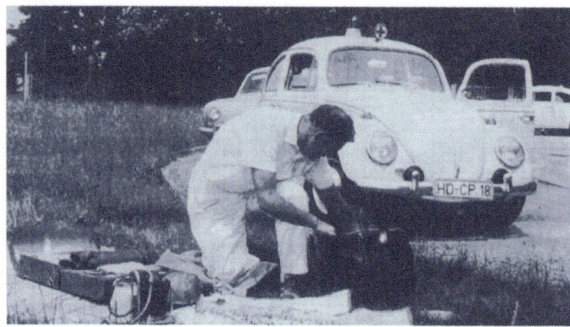

Fig. 2.55. The Heidelberg physician rapid response car (HD 10)

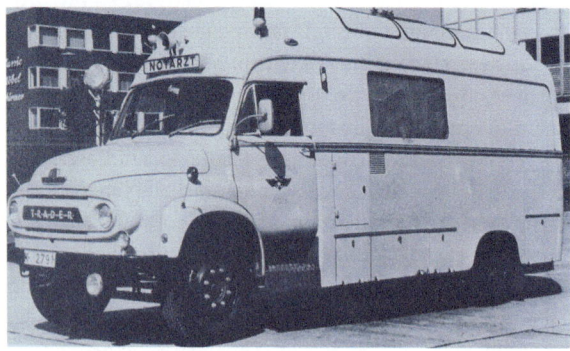

Fig. 2.53. The first emergency ambulance unit of Cologne

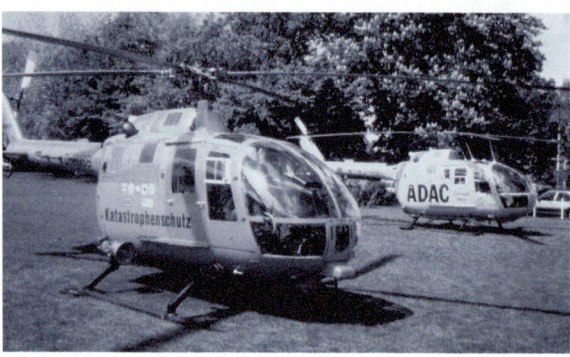

Fig. 2.56. Emergency helicopters (MBB BO 105 CB or CBS-5)

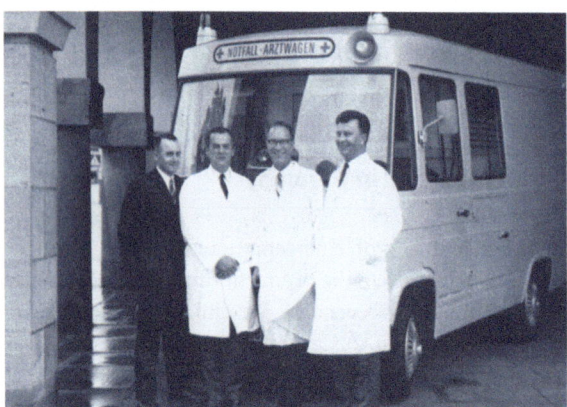

Fig. 2.54. The first emergency ambulance of Mainz (*from right to left*: M. Halmagyi, R. Frey, F.W. Ahnefeld)

were: R. Frey (Mainz), F.W. Ahnefeld (Mainz/Ulm), W. Röse (Magdeburg), G. Hossli (Zurich), H. Bergmann (Linz, Austria). In the early 1960s, additional MLSU systems were initiated, e.g. in Magdeburg (Röse) (▶ Chap. 3.3.26), Mainz (Frey, Ahnefeld, ◘ Fig. 2.54), Ludwigshafen (Gillmann) and Gummersbach (Herzog).

The special physician rapid response car put into operation on 7 April 1964 in Heidelberg (Gögler) (HD 10) was, in principle, the prototype of the first »emergency

physician response unit« working in co-operation with a separate mobile transport unit [28] to meet at the scene as part of a rendezvous system (◘ Fig. 2.55).

In the early 1970s, the ground operating system was supplemented by the introduction of air rescue transport (helicopters). The first helicopter, Christoph 1, started on 29 September 1970 in Munich, to be followed by Christoph 22 in Ulm, Christoph 3 in Cologne and Christoph 2 in Frankfurt (◘ Fig. 2.56).

Prior to these initiatives, pilot studies had been carried out in Frankfurt, Munich, Nuremberg/Erlangen and Mainz in the late 1960s. Ahnefeld launched landmark helicopter studies in Ulm (Military Hospital). Today, more than 60 systems are in operation, covering the entire country in a tight network of primary care helicopters; additional intensive care helicopters complete the system.

One of the main supporters of emergency medicine in the German-speaking countries was the late P. Safar (◘ Fig. 2.57 [4]). Closely associated with his name is the rediscovery and development of mouth-to-mouth ventilation and – together with Knickerbocker – cardiac compression or a combination of both. In a key publication of the time, »**Ventilatory efficacy of mouth-to-mouth artificial respiration**«, Safar wrote: »In coma without a tracheal tube, direct MMV is effective because of the ability of the rescuer to support the head and jaw for upper airway patency

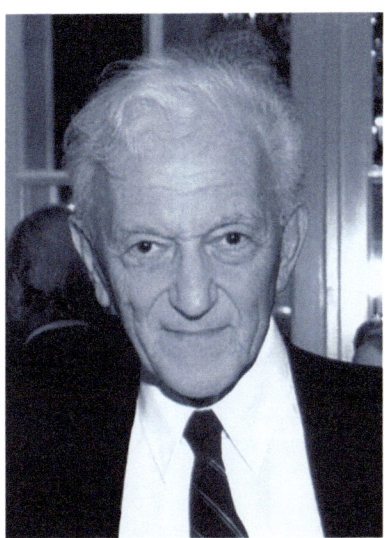

Fig. 2.57. Peter Safar

and because of controllable high inflation pressures and volumes, whereas manual methods frequently fail to ventilate, mainly because of the upper airway obstruction. We recommend that backward tilt of the head plus exhaled air inflation methods be taught for general use in adults and children« [42].

On changing from Heidelberg to Mainz in 1959, R. Frey [21] was already familiar with the »Clinomobil« and its requirements. Together with Ahnefeld, he introduced the first MLSU in Mainz in 1964. The vehicle was originally operated by an anaesthetist in training, an anaesthesia nurse and an emergency medical technician (EMT), who also served as driver. Even the first vehicle was furnished with the necessary equipment to allow external defibrillation to be carried out in patients in VF/VT. However, the majority of patients treated at that time suffered from trauma, tetanus and intoxication, while only a small number of patients with myocardial infarction was treated by the MLSU team.

It was again Frey and Safar [26] who initiated – modelled on the concept of the Club of Rome – the »Club of Mainz« in 1976 and who organized the 1st World Congress on Emergency and Disaster Medicine in Mainz only 1 year later. This was followed by congresses hosted biennially in different countries worldwide; the 10th World Congress was once again held in Mainz in 1997. In 2001 WADEM celebrated, on the occasion of the 12th World Congress in Lyon (France), the 25th anniversary of the Club of Mainz. In 1983 Safar and Frey founded the journal *Disaster Medicine* (the first issue was published in 1985), today's *Prehospital and Disaster Medicine*, the official journal of the World Association for Disaster and Emergency Medicine (WADEM).

In his doctoral dissertation on »Artificial colloids as volume replacement in shock«, Ahnefeld [16] already

described different aspects of emergency medicine, which reflected the experience gained in his work with H. Weese in Wuppertal. At that time, like other future anaesthetists, he worked as a surgeon, but soon left Bochum for the military hospital in Koblenz to study different aspects of burn disease. In Koblenz he developed an interest in anaesthesia. As a member of the Military Health Service and of the Department of Anaesthesiology in Mainz he became a specialist in anaesthesia and established a modern anaesthesia service in Koblenz. His scope of scientific activities comprised the pathophysiology and therapy of shock, fluid losses in severely burned patients, or patients after trauma, uniform design and equipment of ambulances and MLSUs, training of laypersons in CPR, training programmes for paramedics, EMTs, etc. After changing to the University of Ulm, Ahnefeld was able to realize his concepts step by step, with special consideration of national and state emergency legislation.

Another member of the Mainz anaesthesia team was Hans Nolte. Based on the findings of Safar's investigations, he compared mouth-to-mouth/nose ventilation during CPR in sedated and relaxed medical students with conventional procedures used at that time to determine their efficacy and superiority (described e.g. by Silvester, Holger Nielsen, etc.). The resulting postdoctoral thesis remains one of the key publications on CPR to date [39].

Further contributions to the development of modern emergency medicine in Germany after the 1970s were made, e.g. by the anaesthetists Wolfgang Dick (Ulm/Mainz), Dietrich Kettler (Göttingen), Karl Heinz Lindner (Ulm/Innsbruck), Jürgen Schüttler (Bonn/Erlangen) and Peter Sefrin (Würzburg).

2.3.3 Definitions and Concepts

Definitions

In order to understand the development of emergency medicine in Germany, an awareness of the underlying concepts and definitions is essential:

- An **emergency patient** is a patient with severely compromised vital functions or with impending disturbance of vital functions (danger to life)
- An **acutely ill patient** is a patient who is acutely ill or traumatized, whose disease or injury are, however, not life-threatening.

Concepts

The concept of emergency medicine [3] in German-speaking countries is based upon the »chain of rescue« (Fig. 2.59) or »chain of survival« (Fig. 2.60). Although coinage of the term is frequently attributed to US emergency medical experts, it is, in fact, a true »product of Mainz«,

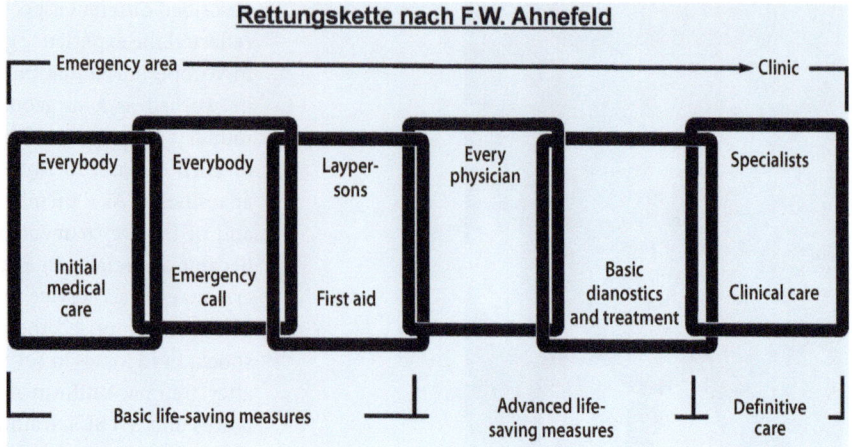

Fig. 2.58. Chain of rescue (Ahnefeld et al. [1])

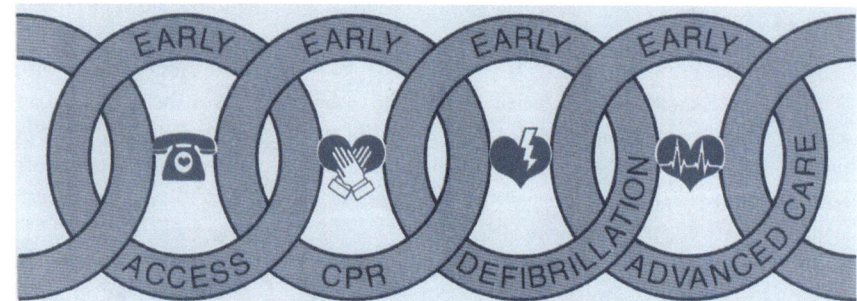

Fig. 2.59. Chain of survival (AHA, [8])

where it was created by F.W. Ahnefeld and developed into the emergency medical service (EMS) system [1]. This fact has always been emphasized by Safar when he used the term himself (e.g. in »Emergency medicine – history and current practice 1991 [2]«). Ahnefeld developed this concept upon the suggestion of R. Frey, and it was later confirmed by similar considerations and findings of P. Safar. In 1968 Safar [42] distinguished between ten components of the US concept of the chain of survival (■ Table 2.1), six of which were identical to the German concept of the chain of rescue (published in 1966) (■ Table 2.2).

In contrast to the US concept of emergency medicine – »The US paramedic-based system was developed in 1963 not because it was thought inherently better, but because of economic reasons and a relative shortage of available physicians« [31] – the German system, i.e. the system established by researchers from German-speaking countries, postulates that a team of qualified emergency physicians and EMTs or paramedics treat emergency patients according to the principles of prehospital intensive care medicine within the shortest time possible, although with a limited spectrum of resources, and subsequently transport the patients under controlled conditions to the nearest appropriate hospital.

Table 2.1. Concepts of emergency medicine in the USA

1. Layperson first aid
2. Universal emergency telephone number
3. Treatment of patients at the scene by qualified personnel (physicians, paramedics)
4. Transport of the patients while sustaining vital functions
5. Treatment of the patients in the hospital emergency unit
6. Treatment in the OR
7. Treatment in the ICU
8. Training of emergency medical personnel
9. Organization including communication and transport of the emergency patient to the appropriate hospital
10. Research and quality assurance

Table 2.2. Requirements for a qualified system of care

1. Trained and ready to help laypersons
2. Rapid alert system, including a uniform emergency telephone number
3. Integrated dispatch system
4. Short delays (intervals without treatment)
5. Physician-guided care for all patients
6. Management of patients in mass casualty situations according to emergency medicine criteria

Time Intervals in the Chain of Survival

Until a few years ago, the interval from receipt of an emergency call at the dispatch centre to the arrival of the first ambulance at the scene was considered as **the** quality criterion of prehospital emergency medicine. Recently, however, the term »interval to treatment« was introduced. It describes the interval from the emergency event to the start of qualified medical care.

Uniformity of the nomenclature was achieved by the Utstein conferences, e.g. the term »times« was replaced by the term »intervals«, etc. (◘ Figs. 2.60 and 2.61) [8, 18, 19].

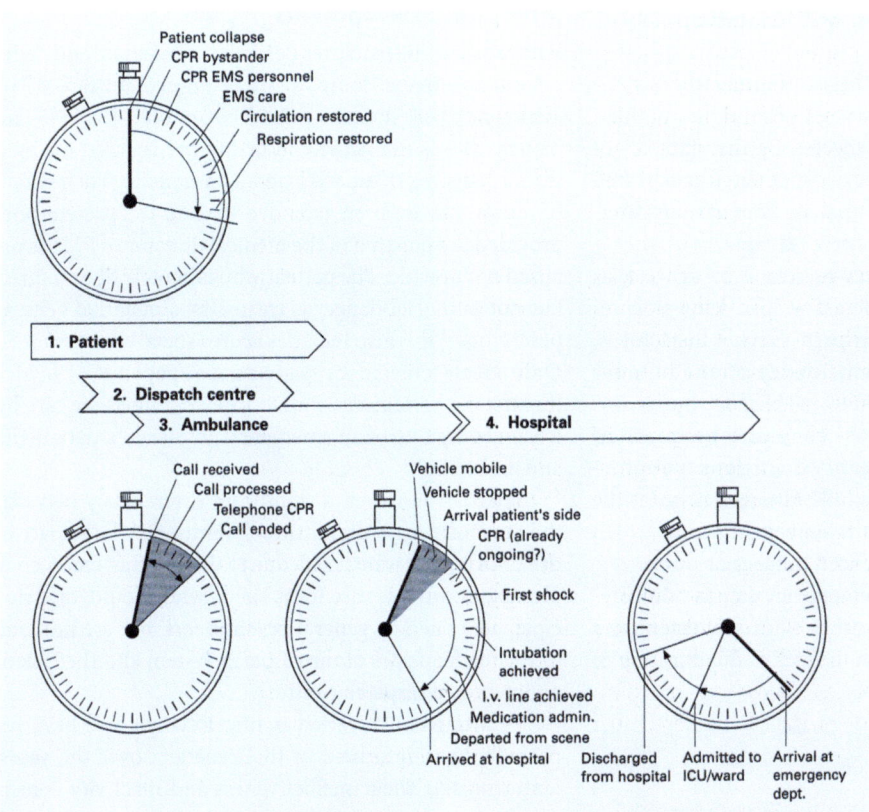

◘ **Fig. 2.60.** The four clocks of sudden cardiac arrest

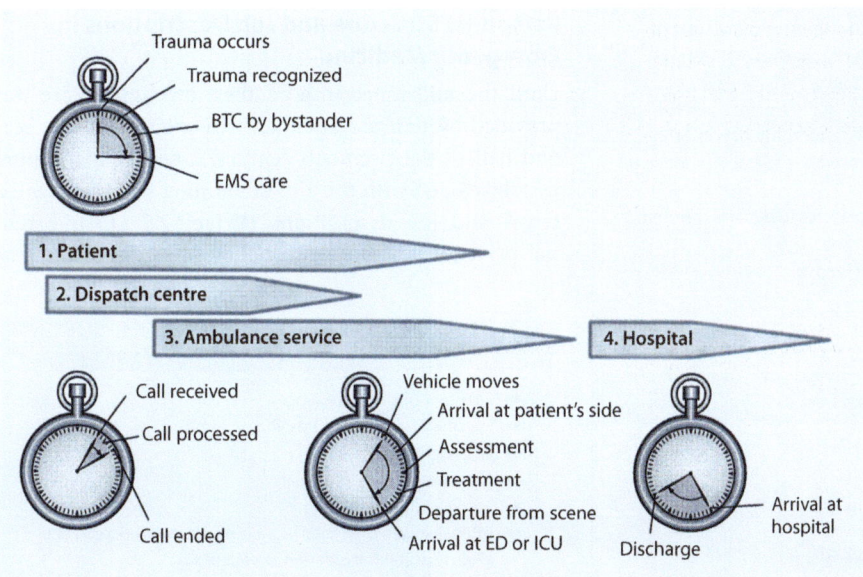

◘ **Fig. 2.61.** The four clocks of trauma

Of equal significance to the »interval to treatment« is the »interval from the emergency event to arrival of the patient at the hospital (emergency unit)« (◘ Table 2.3).

In »Emergency medicine – history and current practice« [42] Safar notes that anaesthesia plays an important role in the concept of the chain of rescue (survival): »The realization of all these components could only be promoted by specialists in resuscitation and intensive care. In many European countries, only anaesthesiologists were equal to this task«.

Meanwhile the »chain of rescue (survival)« has developed into a multimodal concept enabling a multidisciplinary approach. This is reflected by the statistics of the Institute for Emergency Services of the German Red Cross (1995), showing that specialists from various disciplines now provide emergency care (◘ Table 2.4).

The chain of rescue is only as strong or as weak as each of its individual links. The first link, layperson resuscitation, works – at least in part – quite satisfactorily. The second link, a uniform emergency phone number (i.e. 112) has not yet been fully established, but is under preparation. The third link, early care by qualified EMTs, paramedics and emergency physicians is improving progressively. The weakest link, however, remains the diagnosis and treatment in the emergency unit, which is often provided by inexperienced trainees or nurses.

The result of prehospital emergency care is not infrequently counteracted by the care provided by emergency unit teams. This is due to both the lack of qualification of these staff members and the lack of a uniform structure of emergency units. Comparable to the standards of training for the team members of ambulances and MLSUs, the structure of emergency units as well as the qualification of the respective team members need to be defined and realized.

Structural Developments

Future-oriented structures designed to integrate and complete the different components of immediate care of an emergency patient were published in 1999 [3, 13]. The patient who is not acutely ill or injured is cared for by a team consisting of an EMT and a paramedic. Their scope of duties may even be extended beyond the present one, provided the position of the medical director of EMS is realized nationwide. The patient who is acutely ill or injured but not in mortal danger is treated by a qualified general practitioner; this also includes acute »social emergencies«. Only »real« emergency patients, i.e. patients with life-threatening conditions, should receive immediate care by a team consisting of an emergency physician, a paramedic and an EMT.

There is, however, a significant discrepancy between the current situation and these premises. A large part of the EMS budget is misused, due to the fact that emergency physicians provide care for patients who should, on principle, be treated by general practitioners, but are not, due to the inadequacies of the dispatch system and the lack of an integrated dispatch centre.

Politicians with varied political sympathies have repeatedly been informed of these matters over the years. Unfortunately their ineffectiveness and inactivity constitute the reasons for this misuse of the health care budget.

Personnel Structure and Job Descriptions in Emergency Medicine

Until the mid-nineteenth century, preclinical care was provided by first aid attendants (*Sanitäter*). In the second half of the twentieth century, a new nomenclature was developed with the aim of defining quality-oriented terms and job descriptions (◘ Table 2.5 [13]). Essential prerequisites for high quality emergency medicine

---

◘ Table 2.3. Relevant intervals in emergency medicine

- Interval from emergency event (e.g. collapse) to diagnosis of the emergency to start of first aid
- Interval from start of first aid (layperson) to emergency call
- Interval from call ended to vehicle moving
- Interval from vehicle moving to arrival at the scene
- Interval from arrival at the scene to arrival of the emergency team at the patient's side
- Interval from arrival of the team at the patient's side to initial measures(IV access, fluids, medication, intubation, others)
- Interval from end of initial procedures to stabilization (e.g. cardiovascular function)
- Interval from end of initial measures to departure from the scene
- Interval from departure from the scene to arrival at the hospital (emergency unit)

◘ Table 2.4. Specialities of emergency physicians

5,500	anaesthesia
5,000	surgery
5,000	internal medicine
1,200	general practice
400–500	paediatrics/gynaecology

◘ Table 2.5. Job descriptions of EMS personnel

- EMT (6 months of training)
- Paramedic (2 years of training)
- Emergency physician
- Chief emergency physician
- Medical director of EMS
- Intensive care physician in training for intra-hospital and inter-hospital transfer of ICU patients

are undergraduate, postgraduate and continuing medical training programmes. Training of EMTs, and later that of paramedics, as well as postgraduate training of emergency physicians has proved extremely difficult to promote and realize. The curriculum of EMTs previously consisted of a 6-month training course, which was divided into an EMS and a hospital training period. Based upon this curriculum, a 2-year programme was designed for a professional group with the separate job description of paramedic. However, extended transition periods led to significant differences in the level of training achieved by paramedics and those EMTs who had worked in this function for a long period before being promoted to the status of paramedic. The new paramedics were thus characterized by significantly different levels of training. The development of privately organized training programmes which meet only minimal standards of training further aggravated the situation. Even today, despite yearlong efforts, a third year of training for paramedics has not yet been made mandatory, despite the fact that the »Standing Conference on EMS« unanimously called for this additional year of training:

> A third year of training is essential, because practical training needs to be improved and more practical experience is requisite. Those aspects of the 2-year training programme need to be intensified which have not been taught adequately. Aspects of techniques, tactics as well as co-operation with other organizations need to be made an integral of the programme. Comprehensive training in mass disaster situations is urgently required.

Additional qualifications are required for dispatch paramedics, paramedics escorting ICU patients during transfer from one hospital to another, etc.

The discussion on an intensified training programme for emergency physicians has been similarly difficult [13, 14]. The draft curriculum presented at the 1980 congress of anaesthetists met with harsh criticism and subsequent rejection. It was the German Interdisciplinary Association of Critical Care Medicine (DIVI) that, 20 years later, pushed the essentials of the programme through the different State Chambers of Physicians and the German Medical Association [»Qualifications of emergency physicians« (1990) and »Supraspecialty status in emergency and disaster medicine« (1995)]. Even at that time (1995), hospital and health insurance administrators frequently refused to recognize that minimum quality requirements need to be met by their emergency physicians. Against this background, representatives of foreign EMS repeatedly made the claim that Germany does not meet international standards of EMS care.

One problem in this regard should indeed not be overlooked: emergency physicians from different specialties who are integrated into the EMS are characterized by different quality standards, due to the fact that the number of cases they have covered in their daily practical work varies considerably.

Today, however, minimum standards for emergency physicians (1995) and/or uniform requirements for supraspecialty status in emergency and disaster medicine are compulsory. Chief emergency physicians need to obtain recognition as emergency physicians and have to undergo a special training programme for chief emergency physicians. Medical directors of dispatch centres also have to meet the respective criteria. Medical directors of EMS have to fulfil the following requirements: recognition as emergency physician and continuous practical activities, recognition as chief emergency physician, extensive theoretical, practical and administrative experience, including management activities, and experience gained in leadership positions.

A relatively new qualification, i.e. physicians qualified in the transport of intensive care patients, was introduced in 1998 [13]. The prerequisites include 3 years of clinical training in a specialty that includes intensive care as part of its remit, plus 6 months of documented full-time work in an intensive care unit, in addition, a certificate of competence in the emergency services, or in emergency medicine, as well as a 20-h course in intensive care patient transport.

Emergency Medical Services

The organization of emergency medical services (EMS) in Germany has been decisively shaped by the standards set by the occupying forces immediately after the Second World War (e.g. USA, 1948). Differences in emergency legislation still in effect today in a number of Federal States are accounted for by these regulations. Thus, in northern Germany the EMSs are dominated by fire departments and in southern Germany by Red Cross organizations. St. John's Ambulance Service or the Maltese Rescue Service (MHD) and Worker's Samaritan League (ASB) are responsible for patient emergency care. Emergency care in the former German Democratic Republic was provided by the »Immediate Medical Care« and was formally organized as the »Rapid Medical Response System« (SMH) after 1976.

The above-mentioned organizations have contributed substantially to the progress of emergency medicine in Germany, and many of their representatives have been enthusiastically involved in their work over many years. All of these organizations are guided by well-known anaesthesiologists, e.g. the German Red Cross (Ahnefeld), the Bavarian Red Cross (Sefrin), the Maltese Rescue Service (Schüttler), the Workers' Samaritan League (Bartels), the German Fire Fighting Services (Sefrin, Stratmann) and the German Water Rescue Service (Jost).

A great number of additional societies, associations, conferences, etc. are involved in the promotion of emergency medicine, e.g. the Committee of First Aid and Resuscitation of the German Medical Association and similar committees at the regional level, the German Resuscitation Council, the Association of Emergency Physicians of Germany (BAND) and its regional branches, the German Interdisciplinary Association of Critical Care Medicine (DIVI), Section of Emergency and Disaster Medicine, the Federal Committee of First Aid of the EMSS, the Committee of Emergency Services of the Federal Government, the Standing Conference of Disaster Medicine, the Conference of Federal Health Ministers, etc.

The Standing Conference of Emergency Services was initiated in 1996 by W. Dick and formally founded in Bonn. The following organizations are represented: the Workers' Samaritan League, the German Water Rescue Service (DLRG), the German Red Cross (DRK), St. John's Ambulance Service, Maltese Rescue Service, BAND (National Association of Emergency Physicians), the German Heart Foundation, the Professional Association of EMSs, various insurance companies (AOK, VDAK/AEV), the German Automobile Club, Convention of Municipal Authorities, Federal Committee of EMSS, the German Medical Association, the Federal Institute of Highways and Roads, the German Hospital Federation, the Working Group on Emergency Services (Munich), the professional associations BKS, DRF and a large number of renowned emergency physicians and researchers.

Change of the Emergency Disease Spectrum

Over the past years there has been a far-reaching change in the spectrum of diseases and injuries in emergency medicine, which was initially dominated by resuscitation and trauma care. Today, more complex clinical pictures, the »golden hour diseases«, require a short interval to treatment to avert an unfavourable outcome (◘ Table 2.6).

The cited incidence of these emergencies is based on figures provided by the EMS of the University Hospital in Mainz (◘ Table 2.7).

Results obtained in previous studies by Moecke et al. [38] demonstrate that the majority of emergency physicians rate themselves as competent in performing routine procedures, while diagnostic and therapeutic measures in infants and children are felt to require special training programmes and expertise to be adequately performed. Recent data reported by Finteis et al. [24] may serve to explain the above situation: e.g. the average emergency physician practising EM in rural areas is required to perform endotracheal intubation only 1.7 times/year, a figure which ranges significantly below the minimum requirements outlined by the International Liaison Committee on Resuscitation (ILCOR). Only a small number

◘ **Table 2.6.** Golden hour diseases

Emergency situation	Time window	Treatment
Cardiac arrest	3–5 min	CPR/Defibrillation
Polytrauma	30–(60) min	Shock therapy/O_2 [44] Analgesia/ventilation
Acute myocardial infarction	1–2 h	Medication/analgesia [36, 46]
Stroke	1–2 h	Thrombolysis/O_2 Where necessary O_2/medication Normoglycaemia Where necessary thrombolysis

◘ **Table 2.7.** Operations of the MLSU Mainz in 2000 ($n = 4,074$)

Cardiovascular emergencies	44.0%
Central nervous system emergencies	18.4%
Respiratory emergencies	11.3%
Trauma	6.0%
Metabolic emergencies	4.7%
Intoxications	4.3%
Abdominal emergencies	4.2%
Paediatric emergencies	1.3%
Gynaecological/obstetric emergencies	6.0%
Others	5.2%

of emergency physicians practising in rural areas achieve the number of procedures recommended by the ILCOR, while the uniform curriculum of the Federal and State Medical Associations requires the performance of a substantially larger number of procedures.

2.3.4 Undergraduate Teaching in Emergency Medicine

Representation of emergency medicine in the undergraduate medical curriculum is relatively new. Correlated with the high input of anaesthesiology into »medical first aid«, »emergency medicine«, and »hands-on« practical training programmes is the availability of sufficient personnel in research and training. Thus, the number of posts for research and teaching may range from 14 – if high input into undergraduate teaching is provided – to merely 1 – if only basic teaching is supplied. The number of available posts for scientific personnel involved in research projects varies accordingly. The recent amendment to the medical curriculum incorporates the concept of case-orientated multidisciplinary teaching and training of medical students. This represents a tremendous improvement in the provision of both basic theoretical knowledge and practical skills.

2.3.5 Science and Research

It is essential to base the concept of emergency disease management upon scientific evidence in order to meet current resource requirements. However, the results of only a small number of studies on the efficacy and effectiveness of the outlined concept are available to date [15, 17]. For example, it has not yet been scientifically proven by randomized controlled studies whether the prehospital physician-guided »Franco-German« emergency medical system (Germany, France) is superior to the paramedic-guided »Anglo-American« prehospital system, where the patient receives definitive care in the hospital emergency unit.

The cost-effectiveness ratio, incidentally, has not yet been put to the question for either system. Unfortunately, randomized controlled trials comparing both systems are considered to be unethical, impractical and medically impossible in Germany. Although, even from a scientific point of view, the designs of similar studies are somewhat limited [31], even trials based on uniform outcome criteria and definitions of medical emergencies and their treatment concepts are doomed to failure. It is hoped that consideration of the six »outcome *D*'s« (◘ Table 2.8), i.e. outcome criteria following trauma and resuscitation recently described by Cone [10], will lead to an improvement of this situation.

The Mainz Emergency Evaluation Score (MEES) has been found useful in the assessment of the efficacy of prehospital treatment as it enables the comparison of data collected at the scene and upon arrival at the hospital emergency unit [29].

Prehospital Trauma Care and the »Golden Hour Concept«

Anyone attempting to discover how the »golden hour concept« was developed and if the concept is scientifically proven and evidence-based will come across a publication by Lerner and Moscaty [35]. The authors failed to find an accurate definition of the term golden hour in their review of the literature including, e.g. the publications of Trunkey [49, 50], who mentions a period of 4 h as critical in patients with craniocerebral trauma and of 20 min for those suffering from haemorrhage. They found the first

◘ Table 2.8. The six outcome *D*'s (after [52])

Death

Disease: symptom complex, physical signs, abnormal laboratory findings or illness as experienced by the patient

Discomfort: reduced quality of life, symptoms such as pain, nausea, vomiting, dyspnoea, itching and tinnitus

Disability: reduced capacity to carry out general daily activities in the home or at the place of work

Dissatisfaction: discontentment with the situation, emotional reaction to illness and treatment modalities such as sadness or anger

Destitution: financial impact of the illness on the individual patient or society.

mention of the »golden hour concept« in a publication by A. Cowley, although Cowley [11] himself refers to an article by Foster, who states that mortality following trauma increases threefold every 30 min if it remains untreated. Foster, in turn, quotes an article by Baker in *Medical World News* as the source for this correlation, even though Baker himself did not provide any indication of his source. While authorship has to ultimately be assigned to A. Cowley, this remains without definite proof of the background for the new terminology.

Cowley first used the term »golden hour« in an article published in 1976, where he described the Maryland Trauma System and concluded that the first 60 min following trauma are decisive for patient outcome. Cowley concedes, however, that there is no scientific proof for these figures. The conclusion reached by Lerner and Moscaty therefore is that even today there are no major controlled studies in large patient populations to prove the concept of the »golden hour«. This means that the interval from trauma to immediate care which decides on the patient's outcome remains a moot point.

Fluid Replacement and Trauma Care

Until recently, the standard of care postulated that each trauma patient should undergo aggressive fluid therapy. Various animal experiments and clinical studies have, however, demonstrated that a number of experimental prerequisites of this concept were improbable. While these experiments are based on the assumption that the underlying condition is controlled haemorrhagic shock, the patient with severe trauma is, in fact, subject to uncontrolled shock conditions. Experiments taking this factor into consideration show that aggressive fluid treatment counteracts the mechanisms capable of controlling blood loss (e.g. coagulation, decreased blood pressure, etc.) [7]. Today, the number of arguments in favour of abandoning aggressive shock treatment is increasing. Small volume resuscitation (hypertonic/hyperoncotic solutions) and permissive hypotension are recommended instead, especially in patients with penetrating trauma [33, 34, 43, 51]. In fact, Svenson and Hahn [47] have stated that traditional aggressive shock treatment has to be viewed as medical history and is no longer justified due to a lack of scientific evidence proving a mortality-reducing effect of the treatment. Furthermore, there is no conclusive evidence in support of the use of a specific fluid or colloid. The results of a systematic review of randomized trials in the *British Medical Journal* [43] suggest that shock treatment using colloids may be responsible for an increase in the mortality rate of 4%, i.e. 4 additional deaths per 100 patients. The authors therefore conclude that the use of colloids in the treatment of haemorrhagic shock is no longer justified.

Cardiopulmonary Resuscitation

Several years ago, the Resuscitation Research Committee of the **European Academy of Anaesthesiology (EAA)** was founded in Mainz (Germany). This committee presented recommendations for both the standardization of animal experiments in CPR research and the standardization of clinical CPR research [22, 23]. A number of researchers on this committee were later actively involved in the foundation of the **European Resuscitation Council (ERC)**, which – on the basis of the above-mentioned publications (EAA) – came forward with the »Utstein Style« recommendations on CPR research. These recommendations for uniform documentation and coding are essential prerequisites of current CPR research [8, 25]. A comparison of outcome data following CPR obtained by selected German centres [30] shows survival rates from 10 to 20% in witnessed cardiac arrest or VF/VT, respectively, which is comparable to data reported by Anglo-American studies. It is common knowledge today that CPR needs to be started as soon as possible following cardiac arrest. The efforts to introduce a concept of CPR initiated by lay bystanders (developed in the 1980s by Kettler and Bahr, Göttingen) have not yet been realized. Unfortunately, governmental support of extensive training programmes, in particular for schoolchildren, is still insufficient.

Although didactically valuable, the statement that mortality following VF/VT increases by 5% every minute in the absence of treatment has not been confirmed by »hard« data. Until recently, it has been postulated that initial defibrillation might be superior to CPR followed by defibrillation in VF/VT [37]. However, the Seattle group [9] and other researchers have shown that in cases of an interval of more than 4 min from VF/VT to initial first aid, mechanical CPR should be carried out in a first step to be followed by defibrillation. This recommendation is supported by hard data recently published by a number of multicentre studies. Results obtained by the ORCA Study [45] have, unfortunately, not confirmed the superiority of biphasic over monophasic defibrillation with respect to outcome, due to an insufficient number of patients included in the study. Only the initial efficacy of biphasic defibrillation was shown to be significantly superior to the efficacy of monophasic defibrillation. Surprisingly, extensive research efforts of the past have not succeeded in solving the most basic problems: the scientific discussion is still ongoing, although on a higher level. The CPR guidelines need to be modified after a minimum period of 5 years. The most important questions, however, are those related to outcome. The studies required to answer these questions can only by performed on the basis of large prospective randomized controlled multicentre trials including thousands of patients. A prerequisite for these studies remains the availability of sufficient financial support.

Research Funding

In an editorial in the journal *Resuscitation* Ornato [40] writes that in the US – and this also applies to Europe – only limited amounts of money are invested into resuscitation research, currently approximately US $10 million/year. This is independent of the fact that in the USA 200,000–300,000 people die from cardiovascular diseases every year. Considering that a total amount of US $18 billion is spent on research in the USA annually, this means that only 0.1% of public research funding is made available for resuscitation research. Ornato nevertheless believes that a renaissance of prehospital research is forthcoming in the USA.

In Germany, resuscitation research can also be regarded as a stepchild of public research funding (German Research Foundation, Ministry of Research, European Community, etc.). Even pharmaceutical companies are only infrequently interested in funding resuscitation research because drugs for CPR rarely hold the promise of large revenues. A further obstacle to obtaining funding is the »criminalization« of raising »soft« research money in this country. The consequences of this were and still are that considerable sums of research money flow into other countries. Only 6% of all studies carried out in Germany are clinical studies compared to 18% in the UK.

On occasion, a consequence of research support of clinical studies by the respective industries has been that not all results were published (especially those with negative results). This was e.g. the case for the ERNST Study (European Resuscitation Nimodipine Study). The described »**conflict of interest**« can have a devastating effect on the »research landscape«, especially if meta-analyses are later carried out without consideration of previously obtained negative results, simply due to their »prospective unavailability«. All study protocols must therefore be submitted to an ethics committee, and the publication of all results, be they positive or negative, has to be made compulsory.

A special problem for prehospital emergency medicine investigations is created by the fact that e.g. studies comparing different resuscitation techniques with the primary endpoint of return of spontaneous circulation (ROSC) require 1,200–1,500 patients per group (e.g. the Vasopressin Trial). Studies comparing 1-year survival after cardiac arrest as the outcome criterion in patients undergoing treatment with two different strategies require approximately 8,000 patients per group.

Publications Relevant to Emergency Medicine

In 1995, Gervais and Hiller [27] carried out an analysis of international journals relevant to emergency medicine which have been published in Europe, the USA and Canada (◘ Table 2.9). Until only recently, journals relevant to emergency medicine (even English-language ones) were characterized by low impact factors (*Annals of Emergency Medicine*). This has, however, led the Institute for Scientific Information to introduce a separate category »critical care medicine« with its own impact factors.

◘ **Table 2.9.** Publications relevant to emergency medicine. Impact factors (in parentheses) shown are those cited in the ISC 2000 [27]

German-language publications:	*Anaesthesist* (0.7)
	Intensiv- und Notfallmedizin
	Notarzt
	Notfallmedizin
	Notfall & Rettungsmedizin
	Unfallchirurg (0.67)
English-language publications:	*Academic Emergency Medicine* (1.74)
	American Journal of Emergency Medicine (0.94)
	Annals of Emergency Medicine (1.86)
	Circulation (9.76)
	Critical Care Medicine (3.98)
	European Journal of Emergency Medicine
	Intensive Care Medicine (2.4)
	Journal of Trauma (1.75)
	Prehospital Disaster Medicine
	Resuscitation (1.82)
	Trauma Care (ITACCS)

2.3.6 Ethical Aspects of Emergency Medicine

Emergency medicine and especially prehospital emergency medicine is characterized by a number of uncertainties. While emergency medicine requires the immediate initiation of life-saving measures on the one hand, these may severely reduce the patient's quality of life on the other hand. Patients increasingly want to express their wishes, in particular with respect to medical treatment in the presence of terminal illness. These wishes may not be in accordance with the plan of treatment decided upon by the team of doctors and nurses and may thus create considerable conflicts for the health care providers [32].

Furthermore, not all emergency therapies fulfil the criteria of evidence-based medicine. However, especially in emergency medicine, randomized controlled trials can only be planned and performed with great difficulties; this is due to the fact that these studies can only rarely be carried out with the patient's informed consent, and the possibility of study protocol violations needs to be dealt with more frequently than under conditions of in-hospital evaluations. As a result, the performance of prehospital trials was impossible for a number of years in the USA. Similar developments are to be feared in Germany (in particular with a view to the introduction of the new »medical drug legislation«). The conditions under which pre-hospital trials are performed may thus become increasingly difficult in the future. The same is to

be expected for the initiation and termination of resuscitation measures.

With respect to the initiation of CPR, AHA/ILCOR Guidelines 2000 [32] state that reliable criteria to predict outcome following CPR are non-existent. Thus, all patients with unexpected cardiac arrest should be resuscitated, provided no patient declaration prohibiting those measures is available, no definitive signs of death are detected or the presence of progressive diseases (septic or cardiogenic shock) which may be a cause of cardiac arrest can be excluded. The guidelines further suggest a time window of 30 min [from initiation of advanced cardiac life support (ALCS) to return of spontaneous circulation (ROSC)] for the decision to continue or terminate CPR. If ROSC is observed within 30 min, CPR should be continued.

This proposal is supported by results of a retrospective analysis by Aufderheide et al. [52] in 6,235 patients with either unwitnessed cardiac arrest or cardiac arrest without bystander CPR. The researchers found a survival rate of 2.3% in these patients and noted that 18% of these 2.3% (i.e. 15 patients) survived with an acceptable neurological outcome. Based on these figures the authors calculated a probability of acceptable qualified survival of 1% in the group of patients below 70 years of age with cardiac arrest under the conditions outlined above. Although the described criteria for decision-making in patients with acute cardiac arrest may serve as a guide for ethical considerations in patients with other clinical pictures, they also demonstrate the limits for decision-making in general.

2.3.7 Outlook

Emergency medicine in Germany has been promoted and developed thanks to the commitment of respected emergency physicians, politicians and public health officials. While German emergency medicine is regarded as exemplary in many countries, at the beginning of the third millennium it is also characterized by a great number of problems and deficits. These deficits are of a historical or political nature, or they may be matters of principle.

The deficits related to matters of principle are as follows:

- Numerous diagnostic and therapeutic criteria of EM are not evidence-based.
- Over the past 25 years the overall survival rate following cardiac arrest and CPR has remained low, despite significant advances and considerable research activities (VF/VT).
- Principles of optimum trauma care continue to be controversially discussed.
- Modern methods of basic research (molecular biology, etc.) are introduced only gradually into emergency medicine research.
- Urgently needed multicentre research projects are rare or slow in being realized.

Deficits of a political nature include:

- Lack of a uniform emergency phone number
- Lack of integrated dispatch centres
- Lack of a uniform definition of the initial interval to therapy
- Deficits in training programmes for paramedics
- Deficits in establishing the concept of »medical director of EMS«
- Lack of integration of EMS and emergency departments
- Lack of investment into emergency and disaster medicine by government health care programmes

It appears that only »events« such as 11 September 2001 can convince incognizant politicians to become acutely aware of the need for action. It is therefore up to us, anaesthesiologists involved in emergency medicine, to advance EBM concepts for the most important emergencies, as well as to develop therapeutic concepts for all relevant emergencies (ILCOR). In addition, emergency medicine has to identify and to determine those areas which are still characterized by methods, procedures, medications and concepts in need of scientific proof. »The introduction of a scientific approach into the art of emergency medicine« is of importance for the future of our specialty. This path needs to be followed with determination, and reductionistic tendencies have to be counteracted. It is both our responsibility and that of politicians to maintain current as well as to develop new prerequisites for this task.

References

1. Ahnefeld FW, Schröder E (1966) Die Vorbereitungen für den Katastrophenfall aus ärztlicher Sicht (Rettungskette). Med Hyg 24:1084
2. Ahnefeld FW (1991) Notfallmedizin und Rettungsdienst – Ein Rück- und Ausblick. In: Ahnefeld FW, Brandt L, Safar P (eds) Notfallmedizin – Historisches und Aktuelles. Laerdal
3. Ahnefeld FW, Dick W, Knuth P, Schuster HP (1998) Grundsatzpapier Rettungsdienst. Notfall Rettungsmed 1:68–74
4. Baskett PJF (2001) Peter J Safar, the early years 1924–1961; the birth of CPR. Resuscitation 50:17–22
5. Bauer KH (1958) Erste chirurgische Hilfe am Unfallort bei Verkehrsunfällen. Monatsschr Unfallheilk 56:137
6. Beyer CW, Dick WF (2001) Johann Friedrich von Esmarch – a pioneer in the field of emergency and disaster medicine. Resuscitation 50:131–134
7. Bickel WH (1993) Are victims of injury sometimes victimized by attempts at fluid resuscitation? Ann Emerg Med 22:225–226
8. Chamberlain D, Cummins R, Eisenberg M et al (1991) Resuscitation, recommended guidelines for uniform reporting of data from out-of-hospital cardiac arrest: the Utstein Style. Resuscitation 22:1–26
9. Cobb LA, Fahrenbruch CE, Walsh TR, Copas MK, Olsufka M, Breskin M, Hallstrom AP (1999) Influence of cardiopulmonary resuscitation prior to defibrillation in patients with out-of-hospital ventricular fibrillation. JAMA 281:1182–1188
10. Cone DC (2000) Outcomes research and emergency medical services: the time has come. Acad Emerg Med 7:188–191
11. Cowley RA (1975) A total emergency medical system for the state of Maryland. Md State Med J 24:37–45
12. Davis JE, Sternbach GL, Varon J, Froman Jr RE (2000) Paracelsus and mechanical ventilation. Resuscitation 47:3–5
13. Deutsche Interdisziplinäre Vereinigung für Intensiv- und Notfallmedizin (DIVI) (2000) Stellungnahmen, Empfehlungen zu Problemen der Intensiv- und Notfallmedizin, 4th edn
14. Dick W (1980) Qualifikation des Notarztes. Anästhesiol Intensivmed 21:257
15. Dick W (1991) Probleme in der notfallmedizinischen Forschung. Notfallmedizin 17:538–549
16. Dick WF (1994) Friedrich Wilhelm Ahnefeld Citation for Honorary Membership of the ERC. Resuscitation 28:179–180
17. Dick W, Ahnefeld FW, Encke A, Schuster HP (1997) Für die Teilnehmer des Workshops Forschung und Ethik in der Notfallmedizin. Intensivmedizin 34:803–809
18. Dick WF (1997) Uniform reporting in resuscitation. Br J Anaesth 79:241–252
19. Dick WF, Baskett PJF and the Utstein group (1999) Recommendations for uniform reporting of data following trauma – the Utstein style. Resuscitation 42:81–100
20. Dick WF (2000) Friedrich Trendelenburg (1844–1924). Resuscitation 45:157–159
21. Dick WF (2001) Rudolf Frey (1917–1981). Resuscitation 51:109–112
22. European Academy of Anaesthesiology (1990) Animal research in CPR: revised version. Eur J Anaesthesiol 7:83–87
23. European Academy of Anaesthesiology (1991) Recommendations for clinical CPR research. Eur J Anaesthesiol 8:86–87
24. Finteis T, Genzwürker H, Seib H, Kern R, Ellinger K, Kuhnert-Frey B (2001) Intubationsinzidenz in einem ländlichen Notarztsystem. Anästhesiol Intensivmed 42:534 (4-U-42)

25. Fischer M, Fischer NJ, Schüttler J (1997) One-year survival after out-of-hospital cardiac arrest in Bonn city: outcome report according to the ‚Utstein style'. Resuscitation 33:233–243

26. Frey R (1978) The Club of Mainz for improved worldwide emergency and critical care medicine systems and disaster preparedness. Crit Care Med 6:389

27. Gervais HW, Hiller BK (1995) Vorstellung des internationalen, notfallmedizinisch relevanten Zeitschriftenspektrums und Ethik bei Autorenschaft und Publikation. Wien Klin Wochenschr 107(12):357–365

28. Gögler E (1991) Das Rettungswesen der 50er und 60er Jahre. In: Ahnefeld FW, Brandt L, Safar P (eds) Notfallmedizin – Historisches und Aktuelles, Laerdal

29. Hennes HJ, Reinhardt Th, Dick W (1992) Beurteilung des Notfallpatienten mit dem Mainzer Emergency Evaluation Score (MEES). Notfallmedizin 18:130

30. Herlitz J, Bahr J, Fischer M, Kuisma M, Lexow K, Thorgeirsson G (1999) Resuscitation in Europe: a tale of five European regions. Resuscitation 41:121–131

31. Holliman J (2000) International development of emergency medicine, lecture at the 1st International Congress of the Polish Society for Emergency Medicine: Emergency Medicine in Middle and Eastern Europe.: 13–16 September 2000, Wroclaw, Poland

32. International Guidelines 2000 for Cardiopulmonary Resuscitation and Emergency Cardiovascular Care: an International Consensus on Science. Resuscitation 46:1–448

33. Kreimeier U, Lackner C, Stolpe E, Peter K, Meßmer K (2001) Schocktherapie: Kann weniger mehr sein? Anästhesiol Intensivmed 42:366

34. Kwan I, Bunn F, Roberts I, on behalf of the Prehospital Trauma Care Steering Committee (2001) Timing and volume of fluid administration for patients with bleeding following trauma. Cochrane Library 8:1–16

35. Lerner EB, Moscaty RM (2001) The golden hour: scientific fact or medical »urban legend«? Acad Emerg Med 8:758–760

36. Martens U, Lange-Braun P, Langer R, Hochrein H (1987) Systemische Frühlyse des akuten Myokardinfarktes. Vergleich zwischen Klinik und Prähospitalphase. Dtsch Med Wochenschr 112:901–914

37. Mauer D, Schneider T, Diehl Ph, Dick W, Brehmer F, Juchems R, Kettler D, Kleine-Zander R, Klingler H, Rossi R, Schüttler J, Stratmann D, Strohmenger U, Zander J (1994) Erstdefibrillation durch Notärzte oder durch Rettungsassistenten? Eine prospektive, vergleichende Multicenterstudie bei außerklinisch auftretendem Kammerflimmern. Anaesthesist 43:36–49

38. Moecke HP, Moecke C (1993) Notarztqualifikation: Untersuchungen zur Strukturqualität im Rettungs-Dienst: Ergebnisse einer anonymen Umfrage. BAND 1993

39. Nolte H (1968) A new evaluatiuon of emergency methods for artificial ventilation. Acta Anaesthesiol Scand Suppl 29:111–125

40. Ornato JP (2001) Resuscitation on a golden anniversary: an American perspective (editorial).Resuscitation 50:15–16

41. Pantridge JF, Geddes JS (1967) A mobile intensive care unit in the management of myocardial infarction. Lancet 2:271–73

42. Safar P (1991) Aufbau einer Rettungskette und eines Rettungsdienstes – eine persönliche Geschichte In: Ahnefeld FW, Brandt L, Safar P (eds) Notfallmedizin – Historisches und Aktuelles. Laerdal, pp 47–54

43. Schierhout G, Roberts I (1998) Fluid resuscitation with colloid or crystalloid solutions in critically ill patients: a systematic review of randomised trials. BMJ 316:961–969

44. Schmidt U, Frame S, Nerlich M, Rowe D, Enderson B, Maull K, Tscherne H (1992) On-scene helicopter transport of patients with multiple injuries–comparison of a German and an American system. J Trauma 33:548–552

45. Schneider T for the Optimized Response to Cardiac Arrest (ORCA) Investigators (2000) Multicenter, randomized controlled trial of 150-J biphasic shocks compared with 200- to 360-J monoppahsic shocks in the resuscitation of out-of-hospital cardiac arrest victims. Circulation 102:1780–1787

46. Schröder R (1992) Ist die prästationäre Thrombolyse bei akutem Myokardinfarkt als Routinemaßnahme sinnvoll? Z Kardiol 81:199–204

47. Svenson CH, Hahn RG (2000) Prehospital fluid therapy. Curr Anaesth Crit Care 11:16–19

48. Thierbach A (2001) Franz Kuhn, his contribution to anaesthesia and emergency medicine. Resuscitation 48:193–197

49. Trunkey DD (1983) Trauma Sci Am 249:28

50. Trunkey DD (1984) Is ALS necessary for pre-hospital trauma care? (editorial). J Trauma 24:86

51. Vassar MJ, Perry CA, Gannaway WL et al (1991) 7.5% sodium chloride/dextran for resuscitation of trauma patients undergoing helicopter transport. Arch Surg 126:1065

52. Weil MH, Tang W (Organizers) (2001) The Sixth Wolf Creek Conference on CPR-Panel VIII. 4–7 June 2001, Palm Springs, CA

2.4   Pain Therapy

M. Zenz

The Beginnings

Alleviation of pain is without a doubt one of the first tasks of any doctor, and for this reason, has always been attempted irrespective of the specialization of the physician concerned. Pain management as an interdisciplinary task, as treatment of an independent illness, however, has developed only over the last few decades.

The origin of the international development of pain management can be traced back to the life's work of a single pioneer in the field of pain. Faced with the terrible injuries and the resulting pain suffered during the Korean War John J. Bonica began a research and investigation odyssey aimed at throwing light on the little-known subject of pain and its relief. His book »The Management of Pain« was published already in 1953 [3], at the end of the Korean War, and its 1500 pages bear witness to the depth and intensity of his work on all aspects of both chronic and acute pain. In 1960, he was appointed to the first Chair of Anesthesiology at the University of Washington in Seattle. This proved to be the starting point of the development of pain therapy and the establishment of national and international professional societies, as well as the further development of independent pain therapy units.

As dictated by the training, knowledge and skills of the anaesthetist in general, the fundamental tool of pain treatment was the nerve block. Bonica was very impressed by the successes achieved by this approach, in particular with the sympathetic blocks carried out on the Korean War victims with causalgia, and this therapy form long continued to dominate the minds of many anaesthetists.

As early as 1954, Bonica gave a lecture on the role of the anaesthetist in the treatment of chronic pain at the Congress of the Austrian Society of Anaesthesiology. Although he spoke about the central role of the nerve block, he also emphasized the fact that the final goal would be a holistic approach to pain management. Some of the keywords of Bonica's speech were: »Deep knowledge of the patient and his problem, ... neurological examination, ... rehabilitative measures, ... a lot of time and energy, ... specialist knowledge of pain mechanisms, ... experience in the general effects of pain...« [4].

He finished this paragraph by saying:

But if he (the anaesthetist) is that rare personality, who possesses these characteristics and on top of that the capability to withstand repeated demoralisation, then he is capable of taking over the complete therapy of a patient with unbearable pain.

Developments in Germany

The emphasis on regional anaesthetic techniques can also be found in some of the first German publications on the topic of pain, e.g. by Gerbershagen et al. [5] who wrote: »Between 1971 and 1973, in the Pain Clinic in Mainz, anaesthetists performed 5,655 nerve blocks on 834 patients.« Also addressed were the reasons for the disappointing results obtained in pain clinics, due in part to a »deficient knowledge of the mode of action of therapeutic regional anaesthetic techniques«. More than 35 years ago, Gerbershagen et al. not only emphasized the professional potentials of anaesthetists enabled through the use of nerve blocks for the diagnosis and treatment of pain, but also identified the problems and opportunities offered by further developments. Unfortunately, suggestions on how to increase the prestige of anaesthesiology by concentrating much more on pain management, and requiring all German-speaking anaesthetists and their professional associations to make every effort to achieve this aim went unheard at the time and for many years thereafter [5].

At the end of the 1960s, in Mainz, a number of dedicated anaesthetists who had either received part of their postgraduate education abroad (e.g. H.U. Gerbershagen, H. Nolte), or who had acquired more than one specialist qualification (e.g. H. Kreuscher), had gathered around the visionary and innovative Professor Rudolf Frey. Already in 1968 and 1969 in Rhineland Palatinate, H.U. Gerbershagen and H.A. Baar had begun to instruct anaesthetists in the use of anaesthetic techniques for the diagnosis and treatment of chronic pain. In 1969 the Social Insurance Board (LVA) in Rhineland Palatinate supported the establishment of therapy rooms and a documentation system at the Department of Anaesthesiology of the University of Mainz.

Eventually, in 1971, the first German Pain Clinic was set up at the University of Mainz. Multidisciplinary cooperation, pain conferences, interdisciplinary case presentations and CME courses were introduced. Since the establishment of the clinic triggered a first rush of patients that had to be coped with, Gerbershagen, Baar and Kreuscher developed the first German pain questionnaire containing 36 items. From 1972 onwards, lectures on pain therapy were offered. Also in 1972, the first interdisciplinary pain symposium on »Headache and facial pain« was organized by the Department. The great interest in issues of pain therapy was demonstrated by the fact that more than 1,000 participants attended.

Unfortunately, these exemplary beginnings of a qualified pain therapy in Germany long remained without significant follow-through. Although Kreuscher and Nolte, two former consultants from Mainz, soon founded pain clinics in their own hospitals in Osnabrück and Minden, university departments were very slow when it came to establishing pain therapy as an integral aspect of anaesthesiology. In the 1970s, the Departments of Anaesthesiology in Giessen, Göttingen, Bochum (Herne), Hannover (Oststadt Hospital of the Medical School) and Würzburg were among the first to incorporate pain therapy in their spectrum of activities.

In the early 1980s, spinal opioid analgesia gave a major impetus to the treatment of pain therapy in Germany. Fruitful competition between the Departments of Giessen and Hannover (H. Müller and M. Zenz) gave rise to numerous studies and resulted in cooperation in this area. Spinal opioid analgesia was the first generally successful anaesthesiological method for the treatment of acute (postoperative) pain and chronic (cancer) pain. Unlike the sympathetic block it was simple, could be taught and implemented in all relevant anaesthesia departments, and had a compellingly high success rate. From one day to the next it catapulted anaesthetists to a central and accepted leading role in the management of pain. Long-acting opioids had not yet been introduced, and the guidelines for the treatment of severe cancer pain were uniformly focussed on the administration of spinal opioids.

Institutionalisation

Very early on, in 1982, a pain therapy working group was set-up by the colleagues in the German Democratic Republic (GDR). In 1987, this group with its 117 members was incorporated in the specialist society. Due to leadership changes in the respective departments of most universities in the GDR, the actual beginnings of clinical pain therapy in the Medical Schools are now difficult to identify. What we do know of are the early beginnings at the Departments in Berlin (M. Tschirner) and Dresden (K. Siegismund).

In 1989, seven years after the setting-up of the working group in the GDR, a pain therapy working group of the German Society of Anaesthesiology and Intensive Care Medicine (DGAI) was established. The first speaker to be elected was G. Hempelmann (Giessen) who 2 years later was succeeded by M. Zenz (Bochum).

The result of a survey conducted in 1990 in co-operation with the DGAI proved disappointing [12]. Unfortunately, no East German University Department participated in the survey although the beginnings there had been worthy of a comment. Thirty-three Departments in the former Federal States of West Germany responded to the enquiry. In 31 of the 33 an anaesthesiologically managed pain therapy unit was available, 2 departments had no pain therapy unit, while 13 offered such a service for only a limited number of hours each day. 82% of the clinics had an anaesthetist whose sole task was pain management. Only 21 clinics offered lectures and seminars, 22 clinics carried out research into

pain. In 1990 the percentage of publications on the topic of pain in German-language journals was less than 7% of all anaesthetic papers – a very poor reflection of the representation of the specialty. The survey ended with an appeal to the German University Departments to prepare themselves thoroughly for the inclusion of the subject pain therapy in the state medical examination as of 1993 (see below).

The Professional Association of German Anaesthetists (BDA) agreed a number of resolutions on pain therapy. The first was a 1991 agreement with the Professional Association of Orthopaedic and Trauma Surgeons on interdisciplinary co-operation [2]. In 1993 the BDA came to an accord with the Professional Association of German Surgeons on the organization of postoperative pain therapy [1]. The fact that these agreements were adopted so late is witness to the hesitant approach of the professional organisations and associations to interdisciplinary co-operation in the domain of pain therapy.

CME, Postgraduate and Undergraduate Education

In 1992, prompted by the DGAI working group on pain therapy, Zenz initiated the first German refresher course on pain therapy in Bochum. This was one of the preconditions for the introduction in 1994 of »Qualified Education in Specific Pain Therapy« by the DGAI. Numerous colleagues acquired this DGAI certificate, and over 30 departments were accredited by the DGAI as training centres for specific pain therapy. In 1992 pain therapy had been included in the programme of training in anaesthesiology, at that time the only specialty with pain as a requirement of training.

Since 1993, pain therapy has been an integral part of the state medical examination. This development was initiated largely by H.F. Herget, an anaesthetist from Giessen. Ever since, anaesthetists have always been represented in the relevant committee of the Institute for Medical and Pharmaceutical Proficiency Assessment (IMPP). Unfortunately, subsequent revisions of the state examination regulations eliminated pain therapy from the list of compulsory subjects forming part of the examination.

In 1993, the anaesthetist M. Zenz and the pharmacologist I. Jurna brought out the first German textbook on pain therapy, and in 2001 a second edition was published [10]. In 1995 the first German handbook on pain therapy followed, which was to serve as a clinical guide and basis for the refresher course in Bochum. A third edition was published in 2007 [11].

In 1995, the German Interdisciplinary Association for Pain Therapy (DIVS) was founded in co-operation with the DGAI and with the support of Professor Walther Weißauer and modelled on the German Interdisciplinary

Association of Critical Care Medicine (DIVI). The neurologist D. Soyka (Kiel) was elected Founding President, and the anaesthetists M. Zenz and H.U. Hankemeier General Secretary and Treasurer, respectively. The DIVS imparted fundamental impulses to pain therapy. In co-operation with the German Society for the Study of Pain (DGSS) and the German Pain Association (STK) the ground was prepared for approval by the German Medical Assembly in 1996 of the subspecialisation »specific pain therapy«. The regulations applying to this subspecialisation are very similar to those of the 1994 DGAI certification. This, however, meant that the new qualification was open to all other medical specialties, which prompted (or should have prompted) action to defend the leading position of anaesthesiologists.

In 1997, the German Medical Association published an instruction book on specific pain therapy, which represented a cooperative effort by the DIVS and the anaesthetists in the DIVS. This served as a guide for the acquisition of special skills in pain management and was adopted by the majority of State Chambers of Physicians. Also in 1997, Guidelines for the Treatment of Acute Perioperative and Posttraumatic Pain were issued by the DGAI, the DIVS and the German Society of Surgery. The anaesthetists H. Wulf and C. Maier (Kiel) coauthored these recommendations. On the authorisation of the DIVS, the latest revised and updated version was published by Laubenthal et al. [8]. The presidents of the two major German pain societies, are both anaesthetists – H. Laubenthal (Bochum) is President of the DIVS and W. Koppert (Hannover) President of the DGSS.

After the beginnings in the 1970s and the period of spinal opioid analgesia in the 1980s, pain therapy played only a secondary role in academic medicine in Germany. Following the appointment of M. Zenz to Bochum in 1986 the first university chair was designated not merely »Chair of Anaesthesiology« but »Chair of Anaesthesiology, Intensive Care Medicine and Pain Therapy«. In 1989 a Professorship of Pain Therapy was created at the University of Göttingen, and was awarded to the anaesthetist J. Hildebrandt. At the end of the 1990s, a Professorship of Pain Therapy was created in Hamburg and awarded to H. Beck. In 1999 Klaschik in Bonn and Zenz in Bochum succeeded in establishing an endowed Professorship of Palliative Medicine and Pain Therapy sponsored by Mundipharma. E. Klaschik was appointed the first Professor of Palliative Medicine in Germany at the Faculty of Medicine of the University of Bonn. C. Maier from Kiel received an endowed professorship for pain therapy in Bochum. Other universities which made successful efforts to the same end were Kiel, Aachen, Cologne, Heidelberg and Erlangen.

Many major developments were initiated by anaesthetists. In 1986 Gerbershagen laid the foundations for internal and external quality assurance programmes, and made reference to Donabedian´s concept which, however, he failed to publish in an anaesthesia journal [6]. Gockel and Maier played a major role in the development of the documentation system for the pain therapy known as Quast [7]. Although numerous other examples could also be mentioned it must be admitted that support by the DGAI for the activities of anaesthetists in the field of pain medicine was not always optimal. To mention but one instance: the sole DGAI prize for research on pain therapy – the Carl-Ludwig-Schleich Prize – had not been awarded for a number of years until it was revived in 2002 through the committed efforts of H. Laubenthal with support from Janssen Cilag.

The situation of pain therapy in the Departments of Anaesthesiology at German universities has changed but little over the last ten years, and there are still University Departments without a pain clinic, and most do not have a pain therapy unit for inpatient care. Fewer than one half of the Departments have established scientific activities in the field of pain medicine. Just under 50% have a psychologist permanently attached to their pain clinics, and more than 50% regularly hold pain conferences. Only a minority of Departments offer lectures on pain management, and even fewer use the Quast documentation and quality assurance system developed by anaesthetists.

Future Prospects

In conclusion, it may be stated that, from the quantitative point of view, the position of pain medicine within the profession of anaesthesiology has not improved significantly over the last ten years. The quality of care and the multidisciplinary approach have certainly improved, but the involvement of anaesthetists in pain research and treatment still leaves much to be desired. Now that pain therapy has become an integral part of the state medical examination and with an eye to the future role of pain therapy in medical education and training, both teaching and research activities need to be improved. Since other specialties are increasingly concerning themselves with questions of pain medicine, anaesthesiologists should not simply abandon this field to others, but rather make every effort to maintain a leading role. This is not to argue against multidisciplinarity; but for actively preserving what has been achieved over 4 decades. For many years anaesthetists alone presented pregraduate teaching in pain therapy.

All the early institutions for pain therapy were set up by anaesthetists. Paralleling the situation in intensive care medicine the increasing interest in pain therapy being shown by other medical disciplines underlines the need for anaesthesiology to lay claim to this field. This applies with equal force to developments in the field of palliative medicine, where anaesthetists are beginning to be replaced by professors elected from other disciplines. The situation of pain therapy in anaesthesiology is internationally comparable, as noted by Sjøgren et al. in an editorial [9]:

> Concerning chronic pain, anaesthesiologists therefore find themselves at a crossroad. We may take the traditional road where acute pain (postoperative pain) is our mainstay, which probably will limit our future participation in and influence on the new area. Or we can choose another direction and become an active, well-educated and dynamic part of the multidisciplinarity around pain and pain treatment, enabling us to play a major role in the coming years.

It is thus essential that the University Departments of Anaesthesiology make it a top priority to achieve the highest standards of pain treatment based on training, research and continuous professional development. Pain medicine in all its facets, treatment of acute and chronic pain and palliative care, is a pillar of the specialty. It can only be powerful and stable when it has a solid basis in terms of personnel, research, lectures, space and time.

References

1. Berufsverband deutscher Anästhesisten und Berufsverband der deutschen Chirurgen (1993) Vereinbarung zur Organisation der postoperativen Schmerztherapie. Anästh Intensivmed 34:28–32
2. Berufsverband deutscher Anästhesisten und Berufsverband der Ärzte für Orthopädie (1991) Vereinbarung über die interdisziplinäre Zusammenarbeit in der Schmerztherapie. Anästh Intensivmed 32:93
3. Bonica JJ (1953) The management of pain, Lea & Febiger, Philadelphia, London
4. Bonica JJ (1955) Die Rolle des Anaesthesiologen bei der Behandlung schwerster Schmerzzustände. Anaesthesist 4:88-94
5. Gerbershagen HU, Magin F, Scholl W (1975) Die Schmerzklinik als neuer Aufgabenbereich für den Anästhesisten. Anästh Inform 16:41-44
6. Gerbershagen HU (1986) Organisierte Schmerzbehandlung. Internist 27:459-469
7. Gockel HH, Maier C (2000) Quast. Schmerz 14:401-415
8. Laubenthal H, Becker M, Sauerland S, Neugebauer E (eds) (2008) S3-Leitlinie Behandlung akuter perioperativer und posttraumatischer Schmerzen. Köln, Deutscher Ärzte-Verlag
9. Sjøgren P, Højsted J, Eriksen J (2001) The anaesthesiologist and chronic pain. Acta Anaesthesiol Scand 45:1057-1058
10. Zenz M, Jurna I (eds) (2001) Lehrbuch der Schmerztherapie, 2nd ed. Stuttgart, Wissenschaftliche Verlagsgesellschaft
11. Zenz M, Strumpf M, Willweber-Strumpf A (2007) Taschenbuch der Schmerztherapie, 3rd ed. Stuttgart, Wissenschaftliche Verlagsgesellschaft
12. Zenz M, Willweber-Strumpf A, Strumpf M, Mathei J (1991) Zukunftsperspektiven der Schmerztherapie. Anästh Intensivmed 32:348-353

2.5   A View of the Future of Anaesthesiology

J. Schüttler

The future often reveals itself through a look backwards at the past and an analysis of the present.

The classic roots of the scientific armamentarium of anaesthesia derive essentially from physiology and pharmacology, although in recent times this basis has greatly expanded through innovations in medicine and computer technology. The majority of today's chairs of anaesthesia, who have assumed the mantel of the earlier generation of pioneers, had their scientific baptism in the disciplines of physiology and pharmacology in their widest sense.

Through this development the research profile of our specialty has been indubitably strengthened over the last 10–15 years. In order to continue to compete among the wider spectrum of medical specialties however, further efforts are required.

To develop the future prospects of our specialty in research, teaching and hospital care, it would seem appropriate to cast a look backwards and to consider the situation on the 25th anniversary of the foundation of the German Society of Anaesthesiology and Intensive Care Medicine (DGAI).

Then, Karl-Heinz Weis in his presidential address [22] and Erich Rügheimer in his article »Future perspectives in anaesthesia – from narcosis to homeostasis« [15] constructed important concepts in terms of determining both a current position and a future perspective for the specialty. It may be extrapolated that: (1) technical advances and the establishment of clinical routine will permit a modification of the anaesthetists' view of his perceived role, (2) the increasing demands on our specialty will necessarily force significant increases in intensive clinical-scientific research and (3) the school of anaesthesia will mature alongside those of the classic disciplines [15].

The Current Position

With the first proposition, the already increasing significance of the anaesthetist in his key role in perioperative care was anticipated even then:

> Anaesthesiology … signifies today, and even more in the future: preoperative optimization of homeostasis through treatment of essential risk factors, minimizing surgery-associated disorders of homeostasis through selection of the anaesthetic technique … , continuous adaptation of the anaesthetic to the course of surgery … and postoperative recovery of homeostasis through intensive care [15].

It is therefore clear that the significance of the well-founded base of anaesthesia in the wider context of operative medicine was recognized in Germany long before so-called perioperative medicine was discovered by our colleagues in the USA [16]. In the future it will increase in significance if the economic orientation of health care delivery determines the scope of our medical activities on a much greater scale than at present. It therefore is of no consequence whether we see this as desirable from a medical point of view or not, since demographic developments [5] increasingly limit financing the realization of medical advances and compel us to deliver care in a manner which is mindful of the resource required. The discipline of anaesthesiology will be significantly affected if, for example, answers are to be found to the problems of whether and how extensively intensive medicine is to be applied to particular cohorts of patients and where in the future limits for what is both diagnostically meaningful and surgically feasible are to be drawn. Palliative medicine – the youngest discipline to which anaesthetists have brought their expertise, particularly in the treatment of chronic pain – will also have an increasing significance in this procedure with both socio-political and medico-ethical dimensions.

A further consideration with implications for the future relates to the value of modern medical technology in its application to monitoring.

> The rapid development of multidimensional, reliable sensors and of remote, miniaturized and inconceivably powerful processors will not make us the technicians among the physicians, but will give us the freedom to focus our attention not only on the patient's basic physiological parameters but also on his psychological needs [15].

With this assessment two elements were foreseen which have been confirmed by the current position and which in the future will increasingly determine our practice. First, extremely comprehensive monitoring which consists not only of highly developed components but also in the way in which the knowledge, the expertise and the evidence base of generations of anaesthetists are integrated – in other words the expansion of monitoring onto a higher plane.

Second, the focussing not only on basic physiological functions of the patient, but also on his psychological needs. This can be interpreted as an expansion of monitoring to encompass neuro-monitoring in its widest sense rather than the earlier limited cardiorespiratory monitoring, which includes the effects and after-effects of anaesthesia on cognitive and mental functions including the condition of the patient long after a given anaesthetic. At present genuine depth of anaesthesia monitoring as a clinical application is still at an early state of development which may soon be completed and will give the clinical anaesthetist a tool with which he may determine how effectively he has achieved his therapeutic target directly at the end organ in question. In a further step, the future developments will incorporate further insights into its relative value, e.g. of subliminal perception during anaesthesia and further differentiated effects of anaesthesia.

This development exists in a form of interaction between the paradigm change which has been taking place for the last 10 years or so, regarding the definition of depth of anaesthesia based on the MAC concept, which is based upon spinal reflexes, and the differential quantitative representation of anaesthetic effects on extremely diverse cerebral functions. Essential for this novel multi-faceted method of observation is also the fact that in the last decade the unitarian theory of anaesthesia, which was based on a single mechanism of anaesthesia at a single location, has been put to rest. Future anaesthetic treatment will therefore not consist of »giving an anaesthetic« but rather will concentrate on the optimal delivery of the various constituents of anaesthesia using differentially targeted agents.

The concept of homeostasis is being enlarged into what in my opinion is a more rigorous and satisfying form – by the increasingly complex performance of anaesthetists in their most basic primary role of removing stress and pain of the operation through sleep and targeted analgesia; thus the complete delivery of anaesthesia is more comprehensively achieved than before.

Anaesthesia is no longer considered merely as a one-dimensional »all or nothing phenomenon«, but rather must be understood as a differentiated, sophisticated and multifactorial event.

Anaesthetic Research

Nowadays, although we know about the existence of these highly complex processes, we have not yet understood them completely. This requires more targeted research efforts; 25 years ago the future of research was outlined as follows:

> Our research must not deceive through its breadth, rather it should convince through its depth…We need anaesthetists who research in physiology, in pharmacology and in immunology etc…and what to me alone is a guarantee of quality, they should present their results not only at anaesthetic congresses but they should present them to physiologists, pharmacologists and immunologists and there hold their ground [15].

Some years after this exhortation was made, our specialist society founded the scientific working conference of the DGAI in 1987, which subsequently took place in Würzburg at the start of each year. Dietrich Kettler (Göttingen) and Karl-Heinz Weis (Würzburg) were the joint founders of this well-established scientific body whose aim is the support of new scientific blood and the promotion of

anaesthetic science. They thereby created an important precondition for the targeted promotion of the necessary quality of research.

While in 1978 physiology and pharmacology, and in particular cardiovascular physiology and pharmacology, were both the important and essential pillars of anaesthetic research, with the expansion of the spectrum of scientific methodology towards molecular biological techniques in pharmacology, immunology and later physiology, there was a corresponding change of emphasis in research.

Worthy of mention in this regard are the new research tools (mainly of Anglo-American origin), which have been introduced by young anaesthetists who worked overseas. These young researchers from university departments have been supported in the main by research grants donated by the German Research Foundation (DFG).

After initial enthusiasm and considerable success using these methods to examine the smallest functional components, e.g. ion channels, receptors and other functional proteins, the recognition has begun to dawn that in anaesthesia it is necessary to learn to think in terms of networks (with other specialties) and that it is also necessary to understand these networks.

Parallel to this development is the above-mentioned paradigm change in the understanding of the mechanisms of anaesthesia. From this emerges, as a research consideration, the characterization of this complexity and to use or influence this mechanism using drugs in a differential therapeutic fashion.

This has empirically always been the case in clinical practice, although with a much more limited capacity for differential anaesthesia. The classic mono-anaesthetic agents have long been abandoned – thanks mainly to a highly sophisticated anaesthetic armamentarium – and are now able to provide highly differentiated therapy. The main problem confronting anaesthetic research – and here we must fall back on our own scientific achievements – is a quantitative system which guarantees an optimum balance in the pharmacological effects already known. What has been lacking until now is a differential quantitative concept which allows the individual components (e.g. GABA-, opioid-, NMDA-, central α_2 receptor-mediated function) to be used therapeutically in a patient-specific manner and in a way which can be adapted according to patient needs depending on feedback from indicators, which are yet to be defined and recognized, of each individual system.

Thus there is a wider opportunity for medical research in general, to make use of anaesthesia in terms of a model of induced, reversible, functional cerebral damage which can be utilized to develop treatments for the many neurological illnesses which are accompanied by cognitive impairment. Besides the cross-fertilization with other disciplines especially in the fields of neuroscientific research, it is for the specialty of anaesthesia of existential importance for the academic departments to establish research groups dealing with subjects which have wider clinical implications.

Only through setting up departments of anaesthetic research, i.e. experimental anaesthesiology, led by first-rate scientists, can wide-ranging research of the highest order be ensured in the future. This has been impressively demonstrated by the success of academic units of varying seniority.

The change in understanding of anaesthetic mechanisms and effects from a monocausal to multimodal basis will also have a direct effect on the research of pain therapy. The varying differential therapeutic loci for intra-operative pain relief have until now too few known overall effects on pain pathways and neuroplastic events. Herein lies the opportunity to direct prophylactic pain therapy not only towards the intraoperative and immediate postoperative periods but also towards the longer term.

Just as the driving forces directing research which are revealing causes and effects through consideration of bio-medical problems in anaesthesia, the advance of technology and its subsequent implementation in the operating theatre, in the intensive care unit and in the emergency department has opened up important medico-technological fields.

While the anaesthetists' area of activity has expanded more and more in the last 25 years from the head end of the patient into the general perioperative area, so too could the monitoring of the acutely ill patient in the operating theatre, intensive care or ambulance conceivably be extended to the monitoring of a seriously ill or incapacitated person in his own home environment.

The current discussion on telemedicine suggests that in the future anaesthesia will be able to contribute towards important research questions in this area. Anaesthetic care in the operating theatre, acute medical care in intensive care and in emergency medicine as well as postoperative pain therapy on the ward create an almost perfect environment for the exploration of teletherapeutic possibilities outside the hospital. These completely new and perhaps unusual concepts have already been touched upon in the Scandinavian countries [11].

Intensive Care Medicine, Emergency Medicine and Pain Management

In a similar vein to the proposition of Erich Rügheimer, Karl-Heinz Weis, in his presidential address on the 25th anniversary of the DGAI [22] demonstrated that one could regard especially intensive therapy, but even emergency medicine and pain therapy as a natural extension of the activity of the anaesthetist in the operating theatre.

In so doing, at this early juncture, the concept of the specialty of anaesthesia resting on four pillars was confirmed and further strengthened.

> …Thus today, general and regional anaesthesia can be described as a specific form of intensive therapy. The methods remain in principle the same. They vary in the application of medications, the use of equipment and most noticeably in the time span. An anaesthetic is counted in hours, intensive therapy rather in days, weeks, if not in months… [22].

In comparison to the considerations of Weis and Rügheimer, which ascribe to intensive care medicine the task of re-establishing and maintaining homeostasis, today's intensive therapy has become more complex. Beyond respiratory therapy, fluid maintenance and nutritional balance, the temporary replacement of virtually all vital organ function (heart, liver, lung, kidney) has moved to the forefront of intensive therapy. The complexity of the treatments using, for example cardiac assist devices, ECMO, MARS and other procedures, requires a considerable input from other specialties and has to that extent determined the current direction of research in intensive care. In view of the clinical research methods, intensive care assumes a unique position in relation to almost all other medical disciplines, since controlled clinical trials are not feasible in view of the diverse co-morbidities and the resulting therapeutic imperatives. Because of the high degree of interlinking of therapies, focussing a study on a particular therapeutic target is not practical, so that the predictive power of individual studies is difficult to determine. Some have voiced the opinion which predicts the end of the current experimental dogma of the double-blind, randomized, controlled clinical trial as the gold standard and herald the future as one of data mining in data warehouses [2]. Electronic data storage of ever greater amounts of medical data in dedicated structured files permits a systematic application of empirical knowledge for the improvement of treatment which stands in direct competition to or as an extension of the clinical trial. Necessary preconditions for this are corresponding monitoring with on-line data collection and the introduction of high-performance patient data management systems. The implementation of these systems both in the sphere of anaesthesia as well as in intensive therapy documentation will continue unchecked even if one considers that experience from recent years has dampened the initial enthusiasm. The necessity to create improved tools with modern programme structuring has been recognized and the corresponding effort to realize these goals has already been applied. Through this development so-called decision support systems have become a reality which allow both diagnosis and treatment to be made by physicians, overwhelmed by information, on a level which is both comprehensive and more rationally orientated.

A further consideration is that from the analysis of intensive care research in the context of surgical patients, only occasionally is the patient treated for a particular illness, but rather, in the main, organ function is supported for a given period of time. The highly complex sepsis syndrome is a typical exception of this. The scientific debate about this illness, which is still associated with a very high mortality, has in recent years generated a wealth of knowledge from the spheres of immunology, molecular biology and genetics. However, all attempts to ascribe a single aetiology to this condition have not met with success.

It has begun to emerge that just as anaesthesia has a multifactorial basis, so too would a therapy based upon diverse, interrelated factors offer the best chance of success. To evaluate this, multicentred research groups with first-rate treatment and research facilities at their disposal are required. With this in mind, the newly established Deutsche SepNet-Initiative (K. Reinhart, personal communication), which is supported by the Federal Ministry of Education and Research (BMBF), could be developed into a body comparable to established groups such as ARDSNet [6, 20].

Apart from the treatment of sepsis, the transient support of organ function and the classic task of maintenance of homeostasis, analgo-sedation of patients in intensive care has in recent years also attracted much interest. This is recognized as an important therapeutic measure to effectively counteract and prevent the psychological stress to which the patient is exposed as well as the consequences which may occur thereafter. Thus the innovative and organ-protective respiratory strategies which are directed towards independent respiratory function, and respiratory protection, have received considerable attention as a consequence of the alteration of the therapeutic objectives. The search for an optimum analgo-sedative for the patient undergoing intensive therapy leads one back to the question of the best combination of hypnotic and analgesic for each procedure in each respective patient.

This question is relevant for the entire field of perioperative pain control and has important implications beyond acute pain relief for the treatment of chronic pain conditions or those that are in the process of becoming chronic. This is an important area of research for the future which is apparent from the activity of different first-rate research initiatives (clinical research groups, Emmy-Noether Group and special research areas) of which the specialty of anaesthesia is an important part. From the investigation of the transition from acute pain to chronic pain, the facets of neuroplasticity, genetic predisposition and the genetic susceptibility of pain processing systems [13] as well as the connection with the psyche of the patient will in future play a significant role.

Teaching and Continuing Education

The position of anaesthesiology in undergraduate education was summarized on the occasion of the 25th anniversary of the specialist society [15] as follows: »… and in the long term we must strive for a change in the medical licensing regulations which should obligate every medical student to be taught by us« [15].

Since the 9th amendment of the medical licensure regulations was implemented, starting in the winter semester of 2003/2004, this demand has finally been fulfilled, since the specialty of anaesthesia is included in the compulsory group of academic subjects as an independent examinable discipline.

This fills us with satisfaction but entails a certain obligation. We must offer attractive undergraduate teaching in order to engender enthusiasm for our specialty from the very beginning. Until now this has been difficult in view of the issues of patient safety, given practicalities of teaching the specialty in both anaesthetic room and the operating theatre. For a number of years however, there has been the possibility of circumventing these handicaps through the use of patient simulators in the environment of an operating theatre. In the whole of medicine anaesthesia is currently at the forefront of teaching using realistic patient simulators in an authentic environment. The idea of the full-scale anaesthesia simulator dating from the 1960s was brought to a state of virtual perfection in Gainesville and Stanford and has found a place over the last 10 years in many teaching and academic centres, particularly in the universities. It has also found a foothold since 1995 in Germany with the first being introduced in Erlangen [17].

The specialty of anaesthesia could take advantage of the current favourable situation and reinforce its position in teaching not only in the sphere of emergency medicine but considerably expand its position as regards the teaching of anaesthesiology. Therein lies the opportunity to make anaesthesia more accessible by linking up with the basic sciences of physiology and pharmacology and thereby to contribute to a profound learning experience. This was shown in a pilot study involving more than 1,000 students to be highly successful and generated great interest in the practical (pre-reg) year and thereafter.

Anaesthetic simulators have a special significance not only for the teaching of undergraduates but have a role in filling the gaps in postgraduate and continuing medical education of the respective specialty, which until now could only be partially achieved using carefully devised, traditional systems. Simulators deal with the management of difficult situations including incidents and complications. The possible, reproducible and highly realistic involvement with anaesthetic emergencies leads through improved communication and better use of staff – i.e. crisis resource management (CRM) – to outstanding performance when confronted with an actual emergency. Herein lies the key for a long-term guarantee for the so-called high-level of anaesthesia safety (*Anästhesiesicherheit auf hohem Niveau*) [18]. It is still uncertain as to how this *Anästhesiesicherheit* can be precisely quantified. If one considers anaesthetic mortality which has dropped in the 50 years of the existence of our society from about 1:2000 to around 1:200,000, then there is difficulty with both the definition and the period of observation. In most publications there is a connection between anaesthetic-related mortality and the outcome of the patient. The latest research has been able to explain that in addition, the early recognition and the competent management of incidents definitely determine anaesthetic-related mortality [20]. The various closed claim studies from the Anglo-American sphere retrospectively supports this, whereby 80% of the deaths are classified as avoidable, that is, the human factor plays a significant role.

Those demands made 25 years ago on the subject of postgraduate and continuing education have been met – just as the pronouncements of the German Academy of Continuing Education in Anaesthesiology (DAAF). This organization which is supported by the DGAI and the Professional Association of German Anaesthetists (BDA) resolutely and single-mindedly pursues the goal of continuing postgraduate education in anaesthesia, intensive care and emergency medicine as well as pain therapy and thereby ensures, against the background of an explosion of medical information and knowledge, a life time of learning.

Therefore, only in this way can the future challenges to our discipline be met and thus we will be best placed to meet the threat of medical re-certification [1, 7].

Summary

If one considers an analysis of present and recent history and extrapolates to the future, then in the last 55 years from the subspecialty of anaesthesia has grown the discipline of anaesthesiology, a clinical discipline resting on four pillars with an independent school of teaching and a demanding research responsibility.

However, not all of these branches can claim to uniquely belong to anaesthesia, as intensive care and pain therapy continue to remain interdisciplinary areas, to which anaesthesiology can make important, specific contributions, if it succeeds in bringing broad-reaching, independently developed research results together with compatible treatment strategies.

The specialist society has been able to meet the increasing subspecialization with the implementation of ten clinically orientated working groups. Through this structure provisions have been made to maintain a united front but to encourage innovations on a subordinate basis. It should not be overlooked that much has been achieved through the close co-operation and an extremely smooth division of labour between specialist society and professional association – an alliance that will have pivotal significance for the fate of the specialty in the future.

References (selection)

1. Beschlüsse der 75. Gesundheitsministerkonferenz am 20./21.06. 2002 in Düsseldorf zur Rezertifizierung von Ärzten
2. Bothner U, Meissner FW (1999) Data Mining und Data Warehouse – Wissen aus medizinischen Datenbanken. Deutsch Ärztebl 96:A-1336–1338
3. Booij LH (2001) The future of anaesthesiology. Eur J Anaesthesiol 18:131–136
4. Cheney FW, Weiskopf RB (1999) The American Society of Anesthesiologists Closed Claims Project: what have we learned, how has it affected practice, and how will it affect practice in the future? Anesthesiology 91:552–556
5. Clade H (2002) Pflegeversicherung: Handlungsbedarf. Deutsch Ärztebl 99:A-1325
6. de Durante G, del Turco M, Rustichini L, Cosimini P, Giunta F, Hudson LD, Slutsky AS, Ranieri VM (2002) ARDSNet lower tidal volume ventilatory strategy may generate intrinsic positive end-expiratory pressure in patients with acute respiratory distress syndrome. Am J Respir Crit Care Med 165:1271–1274
7. Gerst T (2002) Rezertifizierung: Ärztlicher Kompetenzerhalt ist Sache der Selbstverwaltung. Deutsch Ärztebl 99:A-1940
8. Gisvold SE (1996) After 150 years of anaesthesia – it is time to expand. Acta Anaesthesiol Scand 40:1065–1067
9. Kochs E (2001) Entwicklungen und Perspektiven in der Anästhesie. In:. Kochs E, Krier C, Buzello W, Adams HA (eds) Anästhesiologie. Thieme, Stuttgart, pp 10–12
10. Lenis S (2000) What will be the function of an anesthesiologist in the new millenium? Can J Anaesth 47:1–4
11. Lindahl S (2000) Future anesthesiologists will be as much outside as inside operating theaters. Acta Anaesthesiol Scand 44:906–909
12. Longnecker DE (1997) Navigation in uncharted waters. Is anesthesiology on course for the 21st century? Anesthesiology 86:736–742
13. Mannion RJ, Woolf CJ (2000) Pain mechanisms and management: a central perspective. Clin J Pain 16 (3 Suppl):S144–S156
14. Raeder JC (2000) Anaesthesiology into the new millenium. Acta Anaesthesiol Scand 44:3–8
15. Rügheimer E (1978) Zukunftsperspektiven der Anästhesiologie – Vom Narkotiseur zum Homöostatiker. Anästhesiol Intensivmed 19:450–453
16. Saidman LJ (1995) The 33rd Rovenstine lecture: what I have learned from 9 years and 9000 papers. Anesthesiology 83:191–197
17. Schüttler J (1999) Training im Simulator – Spielerei oder unverzichtbare Komponente ärztlicher Lernprozesse? Anaesthesist 48:431–432
18. Schüttler J, Biermann E (2002) Der Narkosezwischenfall. Thieme, Stuttgart
19. Silber JH, Kennedy SK, Even-Shoshan O, Chen W, Koziol LF, Showan AM, Longnecker DE (2000) Anesthesiologist direction and patient outcomes. Anesthesiology 93:152–163
20. Slutsky AS, Ranieri VM (2000) Mechanical ventilation: lessons from the ARDSNet trial. Respir Res 1:73–77
21. Van Aken H, Gelb A (eds) (2002) Future of departments of anaesthesia. In: Best practice & research – clinical anaesthesiology 16. Elsvier, New York, p 2
22. Weis KH (1978) Ansprache des Präsidenten der DGAI zum 25jährigen Gründungsjubiläum. Anästhesiol Intensivmed 19:581–588

Establishment of Anaesthesiology in Germany

3.1. Specialization at the Universities as Exemplified by Anaesthesiology

Heike Petermann

Up until the middle of the twentieth century anaesthesia in Germany was nothing more than an aspect of surgery, and had not yet developed into a specialty and a profession in its own right. In Great Britain, in contrast, it had already evolved into an independent specialty between 1935 and 1948.

3.1.1 Medicine at Universities

Universities played an important role in the process of specialization in medicine. The first European universities were founded in the twelfth and thirteenth centuries – Bologna (1158), Oxford (1167), Paris (1200), Cambridge (1209), Montpellier (1181/1220) and Padua (1222). They were responsible not only for imparting to their students the latest knowledge in all fields, including medicine, but also for regulating their entry into the profession. Initially, however, the study of ancient literature and antique medical literature was still considered essential, but over time became to be less and less regarded as the sole qualification needed to practice as a physician. During the Renaissance increasing importance was attached to empirical aspects of medical practice and a knowledge of the latest discoveries in anatomy and physiology, both of which were gradually introduced into the curriculum.

During the nineteenth century the universities underwent a reorientation, initiated by such influential reformers as Wilhelm von Humboldt (1767-1835) who in 1820 founded the University of Berlin. He introduced the principle of unity of research and teaching and the German universities adopted this basic concept earlier than did those in other countries. During the course of the century such innovations made them successful and highly attractive leading educational institutions despite the fact that, at the beginning of the century, the continuing influence of romantic natural philosophy was still hampering the development of scientific medicine. Nevertheless, academic medical studies were increasingly acquiring an empirical and scientific basis. The list of medical courses was expanding, new scientific discoveries were being incorporated, and old subjects were being taught in a new way.[1] By the end of the century medical studies required three or four years to complete and were confined not only to the principles of medicine, surgery, anatomy and physiology, but also included such subjects as chemistry, hygiene, obstetrics, ophthalmology and psychiatry (◨ Table 3.1). In many countries

▢ **Table 3.1.** Establishment of disciplines in Bonn, Erlangen and Heidelberg

Subject	Bonn	Erlangen	Heidelberg
Ophthalmology	1862	1872	1859
Obstetrics	1819	1826	1773
Ear, nose and throat specialist	1877	1880	1862
Hygiene	1894	1865	1868
Pharmacology	1862	1876	1890
Physiology	1859	1872	1836
Psychiatry	1881	1849	1827

prior education in the liberal arts was still required of the student before he could begin his medical studies proper.

As a result of increasing specialization, the number of professors employed in the Faculties of Medicine expanded greatly: by 45.6% in the years between 1820 and 1850, by 110% between 1850 and 1880 and by 41.5% between1880 and1910; this represented a tripling in the number of chairs. Beginning in 1850, growth in the number of specialties and the resulting differentiation and expansion of medical knowledge progressed more vigorously in German universities than in those in other countries – for the following reasons:

- neo-humanistic ideology called for more originality and creativity in scientific work,
- the decentralised organisation of the German academic system stimulated more competition between the universities,
- state policy sought to boost national prestige through the advancement of science.

3.1.2 Changes at the Universities: Specialization and Professionalization

In »modern times«, beginning around the year 1900, the universities entered a phase of constant expansion. There was a rational basis for this, as Karl Jaspers noted: »**All human activity is doing based on knowledge, and wherever knowledge is necessary, universities are expected to expand and teach it.**«[2] With regard to the evolution of medicine this is a perfectly natural development of science. »**In the diversification of the whole, each »new« will itself become the whole, in the same way as life produces new life.**«[3] Among those areas of medicine that have evolved into independent specialties, some, such as psychiatry or ophthalmology, are universal, and are therefore on the same hierarchical level as internal medicine or

---

[1] Bonnet (1995), p 35.

[2] Jaspers (1946), p 76f – Translation by the author.

[3] ibid. p 77.

surgery. Others, such as forensic medicine or hygiene, are not properly considered to be specialties in their own right, and this assessment also applies to anaesthesia.

> Today, the position of science as a profession is determined by the need for further specialization – to an extent that was previously unknown and that will continue to persist into the future … The top performance today is always a specialised one.[4]

All those medical specialties that have evolved over the course of time underwent various stages of development before attaining to final professionalization. Paul Unschuld described this as a process of »strategies«, viz. manipulation of knowledge, development of a particular ethic and the formation of professional associations: »The techniques of knowledge manipulation include the creation of a specific terminology comprehensible only to the members of a certain group and restricting general access to the specialised knowledge.«[5]

Professionalization is a lengthy process that also involves the assignment or control of resources. In medicine these latter are »(medical) knowledge, (medical) skills, drugs, (medical) equipment and techniques, material goods (obtained from medical activities) and clientele (patients).«[5]

The process of professionalization is characterized by various aspects, as here exemplified in the case of anaesthesiology on the basis of Unschuld's criteria:

- Acceptance of remuneration for services rendered
- Use of a technical terminology
- Wearing of professional symbols or clothing
- Completion of formal training as bindingly defined in 1953 for anaesthetists in the Postgraduate Training Regulations of the German Medical Association (▶ Chap. 1.1 and 2.1.2)
- Monopoly and professional autonomy – which are of major relevance in the case of anaesthesia and which were accordingly regulated in 1962 in Weißauer's influential report to the Executive Committee of the DGAI entitled »Division of labour and sharing of responsibility between anaesthetist and surgeon«.
- Internationalisation
- Equality of social status with other medical specialties

3.1.3 The Establishment of Anaesthesiology at the Universities

A 1943 brochure providing information for would-be medical students contained the following passage describing surgery:

---

[4] Weber (1991), p 11.
[5] Unschuld (1974), p 259f

For the student, it will be an unforgettable event when, for the first time, he can be present when the surgeon is performing a difficult major procedure, for which the preparatory work, task assignment and operating skills all come together to create, as it were, a work of real art. On such an occasion he will experience that spirit of discipline and camaraderie that is typically prevalent among well-trained soldiers: after the carefully planned and dedicated efforts of all those human resources involved in the areas of diagnostics, indications and pre-operative preparation, the procedure itself will be self-assuredly performed by the responsible surgeon with professional support from medical, anaesthetic and other assistants – one man, is in sole command of the proceedings.[6]

This text from the 1940s reflected the views of many Professors of Surgery during the first half of the twentieth century who did everything they could to prevent the recognition of anaesthesia as an independent medical specialty, even at the universities (◘ Fig. 3.1). However, this situation began to change in the late 1940s. Soon after World War II, the need to further new developments in the practice and teaching of anaesthesiology as a specialty in its own right came to be recognized both by many surgeons and health care authorities in Germany. This change in attitude was strongly supported by the Recommendations oft the German Science Council on the Extension of Scientific Institutions, Part I: Universities (Empfehlungen des Wissenschaftsrates zum Ausbau der wissenschaftlichen Einrichtungen, Teil 1: wissenschaftliche Hochschulen)[7] that set the points for this revolution.[8]

---

[6] Bach (1943), p 10
[7] Wissenschaftsrat (1960).
[8] Wissenschaftsrat (1960).

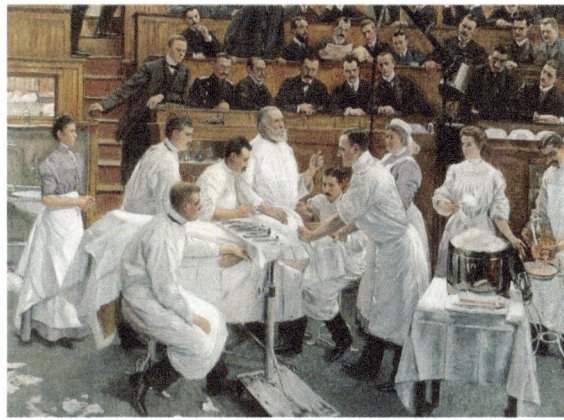

◘ Fig. 3.1. Ernst von Bergmann operating and teaching in the lecture room of the Department of Surgery at the Charité University Hospital, Berlin. Coloured copperplate engraving from a painting by Franz Skarbina (1907)

3.1.4 The Recommendations of the German Science Council of 1960

The universities were called upon to preserve the unity of research and education, with each university offering a certain basic number of subjects in every faculty. At the same time allowance was to be made for individual emphasis to be put on particular objectives, methods and areas of research. It was also noted that, in 1960 despite increasing numbers of students there were fewer universities in the Federal Republic of Germany than in the German Reich (Deutsches Reich) in 1935. Prompted by the fact that in certain disciplines, such as medicine, the numbers of students were overwhelming the available capacity of the universities, three new universities were planned. These were to be established in Munich, in the northern part of Germany, and in the industrial region of North Rhine-Westphalia. To accommodate the increased demand, the number of university posts, academic chairs and professorships also needed to be expanded. In 1960 3,160 professors were responsible for some 200,000 students, while in 1928 the corresponding figures were 3,050 and 111,600.[9] In a recommendation dated 11 March 1960, new permanent associate professorships were to be created only
- for a study course still in the process of evolving but expected to develop into a full-blown discipline requiring an ordinary (full) chair,
- in individual cases for the permanent promotion of more minor special subjects.

Anaesthesiology was identified as such an evolving specialty. The recommendations covered such aspects as the structure of university hospitals and their respective purposes, as well as their equipment and staffing. It was proposed that a central group of anaesthetists should provide anaesthetic services to all those departments providing surgical services.[10] The expected consequences of the recommendations were specified in concrete terms in section D, Suggestions for the Extension of the Universities (◘ Table 3.2). In the case of anaesthesia the recommended establishment of associate professorships was implemented in the following years.

3.1.5 The Recommendations of the German Science Council of 1968

The Recommendations of the German Science Council on Structure and Extension of Medical Research and Teaching Institutions[11] dated March 1968 stated in the preface that the particular role of the Faculties of Medicine should be examined, and ways found to enable them to meet the general demands made on academic institutions more efficiently than in the preceding decades. This aim was rendered more difficult by the need both to impart the clinical experience that is an indispensable requirement, while at the same time adequately promoting research and improving teaching:

> Clinical achievements serve both as a pacemaker and as a check of medical research; any assertion that a high standard of training is provided becomes implausible when poor clinical performance makes it impossible to ascribe the epithet exemplary to the educational institution.[12]

The major progress in modern medicine made possible by new diagnostic techniques, together with innovative surgical procedures and revolutionary advances/discoveries in the natural sciences made it imperative for the Faculties of Medicine to integrate the areas research, education and clinical competence. In addition to the reorganisation of medical studies, further specialization was also needed. Objections raised by clinicians that this would threaten the unity of medicine were disregarded; total individual responsibility for such an extensive field of competence coupled, moreover, with the highest qualification in a special field of expertise and research would put too large a burden of responsibility on a physician. It was clearly pointed out that no arguments were to be found against the specialization of an individual scientist in an area of research. The Faculties of Medicine and their clinical institutions were encouraged to continue moving towards specialization in as far as this proved to be necessary.

With regard to the developments prompted by the 1960 recommendations, two evolutionary trends were noted in 1968: a reduction in the burden on existing departments through the establishment of new independent subspecialties and of specialised divisions within departments. It was also noted that while the creation of new independent subspecialties and new posts for full or associate professors did not necessarily mandate the establishment of new departments, adequate opportunities for relevant work had to be ensured. In the section on Common Clinical Institutions extensive centralisation of anaesthetic services was recommended:[13] »The division

---

[9] Wissenschaftsrat (1960), p 61.

[10] Wissenschaftsrat (1960), p 426.

[11] Empfehlungen des Wissenschaftsrats zur Struktur und zum Ausbau der medizinischen Forschungs- und Ausbildungsstätten.

[12] Wissenschaftsrat (1968), p.8.

[13] Gemeinsame klinische Einrichtungen. In: Wissenschaftsrat (1968).

Table 3.2. Establishment of Anaesthesiology at German Universities

University (Today's Name)	Estraordinary Chair (Associate Professorship)	Chair (Full Professorship)
Aachen, Rheinisch-Westfälische Technical University		1973
Berlin, Humboldt-University, University Hospital Charité		1969
Berlin, Free University, University Hospital Westend	1963	1966
Berlin, Free University, University Hospital Steglitz		1969
Bochum, Ruhr University Knappschaftskrankenhaus University Hospital Bergmannsheil St. Josef-Hospital Marienhospital Herne		1983 1986 1987 1987
Bonn, Rheinische Friedrich-Wilhelms University		1974
Dresden, Technical University		1979
Düsseldorf, Heinrich-Heine University	1962	1966
Erlangen, Friedrich-Alexander University	1966	1970
Essen, Gesamthochschule		1974
Frankfurt, Johann-Wolfgang-Goethe University		1973
Freiburg, Albert-Ludwigs University	1966	1969
Gießen, Justus-Liebig University		1968
Göttingen, Georg-August University	1964	1969
Greifswald, Ernst-Moritz-Arndt University		1977
Halle/Wittenberg, Martin-Luther University		1973
Hamburg, University	1963	1966
Hannover, Medical School		1968
Heidelberg, Ruprecht-Karls University	1963	1967
Homburg, Saarland University	1963	1966
Jena, Friedrich-Schiller University		1979
Kiel, Christian-Albrecht University		1971
Köln (Cologne), University		1971
Leipzig, University		1984
Lübeck, Medical University		1981
Magdeburg, Otto-von-Guericke University		1973
Mainz, Johannes-Gutenberg University	1960	1967
Mannheim, Faculty of Clinical Medicine, University of Heidelberg		1971
Marburg, Philipps University		1967
München, Ludwig-Maximillians University	1967	1970
München, Technical University		1972
Münster, Westfälische Wilhelms University		1976
Regensburg, University		1991
Rostock, University		1972
Tübingen, Eberhard-Karls University		1968
Ulm, University		1974
Witten-Herdecke, University		1995
Würzburg, Julius-Maximilians University	1968	1969

3

has an obligation to make its services available to all surgical departments and is responsible for organizing anaesthetic requirements for the entire hospital.«[14]

To enable the anaesthesiological service to better comply with the specific needs of the surgical subspecialties, such as cardiac surgery or neurosurgery, the concept of »decentralised centralisation« was introduced. Experienced anaesthetists were expected to work for lengthy periods of time in the specialised divisions while remaining on the permanent staff of the central division of anaesthesiology. A priority concern was good co-operation with the various surgical specialties and extensive training in all aspects of anaesthesia. Moreover, adequate opportunities for research, possibly in a centre of clinical research, should also be available to the anaesthetic department.

The 1968 recommendation that 1,518 new clinical positions be created represented a 20.6% increase in the 1967 total of 7,357 positions, included 389 positions for full and associate professors and increased the total number of professors in clinical specialties to 1,090. In 1967, 94 positions for professors were available in the common clinical institutions (including anaesthesiology) and centres of clinical research. The 1968 recommendations of the Science Council aimed to increase this number by 214.

The recommendations made by the Science Council in 1976 proposed establishing a structure comprising centres and divisions. Two alternatives were suggested for anaesthesiology: either to be a part of the surgical centre (with no beds of its own) or to be a central unit of the hospital.

On its establishment at the universities, anaesthesiology was integrated within an overall concept and the general development of medicine. Since the organization and structure of German universities are the responsibility of the individual Federal States, the development of academic medicine in general and of anaesthesiology in particular has not been uniform, but differs from one university to another.

3.1.6 Comparison with Other Surgical Specialties

The evolution of anaesthesiology has been similar to that of neurosurgery, orthopaedics and urology, and the Science Council of 1960 contained the recommended number of professors and chairs. The 1968 recommendations of the Science Council proposed that neurosurgery should be split up into 2 separate subspecialties, with stereotactic surgery as a separate specialty. The number

of surgical subspecialties was defined as five, viz. trauma, cardiac and thoracic surgery and urology. All universities were to establish orthopaedics as urgently as possible as a single separate chair. Anaesthesiology was not considered as properly belonging in the area of surgery, but was defined as a separate central clinical institution.

There was a fundamental difference between the development of anaesthesiology and that of orthopaedics and urology, both of which (but not neurosurgery) were already mentioned as specialties in the **Bremer Richtlinien**[15] approved by the German Medical Assembly in 1924. In 1935, the Bremer Richtlinien were adopted by the **Berufsordnung Deutscher Ärzte**[16] which came into force as of 5 November 1937.

In 1949, the 52nd German Medical Assembly suggested a revision of the **Berufsordnung** that included anaesthesiology as a separate specialty, but the proposal was rejected due to intense opposition by the surgeons, who had not been consulted in advance. A new attempt was undertaken in 1951, and the professional title of specialist in anaesthesiology was finally recognized by the **German Medical Assembly** in 1953; 107 years after the first anaesthesia in Germany the **Narkosearzt**[17] had at last come into his own (Chap. 1.1).

3.1.7 Concluding Remarks

A reform is necessary since the new anaesthetic techniques developed in recent years are so complex and multifaceted that no surgeon – much less a layperson – has the necessary expertise to employ any of them »on the side«, as it were. The induction and maintenance of anaesthesia and pain control requires special knowledge and skills that can be acquired only through systematic and lengthy training. In this respect, foreign, especially Anglo-American, but also the Romanic and Nordic, countries are ahead of us. In those countries, specialists in anaesthesia have long since become well established and recognised.[18]

This comment was made by the surgeon Professor E. Derra in 1952, to emphasise the need to reform anaesthesiology in Germany. However, the path leading to the establishment of an independent academic discipline involved much more than simply the creation of the professional title »specialist in anaesthesia«. In a 1959 over-

---

[14] Wissenschaftsrat (1968), p 34

[15] Basic Principles of Medical Specialization, approved in Bremen. Hoppe (1997).

[16] Professional Code of German Physicians.

[17] Anaesthesiologist.

[18] Derra (1952), p 49.

view of university chairs, the clinical medicine section lists only surgery, orthopaedics and urology as surgical disciplines, but not anaesthesiology. External factors also contributed to the growing need to make anaesthesiology an independent medical discipline at Germany's universities. In the United States of America, at the University of Wisconsin, Ralph M. Waters became the first Professor of Anaesthesiology as long ago as 1933, while in England Sir Robert R. Macintosh was appointed the first Professor of Anaesthetics at the University of Oxford in 1937.

Other milestones in this development were:

- The establishment of the first associate professorships. As early as 1928 the surgeon Helmut Schmidt became the first Lecturer in Anaesthesia at the University of Hamburg. But 25 more years passed before, in 1953, Karl Horatz was appointed to teach the subject »Introduction to anaesthesiology« at the University Hospital Eppendorf in Hamburg. The first (associate) chair was established in 1960 in Mainz and awarded to Rudolf Frey. Six years later, in 1966, Horatz was appointed the first Full Professor of Anaesthesiology in Hamburg. In the following years chairs were established at all German universities (◻ Table 3.2).

- The foundation of a scientific society
  In 1952 the **Deutsche Arbeitsgemeinschaft für Anästhesiologie** (German Working Group on Anaesthesiology) was established, and was followed in 1953 by the **Deutsche Gesellschaft für Anaesthesie** (German Society of Anaesthesia).

- The first publication
  In 1952, *Der Anaesthesist* was founded by O. Mayrhofer (Vienna, Austria), R. Frey (Mainz, Germany) and W. Hügin (Basel, Switzerland) as the official scientific journal of the Austrian Society, and one year later of the German and Swiss Societies, of Anaesthesiology.

»There is no doubt that both surgeon and patient would equally benefit, if the anaesthetist were to be accorded more rights and greater recognition than previously«, maintained the editors of the journal *Der Schmerz* in a 1928 editorial.[19] Since then, anaesthesiology has become recognised throughout Germany as an independent medical specialty, and is now a fully acknowledged academic discipline in its own right. This development was delayed for many years by the need to overcome various hurdles, such as, for example, the conservatism of the dominating surgeons, the complete isolation of Germany from the outside world during World War II, the federal structure of West Germany, and the existence of two German States that lasted for four decades.

References

Bach E (1943) Das Studium der Medizin. Einführungsband. Winter, Heidelberg (Studienführer Gruppe IV: Medizin und Pharmazie)

Bergeat (1924) 43. Deutscher Aerztetag. Münch Med Wochenschr 71: 925-929

Bonnet TN (1995) Becoming a Physician. Medical Education in Britain, France, Germany, and the United States, 1750-1945. Oxford Univ Press, New, Oxford

Buchborn E (1985) Spezialisierung und Integration in der Medizin. Focus MHL 2: 263-268

Derra E (1952) Gedanken zur Neuordnung des Narkosewesens in Deutschland. Das Krankenhaus 44: 49-51

Die Anästhesie (1952). Ciba-Zeitschrift Bd 11, No 130/131. Basel

Eulner HH (1970) Die Entwicklung der Medizinischen Spezialfächer an den Universitäten des deutschen Sprachgebietes. Enke, Stuttgart

Gauß W, von der Porten E (1928) Zur Einführung. Der Schmerz 1: 1-4.

Hochschulverband (Hrsg) (1959): Die Lehrstühle an den wissenschaftlichen Hochschulen in der Bundesrepublik und in Westberlin. Schwartz, Göttingen

Hoppe JD (1997) Die Weiterbildungsordnung. Dtsch Ärztebl 94: A-2483-2491

Huerkamp C (1985) Der Aufstieg der Ärzte im 19. Jahrhundert. Vandenhoeck& Ruprecht, Göttingen

Hunter AR (1949) Moderne Anästhesie in der Bauchchirurgie. Langenbecks Arch Dtsch Z Chir 262: 464-493

Jaspers K (1946) Die Idee der Universität. Springer, Berlin

Maier J (1962) Der historische Ablauf der Emanzipierung neuer Fächer aus der Chirurgie. Diss med, Kiel

Neumann H (1957) Die Entwicklung der deutschen Facharztordnung. Der Nervenarzt 28: 278-279

Röse W (1999) 40 Jahre Anästhesie in Deutschland. Anaesthesiol Reanimat 24: 19-26

Seidler E (1991) Die medizinische Fakultät der Albert-Ludwigs-Universität Freiburg im Breisgau. Grundlagen und Entwicklungen. Springer, Berlin

Toellner, R (1986) Illustrierte Geschichte der Medizin. Bd 3. Andreas & Andreas, Salzburg

Unschuld, P (1974) Professionalisierung im Bereich der Medizin. Saeculum 25: 251-276

Unschuld, P (1978) Professionalisierung und ihre Folgen. In: Schipperges H, Seidler E, Unschuld P (Hrsg) Krankheit, Heilkunst, Heilung. Alber, Freiburg, S 517-555

Weber M (1991) Wissenschaft als Beruf. 8. Aufl., Duncker & Humblot, Berlin

Wissenschaftsrat (ed) (1960) Empfehlungen des Wissenschaftsrates zum Ausbau der wissenschaftlichen Einrichtungen. Teil 1: Wissenschaftliche Hochschulen. Mohr, Tübingen

Wissenschaftsrat (ed) (1968) Empfehlungen des Wissenschaftsrates zur Struktur und zum Ausbau der medizinischen Forschungs- und Ausbildungsstätten. Bundesdruckerei, Bonn

Wissenschaftsrat (ed) (1976) Empfehlungen des Wissenschaftsrates zur Struktur und zum Ausbau der medizinischen Forschungs- und Ausbildungsstätten. Bundesdruckerei, Bonn

Wissenschaftsrat (ed) (1978) Empfehlungen zu Aufgaben, Organisation und Ausbau der medizinischen Forschungs- und Ausbildungsstätten. Köln

---

[19] Gauß, von der Porten (1928), p 2

3.2   History of the Chairs of Anaesthesiology at the German Faculties of Medicine

3.2.1   RWTH Aachen University Department of Anaesthesiology

R. Rossaint, G. Kalff, G. Marx

The Faculty of Medicine of the RWTH Aachen University was founded in 1966. Professor Martin Reifferscheid (Bonn) was appointed Chairman of the Department of Surgery. He was accompanied by Dr. Günter Kalff, Specialist in Anaesthesiology, who was initially responsible for the anaesthesia service of surgical patients, but soon also for that of other surgical departments. In 1970 Kalff qualified as Lecturer in Anaesthesiology. Three years later, he was appointed Full Professor and Chairman of the Department of Anaesthesiology.

Right from the beginning of Kalff's chairmanship the Department was structured as a central service providing anaesthetics for all operative disciplines of the University Hospital except urology. An ICU with 6 beds was created. In 1976 the Department got in charge of the mobile life support units of the City of Aachen. When the University Hospital moved into a new building in 1983 the services were extended by a pain clinic. The number of doctors of the Department increased from 15 in 1973 to 68 in 1989. Besides residency training the Department started an educational programme for specialized anaesthesia nurses as early as in 1969 accompanied by annual international symposia for anaesthesia nurses.

Research activities started in 1967, directed on new relaxants and their application in ophthalmology, problems of controlled hypotension, and the development of new respirators. Another scientific key issue became the pharmacodynamics and pharmacokinetics of analgesics and opioids relating to anaesthesia and pain therapy.

1973–1997 Chairmanship Professor Günter Kalff

Prof. Dr. med. Günter Kalff

Born 5 February 1932 in Aachen; 1952–1957 student of medicine in Bonn, Innsbruck, Düsseldorf and Bonn; 1956–1958 internship at the DVL Institute of Aviation Medicine, Bonn-Bad Godesberg; 1959 doctorate in medicine; 1959–1961 Resident, Departments of Internal Medicine and Surgery, University of Bonn; begin of anaesthesia training; 1961 Department of Gynaecology; 1962 Resident, Division of Anaesthesia; 1965 Specialist in Anaesthesiology; 1966 Senior Physician at the Department of Surgery, RWTH Aachen University, building up of the Division of Anaesthesia; 1970 Lecturer in Anaesthesiology; 1973 Full Professor and Chairman of the Department of Anaesthesiology; 1997 Professor Emeritus.

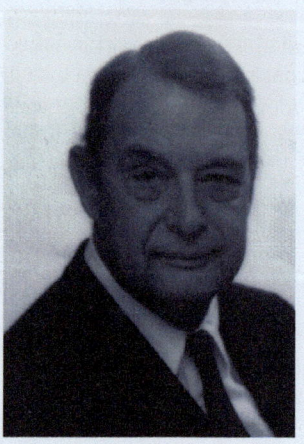

Since 1997 Chairmanship Professor Rolf Rossaint

Prof. Dr. med. Rolf Rossaint

Born 26 June 1958 in Neuss; 1977–1983 student of medicine at Düsseldorf; 1983 doctorate in medicine; 1983–1988 Resident at the Department of Anaesthesiology, University of Düsseldorf; 1987 Specialist in Anaesthesiology; 1988–1997 Deputy Chairman, Department of Anaesthesiology and Surgical Intensive Care Medicine, Rudolf Virchow Hospital, Free University of Berlin; 1993 Lecturer in Anaesthesiology; 1997 Full Professor of Anaesthesiology, RWTH Aachen University, and Chairman of the Department of Anaesthesiology, University Hospital Aachen.

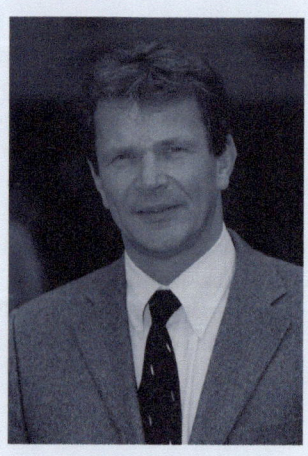

To optimize the clinical organisation and to reduce the expenses for personnel a preanaesthetic clinic was installed in 1998. Owing to Rossaint's scientific focus on the therapy of acute pulmonary failure the personnel of the ICU with 14 beds was increased and in addition to the ICU-patients from the University Hospital also 3 to 4 patients with severe ARDS from all over Germany were treated. In 2001 the Department additionally took the medical and organisational responsibility for the ICU of the Department of Cardiac and Thorax Surgery (14 beds). New fields of research were inaugurated by Rossaint. Main projects were experimental and clinical aspects of ARDS and ventilator-induced lung injury, the use of xenon for inhalation anaesthesia, immunological effects of anaesthetics, development of sepsis, pathomechanisms of SIRS, and development of telemedical devices for emergency medicine.

Due to the positive experience with the management of the cardio-thoracic ICU by the Department of Anaesthesiology, the University Hospital decided to centralize all surgical ICU beds in a separate Department and the Faculty of Medicine established a second Chair of Anaesthesiology with emphasis on Surgical Intensive Care Medicine. In 2005 Professor Ralf Kuhlen, Associate Professor of Anaesthesiology since 2003 and Deputy Chairman of the Department of Anaesthesiology, was appointed Chairman of the Department of Surgical ICM. Since then both Departments formed an integrated whole, both Chairmen substituting one another. These arrangements offer good conditions for common strategies in patient care and provide synergies in education and research.

Between 2005 and 2006 the ICUs of the Departments of Surgery and Neurosurgery were added to the Department of Surgical ICM resulting in a total of 48 beds. Kuhlen's research was mainly focused on therapy of acute lung failure, ventilation and weaning. Kuhlen left the University Hospital Aachen in 2007, and Rossaint assumed the interim Chairmanship from 2007 until October 2008 when Professor Gernot Marx (Jena) was appointed Full Professor of Anaesthesiology, especially ICM, and Chairman of the Department of Surgical Intensive Care Medicine and Intermediate Care.

Since 2008 Additional Chairmanship Professor Gernot Marx

Prof. Dr. med. Gernot Marx

Born 29 January 1966 in Sehnde; 1987–1994 student of medicine in Hannover; 1995 doctorate in medicine; 1995–1999 residency at the Department of Anaesthesiology, Hannover Medical School; 1999 Specialist in Anaesthesiology; 2000 Senior Physician; 2000 Lecturer in Anaesthesiology; 2000–2004 Senior Lecturer, Department of Anaesthesia, Royal Liverpool University Hospital; 2004 Adjunct Professor, Hannover Medical School; 2004 Associate Professor and Deputy Chairman, Department of Anaesthesiology and Intensive Care Medicine, University of Jena; 2008 Full Professor of Anaesthesiology, especially Intensive Care Medicine, and Chairman of the Department of Surgical Intensive Care Medicine and Intermediate Care, RWTH Aachen University.

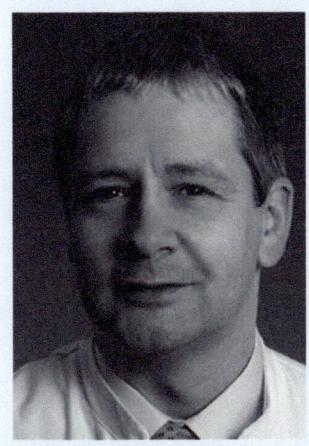

The ICU for burned patients and the surgical intermediate care unit were included into the renamed Department of Intensive Care Medicine and Intermediate Care, then comprising 55 ICU beds and 28 surgical IMC beds. Marx' research interest is directed on systemic inflammation and sepsis with focus on innovative and forward-looking translational research and comprises clinical and experimental studies as well as basic research.

Qualification as Lecturers in Anaesthesiology

Daub, Dieter (1980); Schlimgen, Rita (1982); Lehmann, Klaus Artur (1984); Behrendt, Walter (1986); Schockenhoff, Bernd (1989); Kuhlen, Ralf (2000); Max, Martin (2001); Buhre, Wolfgang (2002); de Rossi, Lothar (2005); Dembinski, Rolf (2006); Rex, Steffen (2008); Schnoor, Jörg (2009); Beckers, Stefan (2010); Coburn, Mark (2010); Fries, Michael (2010); Hein, Marc (2010); Schulz-Stübner, Sebastian (2010)

Professors of Anaesthesiology
Full Professors

Prof. Dr. Wolfgang Buhre (2008), University Medical Center, Utrecht, The Netherlands

Associate Professors

Prof. Dr. Dr. Klaus A. Lehmann (1985), University of Cologne

Prof. Dr. Ralf Kuhlen (2003), RWTH Aachen University

For further information:

www.anaesthesie.ukaachen.de
www.ukaachen.de/sites/opintensivmedizin/
www.operative-intensivmedizin.de

3.2.2 Charité – University Medicine Berlin Department of Anaesthesiology and Surgical Intensive Care Medicine

W.J. Kox

The history of anaesthesia at the university hospitals of Berlin started on 12 February 1847. Johann Friedrich Dieffenbach, Professor of Surgery, operated on a 16 years old boy under ether anaesthesia. Only 5 months later he published one of the most important monographs on ether anaesthesia in Germany. Curt Schimmelbusch who described his famous face mask was lecturer at the Charité. At the end of the 19th century surgeons at the Charité pioneered local anaesthesia, e.g. Carl Ludwig Schleich who in 1894 presented infiltration anaesthesia at the German Congress of Surgeons, and August Bier who had described spinal anaesthesia with cocain in 1899 (at that time still in Kiel) and intravenous regional anaesthesia (»Bier block«) in 1908. From 1928–1949 Ferdinand Sauerbruch, the most influential surgeon in the German speaking parts of Europe, was Professor of Surgery at the Charité. He generally operated his patients under ether anaesthesia and remained a forceful opponent of new methods (e.g. endotracheal intubation) and structures of anaesthesia for his entire life. From 1929–1931 one of his assistants was Werner Forßmann who carried out self-experiments with right heart cathetherization for what he was awarded the Nobel Prize in 1956. In 1950 Professor Willi Felix followed Sauerbruch. He set up an anaesthesia division in 1958 which was at first led by Dr. Horst Bertram who was appointed Head of a Central Anaesthesia Division in 1961. When Professor Hans Joachim Serfling became Felix' successor in 1962 he entrusted Dr. Manfred Schädlich with the development of a Division of Anaesthesia and Intensive Therapy which became an independent Department in 1969.

1969–1990 Chairmanship Professor Manfred Schädlich

> **Prof. Dr. med. habil. Manfred Schädlich**
>
> Born 16 July 1926 in Auerbach/Vogtland; 1948-1954 student of medicine in Halle; 1956 doctorate in medicine, University of Halle; 1954-1957 Resident, Department of Surgery, University of Halle; 1957-1962 Department of Surgery, University of Greifswald; 1960 Specialist in Anaesthesiology; 1960-1962 development of a Division of Anaesthesia and Intensive Care Medicine and Encephalography; 1962-1969 Senior Physician, Department of Surgery of the Charité, Humboldt University Hospital Berlin; 1967 Lecturer in Anaesthesiology; 1969 Full Professor and first University Chairman of Anaesthesiology and Intensive Therapy of the German Democratic Republic; 1990 Professor Emeritus.

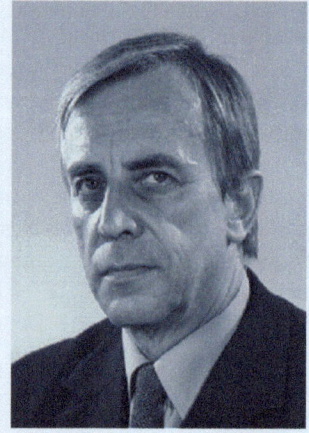

In 1969 Schädlich was appointed Chairman of the new Department and Full Professor of Anaesthesiology. For many years the clinical commitments remained dispersed over several sites, however, an ICU with 12 beds was established as early as 1962. It was not before 1982 that a new surgical centre was put into function what eventually enabled the Department to concentrate the majority of its activities and to increase the number of anaesthetics markedly. Now there were 3 ICUs and an intermediate care unit, a pain clinic and research laboratories could be opened. Main areas of research were electroencepalography and perioperative stress metabolism. After Schädlich's retirement in 1990, Professor Gerhard Zietz, Head of the Division of Intensive Therapy, was entrusted with the interim direction of the Department until 1992.

1993–2004 Chairmanship Professor Wolfgang J. Kox

Prof. Dr. med. Wolfgang J. Kox, PhD, MBA, FRCP, FRCA

Born 6 October 1946 in Berlin; 1966–1973 student of medicine, Free University of Berlin; 1973–1975 housemanship in Nordhorn; 1975–1979 Senior House Officer, Department of Anaesthesiology and Surgical Intensive Care, University Hospital Münster; 1979 Senior Registrar, St.Mary's Hospital Herne, University Hospital of the University of Bochum; 1980 Specialist in Anaesthesiology; 1980 Locum Consultant Anaesthetist, Department of Anaesthesia and Intensive Care, St. Mary's Hospital, Lünen; 1980–1983 Research Fellow at the Cardio-Thoracic-Institute, Midhurst Branch, Midhurst, West Sussex, UK; 1983–1992 Director of Intensive Care Services, Consultant Anaesthetist, Charing Cross Hospital, and Senior Lecturer, Charing Cross and Westminster Medical School, London; 1992 Associate Professor and Deputy Chairman, Department of Anaesthesiology, University Hospital Essen; 1993–2004 Full Professor and Chairman, Department of Anaesthesiology and Intensive Care Medicine, University Hospital Charité, Humboldt University Berlin; 1994 Honorary Fellow of the Royal College of Physicians, London; 2004–2009 Chairman of the Board of Directors and Medical Director, University Hospital Münster; 2006 Honorary Fellow of the Royal College of Anaesthetists, London; 2009 Director of the Institute of Hospital Management, Charité-University Medicine Berlin.

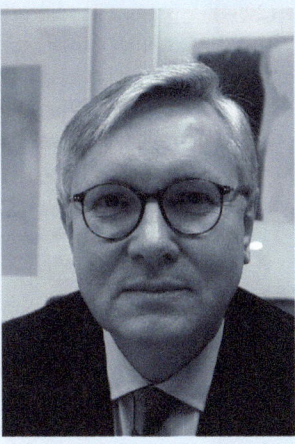

At the end of 1992 Wolfgang J. Kox was appointed Full Professor and Chairman of the Department of Anaesthesiology and Surgical Intensive Care Medicine. He pushed regional anaesthetic techniques, particularly in obstetrics, reorganised and updated both the anaesthesiological service and intensive care, introduced SOPs and could build up a new emergency unit including an emergency ambulance. Twelve research groups were established. Main fields of scientific work were the identification and reduction of perioperative risks as well as experimental studies on shock, sepsis, lung injury and immune deficiency, to a large extent supported by competitive grants. In 1998 the Campus Mitte and the Campus Rudolf Virchow of the Charité were merged and 2003 the amalgamation was extended to the University Hospital Benjamin Franklin of the Free University of Berlin now forming the Charité-University Medicine Berlin but the 3 chairs of Anaesthesiology persisted (▶ Chap. 3.2.3 and 3.2.4). In 2004 Kox was appointed Medical Director of the University Hospital Münster and left the Charité.

Charité – University Medicine Berlin, Campus Charité Mitte and Campus Virchow Klinikum

Department of Anaesthesiology and Surgical Intensive Care Medicine: One Department at Two Sites

W. Boemke, C.D. Spies

Since 2005 Chairmanship Professor Claudia Spies

Prof. Dr. med. Claudia D. Spies

Born 6 April 1961 in Würzburg; 1980–1987 student of medicine in Erlangen and at Harvard University, USA; 1987 doctorate in medicine, University of Erlangen-Nuremberg; 1987–1993 training in anaesthesiology and intensive care (Nuremberg, Berlin); 1993 Specialist in

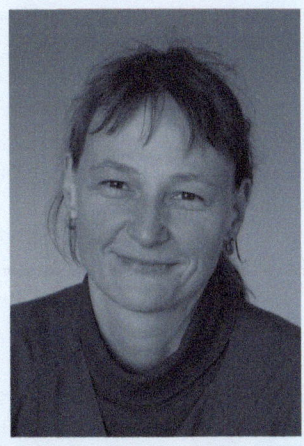

Anaesthesiology; 1994–1997 Resident/Senior Physician in anaesthesiology and intensive care medicine, University Hospital Benjamin Franklin, Berlin; 1996 Lecturer in Anaesthesiology and Intensive Care Medicine, Free University of Berlin; 1997–1999 Senior Consultant, interdisciplinary surgical intensive care medicine, University Hospital Benjamin Franklin; 2000 Professor of Anaesthesiology and Intensive Care Medicine; 1999–2004 Vice Chairperson, Charité Campus Mitte, Berlin; 2005 Full Professor and Chairperson of the Department of Anaesthesiology and Intensive Care Medicine, Charité Campus Mitte and Campus Virchow Klinikum; 2006 Head of the »Charité Centre 7 for Anaesthesiology, Operating-Room Management and Intensive Care Medicine«.

When Professor Wolfgang Kox was appointed Medical Director at the University Hospital of Münster in April 2004, Professor Claudia Spies became his successor as Chairperson of the Department of Anaesthesiology and Surgical Intensive Care Medicine at Charité Campus Mitte. One year later, after the retirement of Professor Konrad Falke as Chairman of the Department of Anaesthesiology and Surgical Intensive Care of the Charité, Campus Virchow Klinikum, Spies successfully applied for his position, and was appointed to his Chair in October 2005. The two departments, finally, were merged into the single new Department of Anaesthesiology and Surgical Intensive Care located at two different sites, Campus Mitte and Campus Virchow Klinikum. In 2006 the Charité – University Medicine Berlin was reorganized. Seventeen Charité Centres were established in order to improve teaching, research, and patient care. In addition to her chair, Spies was appointed Medical Head of the »Charité Centre for Anaesthesiology, Operating-Room Management and Intensive Care Medicine«. Important management tasks of the Centre are the overall organization of both the operating room management and interdisciplinary surgical intensive care medicine at the Charité, and other interdisciplinary management tasks. The Centre comprises the anaesthesiological departments at Campus Virchow Klinikum and Campus Mitte as well as that at Campus Benjamin Franklin chaired by Professor Christoph Stein (▶ Chap. 3.2.4).

The Department of Anaesthesiology and Surgical Intensive Care Medicine with about 200 anaesthesiologists serves all surgical subspecialties. At 68 anaesthesia workplaces it takes care of more than 46,000 anaesthesiological procedures per year. The intensive care facilities of the Department comprise 8 multidisciplinary ICUs as well as intermediate care and post anaesthetic care units with a total of 86 beds. One of the ICUs is a nationally recognized centre of excellence for treatment of severe pulmonary failure (ARDS). In the 2 pain clinics of the Department about 3,000 inpatients and 4,200 outpatients are annually treated. Two physician-staffed-emergency vehicles are equipped by the Department.

Research concentrates on postoperative and posttraumatic risk reduction through preventive anaesthesiologic and intensive care measures, especially complications of alcohol-related disease, delirium, and severe lung injury, as well as the etiology of pain and its management. One of the main fields of interest is patient safety and improvement of perioperative processes and continuous improvement of patient treatment by application of SOPs and evaluation of key performance indicators. The Department covers 5,200 teaching hours per year for medical students. It offers fellowships in intensive care medicine, pain management and emergency medicine and training for physicians from abroad. It organizes the »Simulator Training in Berlin (BeST)«, the »Berlin Regional Anesthesia Intensive Course (BRAIN)« and, on behalf of the German Society of Anesthesiology and Intensive Care Medicine, an annual congress with 3,500 participants.

Qualification as Lecturers in Anaesthesiology

Barth, Lothar (1960, at German Academy of Sciences, Berlin); Schädlich, Manfred (1967); Olthoff, Derk (1973); Schoeppner, Heinz (1975); Jage, Jürgen (1977); Flämming, Isolde (1979); Friis, Erich (1980); Münchow, Renate (1981); Schöntube, Eberhard (1982); Golosubow, Alexander (1983); Schneider, Manfred (1986); Krug, Gisela (1990); Schlame, Michael (1996); Hensel, Mario (2000); Volk, Thomas (2000); Lehmann, Christian (2000); Kern, Hartmut (2001); Rundshagen, Ingrid (2002); Kerner, Thoralf (2003); Keh, Didier (2004); Höhne, Claudia (2005); Braun, Jan Peter (2007); Brack, Alexander (2007); Unger, Juliane (2007); von Heymann, Christian (2007); Vargas-Hein, Ortrud (2007); Birnbaum, Jürgen (2008); Rittner, Heike (2008); Zöllner, Christian (2008); von Dossow-Hanfstingl, Vera (2009); Sander, Michael (2009); Baars, Jan (2010); Deja, Maria (2010)

Professors of Anaesthesiology
Full Professors

Prof. Dr. med. Derk Olthoff (1980), Charité University Hospital, Berlin, and (1984), University of Leipzig
Prof. Dr. Thomas Volk (2009), Saarland University Homburg

Associate Professors

Prof. Dr. Ralf U. Scherer (1997), Berlin
Prof. Dr. Michael Schäfer (2002), Berlin
Prof. Dr. Christian von Heymann (2008), Berlin
Prof. Dr. Michael Sander (2010), Berlin

Adjunct Professors

Prof. Dr. Willehad Boemke; Prof. Dr. Klaus Lewandowski; Prof. Dr. Benno Rehberg-Klug

For further information:

http://anaesthesieintensivmedizin.charite.de/klinik/

3.2.3 Charité – University Medicine Berlin, Campus Virchow Klinikum

Department of Anaesthesiology and Surgical Intensive Care Medicine

K.J. Falke

When in 1951 Professor Fritz Lindner was appointed Chairman of the Department of Surgery of the Klinikum Westend (later renamed Klinikum Charlottenburg) of the Free University of Berlin, Dr. Otto H. Just (Heidelberg) took over the Division of Anaesthesia which he developed further during the following years. In 1962 Just left Berlin and was appointed Full Professor at the University of Heidelberg (▶ Chap. 3.2.19).

1963–1968 Chairmanship Professor Ernst Kolb

(▶ Chap. 3.2.31 for his C.V.)

After an interim period with Dr. Ulrich Henneberg acting as Head, Professor Ernst Kolb from Mainz was appointed to the new chair in 1963. In 1966 the Division was promoted a Department of Anaesthesiology of the Free University and Kolb appointed Full Professor. Two years later, the new University Hospital Steglitz (later University Hospital Benjamin Franklin) of the Free University was put into operation with Kolb as Professor and Chairman. In 1972 Kolb moved to Munich where he was appointed to the new chair at the Technical University (▶ Chap. 3.2.31).

1968–1988 Chairmanship Professor Hans Joachim Eberlein

> ##### Prof. Dr. med. Hans Joachim Eberlein
>
> Born 20 August 1919 at Frankfurt/Main; deceased 27 July 2011; 1937–1945 military service; 1946–1952 student of medicine in Frankfurt; 1952 doctorate in medicine; 1953–1958 anaesthesia training in USA with Robert D. Dripps (Philadelphia) and Henry K. Beecher (MGH, Harvard Medical School, Boston); 1958–1968 Head, Anaesthesia Divisions of

the University Hospitals of Marburg and Cologne, then Research Associate, Department of Physiology, University of Göttingen; 1965 Lecturer in Anaesthesiology; 1968 Full Professor of Anaesthesiology and Chairman of the Anaesthesia Department, Westend Hospital of the Free University of Berlin; 1988 Professor Emeritus.

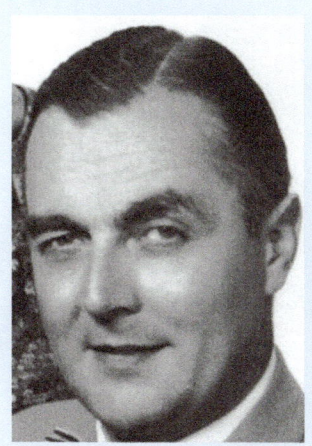

In May 1968 Professor Hans Joachim Eberlein became Kolb's successor. He launched a number of successful research groups, the most renowned being the group under his Deputy Chairman Professor Jürgen Brückner and the group under the physiologist Professor H. Wolfgang Reinhardt who then became Head of a Division of Experimental Anaesthesiology. Brückner's scientific interests were focused on the cardiovascular system, Reinhardt's on the regulation of salt and water balance.

1988–2004 Chairmanship Professor Konrad J. Falke

> ##### Prof. Dr. med. Konrad J. Falke, FRCA
>
> Born 18 August 1939 at Grüna/Saxonia; 1964 doctorate in medicine, University of Munich; Resident, Anaesthesia Division, Department of Neurosurgery, University of Munich; 1968–1971 Resident, Research Fellow und Instructor, MGH, Harvard Medical School, Boston, MA,USA; 1972–1973 General Hospital Hamburg-Altona; 1972 Specialist in Anaesthesiology; 1973–1988 Department of Anaesthesiology, University of Düsseldorf; 1976 Lecturer in Anaesthesiology; 1978–1988 Associate Professor

and Head of ICU; 1988 Full Professor and Chairman of the Department of Anaesthesiology and Surgical Intensive Care Medicine, Free University of Berlin (later University Hospital Charité, Campus Virchow Klinikum, University Medicine Berlin); 1996 Fellow of the Royal Society of Anaesthetists; 2004 Professor Emeritus.

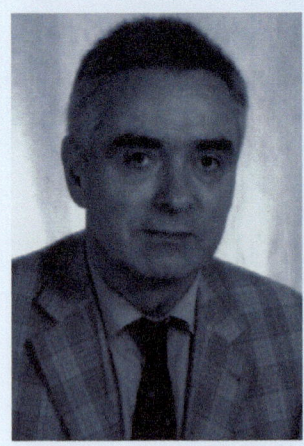

In 1988 Professor Konrad Falke was appointed Eberlein's successor. The University Hospital moved from Charlottenburg to the Virchow Klinikum in Wedding and was subsequently merged with the University Hospital Charité of the Humboldt University (▶ Chap. 3.2.2) but both Departments of Anaesthesiology remained independent. It provided the anaesthesia service for all surgical specialties except cardiac and urological surgery, had an ICU with 14 beds and participated in the intensive care of transplant and neurosurgical patients.

Falke soon made his ICU to a nationwide recognized centre for the therapy of severe acute lung injury. Resulting from an international cooperation with centres in Milan, Stockholm and Marburg he was the first in Germany who treated a young patient with ARDS by extracorporeal gas exchange by means of a heparin-coated artificial membrane lung. On the basis of a close cooperation with the Anesthesia Department of the MGH in Boston (Warren Zapol) and experimental studies carried out by Dr. Ulrich Pison the worldwide first treatment of severe ARDS with inhaled nitric oxide was successfully performed in the same year 1989. This concept of selective pulmonary vasodilatation then became a standard for the therapy of pulmonary hypertension. A large number of clinical and experimental studies on problems of epidemiology, pathophysiology and therapy of ARDS and severe sepsis went along with these clinical commitments.

Qualification as Lecturers in Anaesthesiology:

Just, Otto-Heinrich (1956); Brückner, Jürgen (1970); Patschke, Detlev (1975); Tarnow, Jörg (1975); Kaczmarczyk, Gabriele (1979); Hess, Wolfgang (1980); Schulte-Sasse, Uwe (1985); Veit, Siegfried (1992); Gerlach, Herwig (1994); Rossaint, Rolf (1994); Pison, Ulrich (1996); Pappert, Dirk (1998); Lewandowski, Klaus (1998); Boemke, Willehad (2001).

Professors of Anaesthesiology
Full Professors

Prof. Dr. Jörg Tarnow (1987), University of Düsseldorf
Prof. Dr. Rolf Rossaint (1997), RWTH Aachen University
Prof. Dr. Udo X. Kaisers (2006), University of Leipzig

Associate and Adjunct Professors

Prof. Dr. Jürgen Brückner; Prof. Dr. Herwig Gerlach; Prof. Dr. Wolfgang Hess; Prof. Dr. Gabriele Kaczmarczyk; Prof. Dr. Detlev Patschke; Prof. Dr. Ulrich Pison; Prof. Dr. H. Wolfgang Reinhardt; Prof. Dr. Uwe Schulte-Sasse

For further information:
www.charite.de/rv/anaest/index.htm

3.2.4 Charité – University Medicine Berlin, Campus Benjamin Franklin

Department of Anaesthesiology and Surgical Intensive Care Medicine
C. Griem, J. Link, C. Stein

Since after World War II West Berlin had no university anymore the West Allies founded the Free University of Berlin in 1948. The City Hospital Westend in Charlottenburg served as the main part of the new University Hospital. Two members of the 2nd Department of Surgery, Dr. Rudolf Hellenschmied and Dr. Paul Mellin, introduced the technique of intubation anaesthesia and the former gave a pregraduate lecture on modern anaesthetic methods in summer 1951. Later this year Professor Fritz Lindner (Heidelberg) was appointed Chairman of the Department of Surgery of the Klinikum Westend (later renamed as Klinikum Charlottenburg) and Dr. Otto H. Just (Heidelberg) took over the Division of Anaesthesia which he developed further during the following years. Just was qualified as Lecturer in Anaesthesiology in 1956, left Berlin in 1962 and was appointed Full Professor at the University of Heidelberg in 1963 (▶ Chap. 3.2.19).

1963–1972 Chairmanship Professor Ernst Kolb

(▶ Chap. 3.2.31 for his C.V.)

After an interim period with Dr. Ulrich Henneberg acting as head Professor Ernst Kolb from Mainz was appointed to the new chair in 1963. In 1966 the Division was promoted a Department of Anaesthesiology of the Free University and Kolb became Full Professor in 1967. When in 1969 the new University Hospital Steglitz (in 1994 renamed as University Hospital Benjamin Franklin) of the Free University was put into operation Kolb moved from Charlottenburg to Steglitz as Professor and Chairman of the Department of Anaesthesiology and Surgical Intensive Care Medicine (▶ Chap. 3.2.3). The Department was responsible for a the central surgical unit with 17 tables, 10 more operating tables, a recovery room, diagnostic units, and an ICU with 22 beds. A number of active research groups were established. Due to political changes in Berlin Kolb moved to Munich already in 1972 where he was appointed to the new Chair at the Technical University. During a long interim period lasting from 1972-1978 Professor Ulrich Henneberg acted as Interim Chairman of the Department.

1972–1978 Interim Chairmanship Professor Ulrich Henneberg

Prof. Dr. med. Ulrich Henneberg

Born 28 July1927 in Schlossberg/Ostpreußen; 1949–1955 student of medicine in Heidelberg; 1955 doctorate in medicine; 1956–1957 Assistant, Physiological Department, University of Heidelberg; 1957–1960 residency in thoracic surgery, Heidelberg-Rohrbach; 1961 Resident, Anaesthesia Department, University Hospital Westend, Free University of Berlin; 1967 Lecturer in Anaesthesiology; 1972-1978 Associate Professor and Interim Chairman, Department of Anaesthesiology, University Hospital Steglitz, Free University of Berlin; 1978 Chief Physician, Anaesthesia Department, Hospital Am Urban, Berlin.

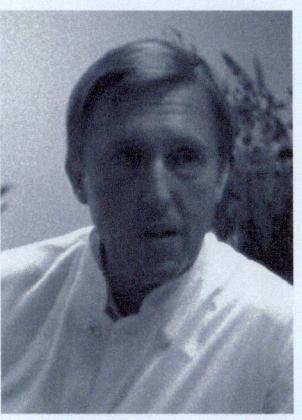

1978–1997 Chairmanship Professor Klaus Eyrich

Prof. Dr. med. Klaus Eyrich

Born 10 January 1927 at Tübingen; 1948–1954 student of medicine in Freiburg; 1954 doctorate in medicine in Freiburg; 1956–1957 Resident in surgery, Stuttgart; 1957–1959 pathology, Hamburg; 1959 ship's doctor; 1959–1960 internal medicine, Heilbronn, and surgery, Stuttgart; 1961–1968 postgraduate training at the Anaesthesia Division, Department of Surgery, University of Freiburg; 1964 Specialist in Anaesthesiology; 1969 Lecturer in Anaesthesiology; 1969–1978 Senior Physician, Department of Anaesthesiology, University of Würzburg; 1978 Full Professor and Chairman of the Department of Anaesthesiology, University Hospital Steglitz, Free University of Berlin; 1997 Professor Emeritus

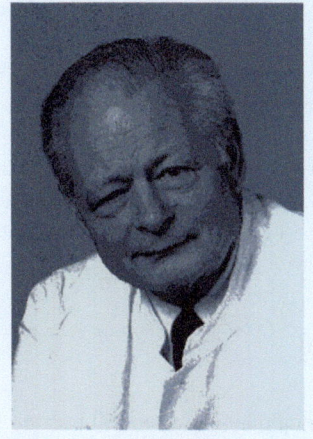

In 1978 Professor Klaus Eyrich (Würzburg) was appointed Full Professor and Chairman of the Department of Anaesthesiology (in 1981 renamed Department of Anaesthesiology and Surgical Intensive Care Medicine). In addition, Rüdiger Dennhardt (Marburg) and Siegfried Piepenbrock (Hannover) were appointed Associate Professors in 1980. With Eyrich the scientific activities went markedly up. Among the manyfold fields of research were circulation and oxygen transport, endocrine system, sepsis, paediatric anaesthesia, brain death and haemodynamic conditioning of braindead organ providers. The number of anaesthestics and intensive care patients steadily increased and from 1987 on anaesthetists were in charge of both the airborne and ground-based rescue services in cooperation with the Department of Internal Medicine.

3

Since 1997 Chairmanship Professor Christoph Stein

Prof. Dr. med. Christoph Stein

Born 30 November 1954; 1976–1982 student of medicine in Munich; 1982 doctorate in medicine; 1982 Resident in anaesthesia, State University of New York, University of California, Los Angeles, and University of Munich; 1988 Specialist in Anaesthesiology; 1992 Lecturer in Anaesthesiology; 1992-1997 Resident, Associate and Full Professor, Anesthesiology and Critical Care Medicine, Johns Hopkins University, Baltimore; 1997 Full Professor and Chairman of the Department of Anaesthesiology and Surgical Intensive Care Medicine; University Hospital Steglitz, Free University of Berlin.

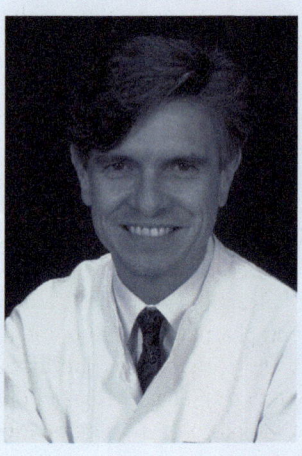

In 1997 Professor Christoph Stein (Baltimore) became Eyrich's successor. He centred the research activities to problems of mechanisms and therapy of pain and analgetic actions of opioids outside the central nervous system. For these projects his team successfully applied for a considerable number of competitive grants. Further problems which were investigated ranged from sepsis, nosocomial infections, artificial O_2 carriers and monitoring of anaesthetic depth to new methods of perioperative pain management.

In 1998 the Department's pain clinic which had been established in 1995 could move into own premises. In 2003 the University Hospital Benjamin Franklin of the Free University was amalgamated with the 2 campuses of the University Hospital Charité to form the Charité-University Medicine Berlin but the 3 Chairs of Anaesthesiology persisted (► Chap. 3.2.2 and 3.2.3).

Qualification as Lecturers in Anaesthesiology

Henneberg, Ulrich (1967); Eckart, Joachim (1972); Link, Jürgen (1983); Reinhart, Konrad (1984); Kretz, Franz-

Josef (1992); Striebel, Hans Walter (1993); Schaffartzik, Walter (1993); Hannemann, Lutz (1994); Papadopoulos, Georgios (1995); Spies, Claudia (1996); Rieger, Armin (1997); Hansen, Diethelm (2000); Schaefer, Michael (2001); Koster, Andreas (2002)

Professors in Anaesthesiology
Full Professors

Prof. Dr. Ernst Kolb (1972), University Hospital Rechts der Isar, Technical University of Munich
Prof. Dr. Siegfried Piepenbrock (1984), Hannover Medical School
Prof. Dr. Konrad Reinhart (1993), University of Jena
Prof. Dr. Georgios Papadopoulos (1995), Ioanina University, Greece
Prof. Dr. Claudia Spies (2004), Charité-University Medicine Berlin – Campus Virchow Klinikum

Associate Professor

Prof. Dr. Rüdiger Dennhardt (1980) Free University of Berlin
Prof. Dr. Siegfried Piepenbrock (1980) Free University of Berlin
Prof. Dr. Halina Machelska (2007), Extraordinary Professor of Experimental Anaesthesiology, Berlin

Adjunct Professors

Prof. Dr. Joachim Eckart, Prof. Dr. Ulrich Henneberg, Prof. Dr. Jürgen Link, Prof. Dr. Michael Schäfer, Prof. Dr. Walter Schaffartzik, Prof. Dr. Martin Welte, Jun. Prof. Dr. Christian Zöllner.

For further information:
http://anaesthesie.charite.de/

3.2.5 University of Bochum

G. Cunitz, H. Laubenthal, C. Puchstein, M. Zenz

The University of Bochum was opened in 1965, and in 1969 the Faculty of Medicine began to teach the first 50 students. For the sake of cost-efficiency the State of Northrhine Westphalia, the City of Bochum and 4 major hospitals agreed on a new way of medical education, i.e. these hospitals became university hospitals while keeping their organizational status unchanged. Consequently there were 4 academic Departments of Anaesthesiology.

Berufsgenossenschaftliche Kliniken Bergmannsheil, Department of Anaesthesiology, Intensive Care, Palliative Care and Pain Medicine

The »Bergmannsheil« was founded in 1890 by the Miners' Professional Association (»Bergbau-Berufsgenossenchaft«) and is the oldest accident hospital of the world. Here, a number of new ways of rescuing and therapy were inaugurated, e.g. a horse and carriage with a doctor (a precursor of a mobile life support unit), a medico-mechanical institute (a precursor of physiotherapy and rehabilitation) in 1892, X-ray diagnostics in 1896, an emergency ambulance in 1930, a blood bank in 1950. In 1958 a Division of Anaesthesia was established which was lead by Dr. Hans-Peter Harrfeldt and became independent in 1965. An intensive care unit was attached in 1960 and an Emergency Doctor's Ambulance introduced in 1968.

1986–2010 Chairmanship Professor Michael Zenz

Prof. Dr. med. Michael Zenz

Born 30 September 1945 in Minden; 1966–1973 student of medicine in Marburg; 1974 doctorate in medicine in Mainz; 1975–1977 Medical Officer, Federal Armed Forces Hospital, Koblenz; 1977–1986 Medical University of Hannover; 1979 Specialist in Anaesthesiology; 1981 Lecturer in Anaesthesiology; 1986 Adjunct Professor; 1986 Full Professor of Anaesthesiology and Chairman of the Department of Anaesthesiology, Intensive Care Medicine and Pain Therapy, University Hospital Bergmannsheil, Bochum; 2001 in addition Chairman of the Department of Anaesthesiology, Intensive Care Medicine and Pain Therapy, University Hospital Bochum-Langendreer; 2010 Professor Emeritus.

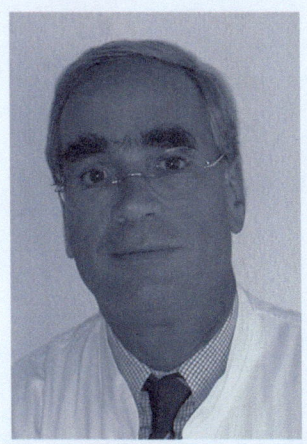

In 1986 Dr. Michael Zenz (Hannover) was appointed Full Professor and Chairman of the Department of Anaesthesiology, Intensive Care Medicine and Pain Therapy of the University Hospital Bergmannsheil which, at that time, was the first academic department carrying pain medicine as part of its name. Zenz reorganised the anaesthetic service, soon introduced an automated anaesthesia record and established an in- and outpatient pain service of great renown. He published textbooks on pain therapy, was founding member of the German Interdisciplinary Association for Pain Therapy (DIVS) which promoted the introduction of a »Certificate of Special Competence in Pain Therapy« by the German Medical Assembly in 1996, and served as Editor-in-chief of the journal »Der Schmerz«. In 1999 he succeeded in attracting an endowed professorship for pain therapy which was assigned to Professor Christoph Maier (Kiel). Research was clinically oriented and focussed on regional anaesthesia and a great variety of problems of pain medicine, e.g. a large project aimed at studying the therapeutic efficacy of acupuncture. In 2006 the Department was renamed Department of Anaesthesiology, Intensive Care, Palliative Care and Pain Medicine. As Zenz retired Professor Peter Zahn (Münster) was appointed his successor on 1 January 2011.

Qualification as Lecturers in Anaesthesiology

Harrfeldt, Hans-Peter (1978); Kulka, Peter-Johannes (1994) Strumpf, Michael (2000); Linstedt, Ulf (2002); Wiebalck, Albrecht (2005)

Professors of Anaesthesiology
Associate Professors

Prof. Dr. Christoph Maier (1999), Endowed Professor of Pain Therapy, Bochum

Ajunct Professors

Prof. Dr. Michael Tryba

For further information

www.anaesthesia.de
www.bergmannsheil.de

Knappschaftskrankenhaus Bochum-Langendreer, Department of Anaesthesiology, Intensive Care Medicine and Pain Therapy

The »Knappschaftskrankenhaus« in Bochum Langendreer was put into operation as a municipal hospital in 1909. As from 1918 it was run by the »Knappschaft«, the Miners' Guild, and developed, in the subsequent decades, to a large general hospital with special emphasis on treatment of miners' accidents. A Division of Anaesthesia and Intensive Therapy was established in 1968 and headed by Dr. E. Chraska until 1979.

1979–2001 Chairmanship Professor Günther Cunitz

Prof. Dr. med. Günther Cunitz

Born 17 November 1936 in Rostock; 1957–1963 student of medicine in Bonn; 1964 doctorate in medicine; 1965–1967 Pharmacological Institute, University of Bonn; 1967–1972 Resident, Department of Anaesthesiology, University of Würzburg; 1973 Lecturer in Anaesthesiology; 1979 Adjunct Professor; 1979 Chairman of the Department of Anaesthesia and Surgical Intensive Care Medicine at the Knappschaftskrankenhaus Bochum Langendreer, University Hospital; 1983 Full Professor of Anaesthesiology, University of Bochum; 2001 Professor Emeritus.

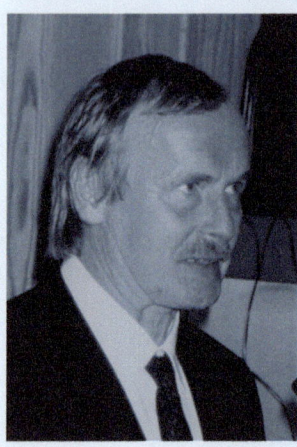

In 1979 Professor Günther Cunitz (Würzburg) assumed chairmanship of the Division which was renamed Department of Anaesthesia and Surgical Intensive Care Medicine. He was appointed Full Professor at the University of Bochum in 1983. He continuously expanded the clinical activities of his team in anaesthesia and intensive care medicine. In 2000, an emergency doctor's ambulance was instituted and alternately operated by anaesthetists and trauma surgeons. Main interests in both patient care and clinical research were multiple and brain trauma and neuroanaesthesia.

On recommendation of the Ministry of Education, Science and Research of the State of Rhineland Westphalia the »Berufsgenossenschaft« and the »Knappschaft« decided that departments should cooperate or even be merged. Therefore Professor Michael Zenz was put into charge when Cunitz retired in 2001. After Zenz' retirement Dr. André Gottschalk became Interim Chairman of the Department.

Qualification as Lecturers in Anaesthesiology:

Singbartl, Günter (1987); Schregel, Werner (1991); Langenstein, Holger (2003).

Professors of Anaesthesiology
Adjunct Professors

Prof. Dr. W. Schregel, Prof. Dr. G. Singbartl

For further information:

http://www.intensivtherapie.de
www.kk-bochum.de/Kliniken/Klinik_fuer_Anaesthesie/Kontakt.htm

St. Josef-Hospital Bochum, Department of Anaesthesiology

The St. Josef Hospital Bochum was founded in 1911. An anesthesiological service was instituted in 1962 and made a Central Division of Anaesthesia in 1967 headed by Dr. Walther Schwiete who retired in 1987.

1987–2007 Chairmanship Professor Heinz Laubenthal

Prof. Dr. med. Heinz Laubenthal

Born 7 January 1942 in Ochtendung/Rheinland-Pfalz; 1966 diploma in agriculture from the University of Bonn; 1966–1972 student of medicine in Munich; 1974–1977 Resident, Anaesthesia Department, Hospital München-Neuperlach; 1975 doctorate in medicine; 1977–1978 Department of Gynaecology, University of Ulm; 1978–1987 Resident (since 1981 Senior Physician), Department of Anaesthesiology, University of Munich; 1979 Specialist in Anaesthesiology; 1984 Lecturer in Anaesthesiology; 1986 Adjunct Professor; 1987 Full Professor and Chairman of the Department of Anaesthesiology, St. Josef University Hospital, Bochum; 2007 Professor Emeritus.

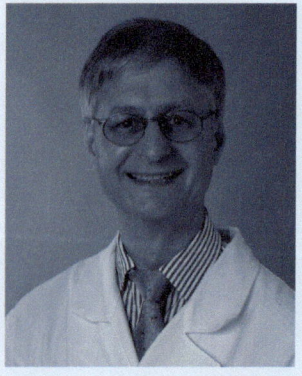

In November 1987 Professor Heinz Laubenthal (Munich) was appointed Full Professor and Chairman of the Department of Anaesthesiology. In 2003 the St. Josef Hospital and the St. Elisabeth Hospital merged so that the number of anaesthetics given by the new Department increased by about 60% to roughly 11,000 per year. Surgical intensive care medicine was a joint commitment of anaesthesiologists and surgeons. A pain clinic was established in 1988 and an emergency doctor's ambulance in 1990. Research was directed on clinical problems, e.g. volume replacement, peripheral actions of local anaesthetics and opioids and regional anaesthesia.

For further information:

www.ruhr-uni-bochum.de/medizin/institute_und_kliniken.htm#klinikum
www.anaesthesie-bochum.de

Marienhospital Herne, Department of Anaesthesiology Surgical Intensive Care Medicine, Pain and Palliative Medicine

The St.Mary's Hospital Herne was founded in 1883, extended in 1902 and 1925 and provided with an ICU in 1931. In 1966 a completely new construction was put into operation. About 5 years later a Division of Anaesthesia was established and headed by Dr. Eva Arlt.

Since 1987 Chairmanship Professor Christoph Puchstein

Prof. Dr. med. Christoph Puchstein

Born 15 March 1951 in Prien; 1969–1975 student of medicine in Munich; 1976 doctorate in medicine; 1977–1979 Research Associate, Department of Pharmacology and Toxicology, Hannover Medical School; 1979–1983 Resident, Department of Anaesthesiology, University of Münster; 1983 Specialist in Anaesthesiology; 1983 Senior Physician; 1984 Lecturer in Anaesthesiology; 1987 Full Professor of Anaesthesiology and Chairman of the Department of Anaesthesiology, St. Mary's Hospital Herne, University of Bochum.

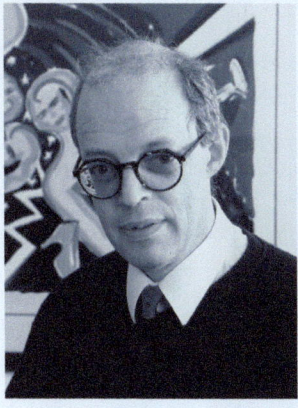

After Arlt's retirement Dr. Christoph Puchstein (Münster) was appointed Full Professor of Anaesthesiology and Chairman of the Department of Anaesthesiology, St. Mary's University Hospital, Herne, in 1987. The Department was in charge of the anaesthesiological service, the surgical ICU and the pain clinic. The latter was extended by an inpatient pain therapy unit of 10 beds and eventually a palliative care unit was added. Therefore the Department was renamed Department of Anaesthesiology Surgical Intensive Care Medicine, Pain and Palliative Medicine. Areas of research are enteral and parenteral nutrition of critically ill and end-stage cancer outpatients, and measurement and treatment of pain in children.

For further information:

www.ruhr-uni-bochum.de/mahe/anaesthesie/anae_index.htm

3.2.6   University of Bonn

Department of Anaesthesiology and Intensive Care Medicine

J. Nadstawek, A. Hoeft

The first ether anaesthesia was given in Bonn in March 1847 by Hermann-Friedrich Kilian, Professor of Obstetrics at the University. In 1902 Oskar Witzel, Associate Professor of Surgery, inaugurated the ether drip application and gave practical courses on this technique. Regional anaesthesia is associated with August Bier, Professor of Surgery at the University from 1903-1907. In 1948 Erich von Redwitz, Professor of Surgery, performed the first thoracic surgical procedure under intubation anaesthesia. In 1965 Dr. Leo Havers, qualified as Lecturer in Anaesthesiology in 1963, was made Senior Consultant, responsible for the anaesthetic service in the Department of Surgery, by the Chairman Professor Alfred Gütgemann. In 1970 he was promoted Associate Professor and Head of the Division of Anaesthesiology of the Department of Surgery. An emergency medical service for the City of Bonn was created in 1971.

1974–1995 Chairmanship Professor Horst Stoeckel

Prof. Dr. Dr. h. c. mult. Horst Stoeckel, FRCA

Born 26 September 1930 in Lodz; 1949–1955 student of medicine, Humboldt University Berlin; 1958 doctorate in medicine; 1955–1956 Research Associate, Department of Pharmacology, Humboldt University Berlin; 1955–1958 residency in Marienberg/Saxonia; 1959–1960 Resident, Division of Anaesthesiology, Hufeland Hospital, Berlin-Buch, 1961 Research Associate, Department of Physiology, Humboldt University, Berlin; 1962–1974 Department of Anaesthesiology, University of Heidelberg; 1962 Specialist in Anaesthesiology; 1969 Lecturer in Anaesthesiology; 1973 Adjunct Professor; 1974 Full Professor and Chairman of the Department of Anaesthesiology, University of Bonn; 1985 Fellow by election of the Royal College of Anaesthetists, London; 1990-1997 Member of the German National Academy of Sciences Leopoldina; Honorary Member of the Polish, Japanese and German Societies of Anaesthesiology and of the Association of University Anesthesiologists of the USA; Corresponding Member of the Finnish Society of Anaesthesiologists; honorary doctorate of the Medical Academy of the University of Lodz, Poland, and of the Faculty of Medicine of the Humboldt University, Berlin; 1995 Professor Emeritus; 2000 Founder of the Horst Stoeckel Museum for the History of Anaesthesiology at the University of Bonn.

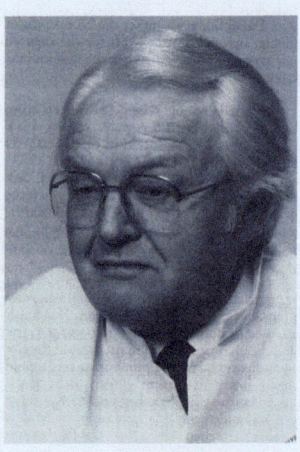

On 1 March 1974 Professor Horst Stoeckel (Heidelberg) became the first Full Professor and Chairman of the Department of Anaesthesiology. First he had to increase the number of doctors and nurses according to the growing demands for providing anaesthesiological services and move towards modern anesthesiology and clinic management. By 1987 Stoeckel had already implemented a computerized documentation of anesthetics, emergency medical services, on-call plans and resident rotations. Modern anaesthetic and monitoring equipment was installed and new anaesthetic techniques were introduced. A pain clinic was opened in 1990. When new premises for the surgical centre were put into operation in 1994, the Department became the Department of Anaesthesiology and Intensive Care Medicine with 10 ICU beds.

Along with the development of an organizational structure a research group was established with its own laboratories. The major research project marking Stoeckel's tenure was the clinical pharmacokinetics and dynamics of general and regional anesthesia which found further development in computer assisted IV anesthesia and the so-called closed loop feedback anesthesia. There was particular interest in the quantification of the depth of anesthesia via EEG, somatosensory and acoustically evoked potentials. As a new research field the molecular pharmacology of IV and inhalation anesthetics was added when Bernd Urban from Cornell University was appointed Associate Professor of Experimental Anesthesiology in 1989. In 1991 Helmut Schwilden became Associate Professor of Clinical Pharmacological Anesthesiology. Many studies on quality assurance in rescue services, traumatic brain injury and resuscitation outcome as well as animal experiments and clinical studies on the endobronchial application of drugs for the purpose of cardiopulmonary resuscitation were carried out. The scientific projects were funded by several major grants from the German Research Foundation, the Ministry of Science and Research in the State of Nordrhein-Westfalen, and the Federal Ministry of Research and Technology. Twelve research prizes were awarded and 31 foreign research fellows hosted by the Department.

Since 1995 Chairmanship Professor Andreas Hoeft

Prof. Dr. med. Andreas Hoeft

Born 22 October 1954 in Bielefeld; 1974–1980 medical school, University of Münster; 1980 doctorate in medicine (MD); 1980–1986 Research Associate, Centre of Physiology and Pathophysiology, University of Göttingen; 1986 PhD in Physiology; 1986–1991 Residency, Department of Anaesthesiology, Emergency and Intensive Care Medicine, University of Göttingen; 1991 Board certification in Anaesthesiology and Intensive Care Medicine; 1991–1992 Visiting Assistant

Professor, Department of Anesthesiology, University of Texas, Houston, TX, USA; 1992 Lecturer in Physiology and Anaesthesiology, University of Göttingen; 1993–1995 Senior Physician, Centre of Anaesthesiology, Emergency and Intensive Care Medicine, University of Göttingen; 1993 Visiting Associate Professor, Department of Anesthesiology, University of Texas; 1995 Full Professor and Chairman of the Department of Anaesthesiology and Intensive Care Medicine, University of Bonn.

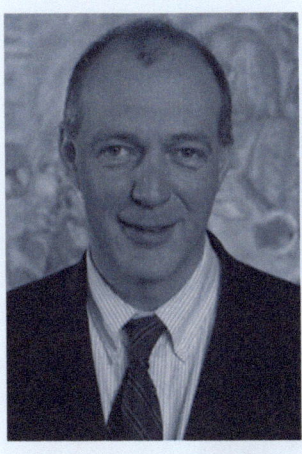

On the 1st of October 1995 Andreas Hoeft was appointed as Full Professor and Chairman of the Department of Anaesthesiology and Intensive Care Medicine at the Faculty of Medicine of the University of Bonn. His first priority was to encourage young physicians to get involved into research in various fields and consequently to undergo professional research trainings in numerous international institutions. Over the years Hoeft has systematically expanded scientific as well as clinical activities in the department. He himself intensified the area of basic as well as clinical studies in cardiovascular research. Complementary he successfully pursued the modernization and optimization of the entire equipment in all anesthesia workplaces and in intensive care units. Moreover, under his supervision the tradition of research on pharmacokinetics and pharmacodynamics of anaesthetics was continued and intensified within the department. In cooperation with Frank Stüber, who currently is Professor and Chairman in the Department of Anaesthesiology at the University Hospital in Bern (Switzerland), Hoeft was able to expand the research focuses of the department to molecular mechanisms of systemic inflammatory reactions and sepsis. Especially in the field of sepsis research the department gained immense expertise within the past years. At present, several academic members and their research groups are working on various areas of sepsis research in Bonn and other recognized international institutions. Furthermore, since decades the Department is a centre for research in the fields of EEG-Monitoring, resuscitation and critical care medicine. Hoeft was entrusted with the guidance of the emergency physician team in the City of Bonn. Dr. Ulrich Heister, one of the senior physicians of the department and an expert in critical care medicine, is in charge of the emergency physician team. The close cooperation between the city authorities as well as the department enabled Hoeft to establish a structured training program in emergency medicine for all residents of the department. After Hoeft became head of the Department, also the organizational responsibility for various surgical ICUs were established as part of the Department for Anesthesia and Intensive Care Medicine. In 1997, Christian Putensen (Innsbruck) was appointed as Associate Professor and Head of the surgical ICUs. Putensen expanded the Department's research interests in ARDS. Currently the Department is in charge of approximately 50 ICU beds (including 8 IMC beds) on 4 ICUs. In 1999, Prof. Joachim Nadstawekk, became head of the pain clinic also including the responsibility for the postoperative pain service of the medical centre of Bonn. Currently the department employs app. 145 physicians, including app. 60 residents. In total the members of the department take care for app. 26.000 anaesthesia procedures, 4.500 intensive care patients, the medical emergency system of the City of Bonn, and allocates a 24 hr pain service including an acute pain service and chronic pain therapy via the outpatient pain treatment clinic.

Qualification as Lecturers in Anaesthesiology

Havers, Leo (1963); Gött, Ulrich (1964); Gabriel, Werner (1972); Schulte am Esch, Jochen (1977); Hack, Guido (1978); Pfeifer, Gerhard (1981); Koenig, Annelie (1983); Lauven, Peter M. (1985); Murday, Harri (1985); Schüttler, Jürgen (1986); Hausmann, Dieter (1986); Rommelsheim, Kuno (1987); Schwilden, Helmut (1988); Hörnchen, Ulrich (1989); Nadstawek, Joachim (1990); Ebeling, Bernd Jörk (1991); Frenkel, Christian (1995); Fischer, Matthias (1997); Stüber, Frank (1999); von Spiegel, Tilman (2002); Röpcke, Heiko (2002); Schröder, Stefan (2002); Bruhn, Jörgen (2002); Wrigge, Hermann (2004); Baumgarten, Klaus (2006); Knüfermann, Pascal (2008); Söhle, Martin (2008); Lehmann, Lutz E. (2009); Weber, Stefan U. (2009); Ellerkmann, Richard (2010)

3

Professors of Anaesthesiology
Full Professors

Prof. Dr. Jochen Schulte am Esch (1982), University of Hamburg
Prof. Dr. Jürgen Schüttler (1995), University of Erlangen-Nuremberg
Prof. Dr. Frank Stüber (2008), University of Bern, Switzerland

Associate Professors

Prof. Dr. Leo Havers (1970), Bonn
Prof. Dr. Bernd Urban (1989), Associate Professor of Experimental Anaesthesiology, Bonn
Prof. Dr. Dr. Helmut Schwilden (1991), Bonn
Prof. Dr. Dr. Helmut Schwilden (1996), University of Erlangen-Nuremberg
Prof. Dr. Christian Putensen (1997), Bonn
Prof. Dr. Hermann Wrigge (2010), University of Leipzig

Adjunct Professors

Prof. Dr. Leo Havers, Prof. Dr. Werner Gabriel, Prof. Dr. Jochen Schulte am Esch, Prof. Dr. Guido Hack, Prof. Dr. Gerhard Pfeifer, Prof. Dr. Dr. Peter M. Lauven, Prof. Dr. Jürgen Schüttler, Prof. Dr. Dieter Hausmann, Prof. Dr. Harri Murday, Prof. Dr. Kuno Rommelsheim, Prof. Dr. Ulrich Hörnchen, Prof. Dr. Dr. Joachim Nadstawek, Prof. Dr. Dr. Bernd Jörk K. Ebeling, Prof. Dr. Christian Frenkel

For further information:

www.meb.uni-bonn.de/institute/kliansint/kliansint.html

3.2.7 Technical University of Dresden, University Hospital Carl Gustav Carus

Department of Anaesthesiology und Intensive Care Medicine

D.M. Albrecht, T. Koch, A. Heller

In 1954, the Medical Academy of Dresden was founded in the City Hospital Dresden-Johannstadt. Since 1961 at least one anaesthetist was employed by the Department of Surgery. In 1963, training in anaesthesia was started and a surgical intermediate care unit run by anaesthesia residents was opened. About one year later, a Division of Anaesthesia was established at the Department of Surgery and headed by Dr. Paul Fritsche until 1967. It was upgraded to a Central Anaesthesia Division of the Medical Academy in 1972 and in 1979 Dr. Karl-Heinz Martin, Head of the Division, was appointed Full Professor and Chairman of the Division of Anaesthesiology and Intensive Therapy of the Medical Academy.

1979–1980 Chairmanship Professor Karl-Heinz Martin

Prof. Dr. med. Karl-Heinz Martin

Born 31 October 1926 in Nuremberg, deceased 1980 in Dresden; 1945–1951 student of medicine in Erlangen; 1952 residency in surgery and anaesthesia, University Hospital Halle (Saale); 1956 Specialist in Anaesthesiology; 1953 Senior Physician and Head of the Division of Anaesthesia; Department of Surgery, University Hospital Halle; 1969 Lecturer in Anaesthesiology; 1978 Senior Lecturer; 1979 Full Professor and Chairman of the Department of Anaesthesiology and Intensive Care Therapy, Medical Academy Dresden.

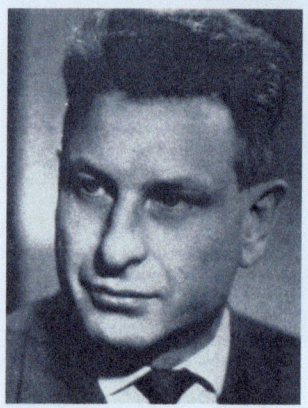

1985–1994 Chairmanship Professor Helga Schiffner

Prof. Dr. med. Helga Schiffner

Born 8 June 1938 in Elsterwerda; 1956–1962 student of medicine in Berlin and Dresden; 1962 doctorate in

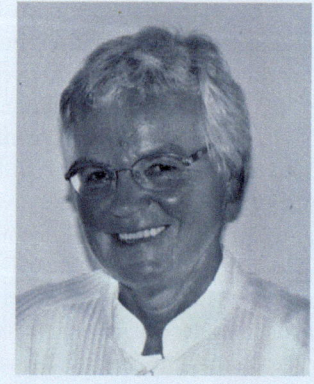

medicine; 1963–1967 training in anaesthesia in Dresden; 1967 Specialist in Anaesthesiology; 1972 Senior Physician;1981 Lecturer in Anaesthesiology; 1982 Chairperson of the Department of Anaesthesiology and Intensive Therapy, Medical Academy Dresden; 1985 appointment as Full Professor of Anaesthesiology.

After Martin's premature death in 1980 an interim direction came into force. In 1982 the Division became the Department of Anaesthesiology and Intensive Therapy and Dr. Helga Schiffner took over the interim chairmanship. In 1985 she was promoted Full Professor and Chairperson of the Department. She adapted the anaesthetic service to the increasing demands and established a pain clinic. In 1993 the Medical Academy became the Faculty of Medicine of the Technical University of Dresden. All Chairs were newly advertised including that of Anaesthesiology.

1994–2002 Chairmanship Professor Detlev Michael Albrecht

Prof. Dr. med. Detlev Michael Albrecht

Born 14 December 1949 in Munich; 1971–1976 student of medicine in Munich; 1977–1978 postgraduate training in Munich, Wolfratshausen, Starnberg, Mühldorf; 1978–1982 residency in surgery and anaesthesia in Mühldorf; 1982 Resident, Department of Anaesthesiology, University of Munich; 1984 Specialist in Anaesthesiology; 1985 doctorate in medicine; 1985 Senior Physician; 1986–1989 Senior Physician, Department of Anaesthesiology, University Hospital Lübeck; 1989 Lecturer of Anaesthesiology; 1989–1990 Interim Chairman;

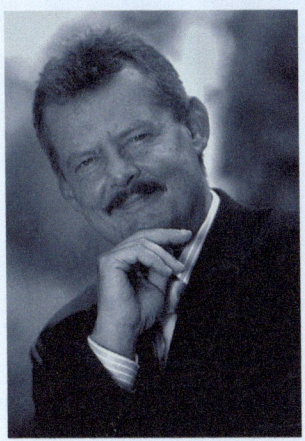

1991 Associate Professor of Anaesthesiology and Senior Physician, Department of Anaesthesiology and Intensive Care Medicine, University Hospital Mannheim; 1994 Full Professor of Anaesthesiology and Chairman of the Department of Anaesthesiology and Intensive Care Medicine, University Hospital Carl Gustav Carus, Technical University of Dresden; 2002 Medical Director of the University Hospital Carl Gustav Carus.

On 1 September 1994 Professor Detlev Michael Albrecht (Mannheim) was appointed Full Professor and Chairman of the Department of Anaesthesiology and Intensive Care Medicine of the Faculty of Medicine Carl Gustav Carus, Technical University of Dresden. He restructured the Department, adjusted the anaesthetic care system to the fast expanding spectrum of surgical activities and established an anaesthesiological ICU. The Department became responsible for the interdisciplinary pain clinic and, in co-operation with internists and surgeons, for the pre-hospital emergency medical service. Albrecht initiated a very active and successful research activity comprising experimental as wells as clinical projects. Main scientific topics were pulmonary perfusion, respiratory and haemodynamic monitoring, prognostic markers after cerebral injury, artificial blood substitutes, development of new oxygenators, inhalational application of perfluorocarbones, endothelin receptors, immunonutrition and new therapeutic approaches to ARDS and sepsis. Collaborative projects were established with the Department of Physiology (perfusion experiments in the isolated rabbit lung) and the Department of Perfusion Technology and Biomaterials of the Technical University (development of new oxygenators). Several competitive grants were obtained from the German Research Council. An association with Harvard Medical School was initiated by Albrecht in 1999 with the aim to reform the undergraduate teaching by implementing the concept of problem-oriented learning.

Since 2002 Chairmanship Professor Thea Koch

Prof. Dr. med. Thea Koch

Born 1 November 1961 in Giessen; 1980-1986 student of medicine in Marburg; 1987doctorate in medicine; 1986-1991 residency in anaesthesia, Universities of Lübeck and Mannheim; 1991 Specialist in Anaesthesiology; 1991-1996 Research Associate, Department of Anaesthesiology and Intensive Care Medicine, University Hospital Mannheim; 1994 Senior Physician; 1995

3

Lecturer in Anaesthesiology; 1996-1998 University Lecturer; 1998 Associate Professor and Senior Physician, Department of Anaesthesiology and Intensive Therapy, University Hospital Carl Gustav Carus, Dresden; 2002 Interim Chairperson; 2006 Full Professor and Chairperson; 2007 President, German Academy of Continuing Education in Anaesthesiology.

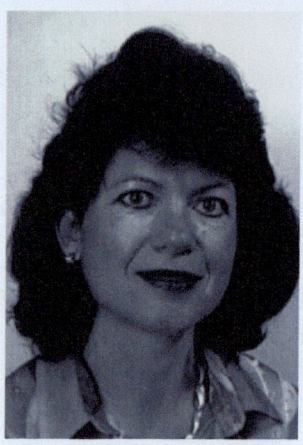

In 2006 Professor Thea Koch who had acted as Interim Chairperson since 2002 was appointed Full Professor and promoted to the position of Chairperson of the Department. She had a leading role in the creation of the Interdisciplinary Simulator Centre Dresden (ISIMED) in 2003 and the foundation of the University Pain Centre (USC) in 2004. In this year, a preanaesthetic clinic was established. Koch continued and markedly expanded the scientific and teaching efforts which had been set up during Albrecht's chairmanship.

Qualification as Lecturers in Anaesthesiology:

Schiffner, Helga (1981); Weber, Friedemann (1985); Siegismund, Kurt (1987); Ragaller, Maximilian (2001); Heller, Axel Rüdiger (2002); Bleyl, Jörg-Uwe (2003); Theilen, Hermann (2003); Gama de Abreu, Marcelo (2004); Hübler, Matthias (2004); Stehr, Sebastian (2010)

Professors of Anaesthesiology
Adjunct Professors

Prof. Dr. Marcelo Gama de Abreu; Prof. Dr. Axel R. Heller; Prof. Dr. Matthias Hübler; Prof. Dr. Maximilian Ragaller; Prof. Dr. Rainer Sabatowski

For further information:

http://www.uniklinikum-dresden.de/das-klinikum/kliniken-polikliniken-institute/ane

3.2.8   University of Düsseldorf

Department of Anaesthesiology
J. Tarnow, B. Pannen

On 15 September 1952, Dr. Martin Zindler, Specialist in Anaesthesiology, was made responsible for the anaesthesia service by Professor Ernst Derra, Chairman of the Department of Surgery of the University of Düsseldorf. In 1959 Zindler became Senior Physician and in 1962, initiated by Derra against the bitter resistance of the surgeon K.H. Bauer (Heidelberg), Associate Professor and Head of the Division of Anaesthesia. Four years later Zindler was appointed Full Professor and Chairman of the Department of Anaesthesiology.

1966–1987 Chairmanship Professor Martin Zindler

Prof. Dr. med. Martin Zindler

Born 28 April 1920 in Straußberg; until 1945 student of medicine in Breslau and Munich; 1949 doctorate in medicine; 1946–1950 residency in surgery at the Hospital München-Schwabing; 1950–1952 residency in anaesthesia, Medical College of Alabama; University of Pennsylvania, Philadelphia; Children's Hospital Philadelphia; 1952 Anaesthesiologist, Department of Surgery, University of Düsseldorf; 1958 Lecturer in Anaesthesiology; 1962 Associate Professor; 1966 Full Professor of Anaesthesiology and Chairman of the Department, University of Düsseldorf; 1987 Professor Emeritus; 1995 Honorary Member of the German Society of Anaesthesiology and Intensive Care Medicine.

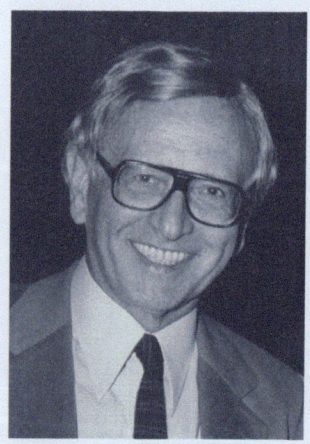

Zindler's Division had a good reputation from the beginning. He introduced surface hypothermia for cardiac procedures with circulatory discontinuity. The first operation carried out using this technique took place on 9 February 1955. Subsequently a large number of anaesthetists from all over the world made visits to Düsseldorf. In order to comply with the fast expanding spectrum of anaesthesiological services, Zindler organized regular lectures which were given twice weekly. In addition, he established a school for anaesthesia nurses in 1970. Intensive care medicine was started when new premises of the Department of Surgery were put into operation in 1958. An agreement was reached stating that ICU patients were treated jointly by surgeons and anaesthesiologists and that an experienced and academically qualified Senior Physician of the Department of Anaesthesiology acted as medical head of this ICU.

The establishment of separate research units dated back to the recommendations published by the German Science Council in 1968. They stated that by involving natural scientists in the respective departments and divisions the efficiency, quality and cost-benefit ratio of clinical research would markedly improve. These political conditions enabled Zindler to establish a Division of Experimental Anaesthesiology and in 1971 the circulatory physiologist Professor Joachim O. Arndt (Berlin) was appointed Professor of Experimental Anaesthesiology. In 1984, a Centre of Anaesthesiology was formed of the Department of Clinical Anaesthesiology and the Division of Experimental Anaesthesiology. Arndt was very successful in establishing a prospering environment for a large number of scientific activities. In the period 1972–1987 four major projects were supported by the German Research Foundation, a large number of original papers, book chapters and doctoral theses were published and several scientific prizes won by members of the Department.

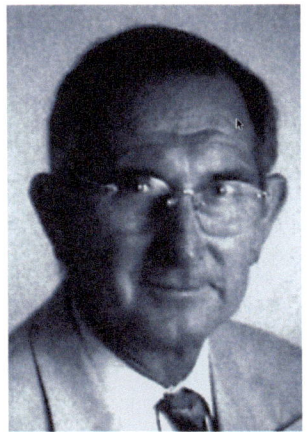

Joachim Arndt

1987–2007 Chairmanship Professor Jörg Tarnow

Prof. Dr. med. Jörg Tarnow, FRCA

Born 22 May 1940 in Wilhelmshaven; 1960–1966 student of medicine in Kiel; 1966 doctorate in medicine; 1966–1968 internship; 1968–1968 Medical Officer; 1970–1973 residency in anaesthesia, Hospital Charlottenburg of the Free University of Berlin; 1973 Specialist in Anaesthesiology; 1975 Lecturer in Anaesthesiology; 1978 Visiting Professor, Department of Anesthesia, Massachusetts General Hospital and Children's Hospital Center, Harvard Medical School, Boston, USA; 1979 Adjunct Professor, Free University of Berlin; 1987 Full Professor and Chairman of the Department of Anaesthesiology, University of Düsseldorf; 1992 Fellow of the Royal College of Anaesthetists, London; 2005 Professor Emeritus.

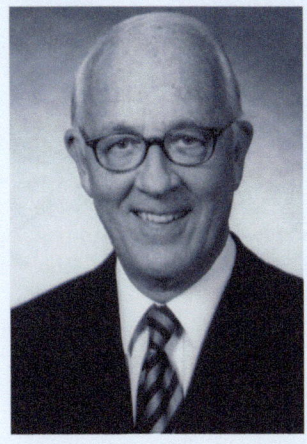

After Zindler's retirement in 1987, Professor Jörg Tarnow (Berlin) was appointed to the Chair of Anaesthesiology. He renovated the departmental rooms, modernized the complete equipment, adapted the human resources to the actual needs and introduced IT-based documentation and data management systems. In 1991 a pain clinic was opened and in 1999 the existing surgical ICU with 15 beds replaced by a new one with 20 beds.

During Tarnow's chairmanship the scientific efforts were again markedly expanded. In the period 1988–2001, 23 projects were supported by external research grants, including 14 supported by the German Research Foundation. A total of 350 papers were published in peer-reviewed journals, the number of scientific prizes added up to 26. Main areas of research were the actions of local anaesthetics on structure and function of nerve fibres, mechanical interactions between respiration and circulation, pulmonary hypertension accompanying acute lung failure, function of nociception, influence of sympathetic blockade on circulatory regulation, blood volume distribution and left ventricular function, relationship between cardiac output and oxygen consumption under various conditions, pulmonary circulation and oxygen consumption of the lung during extracorporeal circulation, influence of anaesthetics on reperfusion injury of the myocardium. After Arndt's retirement in 1999 the Division of Experimental Anaesthesiology was reunified with the Clinical Department, now forming one single Department of Anaesthesiology.

Since 2007 Chairmanship Professor Benedikt Pannen

Prof. Dr. med. Benedikt Pannen

Born 30 May 1962 in Weeze; 1981-1987 student of medicine in Aachen; 1988 doctorate in medicine; 1988-1989 Resident, Department of Pathology, University of Mainz; 1989-1993 residency at the Department of Anaesthesiology, University of Freiburg; 1993 Specialist in Anaesthesiology; 1993-1995 Postdoctoral Fellow, Department of Anesthesia and Critical Care, Johns Hopkins University School of Medicine, Baltimore, USA; 1995 Staff Anaesthesiologist, Department of Anaesthesiology, University of Freiburg; 1999 Lecturer in Anaesthesiology and Senior Physician; 2000-2004 Heisenberg-Scholar of the German Research Foundation; 2004 Associate Professor; 2007 Full Professor and Chairman of the Department of Anaesthesiology, University of Düsseldorf.

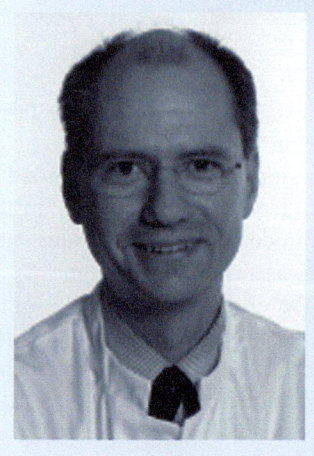

In 2007, Professor Benedikt Pannen (Freiburg) was appointed Full Professor and Chairman of the Department of Anaesthesiology. The annual number of anaesthetics increased to 18,000, that of ICU beds under anaesthesiological responsibility to 40. Eight clinical and experimental research groups cover a large number of problems with special emphasis on translational research.

Qualification as Lecturers in Anaesthesiology

Zindler, Martin (1958); Pulver, Karl-Georg (1966); Dudziak, Rafael (1966); Podlesch, Ingrid (1968); Lennartz, Herbert (1969); Purschke, Reinhard (1974); Falke, Konrad (1977); Huse, Klaus (1977); Siepmann, Hermann Paul (1977); Strasser, Klaus (1978); Freye, Enno (1980); Wüst, Hans Joachim (1981); Inoue, Kazuo (1981); Steinhoff, Heinz-Hagen (1982); Grote, Bernhard (1983); Fournell, Artur (1985); Lipfert, Peter (1989); Peters, Jürgen (1990); Radermacher, Peter (1992); Klement, Wolfgang (1993); Hopf, Hans-Bernd (1994); Stühmeier, Klaus-Dieter (1997); Holthusen, Holger (1998); Schlack, Wolfgang (1998); Scheeren, Thomas Werner (1999); Loer, Stephan A. (1999); Zucker, Tom-Philipp (2000); Hartmann, Matthias (2000); Preckel, Benedikt (2002); Müllenheim, Jost (2003); Zacharowski, Kai (2003); Picker Olaf (2004); Ebel, Dirk (2006); Freynhagen, Rainer (2007); Schwarte, Lothar (2006); Stevens, Markus (2007); Beiderlinden, Martin (2008)

Professors of Anaesthesiology
Full Professors

Prof. Dr. Rafael Dudziak (1972), University of Frankfurt am Main

Prof. Dr. Herbert Lennartz (1976), University of Marburg

Prof. Dr. Konrad Falke (1988), Free University of Berlin

Prof. Dr. Jürgen Peters (1996), University of Essen

Prof. Dr. Stephan A. Loer (2006), University Medical Center, Free University of Amsterdam

Prof. Dr. Wolfgang Schlack, (2006), Academic Medical Center, University of Amsterdam

Prof. Dr. Kai Zacharowski (2006), Department of Anaesthesia and Critical Care, University Hospitals Bristol

Associate Professors

Prof. Dr. Joachim O. Arndt (1971), Associate Professor of Experimental Anaesthesiology, Düsseldorf

Prof. Dr. med. Peter Radermacher (1994), Associate Professor of Clinical Anaesthesiology, University of Ulm

Prof. Dr. Thomas W. Scheeren (2004), University of Rostock

Adjunct Professors

Prof. Dr. Karl-Georg Pulver (1971), Prof. Dr. Reinhard Purschke (1979), Prof. Dr. Klaus Huse (1980), Prof. Dr. Hermann Siepmann (1982), Prof. Dr. Klaus Strasser (1983), Prof. Dr. Enno Freye (1985), Prof. Dr. Hans Joachim Wüst (1986), Prof. Dr. Kazuo Inoue (1989), Prof. Dr. Peter Lipfert (1994), Prof. Dr. Eckhard Müller (1999); Prof. Dr. Wolfgang Schlack (2003); Prof. Dr. Holger Holthusen (2004); Prof. Dr. Stephan A. Loer (2005); Prof. Dr. Artur Fournell (2005); Prof. Dr. Detlef Kindgen-Milles (2008); Prof. Dr. Peter Kienbaum (2009)

For further information:

www.uniklinik-duesseldorf.de/anaesthesiologie

3.2.9 University of Erlangen-Nuremberg

Department of Anaesthesiology

W. Schwarz, H. Schwilden, J. Schüttler

The University Hospital of Erlangen was one of the first places in Germany where on 24 January 1847 ether anaesthesia was introduced by Johann Ferdinand Heyfelder, then Full Professor of Surgery at Erlangen University. He also published the first monograph on ether anaesthesia in Germany in March 1847, 2 months after he had begun to use sulphuric ether.

In 1956 modern anaesthesia was introduced to Erlangen by Dr. Heinz-Otto Silbersiepe who had passed a residency in anaesthesia at the Georgetown Medical Center at Washington D.C. Half a year later he went back to the USA. After several changes of personnel Dr. Erich Rügheimer became Head of the Division of Anaesthesia in 1960. He devoted his further career to the development of anaesthesia in Erlangen.

1970–1995 Chairmanship Professor Erich Rügheimer

Prof. Dr. med. Erich Rügheimer

Born 16 February 1926, in Nuremberg; deceased 24 February 2007 in Erlangen; 1946–1951 student of medicine at the University of Erlangen; 1951 postgraduate training at the Department of Surgery, University of Erlangen; 1953 doctorate in medicine; 1953 Resident at the Department of Surgery; besides surgical training turning more and more to anaesthesia; 1956 Specialist in Anaesthesiol-

ogy; 1958 Specialist in Surgery; 1960 Senior Physician and Head of the Division of Anaesthesia; 1964 Lecturer in Anaesthesiology; 1966 Associate Professor of Anaesthesiology; 1970 Full Professor of Anaesthesiology; 1974 Chairman of the Department of Anaesthesiology; 1994 Honorary Member of the German Society of Anaesthesiology and Intensive Care Medicine; 1995 Professor Emeritus.

During Rügheimer's chairmanship the Department evolved into a central institution providing anaesthesia services for all surgical departments and units of the University Hospital. Rügheimer also established facilities for emergency care (1974), pain therapy (1990), and intensive care medicine (1995). As a legacy he left some innovative ideas to improve patient safety in anaesthesia and intensive care medicine by new training concepts for residency training and CME.

Since 1995 Chairmanship Professor Jürgen Schüttler

Prof. Dr. med. Dr. h.c. Jürgen Schüttler

Born 19 December 1953 in Bonn; 1974–1980 student of medicine in Bonn; 1981 Resident at the Department of Anaesthesiology, University of Bonn; 1982 doctorate in medicine; 1982–1983 Postdoctoral Fellow at the Department of Anesthesia, Stanford University School of Medicine, USA; 1985 Specialist in Anaesthesiology; 1985 Senior Physician at the Department of Anaesthesiology, University of Bonn; 1986 Lecturer in Anaesthesiology; 1990 Senior Consultant; 1991 Adjunct Professor; 1995 Full Professor and Chairman of the Department of Anaesthesiology, University of Erlangen; 2004 honorary doctorate of the Iuliu-Hatieganu University of Medicine and Pharmacy, Cluj-Napoca, Romania; since 2008 Dean of the Faculty of Medicine.

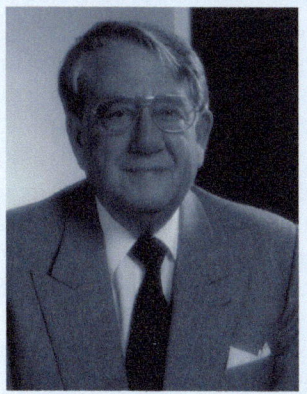

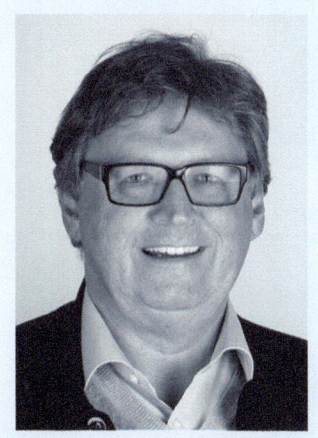

3

In 1995 Professor Jürgen Schüttler (Bonn) was appointed to the Chair of Anaesthesiology. At the beginning of his chairmanship the Department was entrusted with the organisational responsibility for the interdisciplinary surgical ICU with 25 beds which after complete renovation increased to 36 beds. The different units for the treatment of patients with chronic pain in 2004 were joined to an Interdisciplinary Pain Centre at the University Hospital under the direction of the Departments of Anaesthesiology and Neurology. The assumption of new responsibilities in clinical anaesthesia with more than 30.000 anaesthetic procedures, severeal emergency care units and in pain management and palliative care caused further increases of staff.

Schüttler brought great momentum to the development of education and scientific work at the Anaesthesia Department in Erlangen. In 1995 he got to work the first full-scale anaesthesia simulator in Germany. He has contributed considerable to the meanwhile widespread application of simulators in the education of medical students and in residents' training and CME in Germany. To improve the structures for scientific work Schüttler established a unit for experimental anaesthesiology which is directed by an Associate Professor of Experimental Anaesthesiology. A Division of Molecular Pneumology was established in 2009. Prof. Dr. Susetta Finotto was appointed its Head. In 2010 a Division of Palliative Medicine with 10 beds could be created. Prof. Dr. Christoph Ostgathe (Cologne) was appointed its Head.

Associate Professorship of Experimental Anaesthesiology

Prof. Dr. med. Dr. rer. nat. Helmut Schwilden

Born 10 March 1949 in Krefeld; 1967–1973 student of physics and mathematics at Bonn University,

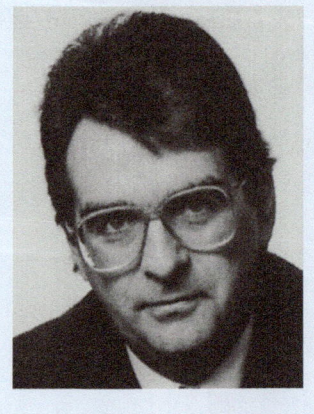

1976 doctorate in physics; 1976–1983 student of medicine; 1978–1988 Resident at the Department of Anaesthesiology, University of Bonn; 1982 doctorate in medicine; 1987 Specialist in Anaesthesiology; 1987 Lecturer in Anaesthesiology; 1988–1991 Chairman of the Paul-Martini-Foundation; 1991 Associate Professor of Clinical Pharmacological Anesthesiology, University of Bonn; 1996 Associate Professor of Experimental Anaesthesiology, University of Erlangen-Nuremberg.

New main areas of scientific research in Erlangen which were initiated by Jürgen Schüttler and Helmut Schwilden lay within the fields of clinical drug research (pharmacokinetics and pharmakodynamics of drugs for anaesthesia, pain therapy, resuscitation medicine or intensive care) and clinical pain research (investigation of approaches to therapy of pain). Based on a variety of approaches in pain research at the University of Erlangen-Nuremberg in 2005 a Clinical Research Unit »Determinants and Modulators of Postoperative Pain« was established at the Department with the support of the German Research Foundation (DFG). It was aimed at pooling the scientific efforts of the various institutions and in 2006 Prof. Dr. Carla Nau was appointed its Head.

Very recently Schüttler initiated more research activities in the field of innovative health technologies that has led to a »Center of Excellence for Medical Technology« under his associate directorship. In January 2010 a victory could be gained in a highly competitive contest, the Leading-Edge Cluster Competition of the Federal Ministry of Education and Research (BMBF). The aim of this cluster is the development of technologies which increase life expectancy, improve quality of life and reduce costs in the public health sector.

Qualification as Lecturers in Anaesthesiology:

Rügheimer, Erich (1964); Opderbecke, Hans Wolfgang (1977); Pasch, Thomas (1978); Grimm, Herbert (1981); Brandl, Martin (1983); Kamp, Johann Dieter (1985); Kraus, Gabriele (1990); Jacobi, Klaus (1991); Götz, Holger (1992); Braun, Günther Giovanni (1993); Mang, Harald (1994): Tschaikowsky, Klaus (1994); Pscheidl, Edgar (1994); Schmitt, Hubert (1995); Dinkel, Michael (1995); Hering, Werner (1997); Albrecht, Sven (1999); Koppert, Wolfgang (2001); Schmitz, Bernd (2002); Nau, Carla (2002); Kirmse, Max (2004); Fechner, Jörg (2005); Bremer, Frank (2005); Schmidt, Joachim (2007); Münster, Tino (2007); Jeleazcov, Christian (2009); Schießl, Christine (2009); Leffler, Andreas (2010); Tzabazis, Alexander (2010)

Professors of Anaesthesiology
Full Professors

Prof. Dr. Thomas Pasch (1987), University of Zurich
Prof. Dr. Michael Georgieff (1992), University of Ulm
Prof. Dr. Wolfgang Koppert (2009), Hannover Medical School
Prof. Dr. Christoph Ostgathe (2010), Endowed Professor of Palliative Medicine, Erlangen

Associate Professors

Prof. Dr. Dr. Helmut Schwilden (1996), Associate Professor of Experimental Anaesthesiology, Erlangen
Prof. Dr. Sven Albrecht (2002), Erlangen
Prof. Dr. Carla Nau (2006), Erlangen
Prof. Dr. Susetta Finotto (2009), Associate Professor of Molecular Medicine Erlangen

Adjunct Professors

Prof. Dr. Martin Brandl, Prof. Dr. Michael Georgieff, Prof. Dr. Herbert Grimm, Prof. Dr. Werner Hering, Prof. Dr. Klaus Jacobi, Prof. Dr. Johann Dieter Kamp, Prof. Dr. Wolfgang Koppert, Prof. Dr. Gabriele Kraus, Prof. Dr. Harald Mang, Prof. Dr. Hans Wolfgang Opderbecke, Prof. Dr. Jürgen Plötz, Prof. Dr. Edgar Pscheidl, Prof. Dr. Hubert Schmitt, Prof. Dr. Klaus Tschaikowsky

For further information:

www.anaesthesie.uk-erlangen.de

3.2.10 University of Essen-Duisburg

Department of Anaesthesiology and Intensive Care Medicine

J. Peters

The Essen University Hospital arose from the Municipal Hospital Essen founded in 1909. This became a Medical School in 1963 according to the recommendations of the German Science Council. The then formed Faculty of Medicine was first affiliated to the University of Münster and in 1967 to the new University of Bochum. In 1973, the Hospital became an institution of the University of Essen (later University of Essen-Duisburg) and is now the Essen University Hospital. In 1961, the anaesthesiologist Dr. Ludwig Stöcker was employed as Senior Physician by Professor Karl Kremer, Chairman of the Department of Surgery of the Municipal Hospital. Six months later, he became Head of the Division of Anaesthesia of the Hospital. In 1974, he was appointed Full Professor and Chairman of the Department of Anaesthesiology.

1974–1995 Chairmanship Professor Ludwig Stöcker

Prof. Dr. med. Ludwig Stöcker

Born 25 April 1930 in Münster; 1951–1956 student of medicine in Würzburg and Frankfurt/Main; 1956 doctorate in medicine at Frankfurt University; 1956–1958 internship, St. Mary's Hospital Witten and St. Louis University, Missouri, USA; surgical Resident, St. Louis University, Missouri, USA; 1959-1960 residency in gynaecology, Bochum and Wuppertal; 1960–1961 residency in anaesthesiology, Medical Academy of Düsseldorf; 1961 Research Fellow in pharmacology, Bayer Werke AG, Wuppertal; 1962 Senior Physician, Surgical Department, Municipal Hospital Essen; 1963 Head, Division of Anaesthesia; 1969 Lecturer in Anaesthesiology; 1972 Adjunct Professor; 1974 Full Professor and Chairman of the Department of Anaesthesiology, University Hospital Essen; 1995 Professor Emeritus.

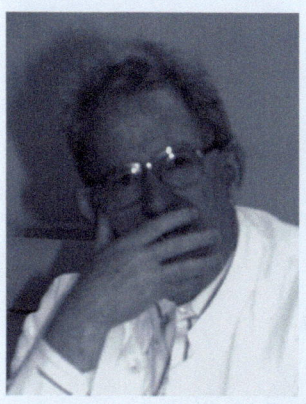

Stöcker was one of the pioneers of German anaesthesiology. From the beginning, his main focus was on the provision of an unexceptionable clinical service irrespective of the deficiency in equipment and personnel he was faced with over a long period of time. He was among those who early turned their attention to the clinical use of neuroaxial blocks and soon introduced the combination of general and regional anaesthesia. The establishment of open heart surgery in 1963 and the development of the University Hospital Essen to a centre of organ transplantation were important steps in which anaesthetists played an important role. Stöcker's manual »Introduction to Anaesthesia« (Narkose. Eine Einführung) was first published in 1967 and favoured as a reference book by students and residents for many years. In 1989, an ICU with 10 beds was made available to the Department

Since 1996 Chairmanship Professor Jürgen Peters

Prof. Dr. med. Jürgen Peters

Born 5 December 1954 in Dortmund; 1973-1979 student of medicine in Bochum und Essen; 1980 doctorate in medicine, University of Essen; 1980 Resident, Department of Anatomy; 1980-1981 Resident in anaesthesia, Municipal Hospital Duisburg; 1981-1985 Resident, Department of Anaesthesiology, University of Düsseldorf; 1984 Specialist in Anaesthesiology; 1985-1987 Attending Anesthesiologist, Department of Anesthesiology and Critical Care Medicine, The Johns Hopkins University Medical School, Baltimore, USA; 1986 Assistant Professor; 1987-1989 Research Associate, Divisions of Experimental and Clinical Anaesthesiology, University of Düsseldorf; 1990 Lecturer in Anaesthesiology and Senior Physician; 1996 Full Professor and Chairman of the Department of Anaesthesiology and Intensive Care Medicine, University Hospital Essen.

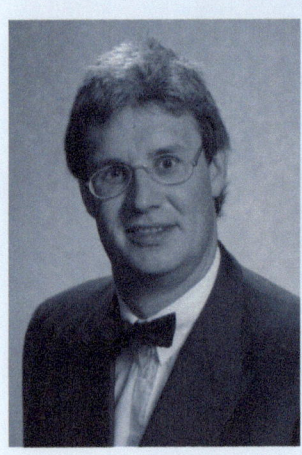

In 1996, Professor Jürgen Peters (Düsseldorf) was appointed to Stöcker's Professorship and Chair. He modernized the anaesthetic service and adapted it to the steadily increasing demands. Until 2001, the annual number of liver transplantations doubled to more than 100 and that of cardiac operations with cardio-pulmonary bypass increased by nearly 70%. In intensive care medicine the emphasis was laid on the treatment on patients with acute lung failure including extracorporeal CO_2 elimination and ventilation with nitric oxide. An acute pain service was established. Starting in 1997, a staff member and a resident of the Department supplemented the team of the interdisciplinary pain clinic. Since September 1998, anaesthetists were regularly involved in the mobile life support unit.

Peters defined 4 main fields of research: the cardiovascular system, physiology and pathophysiology of the lung and airways, neuromuscular transmission and pain therapy. For this purpose, cooperations were established with the Department of Anesthesiology and Critical Care Medicine, The Johns Hopkins University Medical School, Baltimore, USA, and the Department of Clinical Neurophysiology, University of Gothenburg, Sweden. The number of publications markedly increased and a considerable number of research grants and scientific prizes were obtained.

Qualification as Lecturers in Anaesthesiology

Stöcker, Ludwig (1969); Montel, Heinrich (1976); Taube, Hans Detlef (1978); Scherer, Ralf U. (1994); Günnicker, Franz-Michael (1996); Groeben, Harald (1999); Giebler, Reiner (2000); Kienbaum, Peter (2002); Adamzik, Michael (2009); Kottenberg, Eva (2009)

Professors of Anaesthesiology
Full Professors

Professor Dr. Dr. Wolfgang Kox (1993), Charité University Hospital, Berlin

Associate Professors

Prof. Dr. Dr. Wolfgang Kox (1992), Essen
Prof. Dr. med. Ralf U. Scherer (1997), Charité University Hospital, Berlin

Adjunt Professors

Prof. Dr. Harald Groeben, Prof. Dr.Matthias Hartmann; Prof. Dr. Ralf U. Scherer

For further information:

www.uni-due.de/anaesthesiologie

3.2.11   University of Frankfurt am Main

Department of Anaesthesiology, Intensive Care Medicine and Pain Therapy
R. Dudziak, K.-D. Zacharowski

In the early 1950s, a Division of Anaesthesia came into being at the Department of Surgery of the University of Frankfurt am Main. Over a period of 20 years, i.e. until 1972, it was headed by Dr. Helmut Vonderschmitt who qualified as Lecturer in Anaesthesiology in 1965. Due to his interest in anaesthetic technology he committed himself to a variety of innovations of anesthesia machines. In 1970, the Faculty of Medicine decided to make anaesthesiology independent and create a Chair and two associate professorships of Anaesthesiology.

1973–2003 Chairmanship Professor Rafael Dudziak

Prof. Dr. med. Rafael Dudziak

Born 6 February 1935 in Posen; 1951–1957 student of medicine in Posen; 1957 residency at the University Hospital Charité, Humboldt University Berlin; 1961 residency in physiology and anaesthesia in Düsseldorf; 1964 doctorate in medicine; 1964 Specialist in Anaesthesiology; 1966 Lecturer in Anaesthesiology; 1970 Adjunct Professor; 1973 Full Professor of Anaesthesiology and Chairman of the Department of Anaesthesiology, Intensive Care Medicine and Pain Therapy, University of Frankfurt; 2003 Professor Emeritus.

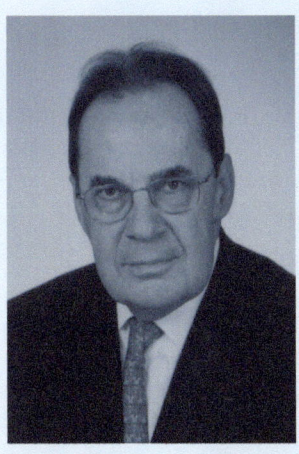

In 1973, Professor Rafael Dudziak (Düsseldorf) was appointed to the new Chair as Full Professor of Anaesthesiology and Chairman of the Centre of Anaesthesiology and Reanimation and to the directorship of Division I of Clinical Anaesthesia of the Centre providing the service for all surgical divisions and urology. Vonderschmitt and Dr. Dieter Böhmer were appointed Associate Professors. Böhmer was made responsible for the anaesthesia services in the Departments of Neurosurgery, Otorhinolaryngology and Ophthalmology (Division II), Vonderschmitt became Head of a new Division of Technical and Experimental Anaesthesia. In the following years, Dudziak and his team had to make every effort to attract a sufficient number of motivated young residents. The clinical tasks markedly increased as a Division of Cardio-Thoracic and Vascular Surgery was created in 1973 and the Division I became responsible for the ICU. When Böhmer was appointed Professor of Sports Medicine in 1976 Divisions I and II were in practice merged, but the final approval of the amalgamation took 6 more years. In 1980, the Division of Technical and Experimental Anaesthesia was renamed in Division of Experimental Anaesthesia and Professor Harald

Förster appointed to the corresponding Professorship. The Division of Clinical Anaesthesia eventually became the Department of Anaesthesiology, Intensive Care Medicine and Pain Therapy in 1997. A pain clinic was established in 1984. In the first year 105 patients were treated, in 2001 this number had increased to 549. Scientific projects were mainly carried out in cooperation with the Division of Experimental Anaesthesia, main topics being pharmacokinetics and pharmacodynamics of volatile and other anaesthetics, blood replacement, histamine, and interactions between carbon dioxide absorbents and volatile anaesthesics. Another research focus was pain medicine with emphasis on actions, side effects and therapeutic use of opioids and local anaesthetics, long-term regional blocks, diagnostic and therapeutic aspects of both acute and chronic pain.

2003–2007 Chairmanship Professor Bernhard Zwißler

(▶ Chap. 3.2.30 for his C.V.)

After Dudziak's retirement in 2003, Professor Bernhard Zwißler (Munich) was appointed Full Professor of Anaesthesiology and Chairman of the Department of Anaesthesiology, Intensive Care Medicine and Pain Therapy. During his chairmanship a new building hosting 16 operating rooms, an emergency centre and a new interdisciplinary ICU (managed by anesthesiologists) at the University Hospital was planned, constructed and opened in 2007. In 2005, the Department introduced a quality management system and was - as one of the first University Departments of Anaesthesiology in Germany - successfully certified according to DIN ISO 9001:2000 and re-certified in 2007. Student education was modernized by instituting a new hands-on training for students in the operating room as well as a full-scale simulator training as an obligatory part of the curriculum. Research focussed on the pathophysiology of respiratory failure and sepsis and the development of new therapeutic strategies for these entities. After Zwißler's move to the Chair of Anaesthesiology at the University of Munich, Professor Paul Kessler was appointed Interim Chairman of the Department.

Since 2009 Chairmanship Professor Kai-Dieter Zacharowski

Prof. Dr. med. Kai-Dieter Zacharowski, PhD, FRCA

Born 3 July 1967 in Kassel; 1989–1995 student of medicine in Mainz; 1995 doctorate in medicine; 1995–1997 Research Associate, Department of Internal Medicine/

Cardiology, University of Mainz; 1997–2001 Clinical Fellow and Lecturer in Clinical Pharmacology and Pharmacology, William Harvey Research Institute, Queen Mary, University of London; 2000 Ph.D. degree in pharmacology, University of London; 2002–2006 Junior Professor, Section of Experimental Anaesthesiology of the Department of Anaesthesiology, University of Düsseldorf; 2003 Lecturer in Anaesthesiology; 2006–2008 Professor and Chairman, Department of Anaesthesia and Critical Care, University Hospitals Bristol; 2009 Full Professor and Chairman of the Department of Anaesthesiology, Intensive Care Medicine and Pain Therapy, University of Frankfurt am Main.

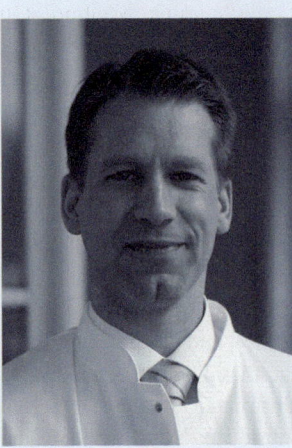

On 1 January 2009 Professor Kai-Dieter Zacharowski (Bristol) was appointed Zwißler's successor. His research, teaching and clinical interests are in both basic and clinical aspects of innate immunity, cardiovascular (myocardial infarction, arrhythmias) and critical care medicine (sepsis and shock). The annual number of anaesthetics has increased to 28,000, nearly 3,000 patients are treated in the anaesthesiological ICU, about 4,000 consultations are carried out in the pain clinic, and the doctors of the Department participate in the mobile life support and helicopter rescue services.

Qualification as Lecturers in Anaesthesiology

Vonderschmitt, Helmut (1965); Böhmer, Dieter (1969); Förster, Harald (1970); Schreiner-Hecheltjen, Josefa (1979); Ottermann, Uwe (1979); Steuer, Armin (1980); Schmidt, Hans (1981); Klein, Gerhard (1985); Ferber, Hubert F. (1985); Vettermann, Jörg (1990); Behne, Michael (1991); Latasch, Leo (1991); Probst, Steffen (1992); Lischke, Volker (1996); Kessler, Paul (1998); Westphal, Klaus (1999); Wissing, Heimo (2000); Bremerich, Dorothee (2001); Byhahn, Christian (2005); Meininger, Dirk (2006); Hofstetter, Christian (2007); Mierdl, Stephan (2007); Breitkreutz, Raoul (2008); Meier, Jens (2009); Scheller, Bertram (2010)

Professors of Anaesthesiology
Full Professors

Prof. Dr. Bernhard Zwißler (2007), Full Professor of Anaesthesiology, University of Munich

Associate Professors

Prof. Dr. Dieter Böhmer (1973), Frankfurt
Prof. Dr. Helmut Vonderschmitt (1973), Associate Professor of Technical-Experimental Anaesthesia, Frankfurt
Prof. Dr. Harald Förster (1980), Associate Professor of Experimental Anaesthesia, Frankfurt
Prof. Dr. Oliver Habler (2004), Frankfurt
Prof. Dr. Peter Rosenberger (2010), Frankfurt

Adjunct Professors

Prof. Dr. M. Behne; Prof. Dr. Dorothee Bremerich; Prof Dr. Christian Byhahn; Prof. Dr. Josefa Schreiner-Hecheltjen; Prof. Dr. Paul Kessler; Prof. Dr. Gerhard Klein, Prof. Dr. Volker Lischke; Prof. Dr. Uwe Ottermann.

For further information:

www.kgu.de/zaw

3.2.12 University of Freiburg

Department of Anaesthesiology and Intensive Care Therapy
K. Geiger

The development of anaesthesiology and intensive care medicine in Freiburg is closely associated with Professor Kurt Wiemers. In 1953 Hermann Krauss, then Professor of Surgery in Freiburg, asked Dr. Wiemers to move to Freiburg to establish anaesthesia care and intensive care medicine within the Department of Surgery. It did not take long before other departments asked for the services of anaesthesia.

1966–1985 Chairmanship Professor Kurt Wiemers

Prof. Dr. med. Kurt Wiemers

Born 6 June 1920 in Cologne; deceased 11 February 2006 in Denzlingen. 1938 student of medicine, University of Freiburg, 1940–1942 Universities of Königsberg, Berlin and Innsbruck; 1944 doctorate in medicine,

University of Munich; 1946–1947 residency in surgery at the Caritas-Krankenhaus, Cologne-Hohenlind; 1947–1950 Postdoctoral Fellow, Department of Physiology, University of Cologne; 1951-1953 Resident in surgery and anaesthesia, Cologne-Merheim; 1953 Anaesthetist, Department of Surgery Freiburg; 1955 Specialist in Anaesthesiology; 1957 Lecturer in Anaesthesiology; 1959 Specialist in Surgery; 1963 Professor and Head of the Anaesthesia Division of the Department of Surgery, University of Freiburg; 1966 Associate Professor and Chairman of the Department of Anaesthesiology; 1969 Full Professor of Anaesthesiology; 1985 Professor Emeritus.

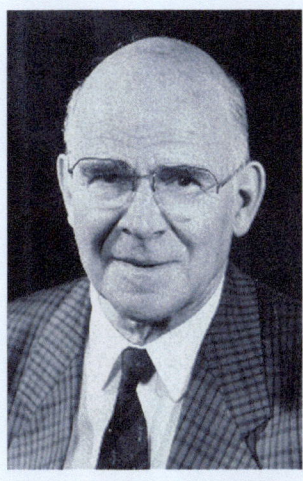

In 1966 Professor Wiemers became Director of an autonomous Department of Anaesthesiology and Intensive Care Medicine. He fostered research in several core areas: the pharmacokinetics and pharmacyodynamics of muscle relaxants, the effect of anaesthesia on liver function, and the pathogenesis and treatment of the shock lung. His efforts led to the establishment of a Division of Experimental Anaesthesiology. Professor Karl Ludwig Scholler, an anaesthetist with a background in biochemistry, was its head. Professor Wiemers belongs to the founding members of the German Society of Anaesthesia (DGA). Under his presidency (1963-1964) and the presidency of Professor Krauss of the German Society of Surgery, both societies agreed upon »Guidelines on the position of the managerial anaesthetist« (► Chap. 1.1). That agreement constituted the basis for the professional and legal autonomy of anaesthesiologists in Germany. Under Wiemers' leadership a curriculum for nurses was introduced, initially lasting one year and later two years. This training significantly improved the quality of anaesthesia care and intensive care medicine.

1986–2008 Chairmanship Professor Klaus Geiger

Prof. Dr.med. Dr. h.c. Klaus Geiger

Born 19 November 1940 in Bamberg; 1960–1966 student of medicine, Universities of Munich and Tübingen; 1967 doctorate in medicine, University of Tübingen; 1966–1968 internship, Karlsruhe and Tübingen; 1968-1970 Resident, Department of Anaesthesiology, University of Basel; 1971 Postdoctoral Fellow, Biological Research Laboratories Ciba-Geigy, Basel; 1972–1973 Resident, Surgical Intensive Care Unit, University Department of Surgery, Basel; 1974 Specialist in Anaesthesiology; 1973–1977 Instructor in Anesthesia, Harvard Medical School, and Senior Anesthetist, Beth Israel Hospital, Boston; 1977–1986 Senior Physician and Deputy Director of the Department of Anaesthesiology and Resuscitation at the Faculty of Medicine Mannheim of the University of Heidelberg; 1979 Lecturer in Anaesthesiology; 1981 Adjunct Professor; 1986 Full Professor of Anaesthesiology and Chairman of the Department of Anaesthesiology and Intensive Care Therapy, University Medical Centre Freiburg; 2001 Honorary Doctor of the University Iasi, Romania; 2008 Professor Emeritus.

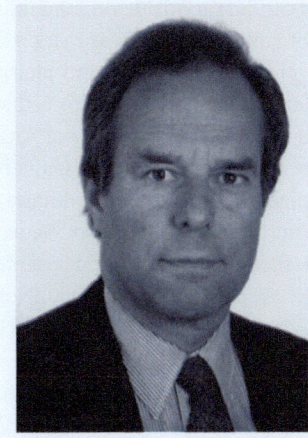

In 1986 Professor Klaus Geiger (Mannheim) was appointed to the Chair of Anaesthesiology and Intensive Care Therapy. His impetus was to expand the clinical and academic activities in order to meet the challenges of the future. In 1994 installation of a preanaesthetic clinic. The ICU became a referral centre for the mechanical and pharmacological treatment of patients with lung failure including those requiring extracorporeal lung support. In 1995 establishment of an acute pain service. In 1991 a »Division of Medical Engineering, Development and Technology« was founded (Head: Dipl.-Ing. Bernd Kristinus). One of the responsibilities is the instant training of all incoming healthcare personnel on the technical equipment and IT-systems. To improve the quality management a PDMS in intensive care medicine and an electronic-based documentation system in anaesthesia were introduced in 2000 so that the Department could participate in an external quality assurance program. Great emphasis was placed on teaching and training. As a result the Department received several times the Teaching Award of the Faculty of Medicine. In 2005 a simulation centre was established, where medical students, doctors and nurses learn basic skills in anaesthesia, intensive care- and emergency medicine, and in pain treatment. The Department is recognized as a postgraduate training centre by the European Academy of Anaesthesiology.

In 1998 Dr. Heike Pahl, a well known molecular biologist from Harvard University, was appointed Extraordinary Professor and Head of a Division of Experimental Anaesthesiology. She was a great promoter of translational research. Several research groups gathered under her leader-participation model studying the effects of anaesthetics and related compounds on immune function, of anaesthesia and ventilation on hepatic and splanchnic microcirculation and their molecular regulation, of respiratory mechanics and energy dissipation in the lungs during different modes of ventilation on ventilator-induced lung injury, of nitric oxide on pulmonary gas exchange, of hydrogen sulfide and carbon monoxide on lung injury; the analysis of exhaled organic compounds as markers for organ dysfunction; the pharmacodynamics and pharmacokinetics of muscle relaxants. In 1999 Professor Gabriele Nöldge-Schomburg was appointed to the Chair of Anaesthesiology and Intensive Care Medicine at the University of Rostock, the first female Full Professor (Ordinaria) of Anaesthesiology in Germany; in 2000 Professor Benedikt Pannen received as the first anaesthetist the Heisenberg Grant of the German Research Council. In 2000 Professor Geiger was elected President of the German Society of Anaesthesiology and Intensive Care Medicine, and Professor Hans-Joachim Priebe served as President of the European Society of Anaesthesiologists from 2002 to 2005.

After an interim chairmanship (Professor Karl-Heinz Kopp) **Professor Hartmut Bürkle** (Münster/Memmingen) was appointed Geiger's successor in 2010.

Qualification as Lecturers in Anaesthesiology

Wiemers, Kurt (1957); Scholler, Karl-Ludwig (1967); Eyrich, Klaus (1969): Burchardi, Hilmar (1971); Vogel, Wolfgang (1972); Buzello, Walter (1974); Metz, Gerhard (1975); Krieg, Norbert (1982); Kopp, Karl-Heinz (1982); Meuret, Gerhard (1983); Kiss, Ivan (1987); Nöldge, Gabriele (1993); Pannen, Benedikt (1999); Benzing, Albert (1999); Mols, Georg (2002); Loop, Thorsten (2006); Hötzel, Alexander (2009); Schmidt, René (2009).

Professors of Anaesthesiology
Full Professors

Prof. Dr. Walter Buzello (1987), Department of Anaesthesiology and Intensive Care Medicine, University Hospital Cologne

Prof. Dr. Gabriele Nöldge-Schomburg (1999), Department of Anaesthesiology and Intensive Care Medicine, University Hospital Rostock;

Prof: Dr. Benedikt Pannen (2007), Department of Anaesthesiology, University Hospital Düsseldorf

Associate Professors

Prof. Dr. Karl Ludwig Scholler (1975), Freiburg
Prof. Dr. Hans-Joachim Priebe (1989), Freiburg
Prof. Dr. Heike Pahl (1998), Professor of Experimental Anaesthesiology, Freiburg
Prof. Dr. Benedikt Pannen (2004), Freiburg

Professors

Prof. Dr. Albert Benzing, Prof. Dr. Dipl. Ing. Josef Guttmann, Prof. Dr. Cornelius Keyl, Prof. Dr. Karl-Heinz Kopp, Prof. Dr. Norbert Krieg, Prof. Dr. Thorsten Loop, Prof. Dr. Gerhard Metz, Prof. Dr. Gerhard Meuret, Prof. Dr. Georg Mols, Prof. Dr. Wolfgang Vogel

For further information:

www.uniklinik-freiburg.de/anaesthesie/live/index.html

3.2.13   University of Giessen

Department of Anaesthesiology and Intensive Care Medicine

G. Hempelmann, M. Weigand, M. Henrich

Compared to other German universities the inauguration of anaesthesiology in Giessen as a separate clinical discipline, independent from surgical disciplines, occurred late. The origin of this new discipline dates from 1948 when Professor Friedrich Bernhard was Chairman of the Department of Surgery. In this year the American anaesthesiologist Dr. Jean Henley demonstrated new anaesthetic methods at several German surgical university departments including Giessen. In 1981, she was awarded honorary membership of the German Society of Anaesthesiology and Intensive Care Medicine (DGAI) for these merits. In 1951 Professor Karl Vossschulte became Bernhard's successor. He early realised the importance of the new specialty anaesthesia so that all his residents were trained in anaesthetic skills. From 1953 on Heinrich L'Allemand, a young Resident in Surgery was exclusively entrusted with anaesthesiological duties. During the following years L'Allemand developed the structures for the eventually founded Department of Anaesthesiology.

During this period he completed his education by studies in physiology at the Kerckhoff Institute for Circulation Research in Bad Nauheim and especially at the Centre Chirurgical Marie Lannelongue in Paris in 1954/55. In 1960 he was certified as Specialist in Anaesthesiology and became Head of an independent Division. In 1964 he acquired his qualification as Lecturer in Anaesthesiology.

1968–1976 Chairmanship Professor Heinrich L'Allemand

Prof. Dr. med. Heinrich L'Allemand

Born 17 September 1924 in Augsburg; deceased 19 December 1976 in Giessen; 1945–1950 student of medicine, University of Munich; 1950 internship, Municipal Hospital Augsburg; 1951 doctorate in medicine, Munich; 1953–1955 residency in anaesthesia, Department of Surgery, University of Giessen; W. G. Kerckhoff Institute of Circulation Research of the Max-Planck-Society, Bad Nauheim; Cardiology, University of Münster; Centre Marie Lannelongue, Paris; 1954 anaesthetist at the Department of Surgery, University of Giessen; 1959 Head of the Anaesthesia Division; 1960 Specialist in Anaesthesiology; 1964 Lecturer in Anaesthesiology; 1968 Full Professor and Chairman of the Department of Anaesthesiology, University of Giessen.

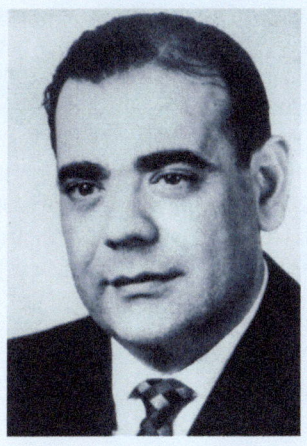

In 1968 L'Allemand was appointed Professor and Chairman of the new Department of Anaesthesiology which, at that time, comprised 8.5 positions. According to the increasing needs the clinical services were expanded and both education of medical students and a research program were started. After Heinrich L'Allemand had passed away very early in 1976 Professor Horst Ferdinand Herget acted as interim Chairman until 1978.

1978–2008 Chairmanship Professor Gunter Hempelmann

Prof. Dr. med. Dr. h.c. Gunter Hempelmann

Born 19 May 1940 in Elmshorn; 1960–1966 student of medicine in Erlangen und Hamburg; 1966 doctorate in medicine; 1966–1967 internship, Halle Hospital in Westphalia; 1967–1968 resident, Department of Anaesthesiology, University Hospital Helsinki, Finland; 1968 Department of Anaesthesiology, Hannover Medical School; 1972 Specialist in Anaesthesiology; 1973 Senior Physician; 1973 Lecturer in Anaesthesiology; 1977 Adjunct Professor; 1978 Full Professor and Chairman of the Department of Anaesthesiology and Surgical Intensive Care Medicine, University of Giessen; 1998 honorary doctorate, Faculty of Medicine, Konya University, Turkey; honorary memberships of the Anaesthesia Societies of Kazakhstan (1997), Hungary (2000), Czech Republic (2000), Bulgaria (2002); 2000 Corresponding Member of the Austrian Society of Anaesthesiology, Reanimation and Intensive Care Medicine; 2008 Professor Emeritus.

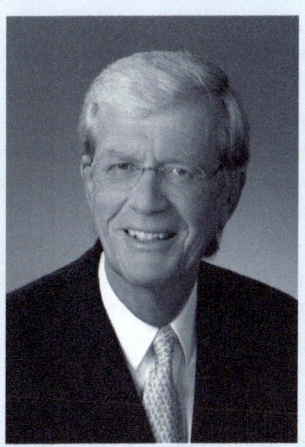

In 1978 Professor Gunter Hempelmann (Hannover) was appointed Full Professor and Chairman of the Department as L'Allemand's successor. During his chairmanship the structure of the Department was further developed, clinical and scientific spectra were expanded. Owing to his intuition the Department experienced a strong growth in staff, clinical aspects and science. The ICU was enlarged, it soon possessed more than 10 beds all equipped with respiratory units. The pain clinic created in 1968 was supplemented by an inpatient ward with 12 beds in 1996 representing the first unit of this kind at a German university hospital for treatment of patients with chronic pain. In 1994 the Department moved into a new extension. This contained a new intensive care unit with 14 modern ventilation facilities and a new section with eight operating theatres. Additionally the department obtained the first university day clinic for outpatient surgery. The Department founded its own IT group that equipped each operating theatre and intensive care unit with an online documentation system. The software was primarily developed by members of the Department. In 2005 the University Hospitals of Giessen and Marburg were merged by the State of Hesse, however, both Faculties of Medicine remained independent. In the following year the University Hospital of Giessen and Marburg was the first that was taken over by a private health care company (Rhön-Klinikum AG) what resulted in a reorganisation of the processes in the operating theatres and intensive care units. In 2007 an intermediate care unit with 10 beds for surgical patients was opened and run by the Department. End of September 2008 Gunter Hempelmann retired.

Since 2008 Chairmanship Professor Markus Weigand

Prof. Dr. med. Markus Alexander Weigand

Born 16 April 1967 in Augsburg; 1986–1993 student of medicine, Ulm and Munich; 1993 doctorate in medicine; 1994 Resident, Department of Anaesthesiology, University of Heidelberg; 1998 Research Fellow, Department of Immunogenetics, German Cancer Research Center (DKFZ), Heidelberg; 2001 Research Fellow, Department of Immunology, University of Basel; 2001 Specialist in Anaesthesiology; 2002 Senior Physician, Department of Anaesthesiology, University Hospital Heidelberg; 2004 Lecturer in Anaesthesiology; 2005 Executive Senior Physician; 2008 Full Professor and Chairman of the Department of Anaesthesiology and Intensive Care Medicine, University Hospital Giessen.

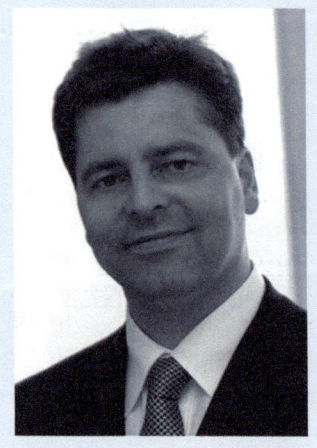

In October 2008 Professor Markus Alexander Weigand (Heidelberg) was appointed to the Chair of Anaesthesiology and Intensive Care Medicine. Subsequently, the intensive care unit was extended, the central operating unit reorganized and a preanaesthetic clinic established. An acute pain service was instituted to achieve a »hospital without pain«. The undergraduate and postgraduate training programmes were updated including case-based and simulator-based learning.

The focus of research interests changed during the past decades. Beside clinical aspects the spectrum covered also pharmacological, immunological and molecular aspects of septicaemia, ion channel investigations and oxygen sensing. When Weigand started in October 2008 the scientific activities were focused on sepsis and inflammation. For this purpose, several patient studies were launched, new organ and cell culture experimental models set up and cooperations with the Departments of Cardiac Surgery, Physiology, Anatomy and Gynaecology brought into being.

Qualification as Lecturers in Anaesthesiology

L'Allemand, Heinrich (1964); Grabow, Lutz (1970); Ehehalt, Volker (1976); Müller, Hermann (1983); Weidler, Burghard (1983); von Bormann, Benno (1985); Biscoping, Jürgen (1986); Börner, Ulf (1987); Boldt, Joachim (1987); Adams, Hans Anton (1988); Kling, Dieter (1989); Russ, Wolfgang (1989); Salomon, Fred (1990); Krumholz, Werner (1992); Thiel, Achim (1994); Bachmann, Bernd (1995); Knothe, Christoph (1997); Zickmann, Bernfried (1997); Heesen, Michael (1999); Bräu, Michael (1999); Dietrich, Gerald (1999); Menges, Thilo (2001); Olschewski, Andrea (2001); Welters, Ingeborg (2002); Sticher, Jochen (2003); Mühling, Jörg (2003); Dehne, Marius (2003); Junger, Axel (2003); Benson, Matthias (2003); Engel, Jörg (2006); Hartmann, Bernd (2006); Gruß, Marco (2007); Harbach, Heinz (2007); Matejec, Reginald (2007); Müller Matthias (2007); Wolff, Matthias (2007); Henrich, Michael (2008).

Professors of Anaesthesiology
Adjunct Professors

Prof. Dr. Jürgen Biscoping, Prof. Dr. Benno von Bormann, Prof. Dr. Volker Ehehalt, Prof. Dr. Jörg Engel, Prof. Dr. Lutz Grabow, Prof. Dr. Horst Herget, Prof. Dr. Axel Junger, Prof. Dr. Werner Krumholz, Prof. Dr. Thilo Menges, Prof. Dr. Jörg Mühling, Prof. Dr. Hermann Müller, Prof. Dr. Detlev Patschke, Prof. Dr. Achim Thiel, Prof. Dr. Burghard Weidler, Prof. Dr. Ingeborg Welters

For further information:

www.ukgm.de/ugm_2/deu/ugi_ana/index.html

3.2.14   University of Göttingen

Centre of Anaesthesiology, Emergency and Intensive Care Medicine

J. Bahr, P. Ahrens, D. Kettler, M. Quintel

In 1949, Professor Hans Hellner, Chairman of the Department of Surgery of the University of Göttingen, established a group of 5 residents who gave anaesthetics. Among them was Dr. Sverre Loennecken, later neuroanaesthetist at the University of Cologne. In 1957, Dr. Jürgen Stoffregen (Heidelberg) joined this group. One year later, he was made Head of a Division of Anaesthesia of the Department of Surgery and qualified as Lecturer in Anaesthesiology. Until 1961, he resumed the anaesthetic service to all surgical departments. Supported by Hellner, he was appointed Associate Professor and Head of an independent Division of Anaesthesia in 1964, which was upgraded to a Department of Clinical Anaesthesia in 1969 as Stoffregen was appointed Full Professor and Chairman.

1969–1974 Chairmanship Professor Jürgen Stoffregen

Prof. Dr. med Jürgen Stoffregen

Born 29 September 1925 in Braunschweig; until 1951 student of medicine in Hamburg; 1952 doctorate in medicine; 1953-1954 Max Planck-Institute of Physiology, Heidelberg; 1954–1957 Resident, Division of Anaesthesia, University of Heidelberg; 1957 Department of Anaesthesia, University of Chicago, USA; then Head of the Anaesthesia Unit, Department of Surgery, University of Göttingen; 1958 Lecturer in Anaesthesiology; 1964 Associate Professor and Head of the Division of Anaesthesia, University of Göttingen; 1969 Full Professor and Chairman of the Department of Clinical Anaesthesia; 1974 resignation and Head Physician, Central Department of Anaesthesia, Hagen/Westphalia.

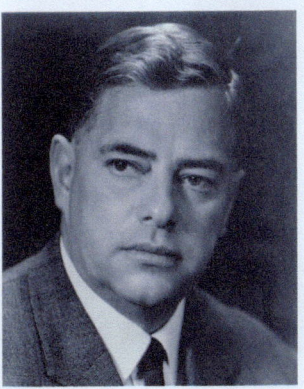

Until 1967, Stoffregen provided the anaesthesia service not only for the University Hospital but also for the other hospitals of Göttingen. He also gave daily support and advice to up to 20, i.e. virtually all, hospitals in the surrounding area. This was only possible by close cooperation with qualified and motivated anaesthesia nurses. As the Faculty of Medicine decided that the Department was restructured into 4 Divisions, Stoffregen resigned from his academic and clinical positions and moved to Hagen, where he became Head of a new Central Anaesthesia Department of 3 hospitals on 1 February 1974. In 1973, Dr. Dietrich Kettler, Dr. Hilmar Burchardi and Dr. Hans Sonntag were appointed Associate Professors and Heads of one of the newly created Divisions of the Department. The 4th Division was entrusted to Dr. Ulrich Braun (Tübingen) in 1977.

1975–2004 Chairmanship Professor Dietrich Kettler

Prof. Dr. med. Dr. h.c. Dietrich Kettler, FRCA

Born 16 June 1936 in Waren-Müritz; 1955–1960 student of medicine, Humboldt-University Berlin; 1962 doctorate in medicine; 1961-1963 internship (Berlin, Stuttgart, Darmstadt); 1964–1965 Resident, Department of Clinical Anaesthesia, University of Göttingen; 1966–1967 Fellowship in Cardiovascular Anesthesia, Department of Anesthesiology, Baylor University, Houston, TX, USA; 1968 Specialist in Anaesthesiology; 1968–1973 Research Associate, Department of Physiology I, University of Göttingen; 1971 Lecturer in Anaesthesiology; 1973 Associate Professor and Head of Division I of the Department of Clinical Anaesthesia, University of Göttingen; 1975 Full Professor and Chairman of the Department of Clinical Anaesthesia (then Centre of Anaesthesiology, Emergency and Intensive Care Medicine); 1996 honorary doctorate, Pomeranian Medical Academy, Szczecin, Poland; 2003 Honorary Member of the German Society of Anaesthesiology and Intensive Care Medicine; 2004 Professor Emeritus.

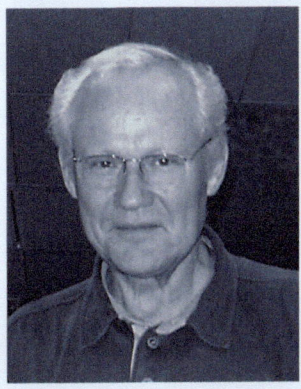

In 1975, Kettler was appointed Full Professor and Chairman of the Department. The cooperation of the 4 Division Heads was always good and trustful. Until 1986, they alternated with each other in their clinical responsibilities. Thereafter this rotation was given up in order to enable better development of clinical and scientific excellence in their respective fields of competence. Until Sonntag's retirement in 2001, the clinical responsibilities were distributed as follows.

- Division I (Kettler): general, trauma, orthopaedic and paediatric surgery, urology, gynaecology, radiology, emergency care, and pain therapy
- Division II (Burchardi): intensive care units
- Division III (Braun): neurosurgery, otorhinolaryngology, dentistry and maxillo-facial surgery, ophthalmology
- Division IV (Sonntag): cardio-thoracic and vascular surgery

In addition, a Division of Anaesthesiological Reasearch was created and headed by Professor Gerhard Hellige.

Prof. Dr. med. Ulrich Braun

Born 1 Oktober 1939 in Memel/East Prussia; 1959–1964 student of medicine in Hamburg; 1964 doctorate in medicine; 1965–1967 internship in Bad Reichenhall, Hamburg, Luzern (Switzerland); 1967–1968 Resident, Anaesthesiology, Cantonal Hospital Luzern and Federal Armed Forces Hospital, Koblenz; 1969–1971 Research Associate, Department of Physiology I, University of Göttingen; 1971–1977 Resident, Central Department of Anaesthesiology, University of Tübingen; 1971 Specialist in Anaesthesiology; 1974 Lecturer in Anaesthesiology; 1975–1977 Senior Physician; 1978 Associate Professor and Head of Division III of the Department of Clinical Anaesthesia, University of Göttingen; 2004 Professor Emeritus.

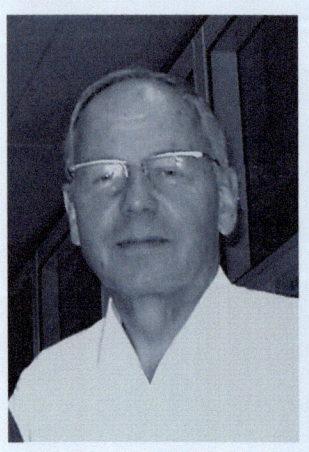

Prof. Dr. med. Hilmar Burchardi, FRCA

Born 19 April 1937 in Tondern, Denmark; student of medicine in Tübingen, Freiburg, Berlin and Hamburg; 1968 doctorate in medicine; until 1970 residency, Division of Anaesthesia, Municipal Hospital Hamburg-Altona; Department of Internal Medicine II, University Hospital Hamburg-Eppendorf; Department of Anaesthesiology, University of Freiburg; 1969 Specialist in Anaesthesiology; 1970–1973 Anaesthetist, German Diagnostic Clinic, Wiesbaden; 1971 Lecturer in Anaesthesiology, University of Freiburg; 1973 Associate Professor and Head of Division II of the Department of Clinical Anaesthesia, University of Göttingen, and Head of the Surgical ICUs; 2003 Professor Emeritus.

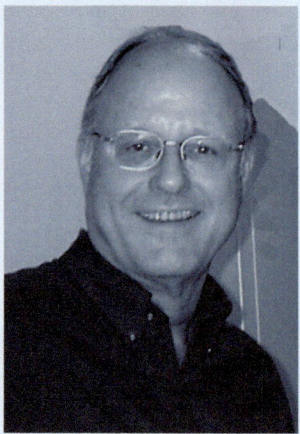

Prof. Dr. med. Hans Sonntag, FRCA

Born 2 February 1936 in Nordhausen/Harz, deceased 7 May 2011 in Charleston, SC, USA; 1957–1963 student of medicine in Göttingen; 1963–1965 internship in Göttin-

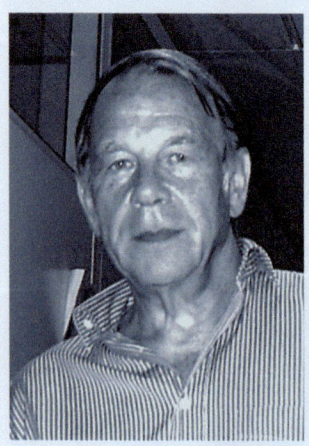

gen-Weende, Witzenhausen and Salzgitter-Lebenstedt; 1965 doctorate of medicine; 1965–1966 Resident, Division of Anaesthesia, University of Göttingen; 1966–1968 Resident, Divisions of Internal Medicine and Surgery, Mission Médicale Allemande in Annaba ex Bone, Algeria; 1968–1970 Resident, Division of Anaesthesia, University of Göttingen; 1970 Specialist in Anaesthesiology; 1970–1973 Research Associate, Department of Physiology I, University of Göttingen; 1973 Lecturer in Anaesthesiology; 1973 Associate Professor and Head of Division IV of the Department of Clinical Anaesthesia; 2001 Professor Emeritus and Order of Merit in Gold of the Republic of Poland.

In 1980, the Department was renamed Centre of Anaesthesiology, Emergency and Intensive Care Medicine and Kettler was appointed acting Chairman. The Centre provided the anaesthetic service for all surgical and interventional specialties of the University Hospital. Postoperatively, all patients were transferred to the post-anaesthesia care unit with 20 beds unless requiring intensive care. The preanaesthetic Clinic was gradually expanded. The operating room management was established as a task of the Centre.

The beginnings of ICM in the University Hospital Göttingen date back to the period around 1960. In 1969, a real ICU was established. The Hospital moved into new premises in 1978 and the Centre became responsible for 2 ICUs with a total of 16 beds. In the following years, ICM of Göttingen achieved an outstanding role under Burchardi's leadership in both a national and European perspective. Clinical research was focussed on the pathophysiology of the respiratory system, treatment of acute lung injury and outcome. A mobile life support unit was put into operation in 1970 and a helicopter rescue service 10 years later.

In 1975, the first patients suffering from chronic pain were treated by Professor Hans Sonntag und Dr. Jan Hildebrandt. A pain clinic came into being 3 years later and developed to one of the leading centres for pain therapy. In 1989, Hildebrandt was appointed to a special professorship of algesiology. He was a renowned expert of chronic back pain and received several large research grants. In 2006, Professor Michael Stumpf (Bremen) succeeded Hildebrandt, but unexpectedly passed away one year later. He was succeeded by Dr. Frank Petzke. On Kettler's initiative, a unit of palliative medicine was created already in the early 1980s. It was initially located in the Hospital Göttingen-Weende and moved to the University Hospital in 1999. In 2006, Friedemann Nauck (Bonn) was appointed Endowed Professor of Palliative Medicine and, in 2007, Chairman of the newly created Centre of Palliative Medicine which since then is one of the 2 divisions of the Centre of Anaesthesiology, Emergency and Intensive Care Medicine.

In the 1970s, research was to a large extent carried out with the support of, and in cooperation with, the Department of Physiology I of the University of Göttingen which was chaired by the ingenious Professor Hans-Jürgen Bretschneider. He introduced many Professors of Anaesthesiology into cardiovascular science, among them Bonhoeffer (Cologne), Brückner and Eberlein (Berlin), and from Göttingen Hensel, Hoeft (later Bonn), Kettler, Radke (later Halle) and Sonntag. The Centre had a major part in several Collaborative Research Centres which were funded by the German Research Foundation. Cardiovascular pathophysiology and pharmacology were the main research fields during many years rounded off by questions of effects and side effects of anaesthesia and operation on organ functions, various pharmacological aspects and problems and methods of ventilatory support.

2005–2009 Chairmanship Professor Bernhard M. Graf

(▶ Chap. 3.2.33 for his C.V.)

In the years 2003-2008, a number of changes in the Professors and Chairpersons of the Centre took place. After Burchardi's retirement, Professor Michael Quintel (Mannheim) became his successor as Head of Division II of the Centre and Head of the Surgical ICUs. As Kettler stepped down on 31 January 2005 Quintel acted as Interim Head of Division I until Bernhard Graf was appointed Full Professor of Anaesthesiology and Head of Division I of the Centre on 20 June 2005. After Graf's change to the University of Regensburg Quintel was appointed Full Professor and Chairman of the Division of Anaesthesiology amalgamated from the previous Divisions I and II. This new Division and the Division of Palliative Medicine then formed the Centre of Anaesthesiology, Emergency and Intensive Care Medicine. Hensel, Head of the Division of Anaesthesiological Research, retired in 2008.

Since 2010 Chairmanship Professor Michael Quintel

Prof. Dr. med. Michael Quintel

Born 4 march 1954; 1978–1985 student of medicine in Heidelberg; 1985–1990 residency in anaesthesiology; 1992 Research Fellow, Department of General and Thoracic Surgery, University of Michigan, Ann Arbor, MI, ISA; Senior Physician, Department of Anaesthesiology, Faculty of Clinical Medicine Mannheim, University of Heidelberg; 1994 Head, Surgical ICU, Department of Anaesthesiology; 1997 Lecturer in Anaesthesiology;2001 Vice Chairman, Department of Anaesthesiology; 2003 Associate Professor and Head of Division II (Surgical ICUs), Centre of Anaesthesiology, Emergency and Intensive Care Medicine, University of Göttingen; 2004 and 2008–2010 in addition Interim Head, Division I, Centre of Anaesthesiology, Emergency and Intensive Care Medicine; 2010 Full Professor and Chairman of the now amalgamated Division of Anaesthesiology, Centre of Anaesthesiology, Emergency and Intensive Care Medicine.

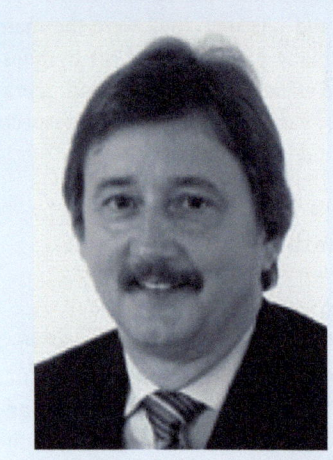

Under Quintel's chairmanship the total number of physicians approached 100, among them about 40 certified specialists, the quality management was extended and a staff section of OR management became part of the Centre. Main areas of research are: diagnosis and therapy of acute lung injury, airway management and simulation, electrical impedance tomography, molecular mechanisms of anaesthetics, emergency medicine, organ protection, infection and sepsis, diagnosis and treatment of low back pain.

Qualification as Lecturers in Anaesthesiology

Schorer, Rudolf (1964); Meyer-Burgdorff, Christoph (1972); Hensel, Ingo (1973); Teichmann, Jens (1974); Kontokollias, Joannis (1977); Larsen, Reinhard (1980); Schenk, Helge (1980); Hilfiker, Otto (1983); Stokke, Trond (1985); Turner, Ernst (1985); Radke, Joachim (1986); Hildebrandt, Jan (1987); Seyde, Walter (1987); Stephan, Heidrun (1988); Crozier, Thomas (1989); Lange, Harald (1991); Rieke, Horst (1991); Hoeft, Andreas (1986/1992); Sydow, Michael (1994); Weyland, Andreas (1994); Weyland, Wolfgang (1994); Schröder, Thomas (1995); Zielmann, Siegfried (1995); Rathgeber, Jörg (1997); Saur, Petra (1997); Klockgether-Radke, Adelbert (1998); Mohr, Michael (1998); Kietzmann, Daniela (2000); Frerichs,

Inez (2001); Pfingsten, Michael (2001); Neumann, Peter (2002); Mielck, Frank (2004); Bräuer, Anselm (2006); Hinz, José (2007); Kazmaier, Stephan (2007); Timmermann, Arnd (2007); Eich, Christoph (2010); Mörer, Onnen (2010); Pavlaković, Goran (2010)

Professors of Anaesthesiology
Full Professors

Prof. Dr. Rudolf Schorer (1968), University of Tübingen
Prof. Dr. med. Reinhard Larsen (1990), Saarland University Hospital, Homburg
Prof. Dr. med. Joachim Radke (1992), University of Halle-Wittenberg
Prof. Dr. med. Andreas Hoeft (1995), University of Bonn
Prof. Dr. Friedemann Nauck (2006), Endowed Professor of Palliative Medicine, Göttingen
Prof. Dr. Bernhard M. Graf (2008), University of Regensburg

Associate Professors

Prof. Dr. Jan Hildebrandt (1989), Associate Professor of Algesiology, Göttigen
Prof. Dr. Gerhard Hellige (1992), Associate Professor of Experimental Anaesthesiology, Göttingen
Prof. Dr. Dr. Martin Bauer (2003), Associate Professor of Anaesthesiological Patient Care Research, Göttingen
Prof. Dr. Michael Stumpf (†) (2008); Associate Professor of Experimental and Clinical Pain Therapy, Göttingen

Adjunct Professors

Prof. Dr. Thomas Crozier; Prof. Dr. Klaus Fischer; Prof. Dr. Walter Henschel; Prof. Dr. Ingo Hensel; Prof. Dr. Adelbert Klockgether-Radke; Prof. Dr. Joannis Kontokollias; Prof. Dr. Werner Kuckelt; Prof. Dr. Christoph Meyer-Burgdorff; Prof. Dr. Peter Neumann; Prof. Dr. Michael Pfingsten; Prof. Dr. Jörg Rathgeber; Prof. Dr. Petra Saur; Prof. Dr. Helge Schenk; Prof. Dr. Heiko Stellpflug; Frau Prof. Dr. Heidrun Stephan; Prof. Dr. Jens Teichmann; Prof. Dr. Ernst Turner; Prof. Dr. Andreas Weyland; Prof. Dr. Wolfgang Weyland

For further information:

www.zari.med.uni-goettingen.de/

3.2.15   University of Greifswald

Department of Anaesthesiology und Surgical Intensive Care Medicine
M. Wendt

The University of Greifswald was founded in 1456, only 6 German universities are older: Heidelberg (1386), Cologne (1388), Erfurt (1392), Würzburg (1402), Leipzig

(1409) and Rostock (1419). At the end of the 19th century, two surgeons who later made important contributions to the development of local and regional anaesthesia lived and worked in Greifswald: Carl Ludwig Schleich and August Bier. In the 1960s especially qualified doctors became responsible for the anaesthetic service. One of those was Manfred Schädlich who moved to the Charité University Hospital, Berlin, in 1962. On 1 October 1971 a Central Division of Anaesthesia was created and Dr. Henning Ritzow (Berlin) hired to fill the leading position. He cared for the acquisition of new equipment and the introduction of modern anaesthetic techniques, but left Greifswald in 1975. He was succeeded by Dr. Erwin Kasper who had already been the leader of the anaesthesia team from 1965–1968 and from 1970–1971, until, in 1977, Dr. Klaus Borchert (Rostock) was appointed to the new Chair of Anaesthesiology and Intensive Therapy.

1977–1991 Chairmanship Professor Klaus Borchert

Prof. Dr. med. habil. Klaus Borchert

Born 27 June 1937 in Stettin; 1957–1963 student of medicine in Rostock; 1963–1966 Resident in surgery, Wolgast County Hospital; 1966–1977 Resident, Senior Physician and Lecturer in Anaesthesiology, Division of Anaesthesiology and Intensive Therapy, University of Rostock; 1977–1991 Full Professor and Chairman, Department of Anaesthesiology and Intensive Therapy, University of Greifswald; since 1992 anaesthetist and pain therapist in medical practice.

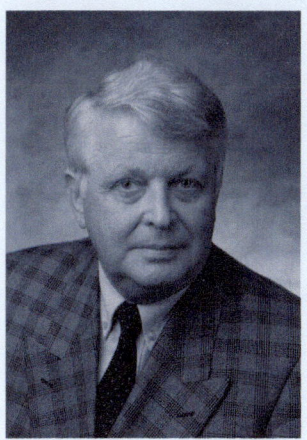

In order to keep up with the growing activities of the surgical specialties Borchert had to increase the number of doctors and nurses. During his first 10 years the number of anaesthetics increased by 30%, and that of doctors by

40%. In 1981 the Division was made the Department of Anaesthesiology and Intensive Therapy by the Ministry of Higher Education. In January 1983, the Department became responsible for a small interdisciplinary ICU. It began to coordinate and guide the emergency medical service of the Greifswald area in the early 1980s. Research efforts were focussed on clinical problems, particularly in neurosurgery. As Borchert left the University, first Dr. Gisela Cierpka and then, on 15 September 1992, Professor Michael Wendt (Münster) assumed interim chairmanship.

Since 1992 Chairmanship Professor Michael Wendt

Prof. Dr. med. Michael Wendt

Born 1 March 1948 in Bielefeld; 1966–1972 student of medicine in Marburg and Frankfurt; 1972–1973 internship in Marburg und Berlin; 1973 doctorate in medicine in Frankfurt; 1973–1975 Resident and Medical Officer in Berlin and Stade; 1975–1980 residency in anaesthesiology in Hamburg and Münster; 1980 Specialist in Anaesthesiology; 1984 Lecturer in Anaesthesiology, University of Münster; 1978–1992 Senior Physician, Department of Anaesthesiology and Surgical Intensive Care Medicine, University Hospital Münster; 1992 Interim Chairman, Department of Anaesthesiology and Intensive Care Medicine, University Hospital Greifswald; 1993 Full Professor and Chairman.

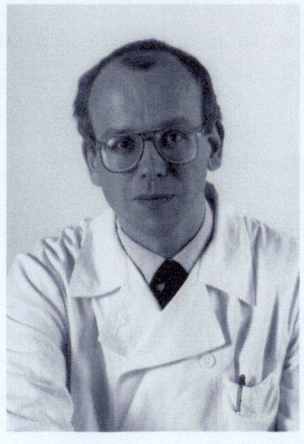

On 1 April 1993, Wendt was appointed Full Professor and Chairman of the Department of Anaesthesiology and Intensive Care Medicine. In order to comply with both the legal requirements and recent developments of anaesthesia and ICM, the technical equipment was completey modernized. In 2002, nearly 50 doctors were employed

by the Department and 16,000 anaesthetics were given; about 15% were regional anaesthesias. The daily clinical work was markedly affected by the spatial spread of the operating departments over the city. This challenged the anaesthetists to inaugurate an operating theatre management system including an Intranet system coping with these needs. The surgical ICU was expanded to 11 beds and remained an area of responsibility of the Department of Anaesthesiology. Another small ICU with 2 beds was added in 1994, an electronic patient data management system introduced in 1995 and then continuously updated. Since 1990, anaesthetists participated to an increasing extent in the emergency medical service. Doctors as well as nurses of the Department are preferentially involved in the operation of mobile life support units and rescue helicopters. In 1993 a pain clinic was established.

Clinical and experimental research is focussed on respiratory and vascular responses to trauma and inflammation (sepsis), and to agents used in the management of multiple organ failure. The basic investigations are done in the Anaesthesia Research Laboratory headed by Dr. Dragan Pavlovic, and involve cardiovascular and pulmonary responses to trauma, inflammation and anaesthetic agents, including enteral microcirculation, pulmonary circulation and airway motility. Clinical investigations incorporate clinical drug studies, pathophysiological mechanisms of diseases and evaluation of techniques applied in ICM.

Qualification as Lecturers in Anaesthesiology:

Cierpka, Gisela (1983); Freitag, Bernd (1984); Thiele, Christa (1984); Rosolski, Tanja (1990); Feyerherd, Frank (1993); Meissner, Konrad (2007); Pavlovic, Dragan (2007); Usichenko, Taras (2007); Mathes, Alexander (2010)

Professors of Anaesthesiology
Full Professors

Prof. Dr. Thomas Hachenberg (2001), University of Magdeburg

Associate Professors

Prof. Dr. Thomas Hachenberg (1994), Greifswald
Prof. Dr. Christian Lehmann (2002), University of Magdeburg
Prof. Dr. Konrad Meissner (2011), Greifswald

Adjunct Professors

Prof. Dr. Frank Feyerherd; Prof. Dr. Bernd Freitag; Prof. Dr. Konrad Meissner

For further information:

www.medizin.uni-greifswald.de/intensiv/

3.2.16   University of Halle-Wittenberg

Department of Anaesthesiology and Surgical Intensive Care Medicine
J. Radke, M. Bucher

In 1953, a Division of Anaesthesia was established at the Department of Surgery of the University of Halle as the first academic anaesthesia unit of the German Democratic Republic and Dr. Karl-Heinz Martin was nominated its Head (▶ Chap. 3.2.7 for his C.V.). As an excellent clinician he was held in great esteem. Many of the early leading university anaesthetists of the GDR were trained in his Division, e.g. Manfred Schädlich (Berlin-Charité), Gottfried Benad (Rostock), Paul Fritsche (Dresden, then Homburg/Saar) and Günter Baust (Halle). He introduced a preoperative assessment scheme for cardiac risk patients and built up a respiratory gas lab for monitoring of ventilated patients. Since there was no opportunity to purchase a heart-lung machine from the USA patients requiring open-heart surgery had to be operated abroad. This prompted Professor K.L. Schober, Chairman of the Department of Surgery, to develop such a machine in Halle with the participation of the physicist F. Struss and the anaesthetist Baust. The first procedure with this cardio-pulmonary bypass device was carried out in 1962. In 1971, the Division became independent of the Surgical Department as Division of Anaesthesia and Reanimation and, ignoring Martin's merits, Baust was appointed to the position of Head of the Division.

1973–1992 Chairmanship Professor Günter Baust

Prof. Dr. sc. med. Günter Baust
Born 25 November 1929 in Halle (Saale); 1950–1956 student of medicine in Halle-Wittenberg and Greifswald; 1958 doctorate in medicine; 1960 residency in anaes-

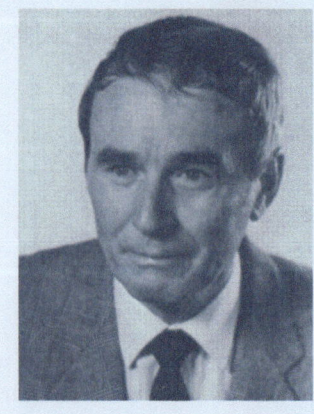

thesia, Department of Surgery, University of Halle-Wittenberg; 1963 Specialist in Anaesthesiology; 1968 Senior Physician, Department of Surgery; 1969 Lecturer in Anaesthesiology; 1971 Head of the Division of Anaesthesiology and Reanimation; 1973 Full Professor and Chairman, Department of Anaesthesiology and Intensive Therapy, University of Halle-Wittenberg; 1992 Professor Emeritus.

ate, Department of Physiology, University of Göttingen; 1977-1980 Resident, Department of Clinical Anaesthesia, University of Göttingen; 1980 Specialist in Anaesthesiology; 1985 Senior Physician; 1987 Lecturer in Anaesthesiology; 1991 Adjunct Professor; 1992 Interim Chairman and 1993 Full Professor and Chairman, Department of Anaesthesiology and Surgical Intensive Care Medicine, University of Halle-Wittenberg; 2009 Professor Emeritus.

In 1973, the Division became the Department of Anaesthesiology and Intensive Therapy and Baust was appointed Full Professor and Chairman. During his entire term of office he made every effort to recruit young doctors and nurses with the aim to meet the steadily increasing demands for providing adequate anaesthesiological services. The postgraduate education of residents was improved by introducing a rota system the adherence to which was binding irrespective of any shortage of personnel. The teaching of medical students in anaesthesiology was optimized too by offering lectures and clinical courses. On Martin's initiative, an ICU had been put into operation in 1972 and was then adapted to the continuing progress in medical diagnostics and therapy. In the context of the German reunification, changes in the composition of academic staff took place in Halle and Professor Joachim Radke (Göttingen) was appointed to the Interim Chairmanship of the Department in 1992.

After one year as Interim Chairman, Radke was appointed Full Professor and Chairman of the Department of Anaesthesiology and Intensive Care Medicine in 1993. From the beginning, he was wholeheartedly committed to the reorganization and further development of not only his Department but also the Faculty of Medicine and the University as a whole. On the basis of his academic experiences obtained in Göttingen and together with a small but highly motivated team of doctors and nurses he soon succeeded in establishing the Department as a competent partner of the surgical specialties. Two interdisciplinary surgical ICUs with 22 beds were newly equipped and run by the Department. Anaesthetists were included into the mobile emergency service. A pain clinic, a preanaesthetic clinic, a service for autologous blood donation and a unit for hyperbaric oxygenation were established. The departmental research activities were continuously extended.

1992–2009 Chairmanship Professor Joachim Radke

Since 2009 Chairmanship Professor Michael Bucher

Prof. Dr. med. Joachim Radke

Born 21 September 1942 in Stolp (Pommern); 1969–1973 student of medicine in Göttingen; 1974 internship; 1974 doctorate in medicine; 1975-1976 Research Associ-

Prof. Dr. med. Michael Bucher

Born 1967 in Straubing; 1986–1992 student of medicine in Regensburg, Munich and Johannesburg (South Africa); 1995-2002 Resident, Department of Anaesthe-

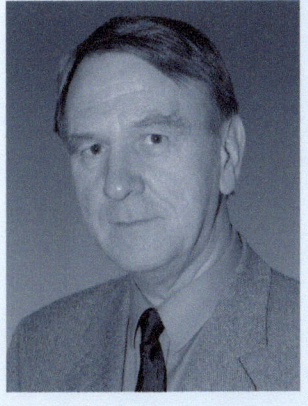

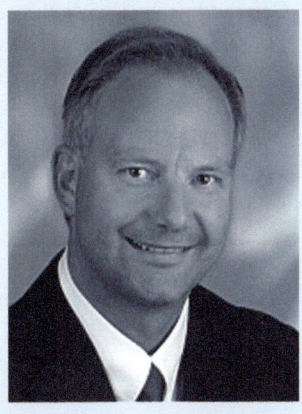

siology, University of Regensburg; 2002 Specialist in Anaesthesiology; 2003 Lecturer in Anaesthesiology and Senior Physician; 2009 Associate Professor; 2009 Full Professor and Chairman, Department of Anaesthesiology and Surgical Intensive Care Medicine, University of Halle-Wittenberg.

After Radke's retirement in 2009, Professor Michael Bucher (Regensburg) was appointed Full Professor and Chairman of the Department. The number of doctors increased to 75, the annual number of anaesthetics was more than 19,000, and up to 2,000 patients were treated in the 2 ICUs with now 30 beds. The activities in out-of-hospital emergency medical services including the helicopter rescue service were markedly expanded. Bucher focused the experimental and clinical scientific efforts on organ failure caused by severe systemic inflammatory disease.

Qualification as Lecturers in Anaesthesiology:

Martin,Karl-Heinz (1969); Baust, Günter (1969); Brähne, Ingrid (1979); Müller, Winfried (1990); Menzel, Matthias (1999); Sablotzki, Armin (2002); Clausen, Tobias (2007); Fritz, Harald (2008); Czeslick, Elke (2007); Soukup, Jens (2010).

For further information:

www.medizin.uni-halle.de/kai/

3.2.17   University of Hamburg

Department of Anaesthesiology

J. Schulte am Esch, A.E. Goetz, M. Goerig

The new Hospital Hamburg-Eppendorf was put into operation in 1889 then being one of the most modern medical institutions in Germany. It had a leading role in clinical anaesthesia until the 1930s. Under Professor Hermann Kümmell, Head of the Department of Surgery, anaesthesias by means of anaesthetic devices must be given only by doctors even before 1900. He expanded the anaesthetic armamentarium by techniques like premedication, intravenous application of anaesthetics and fluids and local anaesthesia. A major step forward was made since 1924 when Professor Paul Sudeck, Kümmell's successor, and his co-worker Dr. Helmut Schmidt began to develop an anaesthesia machine for the application of nitrous oxide-oxygen in cooperation with Dräger Company. This was the first device with a circle system and became worldwide known as the »Modell A«. Schmidt gave theoretical lectures and practical courses in anaesthesia for

students and was founding editor of the first German anaesthesia journals. He qualified as Lecturer in Surgery at the University of Hamburg in 1928 having presented a thesis on an anaesthesiological topic. After Schmidt had left Hamburg in 1932 and Sudeck had retired Hamburg lost its position as forerunner of German anaesthesia.

After World War II Dr. Karl Horatz became Resident at the Department of Surgery and was educated in both surgery and anaesthesiology. He gradually became responsible for the anaesthetic service of this Department, in the period 1955-1960 as Senior Physician. In 1953 he became Instructor for medical students and qualified as Lecturer in 1957. In 1960 he was appointed Head of the Division of Anaesthesia, in 1963 Associate Professor and in 1966 Full Professor of Anaesthesiology.

1966–1982 Chairmanship Professor Karl Horatz

Prof. Dr. med. Karl Horatz

Born 14 January 1913 in Cologne; deceased 16 May 1996 in Hamburg; student of medicine in Cologne, Munich and Königsberg; 1939 doctorate in medicine in Cologne; 1939 internship in Berlin; 1939–1944 Medical Officer; 1944–1945 residency in surgery, University of Göttingen; since 1945 residency in surgery and anaesthesia, Department of Surgery, University Hospital Hamburg-Eppendorf; 1948 Specialist in Surgery; 1954 Specialist in Anaesthesiology; 1957 Lecturer in Anaesthesiology; Head of the anaesthetic team of the Department of Surgery; 1960 Head, Division of Anaesthesia; 1963 Associate Professor; 1966 first Full Professor of Anaesthesiology in Germany and Chairman of the Department of Anaesthesiology at the University Hospital Hamburg-Eppendorf; 1981 Professor Emeritus; 1982 Honorary Member of the Professional Association of German Anaesthetists.

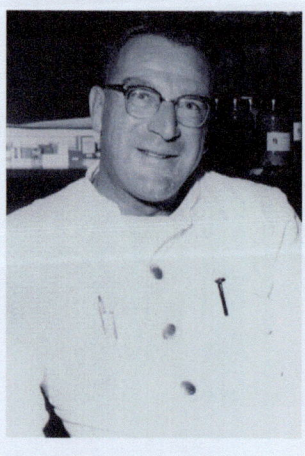

After his appointment Horatz was responsible for the anaesthetic care in the Department of Surgery. In the following years he took over that for the other operative departments which were located in various buildings of the Hospital campus. A surgical ICU was created in the early 1960s, a recovery room in 1972. Horatz was particularly committed to the promotion of professional matters of the specialty. Research activities were focussed on clinical problems, among them studies on organ function of potential organ donors, cerebral monitoring, haemodynamic effects of cardio-pulmonary resuscitation, long-term intubation, parenteral nutrition, complications of major abdominal procedures. In 1982 the annual number of anaesthetics was 16,400.

1982–2005 Chairmanship Professor Jochen Schulte am Esch

Prof. Dr. med. Dr. h.c. Jochen Schulte am Esch

Born 5 October 1939 in Leipzig; 1960–1966 student of medicine in Bonn and Vienna; 1966–1967 internship in Düsseldorf, Krefeld and Lindlar; 1967 doctorate in medicine in Bonn; 1968–69 Research Associate, Department of Pharmacology, University of Bonn; 1969–1974 residency in anaesthesia, Departments of Surgery and Neurosurgery; 1974-1982 Senior Physician, Department of Anaesthesiology; 1973 Specialist in Anaesthesiology; 1977 Lecturer in Anaesthesiology; 1980 Adjunct Professor; 1982 Full Professor and Chairman of the Department of Anaesthesiology, University Hospital Hamburg-Eppendorf; 1998 Honorary Member of the Romanian Society of Anaesthesia and Intensive Care; 2001 honorary doctorate of the Iuliu-Hatieganu University of Medicine and Pharmacy, Cluj-Napoca, Romania; 2005 Honorary Member of the German Society of Anaesthesiology and Intensive Care Medicine; 2005 Professor Emeritus.

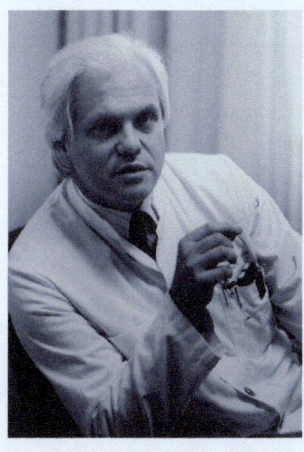

In 1982 Professor Jochen Schulte am Esch (Bonn) was appointed Full Professor and Chairman of the Department of Anaesthesiology. He continuously increased the number of doctors and nurses and made every effort to centralize and integrate all single units of the Department including the ICU and newly created PACUs. Modern monitoring and anaesthetic equipment could be provided. New anaesthetic methods were more and more employed, e.g. closed-system anaesthesia, central and peripheral neuronal blocks. Paediatric surgery (about 4,000 procedures per year) and hepatic transplantation developed to core areas. Already in 1987 an automated anaesthesia record was introduced. In addition to the ICU with 8 beds already existing, a new one with 10 beds was made available to the Department in 1992 in the newly built surgical centre of the Hospital. In the same year the anaesthetists could fill an additional mobile life support unit of the Fire Department of Hamburg which then came into operation in far more than 4,000 cases per year. In 1987 a pain clinic was established which was moved into new premises in 1995 and since then was operated as a modern pain unit for inpatients as well and served also as unit of palliative medicine.

Schulte am Esch established a strong commitment to scientific work. Numerous clinical and experimental research groups came into being and were successful in terms of grant acquisition, high-ranking publications, academic advancement and organization of a large number of congresses, meetings and symposia. Main fields of research were cerebral function and perfusion, cerebral monitoring and anaesthetic depth, malignant hyperthermia, transoesophageal echocardiography, tissue oxygenation, artificial haemoglobin, molecular actions of anaesthetic agents and, last but not least, history of anaesthesia.

Since 2005 Chairmanship Professor Alwin E. Goetz

Prof. Dr. med. Alwin E. Goetz

Born 9 April 1955 in Bayreuth; 1976–1982 student of medicine in Munich; 1987 doctorate in medicine in Munich; 1982–1990 Research Associate, Institute of Surgical Research, University of Munich; since 1991 residency at the Department of Anaesthesiology, University of Munich; 1995 Lecturer in Anaesthesiology 1997 Senior Physician; 1999 Specialist in Anaesthesiology; 2002 Senior Consultant; 2003 Adjunct Professor; 2005 Full Professor and Chairman of the Department of Anaesthesiology, University Hospital Hamburg-Eppendorf.

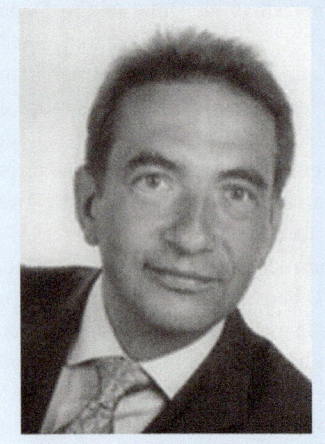

When Schulte am Esch retired in 2005 Professor Alwin Goetz (Munich) was appointed his successor as Full Professor and Chairman of the Department. He gave additional input to the clinical as well as experimental research activities. New scientific projects were funded by the German Research Foundation, e.g. molecular mechanisms of acute lung injury and mechanisms of opioid analgesia.

Qualification as Lecturers in Anaesthesiology

Horatz, Karl (1957); Giebel, Ortwin (1967); Rittmeyer, Peter (†) (1967); Lawin, Peter (†) (1971); Doehn, Manfred (1976); Pokar, Helmut (1981); Brandt, Ludwig (1985); Bause, Hanswerner (1989); Kochs, Eberhard (1989); Beck, Helge (1989); Roewer, Norbert (1989); Scholz, Jens (1992); Werner, Christian (1994); Standl, Thomas (1997); Tonner, Peter (1998); Steinfath, Markus (1998); von Knobelsdorff, Georg (1998); Wappler, Frank (1998); Bischoff, Petra (1999); Horn, Ernst-Peter (2000); Friederich, Patrick (2002); Burmeister, Marc-Alexander (2003); Fiege, Marko (2004); Krause, Thorsten (2004); Gottschalk, André (2005); Goerig, Michael (2006); Reissmann, Hajo (2006); Schuster, Martin (2006); Felbinger, Thomas (2007); Freitag, Marc (2008); Kiefmann, Rainer (2010); Kubitz, Jens (2010)

Professors of Anaesthesiology
Full Professors

Prof. Dr. Dr. h.c. Peter Lawin (1976), University of Münster
Prof. Dr. Eberhard Kochs (1993), Technical University of Munich
Prof. Dr. Norbert Roewer (1995), University of Würzburg

Prof. Dr. Jens Scholz (2000), University of Kiel
Prof. Dr. Frank Wappler (2004), Hospital Cologne-Merheim, University of Witten-Herdecke (Chair II)

Associate Professors

Prof. Dr. M. Doehn (1980), Hamburg
Prof.Dr. Eberhard Kochs (1990), Hamburg
Prof. Dr. Hanswerner Bause (1992), Hamburg
Prof. Dr. Jens Scholz (1996), Hamburg
Prof. Dr. Helge Beck (1997), Hamburg
Prof. Dr. Thomas Standl (1999), Hamburg
Prof. Dr. Frank Wappler (2002), Hamburg
Prof. Dr. Daniel A, Reuter (2009), Hamburg

For further information:
www.uke.uni-hamburg.de/kliniken/anaesthesiologie

4.2.18   Hannover Medical School

Department of Anaesthesiology and Intensive Care Medicine
S. Piepenbrock, T. Palmaers, W. Koppert

Hannover Medical School was founded in 1961 and began teaching medical students in 1965. Clinical departments were established at the Municipal Hospital Oststadt. Since there were no certified anaesthesiologists at this time, a scientifically qualified specialist was looked for, resulting in the employment of Dr. Erich Kirchner (Marburg). He began his activities in 1966. In 1967 he was appointed Professor and Head oft the Division of Anaesthesia and one year later Full Professor of Anaesthesiology.

1968–1996 Chairmanship Professor Erich Kirchner

Prof. Dr. med. Erich Kirchner

Born 25 April 1928 in Fürth/Bavaria; 1948–1954 student of medicine in Erlangen; 1955 doctorate in medicine in Erlangen; 1955–1957 Resident in anaesthesia, Department of Surgery, University of Heidelberg; 1957-1958 Head of the Anaesthesia Unit of the Department of Surgery, University of Erlangen; 1958–1959 Resident, Division of Anaesthesia, 2nd Department of Surgery, University Hospital Cologne-Merheim; 1959 Resident, Division of Anaesthesia, University of Marburg; 1961 Research Associate in pharmacology; 1962 Resident in internal medicine; 1963 Specialist in Anaesthesiology; 1965 Lecturer in Anaesthesiology; 1966 Head of the Division of Anaesthesia, Hannover Medical School; 1967 Professor; 1968 Full Professor and Chairman of the Department of Anaesthesiology; 1996 Professor Emeritus.

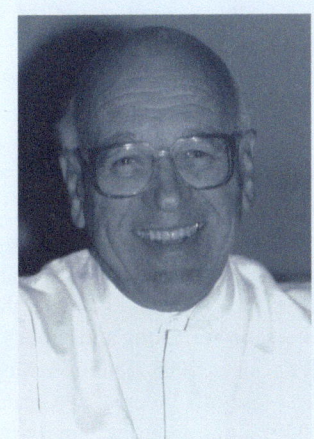

Kirchner introduced modern monitoring equipment and the principle of »deep anaesthesia«, which should, combined with »controlled hypervolaemia«, prevent any stress response of the organism to the surgical trauma. In 1968 cardiac surgery and in 1969 renal transplantation were started. In the following years Hannover Medical School grew to a leading centre of transplant surgery. The new premises of the Central University Hospital were gradually put into operation since October 1971.

Prof. Dr. med. Ina Pichlmayr

Born 24 September 1932 in Wahlstatt/Silesia; 1950–1956 student of medicine in Munich; 1956 doctorate in medicine; 1957–1958 internship; 1959–1963 Resident, Division of Anaesthesia, University Department of

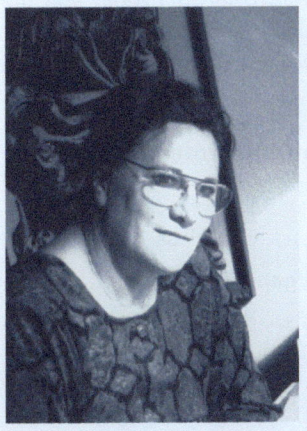

Surgery, Munich; 1963 Specialist in Anaesthesiology; 1968 Lecturer in Anaesthesiology; 1968 Department of Anaesthesiology, Hannover Medical School; 1972 Professor; 1974 Head of the Anaesthesia Service of the Department at the Oststadt Hospital, Hannover; 1977 Head of Division IV of the Centre of Anaesthesiology; 1997 retirement.

Prof. Dr. med. Jürgen Hausdörfer, FACA

Born 29 October 1936 in Munich; 1957–1963 student of medicine in Munich and Vienna; 1963 doctorate in medicine; 1963–1967 internship in the USA and Munich; 1967–1968 Resident, Division of Anaesthesia, University Department of Surgery, Munich; 1968–1971 Resident, Department of Anesthesiology, University of Pennsylvania, Philadelphia, PA, USA; 1971 Fellow of the American Board of Anesthesiology and Specialist in Anaesthesiology; 1971–1979 Senior Physician, Central Department of Anaesthesiology, University of Tübungen; 1976 Lecturer in Anaesthesiology; 1979 Professor and Head of Division III, 1997 in addition Head of Division IV of the Centre of Anaesthesiology, Hannover Medical School; 2000 retirement.

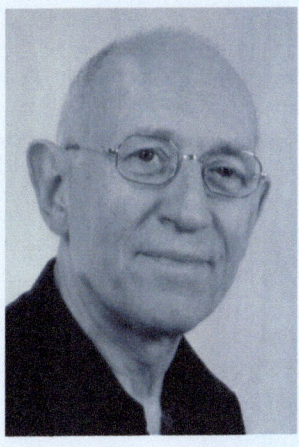

As a new University Law came into effect in 1976, the Department of Anaesthesiology was divided into 4 separate Divisions forming a Centre of Anaesthesiology. The Centre as a whole was entrusted with postgraduate education in anaesthesiology, trainees rotated between the Divisions.

- Kirchner's previous Division became Division I and provided the anaesthesia service for the Department of Surgery with its subdivisions and the anaesthesiological ICU.
- Division II was created in 1984 and headed by Professor Siegfried Piepenbrock (Berlin). It was in charge of

the Departments of Neurosurgery, Otorhinolaryngology, Ophthalmology, Radiology, Radiation Therapy, Nuclear Medicine, a pain clinic, an additional interdisciplinary ICU and pregraduate teaching.

- In 1979 Dr. Jürgen Hausdörfer (Tübingen) was appointed Professor and Head of Division III. He was made responsible for the Departments of Dentistry and Maxillo-Facial Surgery, Paediatrics and Paediatric Surgery.
- Division IV located in the Hospital Oststadt was created in 1977 and Professor Ina Pichlmayr officially appointed Head of the Division. The Division served the Departments or Divisions of General and Plastic and Reconstructive Surgery, Gynaecology and Radiology, and ran an interdisciplinary ICU and a pain clinic.

After Kirchner's retirement in 1996, Piepenbrock became Head of Division I and of Divisions III and IV too, when Hausdörfer retired in 2000. In this year, Piepenbrock was appointed Chairman of the now joint Department of Anaesthesiology.

2000–2009 Chairmanship Professor Siegfried Piepenbrock

Prof. Dr. med. Siegfried Piepenbrock

Born 20 February 1944 in Verl; 1963–1969 student of medicine, veterinary medicine and ethnology in Giessen, Frankfurt, Freiburg and Hamburg; 1969–1971 internship in gynaecology, internal medicine and surgery at the University Hospital Hamburg-Eppendorf; 1971 Resident, Department of Anaesthesiology, Hannover Medical School; 1974 doctorate in medicine; 1975 Specialist in Anaesthesiology; 1975–1980 Senior Physician; 1978 Lecturer in Anaesthesiology; 1980–1984

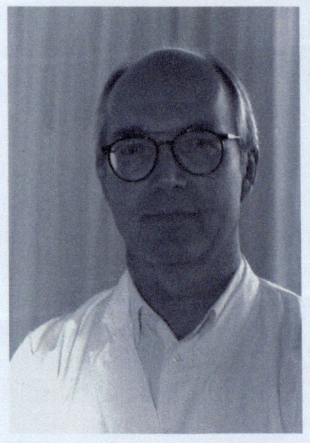

Associate Professor, Department of Anaesthesiology and Intensive Care Medicine, University Hospital Steglitz, Free University of Berlin; 1984 Professor and Head of Division II of the Department of Anaesthesiology, Hannover Medical School; 1996 in addition Head of Division I; 2000 Chairman of the joint Department of Anaesthesiology; 2009 Professor Emeritus.

Under Piepenbrock's chairmanship the Department developed into a very efficient unit with more than 120 physicians and more than 100 nurses. The annual number of anaesthetics approached 30,000. There were a large number of highly complex procedures, e.g. more than 100 liver, more than 40 heart or heart-lung and about 100 lung transplantations per year. In 2008 Hannover Medical School had the highest case-mix index of all German university hospitals. In 2009 a new interdisciplinary ICU with 20 beds was put into operation. The treatment of patients suffering from severe acute lung injuries became a main focus including extracorporeal CO_2 elimination and external negative-pressure ventilation. The doctors of the Department became involved into the emergency medical service outside the hospital and initiated the implementation of the concept of a Chief Emergency Physician into the services of Hannover Medical School. In 2004 the pain clinic of the Hospital Oststadt was merged with that of the Central Hospital. The following courses which are compulsory for the acquisition of additional competences are periodically organized: a course on pain therapy and a course for Chief Emergency Physician candidates every year and a course on emergency medicine twice a year.

With the appointment of Professor Gregor Theilmeier (Münster) to a new professorship of experimental anaesthesiology in 2007 the scientific activities of the Department were expanded to experimental projects with special emphasis on translational research. Main areas of research were perioperative inflammation, lung injury, neurophysiology and neuromonitoring, haemostasis and mechanisms of the development of chronic pain.

Since 2009 Chairmanship Professor Wolfgang Koppert

Prof. Dr. med. Wolfgang Koppert, M.A.

Born 23 February 1964 in Hamburg; 1985–1991 student of medicine in Erlangen; 1991–1993 Research Associate, Department of Physiology and Pathophysiology, University of Erlangen-Nuremberg; 1992 doctorate in medicine; 1993 Resident, Department of Anaesthesiology, University of Erlangen-Nuremberg; 1999 Specialist in Anaesthesiology; 2001 Lecturer in Anaesthesiology and Senior Physician; 2007 Adjunct Professor and Vice Chairman; 2009 Full Professor of Anaesthesiology and Chairman of the Department of Anaesthesiology and Intensive Care Medicine, Hannover Medical School.

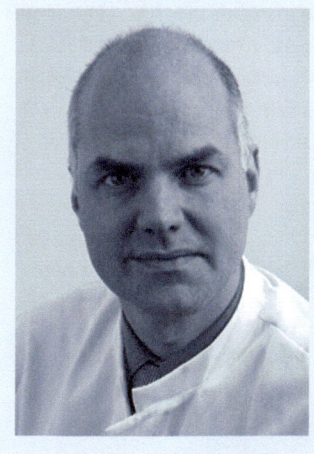

In 2009 Professor Wolfgang Koppert was appointed as Piepenbrock's successor to the Chair of Anaesthesiology. The clinical commitments continued to increase, the number of physicians grew to more than 130 and that of nursing personnel to 150. Experimental pain research became a new field of scientific activities.

Qualification as Lecturers in Anaesthesiology

Hempelmann, Gunter (1973); Helms, Uwe (1977); Piepenbrock, Siegfried (1978); Schaps, Dagmar (1981); Zenz, Michael (1981); Lips, Ulrich (1982); Tryba, Michael (1984); Panning, Bernhard (1987); Seitz, Wolfgang (1987); Fritz, Karl-Wilhelm (1988); Schäffer, Jürgen (1988); Pohl, Sönke (1989); Lübbe, Norbert (1992); Strauß, Jochen (1992); Leuwer, Martin (1994); Schultz, Barbara (1994); Schultz, Arthur (1995); Otto, Klaus (1996); Bund, Michael (1999); Sümpelmann, Robert (1999); Marx, Gernot (2000); Heine, Jörn (2001); Jaeger, Karsten (2001); Haeseler, Gertrud (2001); Münte, Sinikka (2001); Karst, Matthias (2002); Przemeck, Michael (2003); Raymondos, Konstantinos (2005); Scheinichen, Dirk (2005); Grouven, Ulrich (2008); Rahe-Meyer, Niels (2008); Winterhalter, Michael (2008); Ahrens, Jörg (2009); Bernsteck, Michael (2009); Weilbach, Christian (2009); Jüttner, Björn (2010); Osthaus, Alexander (2010).

Professors of Anaesthesiology
Full Professors

Prof. Dr. Gunter Hempelmann (1978), Department of Anaesthesiology and Surgical Intensive Care Medicine, University of Giessen
Prof. Dr. Michael Zenz (1986), Department of Anaesthesiology, Intensive Care Medicine and Pain Therapy, University Hospital Bergmannsheil, Bochum
Prof. Dr. Martin Leuwer (2001), Department of Anaesthesia, Royal Liverpool University Hospital

Associate Professor

Prof. Dr. Gregor Theilmeier, Associate Professor of Experimental Anaesthesiology, Hannover

For further information:

www.mh-hannover.de/anaesthesiologie.html

3.2.19 University of Heidelberg

Department of Anaesthesiology

E. Martin, H.-J. Bender

The University of Heidelberg including a Faculty of Medicine was founded in 1386, it is the oldest German university. Early highlights of anaesthesia in Heidelberg were the first report on the use of cocaine as a local anaesthetic for an ophthalmic operation given by Carl Koller's colleague Josef Brettauer at the Congress of Ophthalmologists on 15 September 1884, and the development of an experimental nitrous oxide-oxygen apparatus with rotameters by Maximilian Neu in 1910. Local anaesthesia was the preferred technique since 1910. Later Professor Karl Heinrich Bauer, Chairman of the Department of Surgery 1942-1962, switched to a barbiturate-nitrous oxide technique. Such combinations became even more favoured after World War II by cooperation with the US Army Hospital in Heidelberg and after visiting professorships of the anaesthetists Dr. Jean Henley (New York) and Dr. Karl Mülly (Zurich). Subsequently, endotracheal intubation and muscle relaxation slowly became routinely used methods at the Department of Surgery. In 1950 Bauer gave a mandate to Dr. Rudolf Frey to bring an anesthesia division into being. When Professor Fritz Linder (Berlin) became Bauer's successor in 1962 he was accompanied by the anaesthetist Dr. Otto Just who had already worked with Frey in the years 1949-1951 and then became Head of the Division of Anaesthesia. Frey had been appointed Associate Professor of Anaesthesiology at the University of Mainz in 1960 (▶ Chap. 3.2.27).

1967–1990 Chairmanship Professor Otto Heinrich Just

Prof. Dr. med. Otto Heinrich Just

Born 27 January 1922 in Lauda (Taubertal); deceased 21 April 2012; 1941 student of medicine in Berlin and Würzburg; 1949 doctorate in medicine, University of Würzburg; 1949–1951 Resident in anaesthesia, University of Heidelberg; 1951 change to the University Hospital, Free University of Berlin, development of an anaesthesia unit; 1956 Specialist and Lecturer in anaesthesiology; 1962 Head of the Division of Anaesthesia, University of Heidelberg; 1963 Associate Professor and Chairman of the Division; 1967 Full Professor of Anaesthesiology; 1990 Professor Emeritus; 1995 Honorary Member of the German Society of Anaesthesiology and Intensive Care Medicine.

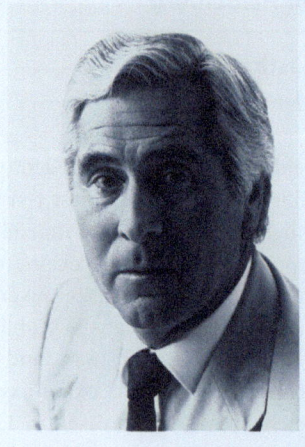

In 1963 Just was appointed Associate Professor and Chairman of the Division of Anaesthesiology and in 1967 advanced to Full Professor of Anaesthesiology and Chairman of the Department of Anaesthesiology. At the beginning he had 2 senior physicians and 13 residents at his disposal, a number that, in order to comply with the ever increasing demands for anaesthetic services, raised to 8 seniors and 45 residents in 1984 and to 9 seniors and 55 residents in 1990 corresponding to an annual number of anaesthetics of 13,800 in 1984 and 18,500 in 1990, respectively. The Department ran a recovery room and, since 1970, an anaesthesiological ICU. In addition, the anaesthesia team was involved in the care of various surgical intermediate care units and ICUs. A pain clinic was started in 1977 and subsequently complemented by a preanaesthetic clinic. In 1970 rooms and equipment for experimental research could be established. The scientific activities were directed at haemorrhagic shock and volume replacement, influence of anaesthetics on the circulation, cerebral metabolism and intracranial pressure, sepsis, apoptosis following cardiac arrest and problems related to hepatic surgery.

Since 1990 Chairmanship Professor Eike Martin

Prof. Dr. med. Eike Martin, FANZCA

Born 1 March 1944 in Waldenburg (Schlesien); 1965–1970 student of medicine in Mainz; 1972 doctorate in medicine; 1974–1977 residency at the Department of Anaesthesiology; Faculty of Clinical Medicine Mannheim; 1976 Specialist in Anaesthesiology; 1977 Lecturer in Anaesthesiology; 1977 Senior Physician, Department of Anaesthesiology, University of Munich; 1980 Associate Professor; 1987-1990 Head of the Department of Anaesthesiology, Municipal Hospital Nuremberg; 1990 Full Professor and Chairman of the Department of Anaesthesiology, University Hospital Heidelberg.

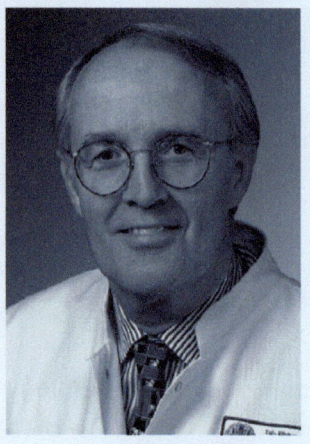

On 1 August 1990 Professor Eike Martin (Nuremberg) was appointed Full Professor and Chairman of the Department of Anaesthesiology. He restructured and expanded the clinical activities in anaesthesia, ICM and pain therapy and soon introduced medical informatics as a tool for both patient data documentation and tasks in clinical practice, research and teaching. The annual number of anaesthetics increased to 24,000 in the year 2000 and approached 30,000 in 2009. The combination of general and regional anaesthesia was introduced and developed to a standard technique for high-risk surgery and postoperative analgesia. An acute pain service was established in 1997. The number of ICU beds under the responsibility of the Department increased. Owing to the great distance between the premises of the surgical departments and the »Kopfklinikum« (»Head Hospital«)

a second combined pain and preanaesthetic clinic was created in the latter. It then was developed to the supra-regional Centre of Pain Therapy and Palliative Medicine, led by Professor Hubert Bardenheuer. Members of the Department were more and more on duty for the mobile life support unit, since 2001 in 50% of all services in the field. The scientific activities were systematically extended under Martin's chairmanship. In 1994, a Section of Clinical-Experimental Anaesthesiology was created and in 1997 a lab for molecular biology put into operation. Main areas of research are apoptosis, sepsis, ischaemia, chronic cerebral oligaemia, pulmonary vasoreactivity, microcirculation, platelet and leucocyte function, mechanisms of neuronal apoptosis caused by cardiac arrest.

Qualification as Lecturers in Anaesthesiology

Frey, Rudolf (1952); Lutz, Horst (1965); Wawersik, Jürgen (1966); Stoeckel, Horst (1969); Dietzel, Werner (1969); Simmendinger, Hans-Joachim (1975); Wiedemann, Klaus (1977); Fischer, Martin Volker (1983); Krier, Claude (1985); Bach, Alfons (1992); Böhrer, Hubert (1992); Graf, Bernhard M. (1996); Böttiger, Bernd W. (1997); Schmidt, Heinfried (1997); Gust, René (2000); Kunst, Gudrun (2000); Weimann, Jörg (2000); Gries, André (2002); Grau, Thomas (2003); Hollmann, Markus W. (2004); Walther, Andreas (2005); Weigand, Markus (2005); Zink, Wolfgang (2005); Schmidt, Werner (2007); Streitberger, Konrad (2007); Bopp, Christian (2009); Hofer, Stefan (2010); Popp, Erik (2010).

Professors of Anaesthesiology
Full Professors

Prof. Dr. Horst Lutz (1971), Faculty of Clinical Medicine Mannheim of the University of Heidelberg
Prof. Dr. Jürgen Wawersik (1971), University Hospital Kiel
Prof. Dr. Horst Stoeckel (1974), University of Bonn
Prof. Dr. Bernhard M. Graf (2005), University of Göttingen
Prof. Dr. Markus W. Hollmann (2005), Experimental and Clinical Experimental Anaesthesiology, Academic Medical Centre, University of Amsterdam, The Netherlands
Prof. Dr. Bernd Böttiger (2007), University of Cologne
Prof. Dr. Markus Weigand (2008), University of Giessen

Associate Professors

Prof. Dr. Rudolf Frey (1960), University of Mainz
Prof. Dr. Hubert J. Bardenheuer (1993), Heidelberg

Adjunct Professors

Prof. Dr. med. Alfons Bach, Prof. Dr. med. Hubert Böhrer; Prof. Dr. Werner Dietzel; Prof. Dr. André Gries; Prof. Dr. Johann Motsch

For further information:

http://www.klinikum.uni-heidelberg.de/Anaesthesie.2364.0.html

3.2.20 Saarland University Homburg

Department of Anaesthesiology, Intensive Care Medicine and Pain Therapy
R. Larsen, T. Volk

In November 1948 Saarland University was founded in Saarbrücken, the capital of Saarland, with the support of the French Government and the University of Nancy. Clinical training courses for medical students had already been introduced at the State Hospital in Homburg/Saar by the »Centre Universitaire d'Études Supérieures de Hombourg« established on 8 May 1947 under the patronage of the University of Nancy. Although the University was located in Saarbrücken the Faculty of Medicine and the University Hospital remained at Homburg. Before the creation of a Division of Anaesthesia at the Department of Surgery and Neurosurgery in 1962, anaesthetics were given by residents or nurses of the surgical departments of the University Hospital. This situation did initially not so much change after 1962 because the number of doctors in the Division did not meet the demands. An improvement did not come about until a Chair of Anaesthesiology was created in 1966.

1964–1988 Chairmanship Professor Karl Hutschenreuter

Prof. Dr. med. Dr. h.c. Karl Hutschenreuter
Born 6 August 1920 in Grünbach/Vogtland; deceased 5 March 1996 in Homburg/Saar; 1940–1946 student

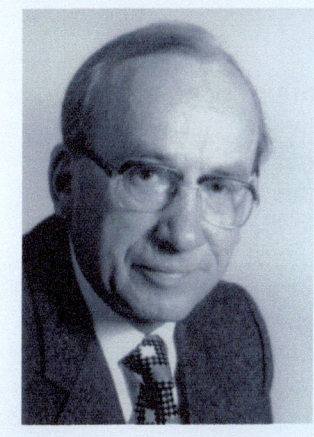

of medicine in Jena; 1946 doctorate in medicine, University of Halle; 1947–1949 Resident in pathology and internal medicine, University of Jena; 1949–1951 Resident, Department of Surgery, University of Jena; 1953 Specialist in Surgery; 1955 Specialist in Anaesthesiology; 1953–1961 Head of the Division of Anaesthesia, University Hospital Jena; 1959 Lecturer in Surgery and Anaesthesiology; 1961–1962 Division of Anaesthesia, University of Heidelberg; 1962 Head of the Division of Anaesthesia, Department of Surgery and Neurosurgery, Saarland University Homburg; 1963 Associate Professor; 1964 Chairman of the Department of Anaesthesiology; 1966 Full Professor of Anaesthesiology; 1983 Honorary Doctorate of the Medical Academy Wroclaw, Poland; 1988 Professor Emeritus.

Dr. Karl Hutschenreuter (Heidelberg) became Head oft he Division of Anaesthesia in 1962 and was appointed Full Professor of Anaesthesiology and Chairman of the Deopartment of Anaesthesiology in 1966. He could augment the number of staff members and residents and gradually become responsible for the entire anaesthesiological service of the University Hospital, e.g. for the Department of Gynaecology and the Emergency Medical Service of the Saarland and Westpfalz in 1968 and the Division of Cardiac and Thoracic Surgery in 1975. In 1974 an anaesthesiological ICU was brought into being and led by Professor Efim Racenberg. Hutschenreuter was wholeheartedly engaged for teaching and training of both anaesthesiologists and nurses. He organized biennial CME courses with renowned speakers from many countries and provided clinical fellowships for colleagues from Poland, Czechoslovakia, Hungary and China. Research was mainly carried out in cooperation with the Departments of Experimental Surgery and Pharmacology.

1990–2009 Chairmanship Professor Reinhard Larsen

Prof. Dr. med. Reinhard Larsen

Born 1 November 1943 in Göttingen; 1965–1970 student of medicine in Göttingen; 1971 doctorate in medicine; 1971–1972 internship, University Hospital Göttingen and Municipal Hospital Herzberg/Harz; 1973–1974 Medical Officer; 1974-1978 Resident, Department of Clinical Anaesthesia, University of Göttingen; 1978 Spe-

cialist in Anaesthesiology; 1978 Senior Physician; 1981 Lecturer in Anaesthesiology; 1986 Adjunct Professor; 1990 Full Professor and Chairman of the Department of Anaesthesiology, Saarland University Homburg; 2009 Professor Emeritus.

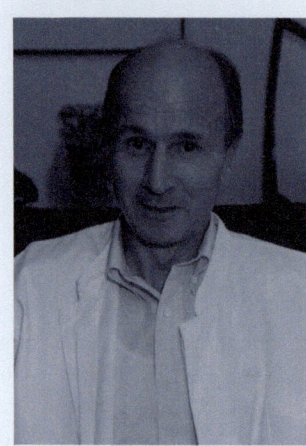

As Hutschenreuter had been retired in 1988 Professor Efim Racenberg became Interim Chairman until Professor Reinhard Larsen (Göttingen) was appointed Full Professor and Chairman of the Department of Anaesthesiology on 1 January 1990. The clinical spectrum covered by the Department pertained to all aspects of anaesthesiology: clinical anaesthesia as well as emergency, intensive care and pain medicine. The number of staff members and residents eventually amounted to 70 doctors. Larsen was author and editor of a number of textbooks and handbooks on anaesthesia and ICM, his comprehensive textbook »Anästhesie« was the most popular one in Germany and the 11th edition was published in 2010. Two research groups were established and were successful in publishing in international peer-reviewed journals and gathering grants. One group worked on molecular mechanisms of organ failure, the second group on neuromuscular transmission and clinical pharmacology of muscle relaxants.

Since 2009 Chairmanship Professor Thomas Volk

Prof. Dr. med. Thomas Volk

Born 24 October 1964 in Koblenz; 1986–1993 student of medicine in Essen; 1994 doctorate in medicine; 1993–1998 Resident, Department of Anaesthesiology and Intensive Care Medicine, University Hospital Charité, Campus Mitte, Berlin; 1998 Specialist in Anaesthesiology; 1999 Senior Physician; 2001 Lecturer in Anaesthesiology; 2005–2009 Deputy Chairman; 2007 Associate Professor; 2009 Full Professor of Anaesthesiology and Chairman of the Department of Anaesthesiology, Intensive Care Medicine and Pain Therapy, Saarland University Homburg.

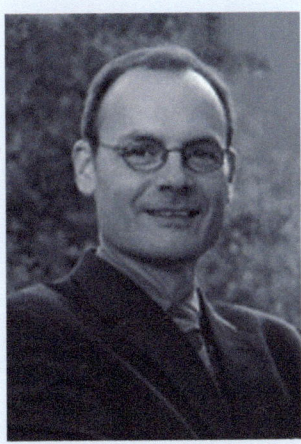

After Larsen's retirement Professor Thomas Volk (Berlin) was appointed Full Professor of Anaesthesiology and Chairman of the Department of Anaesthesiology, Intensive Care Medicine and Pain Therapy in 2009. He established a number of research groups working on the following projects: molecular mechanisms of organ protection, pharmacokinetics and pharmacodynamics of modern anaesthetics and opioids, standards and models for objective assessment of skills on the simulator, airway management, use of ultrasound in anaesthesia, various aspects of chronic pain.

Qualification as Lecturers in Anaesthesiology

Bihler, Karl (1970); Fritsche, Paul (1972); Motsch, Johann (1988); Büch, Uta (1988); Altmayer, Paul (1989); Mertzlufft, Friedrich (1993); Molter, Gerd (1995); Fösel, Thomas (1996); Kleinschmidt, Stefan (1998); Bauer, Michael (1999); Fuchs-Buder, Thomas (1999); Bauer, Clemens (2000); Grundmann, Ulrich (2000); Silomon, Malte (2002); Wilhelm, Wolfram (2002); Biedler, Andreas (2004); Rensing, Hauke (2005); Kreuer, Sascha (2006); Kubulus, Darius (2009)

Professors of Anaesthesiology
Associate Professors

Prof. Dr. Paul Fritsche; Prof. Dr. Efim Racenberg

Adjunct Professors

Prof. Dr. Paul Altmayer; Prof. Dr. Clemens Bauer; Prof. Dr. Michael Bauer; Prof. Dr. Uta Büch; Prof. Dr. Ulrich Grundmann; Prof. Dr. Stefan Kleinschmidt; Prof. Dr. Sascha Kreuer; Prof. Dr. Friedrich Mertzlufft; Prof. Dr. Hauke Rensing; Prof. Dr. Malte Silomon; Prof. Dr. Wolfram Wilhelm

For further information:

www.uniklinikum-saarland.de/de/einrichtungen/kliniken_institute/anaesthesiologie

3.2.21   University of Jena

Department of Anaesthesiology and Intensive Care Medicine

K. Reinhart, T. Uhlig

The development of anaesthesia and intensive care medicine in Jena was pioneered by Dr. Karl Hutschenreuter, who was responsible for the Department from 1953 to 1961, since 1960 in the academic rank of an Associate Professor (▶ Chap. 3.2.20 for his C.V.). He was followed by Dr. Gerhard Endres and Dr. Horst Winkler. Winkler became the first Full Professor of Anaesthesiology in 1979. ICM in Jena started with a small post-surgical care unit in 1958 which was extended in 1964 and made an ICU in 1976.

1979–1987 Chairmanship Professor Horst Winkler

Prof. Dr. sc. med Horst Winkler

Born 2 August 1929 in Bad Lausick; deceased 23 December 1985; 1949–1955 student of medicine at the University of Leipzig; 1955–1956 residency in forensic

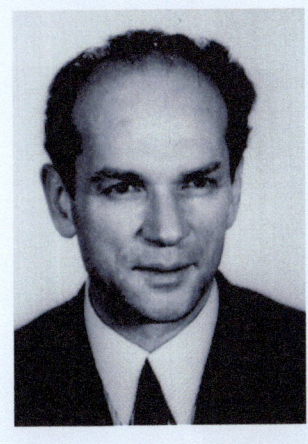

3

medicine in Leipzig; 1956–1962 residency in pathological physiology, University of Jena; 1962–1967 residency in anaesthesiology and ICM; 1967–1970 Chairman of the Anaesthesia Department, Yarmouk University Hospital Bagdad; 1970–1985 Head of the Division of Anaesthesia of the Department of Surgery, University of Jena; 1979 Full Professor of Anaesthesiology; 1985–1987 Chairman of the Department of Anaesthesiology and Intensive Care Medicine.

After Winkler's early death the Department was chaired by Professor Wulf Schirrmeister from 1988-1993, who was very successful in further developing the speciality in all its four main areas.

1987–1993 Chairmanship Professor Wulf Schirrmeister

Prof. Dr. med. Wulf Schirrmeister

Born 29 October 1943 in Jena; 1965–1971 student of medicine at Leipzig and Jena; 1971–1973 Resident, Department of Pathophysiology, University of Jena; 1973–1976 Resident, Division of Anaesthesia of the Department of Surgery; 1973 doctorate in medicine; 1982 Senior Physician; 1983 Lecturer in Anaesthesiology; 1985–1986 postgraduate studies at the Department of Anaesthesiology, University of Prague, Czechoslovakia; 1988 Chairman of the Department of Anaesthesiology and Intensive Care Medicine, University of Jena; 1988 Full Professor of Anaesthesiology and Intensive Therapy; 1995 Head Physician, Department of Anaesthesiology and Intensive Therapy, Municipal Hospital (Wald-Klinikum) Gera.

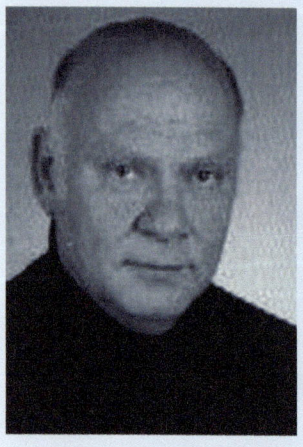

When Schirrmeister had left the University and moved to the nearby Municipal Hospital Gera, Professor Konrad Reinhart (Berlin) was appointed Full Professor and Chairman of the Department of Anaesthesiology and Intensive Therapy in 1993.

Since 1993 Chairmanship Professor Konrad Reinhart

Prof. Dr. med. Konrad Reinhart

Born 26 Oktober 1947 in Bamberg; 1969–1975 student of medicine at Munich and Berlin; 1975–1976 internship, Free University of Berlin; 1976–1977 resident in surgery, Evangelisches Waldkrankenhaus Berlin; 1977–1978 resident in surgery and urology, Franziskus Hospital Berlin; 1978–1982 Resident, Department of Anaesthesiology and Surgical Intensive Care Medicine, Free University of Berlin; 1978 doctorate in medicine; 1982–1985 Senior Physician; 1984 Specialist and Lecturer in Anaesthesiology; 1988–1989 Visiting Associate Professor, Department of Physiology and Biophysics, University of Alabama at Birmingham, USA; 1989 Adjunct Professor; 1993 Associate Professor;1993 Full Professor and Chairman of the Department of Anaesthesiology and Intensive Therapy, University of Jena.

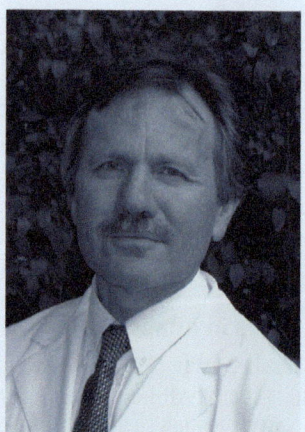

Since 1993 the Department has considerable grown in all fields. It is structured in five sections: anaesthesiology, responsible Professor Michael Bauer who is also Vice Chairman of the Department; ICM, responsible until 2008 Professor Gernot Marx, since then Professor Niels Riedemann; pain medicine, run by Dr. Winfried Meißner; emergency medicine, responsible Dr. Jens Reichel. The section of Experimental Anaesthesiology is headed by Dr. Dr. Ralf A. Claus.

Main research fields are sepsis and pain. Sepsis research is focussed on supportive and adjunctive sepsis therapies, the development and clinical evaluation of innovative sepsis markers. The Section of Experimental Anaesthesia works in the field of the pathogenesis of sepsis related organ failure using systems biology approaches. This research area is led by Bauer. The Department was quite successful in gaining major funding on the regional, national and European levels. The most important ones are listed here:

- From 2001-2010 the Network of competency *SepNet* chaired by Reinhart received € 8 millions funding by the Federal Ministry of Education and Research. SepNet is a clinical trials group that in the meanwhile comprises almost 50 ICUs.
- Since 2008 an interdisciplinary Centre for Innovation Competency *Septomics* was funded by the Federal Ministry of Education and Research and the Federal State of Thuringia with € 19 millions over five years.
- Since 2008 a Centre for Sepsis Control and Care, an interdisciplinary research centre chaired by Bauer, was funded by the Federal Ministry of Education and Research and the University Hospital Jena. A total of 68 academic and 32 technical staff members cover all aspects of sepsis-related clinical, translational and basic research.

Pain medicine is another important field of clinical and scientific activities in Jena. Led by Meißner and in close cooperation with the German Society of Anaesthesiology and Intensive Care Medicine and the Professional Association of German Anaesthetists, a nation-wide registry and benchmark project in postoperative pain management (QUIPS) has been established, meanwhile expanding internationally. Further areas of research comprise opioid-associated gastrointestinal dysfunction and non-pharmacologic approaches in acute pain. Moreover, one of the first outpatient palliative care teams in Germany has been established at the pain unit. Since 2003 the pain medicine section obtained funding by the German Ministry of Health and the European Union that totals over € 3.5 millions for research on quality of care for post-surgical pain control. Since 2008 the Department of Anaesthesia and Intensive Care is ranked number one in the internal research ranking of the Faculty of Medicine of the University of Jena.

Qualification as Lecturers in Anaesthesiology

Schirrmeister, Wulf (1983); Klein, Uwe (1990); Kretzschmar, Michael (1992); Meier-Hellmann, Andreas (1999); Karzai, Waheedullah (1999); Meisner, Michael (2001); Rußwurm, Stefan (2003); Sakka, Samir (2003); Hüttemann, Egbert (2005); Meißner, Winfried (2005); Paxian, Markus (2006); Schreiber, Torsten (2007); Schummer, Wolfram (2007); Schürholz, Tobias (2007); Claus, Ralf (2008); Brunkhorst, Frank Martin (2008); Schwarzkopf, Konrad (2008)

Professors of Anaesthesiology
Full Professors

Prof. Dr. Gernot Marx (2008), Professor of Anaesthesiology and Intensive Care Medicine, University of Aachen
Prof. Dr. Michael Bauer (2010), Professor of Translational Sepsis Research, Jena

Associate Professors

Prof. Dr. Michael Bauer (2004), Jena
Prof. Dr. Gernot Marx (2004), Jena
Prof. Dr. Frank Martin Brunkhorst (2006); Endowed Professor of Clinical Sepsis and Research, Jena

Adjunct Professors

Prof. Dr. Waheedullah Karzai; Prof. Dr. Uwe Klein, Prof. Dr. Andreas Meier-Hellmann; Prof. Dr. Wulf Schirrmeister

For further information:

www.kai.uniklinikum-jena.de/

3.2.22 University of Kiel

Department of Anaesthesiology and Surgical Intensive Care Medicine

J. Wawersik, J. Scholz, M. Steinfath

The University of Kiel represents a milestone in the early history of anaesthesia because August Bier, then Professor of Surgery and Chairman of the Department of Surgery, performed the first surgical procedure under spinal anaesthesia on 16 August 1898. It was not before the end of World War II that individual dedicated physicians began to direct their professional activities towards anaesthesia, but always within the Department of Surgery. In 1955 Dr. Johannes Eichler was employed at the Department with the aim of being trained in anaesthesiology. In 1960, he was entrusted with the responsibility for anaesthetics by the Chairman of the Department, Professor Robert Warnke. After Eichler had left to Lübeck in 1964 (▶ Chap. 3.2.25) Dr. Theodor Schmitz (Düsseldorf) resumed his tasks but deceased already in 1970. He was followed by Dr. Klaus Fischer until, on 1 August 1971, Dr. Jürgen Wawersik (Heidelberg) was appointed Full Professor of Anaesthesiology and Chairman of the Central Division of Anaesthesiology of the University Hospital.

1971–2000 Chairmanship Professor Jürgen Wawersik

Prof. Dr. med. Jürgen Wawersik

Born 20 August 1933 in Beuthen; 1952–1958 student of medicine at Hamburg; 1959 doctorate in medicine; 1958–1961 internship in Wuppertal-Elberfeld, Düsseldorf and Berlin; 1961 Resident, Division of Anaesthesia of the Department of Surgery, University Hospital Berlin-Westend; since 1962 Division of Anaesthesia, Department of Surgery, University of Heidelberg; 1966 Lecturer in Anaesthesiology; 1971 Full Professor and Chairman of the Central Division of Anaesthesiology, University Hospital Kiel; 2000 Professor Emeritus.

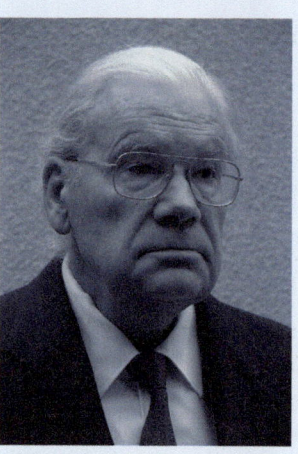

Since 2000 Chairmanship Professor Jens Scholz

Prof. Dr. med. Jens Scholz

Born 7 September 1959 in Osnabrück; 1979–1985 student of medicine at Hamburg; 1985 doctorate in medicine; 1985–1986 Resident, Department of Anaesthesiology, University of Hamburg; 1986–1988 Fellow of the German Research Foundation, Department of Pharmacology, University of Hamburg; 1992 Specialist in Anaesthesiology, Senior Physician and Lecturer in Anaesthesiology; 1996 Associate Professor, University of Hamburg; 2000 Full Professor and Chairman of the Department of Anaesthesiology and Surgical Intensive Care Medicine, University Hospital Kiel; 2009 Medical Director of the University Hospitals Schleswig-Holstein.

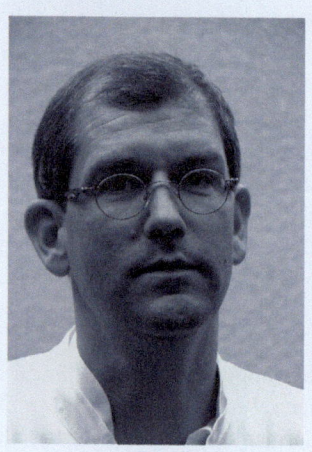

Parallel to the surgical specialties the Division of Anaesthesia expanded markedly during Wawersik's chairmanship. The annual number of anaesthetics increased from 9,849 in 1972 to about 19,500 in the following decade. Balanced anaesthesia and regional anaesthesia became the preferred techniques. The revival of spinal anaesthesia was actively initiated and further developed by Dr. Hinnerk Wulf. The Division became responsible for the surgical and otorhinolaryngological ICUs. Between 1971 and 2000, the number of doctors increased from 8 to 79, that of nurses from 6 to 82. In 1985 an outpatient pain clinic and in 1990 an inpatient pain unit were created and successfully led by Dr. Christoph Maier. In 1990 the Division became the Department of Anaesthesiology and Surgical Intensive Care Medicine. The scientific activities were directed at various pharmacological questions, shock and transfusion related lung injuries, sepsis and pain.

As Professor Jens Scholz (Hamburg) was appointed Full Professor and Chairman of the Department of Anaesthesiology and Surgical Intensive Care Medicine in 2000 he made changes in the organization of the Department. An effective human resource and process management covering the whole Department was established. A global hospital information system as well as a patient data management system in the ICUs were established. The anaesthetic equipment was modernized and extended by the most recent equipment for ventilator support and patient monitoring. The annual number of anaesthetics increased to 24,000 and that of ICU patients by one third. Anaesthetists were enabled to participate in the out-of-hospital emergency medical service. In 2005 a modern ward for pain and palliative medicine was put into service. This unit is located in the completely renewed premises of the Department and is part of the Interdisciplinary Pain and Palliative Centre of the University Hospital, a joint activity of the Departments of Anaesthesiology and Radiotherapy. Scientific labs were made available to various research groups which were staffed with scientists and research assistants. Main projects are ischaemic preconditioning, resuscitation, impedance tomography, automated weaning from the respirator, sepsis, airway management and new monitoring techniques. CME activities were increased, e.g. by courses in TEE, emergency medicine, pain therapy and haemodynamics.

When Scholz became Medical Director of the University Hospitals Schleswig-Holstein, Campus Kiel and Campus Lübeck, in April 2009, Professor Markus Steinfath was appointed acting Chairman of the Department.

Qualification as Lecturers in Anaesthesiology

Eichler, Johannes (1965); Schmitz, Theodor (1969); Fischer, Klaus Jürgen (1977); Harke, Henning (1981); Marquort, Hermann Walter (1981); Schuh, Friedrich Theodor (1981); Wulf, Hinnerk (1994); Maier, Christoph (1995); Petry, Andreas (1998); Bauer, Martin (2004); Bein, Berthold (2006); Hanß, Robert (2006); Ledowski, Thomas (2008); Paris, Andrea (2009); Renner, Jochen (2009), Meybohm, Patrick (2009).

Professors of Anaesthesiology
Full Professors

Prof. Dr. Hinnerk Wulf (2001), University of Marburg

Associate Professors

Prof. Dr. Christoph Maier (1999), Endowed Professor of Pain Therapy, University of Bochum
Prof. Dr. Peter H. Tonner (2002), Kiel
Prof. Dr. Norbert Weiler (2002), Kiel
Prof. Dr. Markus Steinfath (2003), Kiel

Adjunct Professors

Prof. Dr. Berthold Bein; Prof. Dr. Volker Dörges; Prof. Dr. Klaus J. Fischer; Prof. Dr. Inez Frerichs; Prof. Dr. Henning Harke; Prof. Dr. Ulf Linstedt; Prof. Dr. Friedrich T. Schuh

For further information:

www.uni-kiel.de/anaesthesie/

3.2.23 University of Cologne

Department of Anaesthesiology and Surgical Intensive Care Medicine

S.-M. Kasper, K. Bonhoeffer, W. Buzello, B.W. Böttiger

As in many other university hospitals, the University Hospital Cologne had no separate anaesthesia division up to the 1970s. Anaesthetics were given by specially trained doctors of the Department of Surgery. During the 1960s, modern anaesthesia was initiated and performed by Dr. Hans-Joachim Eberlein, Dr. Karl Bonhoeffer, and Dr. Hans-R. Rümmele. With the increasing requirement of anaesthesiologists and the anaesthesia techniques becoming more and more complex, the Faculty of Medicine decided in June 1967 to create an independent Chair of Anaesthesiology. Bonhoeffer who had been qualified as Lecturer in Anaesthesiology in 1965 was nominated for this position and appointed Head of a Division of Anaesthesia of the Department of Surgery in 1969. It then took 4 more years until the first Chair of Anaesthesiology was established at the University Hospital Cologne-Lindenthal.

1971–1987 Chairmanship Professor Karl Bonhoeffer

Prof. Dr. med. Karl Bonhoeffer

Born 10 January 1931, in Frankfurt/Main, 1948–1954 student of medicine in Göttingen; 1954 doctorate in medicine; 1954–1956 internal medicine, University of Heidelberg; 1956–1958 physiology, University of Göttingen; 1958–1959 surgery and anaesthesia, University of Marburg; 1959–1963 surgery, anaesthesia and experimental surgery in Cologne-Merheim; since 1963 anaesthesiology, University Hospital, Cologne-Lindenthal; 1965 Lecturer in Anaesthesiology; 1969 Adjunct Professor; 1971 Full Professor of Anaesthesiology and Chairman of the Department of Anaesthesiology and Surgical Intensive Care Medicine, University of Cologne; 1987–1996 on leave; 1996 Professor Emeritus.

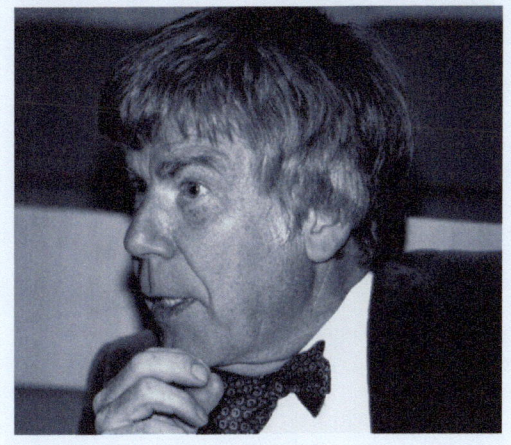

Bonhoeffer was appointed Full Professor of Anaesthesiology on 30 August 1971 and Chairman of the Department of Anaesthesiology in February 1972. At that time, the team comprised 18 doctors and 12 nurses. A new ICU was planned and put into existence, but not yet as-

3

sociated to the Department. Bonhoeffer established a preanaesthetic clinic in 1976 and a Pain Clinic in 1983. In 1985, Klaus A. Lehmann (Aachen) and Walter Buzello (Freiburg) joined the team and promoted scientific activities in pain medicine and pharmacology of neuromuscular blockade. Bonhoeffer left the Department on his own request in 1987 in order to devote all his energies and enthusiasm to the Organization »International Physicians for the Prevention of Nuclear War« (IPPNW).

1988–2007 Chairmanship Professor Walter Buzello

Prof. Dr. med. Walter Buzello

Born 29 July 1939 in Völklingen/Saar; 1957–1963 student of medicine in Frankfurt/Main; 1965 doctorate in medicine; 1966–1967 Medical Officer; 1967–1968 pharmacology in Homburg/Saar; 1968–1970 Resident in internal medicine in Saarbrücken; 1970–1973 Resident, Department of Anaesthesiology, University Hospital Freiburg; 1973 Specialist in Anaesthesiology; 1974 Lecturer in Anaesthesiology; 1979 Adjunct Professor; 1983–1984 Visiting Professor at the Department of Anesthesiology, Texas Tech University, School of Medicine, El Paso, Texas; 1985 Associate Professor of Anaesthesiology, University of Cologne; 1987 Interim Chairman; 1988 Full Professor and Chairman of the Department of Anaesthesiology and Surgical Intensive Care Medicine; 2007 Professor Emeritus.

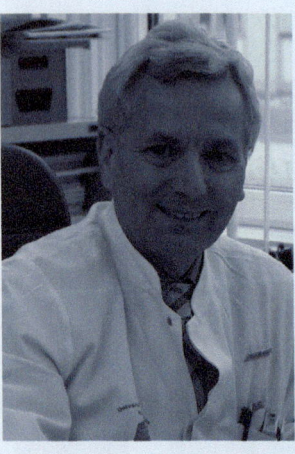

Walter Buzello became Full Professor of Anaesthesiology and Chair of the Department in March 1988. During his chairmanship clinical activities were extended what was made visible in 1991 by the new name Department of Anaesthesiology and Surgical Intensive Care Medicine. Starting in 1990, the University Hospital became a new location of a physician-staffed emergency ambulance

car (»NEF3«) which was operated by the Department in cooperation with the Municipal Fire Department. The new ICU was opened in 1991 but separated from the Department in 2007. From 1991 to 2007, the Emergency Department of the Hospital was run by the Department of Anaesthesiology. Main areas of research were pain medicine research and neuromuscular blocking agents.

Since 2007 Chairmanship Professor Bernd W. Böttiger

Prof. Dr. med. Bernd W. Böttiger

Born 11 June 1958 in Pfungstadt; 1979–1986 student of medicine in Heidelberg; 1988 doctorate in medicine; 1986–1990 Resident in anaesthesia, Enzkreis Hospital; 1990–1992 Resident, Department of Anaesthesiology, University Hospital, Heidelberg; 1992 Specialist in Anaesthesiology; 1994 Senior Physician; 1997 Lecturer in Anaesthesiology; 2002 Vice Chairman; 2004 Adjunct Professor; 2007 Full Professor of Anaesthesiology and Chairman of the Department of Anaesthesiology and Intensive Care Medicine, University Hospital Cologne; 2008 Chairman of the European Resuscitation Council (ERC).

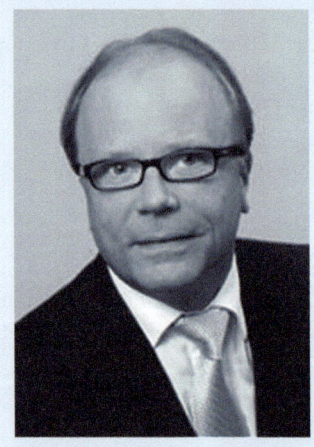

Professor Bernd W. Böttiger (Heidelberg) was appointed Full Professor of Anaesthesiology and Chair of the Department in September 2007. Even though made an own Department before his chairmanship, ICM could again be reunited with anaesthesiology by Böttiger within the Department of Anaesthesiology and Surgical Intensive Care Medicine. Extensive restructuring activities were initiated within the Department to develop a modern academic anaesthesiology. For anaesthesiologists a training curriculum was established. A critical incident reporting system (CIRS) was designed to enhance safety. Owing to

Böttiger's outstanding expertise in the field of emergency medicine and resuscitation, the scientific activities were extended to cardio-pulmonary resuscitation.

Qualifications as Lectureres in Anaesthesiology

Sverre Johan Loennecken (1963); Hans-Joachim Eberlein (1965); Karl Bonhoeffer (1965); Hans Matthes (1970); Klaus Standfuss (1971); Jörg Busse (1976); Hermann Kämmerer (1976); Eberhard Klaschik (1981); Christoph Diefenbach (1996); John Lynch (1996); Stefan Grond (1996); Stefan-Mario Kasper (2000); Lukas Radbruch (2000); Sandra Kampe (2004); Matthias Paul (2004); Michael Dück (2005); Thomas Meuser (2005); Frank Petzke (2005); Thorsten Giesecke (2007); Henning Krep (2008); Stefan Soltész (2009); Fabian Spöhr (2010); Peter Teschendorf (2010); Stephan A. Padosch (2010); Jochen Hinkelbein (2010)

Professors of Anaesthesiology
Full Professors

Prof. Dr. Lukas Radbruch (2002), Endowed Professor of Palliative Medicine, RWTH Aachen University

Associate Professors

Prof. Dr. Dr. Klaus A. Lehmann (1985), Cologne
Prof. Dr. Stephan A. Schug (1994), Associate Professor, Section of Anaesthetics, Department of Pharmacology and Clinical Pharmacology, University of Auckland, New Zealand
Prof. Dr. Christoph Diefenbach (1997), Cologne
Prof. Dr. Eberhard Klaschik (1999), Endowed Professor of Palliative Medicine, University of Bonn
Prof. Dr. Stefan Grond (2001), University of Halle-Wittenberg

Adjunct Professors

Prof. Dr. Manfred Abel, Prof. Dr. Jörg Busse, Prof. Dr. Hermann Kämmerer, Prof. Dr. Stefan-Mario Kasper, Prof. Dr. Eberhard Klaschik, Prof. Dr. Georg Loeschcke, Prof. Dr. Klaus Standfuss

For further information:

http://anaesthesie.uk-koeln.de/

3.3.24 University of Leipzig

Department of Anaesthesiology and Intensive Therapy

H. Rüffert, T. Busch, U.X. Kaisers

The University of Leipzig has been founded in 1409, its Faculty of Medicine is one of the oldest Medical Schools in German speaking countries. In Leipzig, the first ether anaesthetic was given in the Municipal Hospital St. Jakob by the auxiliary doctors Johann Carl Friedrich Eduard Obenaus and Heinrich Eduard Karl Weickert for a tooth extraction on 24 January 1847, i.e. on the same day as in Erlangen (▶ Chap. 3.2.9). In the years before and after 1900 two renowned pioneers of anaesthesia in Germany, Professor Heinrich Braun and Dr. Arthur Läwen, acted as surgeons in Leipzig. Irrespective of this early progress, anaesthesia was considered a simple technical procedure for many decades by surgeons in Leipzig. New anaesthetic techniques like orotracheal intubation were first used in the Division of Thoracic Surgery in 1952 by the staff surgeon Dr. Claus Kerrinnes. Three residents of this Division joined him and decided to become full-time anaesthetists as the specialist status in anaesthesiology was created in East Germany in 1956. As Kerrinnes moved to West Germany in 1960 Dr. Harry Hartmann became Head of a Division of Anaesthesia of the Department of Surgery which eventually developed into a more or less independent unit as Central Division of Anaesthesia in 1974. In 1983, Hartmann had to leave due to illness and Dr. Hans-Jürgen Rehnig became his successor for a short interim period.

1984–2006 Chairmanship Professor Derk Olthoff

Prof. Dr. med. habil. Derk Olthoff

Born 17 March 1941 in Lychen/Uckermark; 1959–1965 student of medicine at the Humboldt University, Berlin; 1966 doctorate in medicine; 1966–1970 Resident. Department of Anaesthesiology and Intensive Therapy, University Hospital Charité, Berlin; 1972 Lecturer in Anaesthesiology, 1973 Senior Physician; 1976–1978 Head of the Department of Anaesthesiology of the University

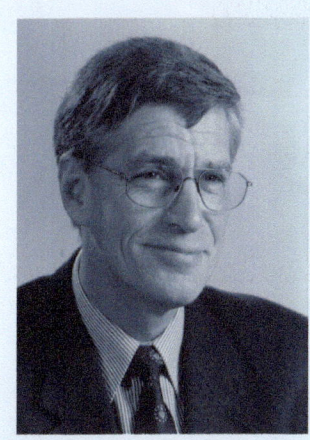

Hospital »Americo Boavida« in Luanda, Angola; 1980 Full Professor of Anaesthesiology, University Hospital Charité, Berlin; 1983–1984 Visiting Professor, University of Havanna, Cuba and Teikyo-University, Tokio, Japan; 1984 Full Professor and Chairman of the Department of Anaesthesiology and Intensive Therapy, University of Leipzig; 2006 Professor Emeritus.

It was only in 1984 that a Chair of Anaesthesiology was created at the Faculty of Medicine. Professor Derk Olthoff (Berlin) was appointed Full Professor of Anaesthesiology and Chairman of the Department of Anaesthesiology and Intensive Therapy on 1 March 1984. He immediately restructured the service and introduced strict standards. In 1986 an own interdisciplinary ICU, in 1987 a pain clinic and in 1988 a preanaesthetic clinic were established. In 1995, a second interdisciplinary ICU was added. Since 1994 the Department organised on behalf of the Saxonian Chamber of Physicians resuscitation courses compulsory for every doctor. Main areas of research were assessment and therapy of compromised haemodynamics, neuromonitoring, measurement of blood flow during anaesthesia by means of MRT and malignant hyperthermia (MH). The Department became a recognised centre for screening patients for MH.

Since 2006 Chairmanship Professor Udo X. Kaisers

Prof. Dr. med. Udo X. Kaisers

Born in 1962 in Nettetal; 1959–1965 student of German language and medicine Bonn, Vienna and Berlin; 1991 doctorate in medicine; 1988–1991 Resident,

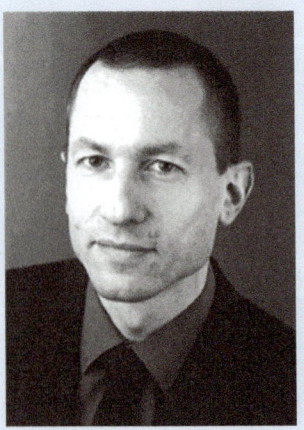

Berlin Centre of Burn Injuries, Hospital Am Urban; 1991–1994 Resident, Department of Anaesthesiology and Surgical Intensive Care Medicine, Campus Virchow-Klinikum, University Hospital Charité, University Medicine Berlin; 1994 Specialist in Anaesthesiology and Senior Physician; 1998 as Lecturer in Anaesthesiology; 2003 Vice Chairman and Associate Professor; 2006 Full Professor and Chairman of the Department of Anaesthesiology and Intensive Therapy, University of Leipzig.

After Olthoff's retirement in 2006 Professor Udo X. Kaisers (Berlin) was appointed Full Professor and Chairman of the Department. He adapted the infrastructure to the changing needs. The annual number of anaesthetics increased from 20,000 in the year 2000 to 28,000 in 2009. Already in 2006, he established a central resuscitation service and in 2008 an acute pain service for the whole University Hospital. In 2007, the Department could assume responsibility for a newly formed interdisciplinary ICU with 58 beds developing the treatment of severe acute lung injuries to a core area of competence far beyond the region of Leipzig. The Department was instrumental in forming a concept of palliative medicine and took the lead of this unit that was put into operation in 2009. Research is focussed on diagnosis and therapy of severe, acute lung injury, perioperative management in liver surgery including transplantation, cerebral actions of anaesthetic drugs, means of organ replacement, postoperative nausea and vomiting, and malignant hyperthermia.

Qualification as Lecturers in Anaesthesiology

Kerrines, Claus (1959); Meyer; Manfred (1963); Lüder, Manfred (1968); Langanke, Dieter (1969); König, Fritjoff (1984); Wild, Lina (1988); Adam, Horst (1989); Deutrich, Christine (1990); Burkhardt, Ulrich (1999); Schaffranietz, Lutz (2001); Rüffert, Hendrik (2003); Heinke, Wolfgang (2004); Wallenborn, Jan (2010).

Professors of Anaesthesiology
Associate Professors
Prof. Dr. Hermann Wrigge (2010)

Adjunct Professors
Prof. Dr. Claudia Philippi-Höhn, Prof. Dr. Dieter Langanke; Prof. Dr. Lutz Schaffranietz

For further information:
www.kai.uniklinikum-leipzig.de/

3.2.25 University of Lübeck

Department of Anaesthesiology and Intensive Care Medicine

M. Strätling, A. Schneeweiß, P. Schmucker

The Medical Academy of Lübeck was founded on 3 November 1964 as the 2nd Faculty of Medicine of the University of Kiel. In 1973 it became the Medical School and in 1985 the Medical University of Lübeck and was extended to the University of Lübeck in 2002. One year later, the Hospital of the University became the Campus Lübeck of the University Medical Centre Schleswig-Holstein, but the Faculty of Medicine continued to be affiliated to the University of Lübeck. Dr. Johannes Eichler, Specialist in Anaesthesiology since 1959 and Senior Physician at the University Hospital of Kiel, began to establish a Division of Anesthesia at the new Medical Academy since 1964 which, however, remained part of the Department of Surgery until 1970. In this year, it was made independent as Central Division of Anaesthesia and Eichler became Professor of Anaesthesia. In 1981, he was promoted Full Professor and Chairman of the Department of Anaesthesiology.

1964–1985 Chairmanship Professor Johannes Eichler

Prof. Dr. med. Johannes Eichler

Born 19 April 1920 in Gelenau/Erzgebirge; deceased 3 April 1998; 1947–1952 student of medicine in Kiel, 1951 doctorate in medicine, 1952–1954 Resident at the Department of Surgery, University of Kiel; 1954–1955 Resident in surgery at Bad Segeberg; 1955–1957 Resident in anaesthesia, University of Kiel; 1957–1958

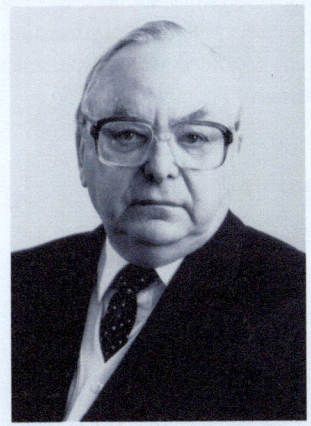

Resident in pharmacology, University of Kiel; 1959 Specialist in Anaesthesiology; 1965 Lecturer in Anaesthesiology; since 1964 Head of the Division of Anaesthesia, Medical University of Lübeck; 1970 Associate Professor, 1981 Full Professor and Chairman of the Department of Anaesthesiology; 1985 Professor Emeritus.

From the beginning, Eichler's scientific interests were focused on technological aspects of anaesthesia like monitoring, artificial ventilation, hypothermia and hyperthermia, medical telemetry and aviation medicine, supported by a close cooperation with the Dräger Company in Lübeck. He contributed to the establishment of a helicopter rescue service in the Federal State of Schleswig-Holstein as early as 1958.

1986–1989 Chairmanship Professor Klaus van Ackern

(▶ Chap. 3.2.28 for his C.V.)

1989–1990 Interim Chairmanship Privatdozent Dr. Detlev Michael Albrecht

(▶ Chap. 3.2.7 for his C.V.)

On 1 January 1986 Professor Klaus van Ackern (Munich) was appointed Full Professor of Anaesthesiology and Chairman of the Department of Anaesthesiology of the Medical University of Lübeck. He adapted the structure of the Department, the organisation of the anaesthesiological service and the technical equipment to the rapidly growing needs. The number of physicians increased from 30 to 48, that of the nurses even more. The scientific efforts were intensified. The existing research fields were continued but complemented by a number of new immunological projects. As van Ackern moved to the Faculty of Medicine Mannheim of the University of Heidelberg already in 1989, his Deputy Chairman Dr. Detlev Michael Albrecht acted as Interim Chairman until Professor Peter Schmucker (Berlin) was appointed van Ackern's successor in 1990.

Since 1990 Chairmanship Professor Peter Schmucker

Prof. Dr. med. Peter Schmucker

Born 9 October 1947 in Nuremberg; 1967-1973 student of medicine, University of Munich; 1973-1974 internship at Munich; 1974-1976 Medical Officer, Munich;

3

1975 doctorate in medicine, University of Munich; 1975-1985 Resident, Department of Anaesthesiology, University Hospital Grosshadern, Munich; 1980 Senior Physician; 1984 Lecturer in Anaesthesiology; 1985 Full Professor of Anaesthesiology, Free University/German Heart Centre, Berlin; 1990 Full Professor and Chairman of the Department of Anaesthesiology, Medical University of Lübeck.

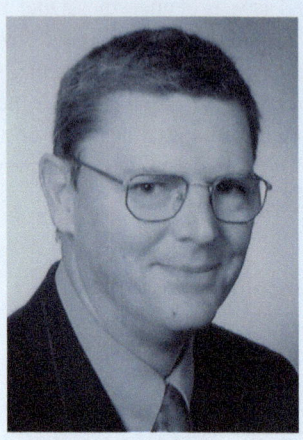

As in the years before, Schmucker had to make sure that the service provided by the Department met the steadily increasing demands. The number of anaesthetics delivered annually increased to 24,000, that of doctors to 75 and that of non-physician personnel to 120. In 1998 a preanaesthetic clinic was established and in 1991 an anaesthesiological ICU was opened which could be expanded to 15 beds within the following 4 years. A pain clinic had been opened in 1986; it was supplemented by a small unit of palliative medicine in 1991 and recognized as training centre for the subspecialisation in »specific pain therapy« in 1994. Main areas of research are medical technology, cardio-circulatory problems in anaesthesia and ICM with particular emphasis on immunological and endocrinological mechanisms underlying specific procedure- or anaesthesia-related disorders, effects of anaesthesia-related phenomena on psychomotor functions and the patient's mental state, and various aspects of emergency medicine, e.g. the SARRAH project (search and rescue, resuscitation and rewarming in accidental hypothermia).

Qualification as Lecturer in Anaesthesiology

Albrecht, Detlev Michael (1989); Klotz, Karl Friedrich (1997); Gehring, Hartmut (1998); Uhlig, Thomas (1999); Dörges, Volker (2000); Wagner, Klaus (2001); Roth-Isigkeit, Angela (2002); Stamme, Cordula (2003); Stephan, Klaus (2003); Bahlmann, Ludger (2004); Gerlach, Klaus (2004); Heringlake, Matthias (2004); Schumacher, Jan (2004); Brandt, Jörg-Matthias (2005); Eichler, Wolfgang (2005); Strätling, Meinolfus (2006); Heinze, Hermann (2009); Meier, Torsten (2009).

Professors of Anaesthesiology
Adjunct Professors

Prof. Dr. Ludger Bahlmann; Prof. Dr. Wolfgang Eichler; Prof. Dr. Hartmut Gehring; Prof. Dr. Matthias Heringlake; Prof. Dr. Cordula Stamme; Prof. Dr. Klaus Stephan.

For further information:

www.anae.uni-luebeck.de/

3.2.26 University of Magdeburg

Department of Anaesthesiology and Intensive Therapy

W. Röse, T. Hachenberg

The Medical Academy Magdeburg was founded in 1954. In this year a small Division of Anaesthesia was established within the Department of Surgery. This was mainly owing to the far-sightedness of Professor Werner Lembcke, then Chairman of this Department. In 1955, he attended the founding Congress of the World Federation of Societies of Anaesthesiologists in Scheveningen, The Netherlands, and was reinforced in his conviction that surgical progress was dependent on modern, academic anaesthesia. Lembcke supported the academic careers of Dr. Lisa Wilken and Dr. Wolfgang Röse and enabled them to achieve the qualification as Lecturer in Anaesthesiology in 1965 and 1969, respectively. Both had partly been trained abroad. They introduced modern anaesthetic methods, established an emergency doctor's ambulance as early as in 1960 and took care of patients requiring respiratory support, e.g. due to tetanus. In 1969, an independent Division of Anaesthesiology was created which was upgraded to the Department of Anaesthesiology and Intensive Therapy in 1981.

1969–2001 Chairmanship Professor Wolfgang Röse

Prof. Dr. med. habil. Wolfgang Röse

Born 23 January1936 in Burg near Magdeburg; 1952–1958 student of medicine in Berlin and Magdeburg; 1958 doctorate in medicine; since 1958 residency in anaesthesia at the Medical Academies of Magdeburg and Düsseldorf; 1964 Specialist in Anaesthesiology; 1969 Lecturer in Anaesthesiology and Chairman of the Division of Anaesthesiology, Medical Academy Magdeburg; 1973 Full Professor of Anaesthesiology; 1977 Honorary Member of the Hungarian Society of Anaesthesiology and Intensive Care Medicine; 1989 Honorary Member of the Soviet Society of Anaesthesiologists and Reanimatologists; 2001 Professor Emeritus.

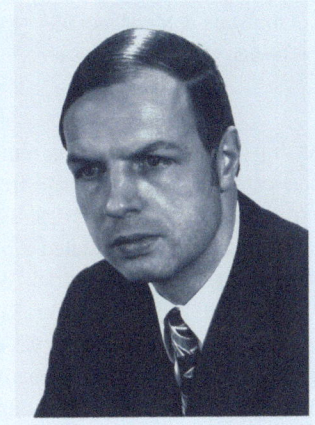

Dr. Röse was appointed Chairman of the Division of Anaesthesiology in 1969 and became Full Professor of Anaesthesiology in 1973 after a Chair had been created at the Academy. Although there was a clear mismatch between workload and manpower during the following 20 years he made every effort to arrange the regular clinical service in anaesthesia, ICM, preclinical emergency medicine and pain therapy and to adapt it to the steadily increasing needs. This was only possible on the basis of a highly sophisticated organisation because the operating departments were spread over various buildings. An ICU was not established before 1975. In the mid-1980s, consultations for patients suffering from chronic pain were started which could be transferred to premises of an anaesthesiological pain clinic in 1989. Pregraduate and postgraduate teaching as well as CME were always an important activities of the Department. Resources for scientific efforts were virtually not available so that only a limited number of goals oriented toward neurophysiological problems in ICM could be pursued. In 1993, the Medical Academy was incorporated into the newly founded University of Magdeburg.

Since 2001 Chairmanship Professor Thomas Hachenberg

Prof. Dr. Dr. med. Thomas Hachenberg

Born 17 May 1957 in Paderborn; 1977–1983 student of medicine in Münster; 1984 doctorate in medicine; 1984–1990 Resident, Department of Anaesthesiology and Surgical Intensive Care Medicine, University of Münster; 1989 Specialist in Anaesthesiology; 1990 Senior Physician; 1990 Lecturer in Anaesthesiology; 1994 Associate Professor of Anaesthesiology and Intensive Care Medicine, University of Greifswald; 1995 Doctor of Medical Science, University of Uppsala, Sweden; 2001 Full Professor and Chairman of the Department of Anaesthesiology and Intensive Therapy, University of Magdeburg.

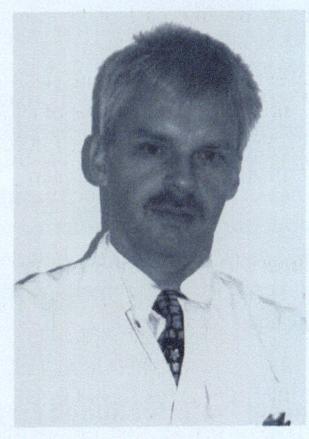

Professor Thomas Hachenberg (Greifswald) was appointed Full Professor and Chairman of the Department after Röse's retirement in 2001. He particularly looked at refining the interdisciplinary cooperation and adapted the organization of the service to the changing requirements in terms of adequate technical infrastructure, planning and management of surgical programmes, quality improvement and economic efficiency, e.g. when the new surgical centre of the Hospital was put into operation. Subsequently to a move into a new building in 2003 the Department could establish a preanaesthetic clinic and 2 PACUs and expand the number of ICU beds to 12. Various scientific projects were initiated. In close cooperation with the University of Uppsala the interaction of anaesthesia or sepsis with the respiratory system became a main field of investigation. Experimental studies on the function of membrane-bound transport proteins of the intestinal mucosa and the CNS and on therapeutic concepts after heart-lung-brain resuscitation by means of an asphyxia cardiac arrest rat model were launched.

Qualification as Lecturers in Anaesthesiology

Wilken, Lisa (1965); Röse, Wolfgang (1969); Mühlnickel, Bernd (1988); Ebmeyer, Uwe (2003); Schneemilch, Christine (2006); Weß, Günter (2007)

Professors of Anaesthesiology

Adjunct Professors

Prof. Dr. Lisa Wilken

For more information

www.med.uni-magdeburg.de/kait.html

3.2.27 University of Mainz

Department of Anaesthesiology

W. Dick, C. Werner

In 1959, the anaesthetist Dr. Rudolf Frey (Heidelberg) gave his first guest lectures in Mainz. At the same time the Division of Anaesthesia was founded and was ultimately established as an independent Department of Anaesthesiology in 1962. Professor Frey became the first »Extraordinarius« (Associate Professor with tenure) in Anaesthesiology. This associate professorship was transferred to a full professorship in 1967. Thus, in 2010 anaesthesiology in Mainz existed for 51 years, the autonomous department for 48 years and the chair for 43 years.

1962–1981 Chairmanship Professor Rudolf Frey

Prof. Dr. med. Rudolf Frey, FFARCS

Born 22 August 1917 in Heidelberg; deceased 23 December 1981 in Mainz. 1938–1943 student of medicine in Heidelberg; 1944 doctorate; postgraduate training in surgery at the Department of Surgery, University

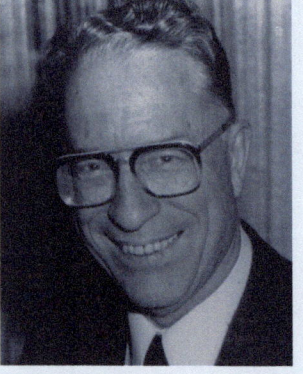

of Heidelberg; 1949 Specialist in Surgery; residency programs in anaesthesiology in Heidelberg, the USA, Switzerland and France; 1952 Specialist and Lecturer in Anaesthesiology; 1956 Adjunct Professor and Head, Division of Anaesthesia of the Department of Surgery, University of Heidelberg; 1960 Associate Professor of Anaesthesiology, University of Mainz; 1962, Chairman of the Department of Anaesthesiology; 1967 Full Professor; recipient of numerous honorary awards and positions (Chief Physician of the German Red Cross ; many honorary memberships of societies and associations; Officer's Cross of the German Order of Merit; honorary citizenship of the State of Maryland, USA; honorary medal of the Taiwan Medical College, etc.).

During Frey's chairmanship clinical anaesthesia, emergency medicine, intensive care medicine, and pain treatment were developed simultaneously. As early as 1961 intensive care patients were treated. Frey initiated a prehospital emergency system along with Dr. Friedrich Wilhelm Ahnefeld. In 1972, Rudolf Frey and Peter Safar founded the Club of Mainz (an unincorporated, yet exquisitely influential expert group that was later renamed to become the World Association for Disaster and Emergency Medicine, WADEM). One of the first pain therapy units in Germany was established together with Professor Hans-Ulrich Gerbershagen.

1983–2004 Chairmanship Professor Wolfgang F. Dick

Prof. Dr. med. Dr. h.c. Wolfgang F. Dick, FFARCS

Born 3 July 1936 in Wesel, Germany. 1957–1963 student of medicine in Cologne; 1963 doctorate; postgraduate training in anaesthesiology in Mainz and Los Angeles; 1969 Specialist in Anaesthesiology; 1970 Lecturer in Anaesthesiology; 1971 Professor and Head of the Division of Anaesthesiology, University of Ulm; 1972 Head of the Division of Anaesthesiology II, Department of Anaesthesiology; 1973–1977 Dean of the Faculty of Clinical Medicine; 1976 Medical Director of the University Hospital; 1983 Full Professor and Chairman of the Department of Anaesthesiology, University of Mainz; 1987–1991 Medical Director of the University Hospital; 1991–1994 President of the European Academy of Anaesthesiology; 1992 Honorary Doctor, University of Poznan, Poland; Honorary Member of national and international scientific and professional societies (DGAI, DIVI, EAA, ERC, etc); 2004 Professor Emeritus.

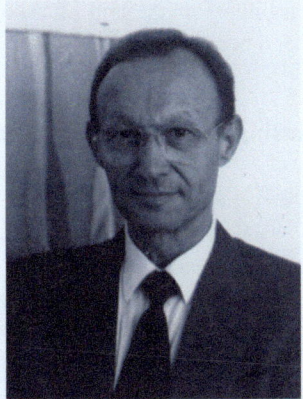

In 1983 Professor Wolfgang Dick (Ulm) was appointed Frey's successor. During his chairmanship he initiated the clinical section of cardiovascular and thoracic anaesthesia in 1984 and anaesthesia for transplant surgery in 1999. Equally important was the establishment of two full-time preoperative patient assessment units. After severe damages caused by a fire the surgical building was renovated and Dick could realize a new 14-bed ICU in 1995. Extensive invasive and non-invasive monitoring, organ replacement procedures and thorough standards were introduced at that time. The clinical expertise and regional importance of the ICU was reflected by multiple admissions of patients with organ failure from other hospitals.

Dick's name will always be connected with an elaborated pre-clinical emergency medicine program based on vehicle as well as helicopter transportation and accompanied and improved by many research projects. Likewise, a distinguished program of acute and chronic pain medicine was continued during his chairmanship. The implementation of basic science laboratory facilities and the establishment of one of the first German full scale human patient simulation centres was the ultimate proof that academic anaesthesiology at the University of Mainz represented a strong clinical, scientific and teaching endeavour in favour of patient care.

Since 2004 Chairmanship Professor Christian Werner

Prof. Dr. med. Christian Werner

Born 7 April 1958 in Bonn; 1980–1986 student of medicine in Bonn; 1987 doctorate in medicine; since 1986 Resident, Department of Anaesthesiology, University Hospital Hamburg-Eppendorf; 1989–1990 neuroanaesthesia research fellowship at Michael Reese Hospital Medical Center, Chicago IL, USA; 1993 Specialist in Anaesthesiology; 1994 Lecturer in Anaesthesiology, University of Hamburg; 1996 Associate Professor of Anaesthesiology and Vice Chairman, Department of Anaesthesiology, Technical University of Munich; 2004 Full Professor and Chairman of the Department of Anaesthesiology, University of Mainz; Past President of the German Neuroanaesthesia Research Group and the Society of Neurosurgical Anesthesia and Critical Care, a subspecialty group of the American Society of Anesthesiologists.

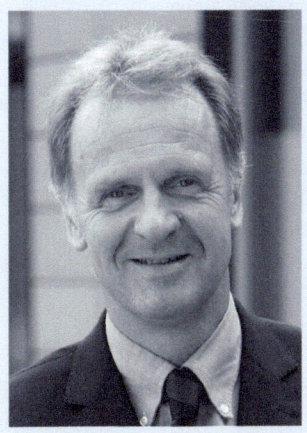

Today, the Department of Anaesthesiology covers the entire spectrum of anaesthesia and perioperative care with pre-clinical emergeny medicine, emergency department service, clinical anaesthesia, intensive care medicine, acute and chronic pain medicine, and palliative care. In recent years, the clinical service as well as basic science and clinical research were expanded in depth and dimension based on hospital growth and the distinctive philosophy that the art and science of anaesthesiology is relevant to patient outcome and can no longer merely be regarded as a »service provider«. Core research areas are organ protection of the brain and the lung, resucitation, airway management and haemodynamic monitoring and funded by the German Research Foundation and nationwide trusts. Research is performed in a serious approach towards translational science.

Qualifications as lecturers in Anesthesiology

Kolb, Ernst (1963); Ahnefeld, Friedrich Wilhelm (1964); Weis, Karl-Heinz (1964); Kreuscher, Hermann (1966); Nolte, Hans(1967); Halmágyi, Miklós (1968);Dick, Wolfgang (1970); Gerbershagen, Hans Ulrich (1972); Erdmann, Wilhelm (1973); Stosseck, Klaus (1976); Sehati Chafai, Gholam (1977); Abdulla, Walied (1979); Lanz, Egon (1980); Kleemann, Peter-Paul (1989); Jantzen, Jan-Peter A.H. (1990); Heinrichs, Wolfgang (1991); Lipp, Markus (1993); Duda, Dorothea (1996); Gervais, Hendrik (1997); Weiler, Norbert (1999); Fauth, Ulrich (2000); Latorre, Federico (2001); Eberle, Balthasar (2001); Mauer, Dietmar (2001); Brambrink, Ansgar (2002); Markstaller Klaus (2004); David, Matthias (2006); Rümelin, Andreas (2007); Pestel, Gunther (2009); Heid, Florian (2010)

Professors of Anaesthesiology
Full Professors

Prof. Dr. Ernst Kolb (1967), Free University of Berlin
Prof. Dr. Abbas Madjidi (1967), University of Teheran, Iran
Prof. Dr. Friedrich Wilhelm Ahnefeld (1968), University of Ulm
Prof. Dr. Karl-Heinz Weis (1968), University of Würzburg
Prof. Dr. Wilhelm Erdmann (1976), University of Rotterdam, The Netherlands
Prof. Dr. Ludwig Brandt (1995), Hospital Wuppertal of the University of Witten-Herdecke
Prof. Dr. Klaus Markstaller (2010), Medical University of Vienna

Associate and Adjunct Professors

Prof. Dr. Hermann Kreuscher; Prof. Dr. Hans Nolte; Prof. Dr. Miklos Halmagyi; Prof. Dr. Hans-Ulrich Gerbershagen; Prof. Dr. Gholam Sehati Chafai; Prof. Dr. Michael Stanton-Hicks; Prof. Dr. Egon Lanz; Prof. Dr. Klaus Stossek; Prof. Dr. Walid Abdulla; Prof. Dr. Peter-Paul Kleemann; Prof. Dr. Jan-Peter Jantzen; Prof. Dr. Wolfgang Heinrichs; Prof. Dr. Jürgen Jage; Prof. Dr. Dr. Markus Lipp, Prof. Dr. Hendrik Gervais, Prof. Dr. Kristin Engelhard, Prof. Dr. Joachim Schmeck

For further information:

www.unimedizin-mainz.de/anaesthesiologie/

3.2.28 Faculty of Clinical Medicine Mannheim, University of Heidelberg

Department of Anaesthesiology and Surgical Intensive Care Medicine

J.-P. Striebel, K. van Ackern, H.-J. Bender

The University Hospital Mannheim developed from the former Municipal Hospital which had been founded in 1922. In 1956 Dr. Elisabeth-Margarethe Gräfin (Countess) von Lüttichau became the first Specialist in anaesthesia and was replaced by Dr. Fiebig in 1958. In consequence of the foundation of the Faculty of Clinical Medicine Mannheim of the University of Heidelberg in 1964 Dr. Horst Lutz (Heidelberg) was appointed Head of the Division of Anaesthesia of the Hospital. He immediately began to expand the clinical service and to establish teaching and research facilities. At the end of 1969, an anaesthesiological ICU of 6 beds was established.

1971–1987 Chairmanship Professor Horst Lutz

Professor Dr. med. Horst Lutz

Born 25 June 1927 in Dessau; deceased 17 January 1987 in Heidelberg; 1947–1953 student of medicine in Halle/Saale; 1953 doctorate in medicine; 1953–1954 internship in Dessau, 1959 Specialist in Surgery; 1961 residency in anaesthesia; 1964 Specialist in Anaesthesiology, Senior Physician at the Department of Anaesthesiology, University of Heidelberg; 1967 Lecturer in Anaesthesiology; 1968 Head of the Division of Anaesthesia, Municipal Hospital Mannheim, 1971 Full Professor and Chairman of the Department of Anaesthesiology and Reanimation, Faculty of Clinical Medicine Mannheim of the University of Heidelberg.

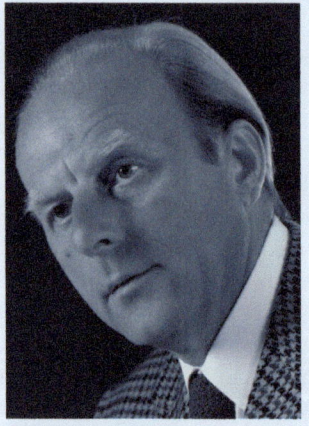

As a Chair of Anaesthesiology was created Lutz was appointed Full Professor and Chairman of the Department of Anaesthesiology and Reanimation at the end of 1970. A recovery room was opened, and the responsibility for the anaesthetic service of the Trauma Hospital including a Division of Severe Burns in Ludwigshafen, just across the Rhine, was taken until 1983 when Dr. Roderich Klose, Senior Physician of the Department, became Head of this service. In 1974 a new surgical centre and a new ICU with 18 beds were put into operation. Physicians of the Department were involved in the operation of the mobile life support unit which was transferred to the exclusive responsibility of the Department in 1980. A pain clinic was opened in 1982.

The blood bank of the Hospital was part of the Department of Anaesthesiology from 1968 to 1989. Lutz initiated and supported numerous research projects, among those were: trauma and shock, volume replacement therapy, haemodilution, cardio-circulatory actions of anaesthetics, clinical nutrition, risk assessment, patient data management in anaesthesia and ICM, surfactant, ARDS and respiratory support.

1987–1989 Interim Chairmanship Professor Jens-Peter Striebel

Prof. Dr. med. Jens-Peter Striebel

Born 20 April 1943 in Mannheim; 1962–1968 student of medicine in Heidelberg; 1968-1969 internship at the Municipal Hospital Mannheim; 1969–1970 residency in gynaecology, Hospital Germersheim; 1970 residency in anaesthesia, Municipal Hospital Mannheim; 1972 doctorate in medicine; 1974 Specialist in Anaesthesiology, Staff Physician; 1977 Lecturer in Anaesthesiology; 1984 Adjunct Professor; 1987–1989 Interim Chairman; 1989 Vice Chairman of the Department of Anaesthesiology and Surgical Intensive Care Medicine.

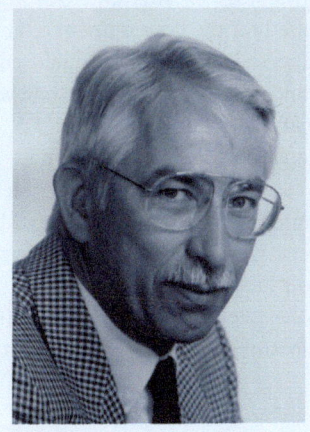

1989–2009 Chairmanship Professor Klaus van Ackern

Prof. Dr. med. Dr. h.c. Klaus van Ackern

Born 12 September 1941 in Essen; 1962–1968 student of medicine in Heidelberg; 1969 doctorate in medicine; 1968–1972 Research Associate, Division of Experimental Surgery, University of Heidelberg; 1972 residency in anaesthesia, Municipal Hospital

Mannheim; 1975 Specialist in Anaesthesiology and Senior Physician; 1975 Lecturer in Anaesthesiology, 1977 Senior Physician, Department of Anaesthesiology, University of Munich; 1980 Associate Professor of Anaesthesiology; 1986 Full Professor and Chairman of the Department of Anaesthesiology, Medical University of Lübeck; 1989 Full Professor and Chairman of the Department of Anaesthesiology, Faculty of Clinical Medicine Mannheim, University of Heidelberg; 1999 Honorary Doctorate, University of Cluj-Napoca, Romania; 2001 Order of Merit in Gold of the Republic of Poland; 2007 Honorary Member of the German Society of Anaesthesiology and Intensive Care Medicine; 2009 Professor Emeritus.

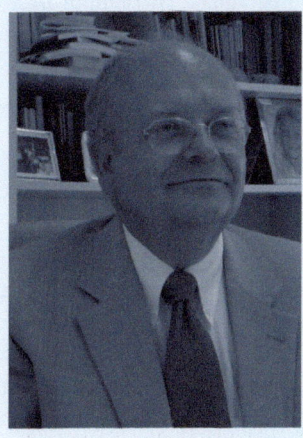

Following the premature death of Lutz on 17 January 1987 Professor Jens-Peter Striebel, Senior Physician at the Department, became Interim Chairman for 2½ years. On 1 June 1989 Professor Klaus van Ackern (Lübeck) was appointed Full Professor of Anaesthesiology and Chairman of the Department of Anaesthesiology and Surgical Intensive Care Medicine where he had been trained in anaesthesiology and qualified as Lecturer in 1975. Under his chairmanship the Department developed into a central service unit of the University Hospital, the concept of perioperative medicine increasingly determining the professional policy. The total number of anaesthetics was 27,000 per year, 26 surgical ICU beds and 3 PACUs were eventually run by the Department, and 2,000 patients were seen in the pain clinic. Particular competence lay on the treatment of, and research on, multiple and neurotrauma, neurosurgical patients, sepsis, multiple organ failure and severe acute lung injury or ARDS including extracorporeal membrane oxygenation. Further research subjects were cardiovascular, cerebral and pulmonary problems in anaesthesia and ICM. Divisions of Experimental Anaesthesiology (Professor Siegfried Labeit) and Clinical Pain Research (Professor Martin Schmelz) were created with the aim of establishing modern microbiological and other experimental methodology within the Department. Special attention was paid to contacts with anaesthestists of Eastern European countries. Young doctors from Romania and Poland had the opportunity to take up a fellowship in Mannheim. After van Ackern's retirement as Chairman in 2009, **Professor Manfred Thiel** (Munich) was appointed Full Professor of Anaesthesiology and Chairman of the Department.

In his function as Dean of the Faculty of Medicine during the periods 1991-1999 and 2001-2011 van Ackern initiated a Centre of Medical Research, a Centre of Computer-aided Medicine and a Centre of Biomedicine and Medical Technology thus enabling medical students to complete the entire pregraduate curriculum in Mannheim. In addition, 10 endowed chairs could be established.

Qualification as Lecturers in Anaesthesiology

Peter, Klaus (1972); Klose, Roderich (1975); van Ackern, Klaus (1975); Martin, Eike (1977); Striebel, Jens-Peter (1977); Geiger, Klaus (1979); Osswald, Peter Michael (1982); Tolksdorf, Werner (1983); Hartung, Hans-Joachim (1985); Georgieff, Michael (1986); Bender, Hans-Joachim (1987); Albrecht, Michael (1989); Koch, Thea (1995); Segiet, Wolfgang (1995); Waschke, Klaus F. (1995); Ellinger, Klaus (1996); Quintel, Michael (1997); Kerger, Heinz (1997); Schmeck, Joachim (2000); Fiedler, Fritz (2001); Konrad, Christoph (2001); Frietsch, Thomas (2003); Krieter, Heiner (2003); Beck, Grietje (2004); Lücke, Thomas (2005); Meinhardt, Jürgen (2005); Piper, Sven (2006); Schleppers, Alexander (2006); Ruckwied, Roman (2007); Suttner, Stefan (2007); Münch, Elke (2008); Witt, Christian (2008); Genzwürker, Harald (2009); Hinkelbein, Jochen (2010).

Professors of Anaesthesiology
Full Professors

Prof. Dr. Klaus Peter (1976), University of Munich
Prof. Dr. Klaus Geiger (1986), University of Freiburg
Prof. Dr. Detlev Michael Albrecht (1994), Technical University of Dresden
Prof. Dr. Michael Quintel (2003/2010), University of Göttingen

Associate Professors

Prof. Dr. Siegfried Labeit (2002), Professor of Experimental Anaesthesiology, Mannheim
Prof. Dr. Martin Schmelz (2003), Professor of Clinical Pain Research, Mannheim

Adjunct Professors

Prof. Dr. Grietje Beck; Prof. Dr. Dr. Hans-Joachim Bender; Prof. Dr. Klaus Ellinger; Prof. Dr. Fritz Fiedler; Prof. Dr. Thomas Frietsch; Prof. Dr. Klaus Geiger; Prof. Dr. Hans-Joachim Hartung; Prof. Dr. Christian Hofstetter; Prof. Dr. Heinz Kerger; Prof. Dr. Roderich Klose; Prof. Dr. Christoph Konrad; Prof. Dr. Thomas Lücke; Prof. Dr. Peter Michael Osswald; Prof. Dr. Sven Piper; Prof. Dr. Jens-Peter Striebel; Prof. Dr. Werner Tolksdorf; Prof. Dr. Klaus Waschke

For further information:

www.ma.uni-heidelberg.de/inst/anae/
www.umm.de

3.2.29   University of Marburg

Department of Anaesthesiology and Intensive Therapy
H. Lennartz, H. Wulf

In 1954 Professor Rudolf Zenker, Chairman of the Department of Surgery, put Dr. Rüdiger Beer in charge of the anaesthesia service. Beer had worked 2.5 years at the Departments of Physiology in Kiel and Göttingen and thus was best qualified for the development of anesthesia for cardiac surgery. In 1958 Beer was qualified as Lecturer in Anaesthesiology and moved, together with Zenker, to the University of Munich (cf. Ch. 3.2.30). Zenker's successor Professor Max Schwaiger had cooperated in Cologne with the anaesthetist Dr. Heinz Oehmig who accompanied him when moving to Marburg. Oehmig had been trained 1952-1956 in Heidelberg by Professor Rudolf Frey. In 1962 he was qualified as Lecturer in Anaesthesiology and promoted Head of the Division of Anaesthesia of the Department of Surgery.

1967–1973 Chairmanship Professor Heinz Oehmig

Prof. Dr. med. Dr. Heinz Oehmig

Born 30 October 1919 in Baden-Baden; 1940–1945 student of medicine in Freiburg; 1945 doctorate in medicine; 1946–1949 general practitioner in Bremen; 1949–1952 residency in surgery in Bremen; 1952–1956 residency in anaesthesia in Heidelberg; 1956 Specialist in Anaesthesiology; 1956–1959 anaesthetist at the University of

Cologne; 1959 Head of the Anaesthesia Division, University of Marburg; 1967 Full Professor and Chairman of the Department of Anaesthesiology; 1973–1977 Institute of Hospital Science, Cologne; 1977–1984 Head Physician of the Department of Anaesthesiology and Intensive Care Medicine, Hospital Baden-Baden.

1977 Full Professor and Chairman of the Department of Anaesthesiology, University of Marburg; 2001 Professor Emeritus.

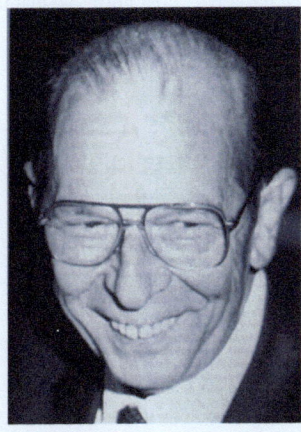

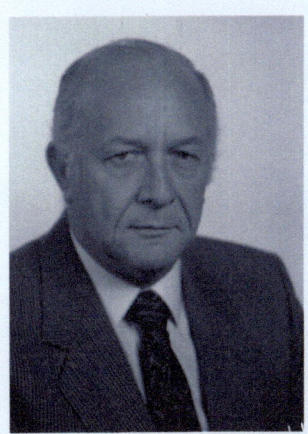

In June 1967 Heinz Oehmig was appointed to the new Chair of Anaesthesiology. The former Division was renamed Anaesthesia Centre and became responsible for the anaesthetic care for all surgical specialities. Oehmig successfully promoted new methods of patient monitoring. Around 1960 he designed one of the first integrated aneasthesia workstations including an automated ventilator and recording of minute ventilation, cardiac and peripheral pulse frequency, minute ventilation, in- and expiratory CO_2 and inspiratory O_2 concentrations. He gave up his academic appointment already in 1973.

1977–2001 Chairmanship Professor Herbert Lennartz

Prof. Dr. med. Herbert Lennartz

Born 8 November 1932 in Grevenbroich; 1954–1960 student of medicine at Cologne; 1960–1962 internship; 1962–1968 residency in anaesthesia, University of Düsseldorf; 1964 doctorate in medicine, University of Cologne; 1968 Specialist in Anaesthesiology; 1969 Lecturer in Anaesthesiology, University of Düsseldorf; 1971–1977 Senior Physician; 1973 Adjunct Professor;

After an interim period of 4 years Herbert Lennartz (Düsseldorf) was appointed Full Professor and Chairman of the Anaesthesia Centre on 2 May 1977. He expanded the anaesthesiological activities with special attention on surgical specialties which were added to those already existing in Marburg, i.e. neurosurgery (1978), maxillary and orofacial surgery (1982), cardiac surgery (1994). He introduced epidural anaesthesia in obstetrics, pulmonary artery catheterization and veno-venous haemofiltration in intensive care patients and founded a preanaesthetic clinic. The influence of epidural opioids on respiration was thoroughly investigated. In 1980 the Centre was renamed Department of Anaesthesia and Intensive Therapy and completed by an ICU with 8 beds in 1984. Special emphasis was laid on the treatment of all advanced forms of severe acute lung injury and the unit became a reference centre for extracorporeal lung support therapy.

Since 2001 Chairmanship Professor Hinnerk Wulf

Prof. Dr. med. Hinnerk F. W. Wulf

Born 28 January 1959 in Kiel; 1977–1984 student of medicine in Würzburg and Kiel; 1984 doctorate in medicine; 1984–1989 residency in anaesthesiology, University of Kiel; 1989 Specialist in Anaesthesiology; 1994 Lecturer in Anaesthesiology; 1991 Senior

3

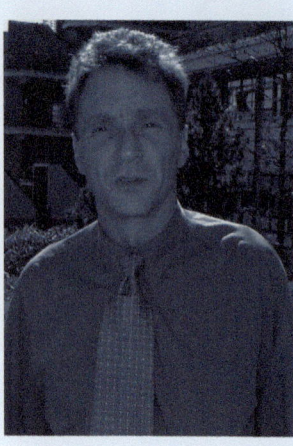

Physician; 1999 Adjunct Professor; 2001 Full Professor and Chairman of the Department of Anaesthesiology and Intensive Therapy, University Hospital Marburg.

On 1 April 2001 Professor Hinnerk F. W. Wulf (Kiel) took over the Chair from Lennartz. His main areas of research were clinical pharmacology of intravenous and local anaesthetics, regional anaesthesia as well as acute and chronic pain therapy. He soon introduced modern anesthetic techniques such as TIVA, laryngeal mask and fibreoptic intubation, regional anesthetic techniques, etc. and new monitoring methods, e.g. TEE. The concepts of complete perioperative management and operating theatre organization were updated and scientifically surveyed. New areas of clinical research were perioperative risk, side effects of anaesthetics, quality of life of oncologic patients and sepsis. For this purpose, a cooperation with the Division of Surgical Research was established. Further development of all clinical facets of pain medicine was another goal of Wulf's endeavours. In 2005, the State of Hesse merged the University Hospitals of Marburg and Giessen and transmitted the economic and administrative management of the now joint University Hospital to a private company (Rhön-Klinikum AG) in 2006.

Qualification as Lecturers in Anaesthesiology

Beer, Rüdiger (1958); Oehmig, Heinz (1962); Kirchner, Erich (1965); Dennhardt, Rüdiger (1978); Konder, Heribert (1987); Kroh, Udo (1991), Müller, Eckard (1991); Knoch, Michael (1991); Höltermann, Walter (1998); Torossian, Alexander (2005); Morin, Astrid (2006); Goldmann, Kai (2006); Graf, Jürgen (2007); Rolfes, Caroline (2008); Haas, Thorsten (2009); Rüsch, Dirk (2009); Maybauer, Dirk (2009); Maybauer Marc (2009)

Professors of Anaesthesiology
Full Professors
Prof. Dr. Erich Kirchner (1968), Hannover Medical School

Associate Professors
Prof. Dr. Martin Max (2003) Extraordinary Professor of Intensive Care Medicine, Marburg

Adjunct Professors
Prof. Dr. Leopold Eberhart, Prof. Dr. Thomas Frietsch, Prof. Dr. Udo Kroh, Prof. Dr. Eckard Müller, Prof. Dr. Alexander Torossian

For further information:
www.ukgm.de/ugm_2/deu/umr_ana/index.html

3.3.30   University of Munich

Department of Anaesthesiology
U. Kreimeier, G. Schelling, K. Peter, B. Zwißler

At the University of Munich a Division of Anaesthesia was founded as a component of the Department of Surgery in 1951 and headed by Dr. Ludwig Zürn who qualified as Lecturer in Anaesthesiology in 1955. In 1967 Dr. Rüdiger Beer was appointed Associate Professor of Anaesthesiology and promoted Full Professor and Chairman of the Department of Anaesthesiology in 1970. During those years, Dr. Alfred Doenicke was head of the Division of Anesthesia of the 2nd Department of Surgery (later University Department of Surgery Munich-Innenstadt) and became Professor in 1970. After Beer's early death in 1970 Professor Udilo Finsterer acted as Interim Chairman of the Department and began to organize the establishment of anaesthesiology in the new University Hospital Großhadern which from now on was the second campus of the University Hospital in addition to the »classical« location in the city centre (»Innenstadt«). The Department's first section in Großhadern was the Division of Neuroanaesthesia which was headed by Professor Robert Enzenbach.

1970–1975 Chairmanship Professor Rüdiger Beer

Prof. Dr. med. Dr. Rüdiger Beer

Born 3 June 1925 in Königsberg; deceased 18 February 1975 in Munich. 1948–1954 student of medicine in Berlin, Freiburg and Kiel; 1954 Resident at the Department of Surgery, University of Marburg; 1958

▼

Lecturer in Anaesthesiology, change to the Department of Surgery, University of Munich; 1967 Associate Professor and Head of the Department of Anaesthesiology; 1970 Full Professor and Chairman of the Department.

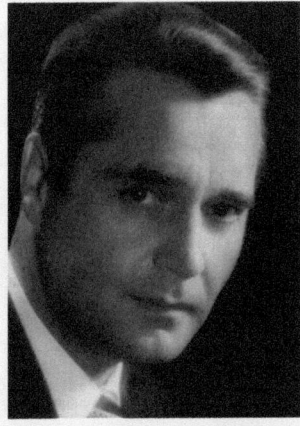

Prof. Dr. med. Alfred Doenicke

Born 1. August 1928 in Göttingen; 1948–1954 student of medicine in Erlangen; 1954 doctorate in medicine; 1954–1955 internship in Miltenberg; 1955–1959 Resident in surgery and anaesthesiology in Würzburg; 1959–1961 internal medicine, surgery, anaesthesiology and pharmacology in Hannover; 1961 Specialist in Anaesthesiology;1964 Lecturer in Anaesthesiology, University of Munich; 1970 Professor, University of Munich; 1961–1993 Head, Anaesthesia Division, University Department of Surgery, Munich-Innenstadt. 1977–1994 Editor-in-Chief of the journal »Der Anaesthesist«. 2004 Honorary Member, German Society of Anaesthesiology and Intensive Care Medicine.

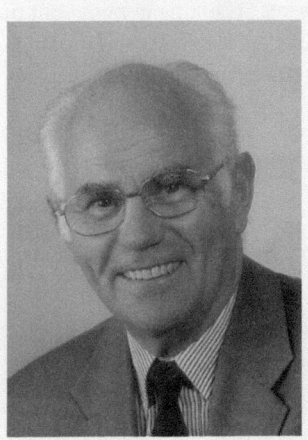

1975–1976 Interim Chairmanship Professor Udilo Finsterer

Prof. Dr. med. Udilo Finsterer

Born 6 March 1939 in Stettin; 1958–1964 student of medicine in Munich und Freiburg; 1964–1966 internship in Munich and Mühldorf am Inn; 1965 doctorate in medicine; 1968–1972 Resident at the Department of Anaesthesiology, University of Munich, 1972–1973 Department of Physiology, University of Munich; 1972 Specialist in Anaesthesiology; 1974 Lecturer in Anaesthesiology; 1975–1976 Interim Chairman, Department of Anaesthesiology, University of Munich; since 1976 Senior Consultant; 2002 retirement.

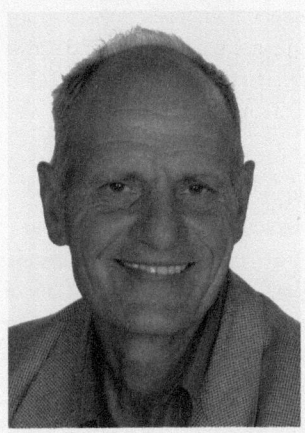

Prof. Dr. med. Robert Enzenbach

Born 15 June 1927 in Munich; deceased 28 December 2004 1945–1951 student of medicine in Munich; 1953 doctorate in medicine; 1951–1953 Resident, Department

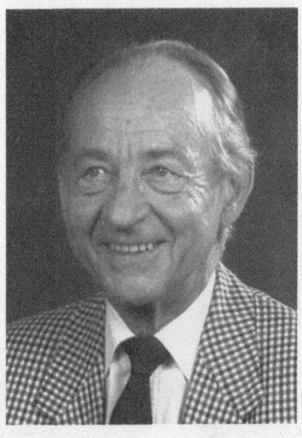

of Surgery, University of Munich; since 1953 training in the Division of Anaesthesia; 1957 Specialist in Anesthesiology; 1963 Lecturer in Anaesthesiolgy; 1964 Head, Division of Anaesthesia, City Hospital Wiesbaden; 1965 Head, Division of Anaesthesia, Department of Neurosurgery, University of Munich; 1970 Adjunct Professor; 1974–1976 Head, Department of Anaesthesiology, University Hospital Munich, Campus Großhadern; 1976 Head, Division of Neuroanaesthesia, Department of Anaesthesiology; 1978 Associate Professor; 1992 retirement.

1976–2007 Chairmanship Professor Klaus Peter

Prof. Dr. med. Dr. h.c. Klaus Peter

Born 14 September 1938 in Zobten/Breslau; 1960-1966 student of medicine in Heidelberg; 1967 doctorate in medicine; 1968–1972 Resident, Department of Anaesthesiology, University of Heidelberg; 1972 Specialist in Anaesthesiology; 1972 Lecturer in Anaesthesiology; 1972–1976 Senior Physician at the Department of Anaesthesiology und Reanimation, Faculty of Clinical Medicine Mannheim, University of Heidelberg; 1974 Adjunct Professor; 1976 Full Professor and Chairman of the Department of Anaesthesiology, University Hospital Munich; 1988 honorary doctorate of the Medical Academy, University of Wroclaw, Poland; 1989-2005 Dean of the Faculty of Medicine, University of Munich; 2001 Honorary Member of the German Society of Surgery; Honorary Member of the Polish (1986), German (2003) and Austrian (2006) Societies of Anaesthesiology and Intensive Care Medicine; 2005-2007 Medical Director of the University Hospital; 2007 Professor Emeritus.

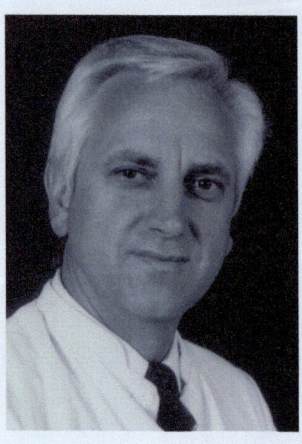

On 1 October 1976 Professor Klaus Peter (Mannheim) was appointed Full Professor of Anaesthesiology and Chairman of the Department of Anaesthesiology which was put in charge of specialist responsibility for both clinical campuses. The anaesthesiological duties expanded markedly and as of 1995 a third location was added, the cardio-surgical centre of the Hospital »Stiftsklinik« Augustinum. As a result of the steadily increasing cooperation the Division of Paediatric Anaesthesia, Dr. von Hauner Children's Hospital of the University, which had been developed by Professor Karl Mantel was included in the Department in 2002. ICM was an integral part of responsibility from the beginning in the fifties. In 2001 the Department was responsible for 48 ICU beds (and 16 beds were added in 2008, see below) and took care for 20 more beds. A core activity was the treatment of severe ARDS including extracorporeal membrane oxygenation. A pain clinic was established in Großhadern in 1980 and in Innenstadt in 2001. Peter and his successor Zwißler were and are members of the Board of Directors of the interdisciplinary Institute of Emergency Medicine and Medical Management of the University founded in 2002. This had emerged from the Working Group Emergency and Rescue Medicine of the University which had been formed in 1993. Peter was, in his functions as Dean of the Faculty of Medicine and Chairman of the Department of Anaesthesiology, one of the founders of the Munich Harvard Educational Alliance. This was aimed at implementing new forms of teaching and learning, was very successful and eventually exemplary for many German faculties.

Under the aegis of Peter the number of research groups and scientific projects was very large. He instituted a close cooperation with the Department of Experimental Surgery and many other national and international researchers. Main topics were systemic and pulmonary microcirculation, perioperative myocardial ischaemia, haemodilution, volume replacement, pharmacology of, and pharmacotherapy with, volatile and intravenous anaesthetics, neuromuscular blockers, opioids and corticosteroids, anaesthetic depth, trauma, shock, sepsis, acute lung injury, ischaemia and reperfusion injuries, etc., resulting in numerous publications, large amounts of external grants and fundings and ten appointments to external full professorships.

Since 2007 Chairmanship Professor Bernhard Zwißler

Professor Dr. med. Bernhard Zwißler

Born 4 April 1960 in Munich; 1978–1984 student of medicine at the University of Munich; 1985 doctorate in medicine; 1985–1986 Medical Officer; 1986–1987 and 1990–1995 residency at the Department of Anaesthesiology of the University of Munich; 1988–1990 Research Fellow at the Department of Experimental Surgery, University of Heidelberg; 1992 Lecturer in Anaesthesiology; 1995 Specialist in Anaesthesiology; 1997 Associate Professor; 2003–2007 Full Professor and Chairman of the Department of Anaesthesiology, Intensive Care Medicine and Pain Therapy, University Hospital Frankfurt; 2005 Member of the German National Academy of Sciences Leopoldina; 2007 Full Professor and Chairman of the Department of Anaesthesiology, University Hospital Munich.

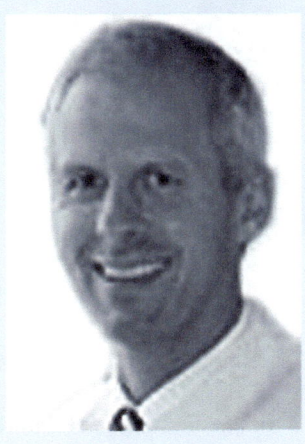

Zwißler's initial focus as Chairman was the institution of a quality management (QM) system in the Department of Anaesthesiology, including anaesthesia, intensive care medicine, pain therapy, and emergency medicine. As a consequence, the Department could be successfully certified according DIN ISO 9001:2008 in 2009. In 2003 the Department of Anaesthesiology, together with the Departments of Neurology and Internal Medicine III (Hemato-oncology), founded the Interdisciplinary Centre of Palliative Medicine (IZP) with 10 beds at the Campus Großhadern. Also in 2003 a new pain clinic was opened at the Campus Innenstadt. In addition, a new 16 bed ICU run by the Department of Anaesthesiology, Campus Großhadern, was opened in 2008. Approximately 200 specialists and residents are now working at the Department. A full scale simulation centre was established in 2005, providing regular crew resource training courses for physcians, nurses and students.

In recent years research focussed, among other topics, on the impact of stress, trauma and sepsis on immune function, endocrine response and coagulation; the role of the endocannabinoid system in memory and pain; the pathophysiology of the endothelial glycocalix and perioperative volume balance; mechanisms of periph-

eral nociception and complex regional pain syndromes; therapeutic options in acute respiratory failure; and mass spectrometer analyses of narcotics.

Qualification as Lecturers in Anaesthesiology

Zürn, Ludwig (1956); Enzenbach, Robert (1963); Doenicke, Alfred (1964); Gürtner, Thomas (1966); Pichlmayr, Ina (1968); Beer, Dubravka (1971) Loeschcke, Georg (1971); Finsterer, Udilo (1974); Götz, Eberhard (1975); Jesch, Franz (1981); Franke, Niels (1983); Laubenthal, Heinz (1984); Schmucker, Peter (1984); Taeger, Kai (1985); Jensen, Ute (1986); Unertl, Klaus (1987); Schmitz, Eberhard (1988); Forst, Helmuth (1989); Kellermann, Wolfgang (1989); Madler, Christan (1989); Vogel, Johann (1989); Conzen, Peter (1990); Hobbhahn, Jonny (1990); Bardenheuer, Hubert (1991); Schwender, Dierk (1992); Stein, Christoph (1992); Zwißler, Bernhard (1993); Weber, Werner (1994); Goetz, Alwin (1995); Kreimeier, Uwe (1995); Schelling, Gustav (1995); Adolph, Michael (1996); Groh, Joachim (1996); Häßler, Reinhard (1996); Welte, Martin (1997); Briegel, Josef (1998); Thiel, Manfred (1998); Christ, Frank (1999); Haller, Mathias (1999); Habler, Oliver (2000); Kleen, Martin (2000); Kuhnle, Gerhard (2001); Heindl, Bernhard (2003); Spannagel, Michael (2003); Kilger, Erich (2004); Rehm, Markus (2005); Azad, Shahnaz-Christina (2006); Irnich, Dominik (2006); Kemming, Gregor (2006); Chouker, Alexander (2008)

Professors of Anaesthesiology
Full Professors

Prof. Dr. Klaus van Ackern (1986), Medical University of Lübeck
Prof. Dr. Heinz Laubenthal (1987), St. Josef University Hospital, Bochum
Prof. Dr. Eike Martin (1990), University of Heidelberg
Prof. Dr. med. Peter Schmucker (1985), German Heart Institute, Berlin; (1990), Medical University of Lübeck
Prof. Dr. med. Kai Taeger (1991), University of Regensburg
Prof. Dr. med. K. Unertl (1994), University of Tübingen
Prof. Dr. med. Christoph Stein (1997), Free University of Berlin
Prof. Dr. Bernhard Zwißler (2003), University of Frankfurt
Prof. Dr. Alwin E. Goetz (2005), University Hospital Hamburg-Eppendorf
Prof. Dr. Manfred Thiel (2009), Faculty of Clinical Medicine Mannheim, University of Heidelberg

Associate and Adjunct Professors

Prof. Dr. Shahnaz Azad; Prof. Dr. Josef Briegel; Prof. Dr. Frank Christ; Prof. Dr. Peter Conzen; Prof. Dr. Alfred

Doenicke; Prof. Dr. Robert Enzenbach; Dr. Udilo Fin-
sterer; Prof. Dr. Helmuth Forst; Prof. Dr. Niels Franke;
Prof. Dr. Alwin Goetz; Prof. Dr. Mathias Haller; Prof.
Dr. Bernhard Heindl; Prof. Dr. Uwe Helms; Prof. Dr.
Ute Jensen; Prof. Dr. Franz Jesch; Prof. Dr. Wolfgang
Kellermann; Prof. Dr. Christian Madler; Prof. Dr. Karl
Mantel; Prof. Dr. Eike Martin; Prof. Dr. Heinz Lauben-
thal; Prof. Dr. Jürgen Riemer; Prof. Dr. Gustav Schell-
ing; Prof. Dr. Dierk Schwender; Prof. Dr. Kai Taeger;
Prof. Dr. Manfred Thiel; Prof. Dr. Klaus Unertl; Prof.
Dr. Klaus van Ackern; Prof. Dr. Martin Welte; Prof. Dr.
Bernhard Zwißler.

For further information:

www.ana.klinikum.uni-muenchen.de/index.html

3.2.31   Technical University of Munich

Department of Anaesthesiology, Hospital Rechts der Isar

G. Tempel, E. Kochs

Initiated by Professor Georg Maurer, Chairman of the
Department of Surgery of the Municipal Hospital Rechts
der Isar, a Division of Anaesthesia was established as part
of the Department in 1954. He later, in 1967, became
the founder and first Dean of the Faculty of Medicine at
the Technical University of Munich. Dr. Charlotte Lehmann, an anaesthesiologist, headed this Division which
was responsible for all anaesthetics administered in the
surgical departments. Within the next years the Division
was expanded to serve all surgical disciplines within the
hospital. It was also responsible for running the blood
bank. An ICU was opened in 1958 under the auspices of
the Division which remained under the umbrella of the
Department of Surgery until 1972.

Department of Anaesthesiology; 1969 Full Professor of
Anaesthesiology at the newly founded University Hospital Steglitz of the Free University; 1972 Full Professor
of Anaesthesiology at the newly founded Department
of Anaesthesiology of the Technical University of Munich, Hospital Rechts der Isar; 1975–1979 Dean of the
Faculty of Medicine; 1992 Professor Emeritus.

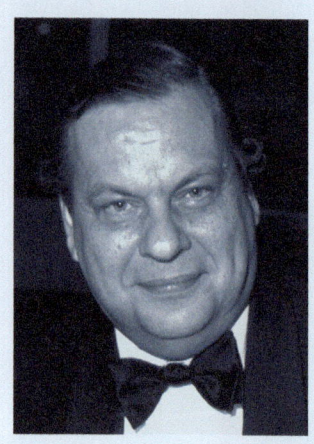

The Department of Anaesthesiology of the Technical
University of Munich at the Hospital Rechts der Isar was
founded on 1 July 1972 with Professor Ernst Kolb (Berlin, cf. Ch. 3.2.4) as its first Chairman. At that time the
Department was in charge of anaesthesia services for the
entire Hospital and had 16 anaesthesiologists on staff. A
pain clinic was established in 1979 which was run in co-
operation with the Department of Neurology. A unit for
blood transfusions was added in 1986. The Department
etablished its own preanaesthetic clinic in 1988 where
approximately 80% of all patients scheduled for elective
surgery were evaluated.

1972–1992 Chairmanship Professor Ernst Kolb

Prof. Dr. med. Ernst Kolb

Born 25 December 1930 in Mainz; student of medicine
in Heidelberg and Innsbruck; 1955 doctorate in medicine; 1955–1959 Resident at the Division of Anaesthesia, University of Heidelberg; 1959 Head of the Division;
1961 Division of Anaesthesia, University of Mainz; 1962
Specialist in Anaesthesiology; 1963 Lecturer in Anaesthesiology, Associate Professor and Chairman of the
Division of Anaesthesia, Free University of Berlin; 1967
Full Professor of Anaesthesiology and Chairman of the

1992-1994 Interim Chairmanship Professor Gunter Tempel

Prof. Dr. med. Gunter Tempel

Born 2 February 1940 in Worms; 1959–1965 student of
medicine, Heidelberg, Berlin, Düsseldorf; 1965–1966
internship in Rheinberg and Berlin; 1965 doctorate
in medicine; 1967-1971 Resident in Anaesthesiology,
Berlin; 1971 Specialist in Anaesthesiology; 1972 Senior
Consultant, Department of Anaesthesiology, Technical
University of Munich, Hospital Rechts der Isar; 1977
Lecturer in Anaesthesiology; 1978 Associate Professor;

1992-1994 Interim Chairman; 1994 Honorary Member of the Romanian Society of Anaesthesiology; 2005 retirement.

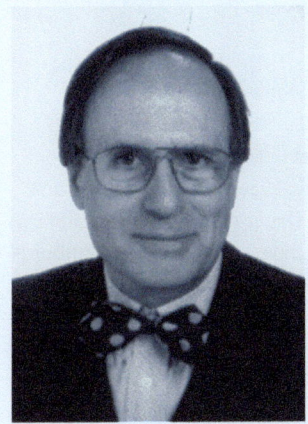

Since 1994 Chairmanship Professor Eberhard Kochs

Prof. Dr. med. Dipl.-Phys. Eberhard Kochs

Born 9 June 1948 in Fulda; 1969-1974 student of physics (Bonn), 1974–1975 Research Associate at the Department of Electrical Engineering, RWTH Aachen University, 1975–1980 student of medicine (Bonn, Lübeck); 1975–1977 Resident, Department of Forensic Medicine (Bonn); 1981–1982 Resident in Anaesthesia, St. Petrus Hospital Bonn; 1982-1985 Resident, Department of Anaesthesiology, University Hospital Hamburg Eppendorf; 1983 doctorate in medicine; 1985 Specialist in Anaesthesiology; 1987 Senior Physician; 1989

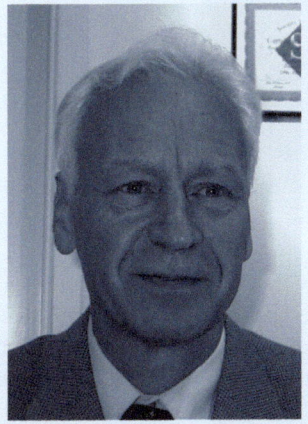

Lecturer in Anaesthesiology; 1990 Associate Professor; 1990 Sabbatical at the University of Illinois, Chicago; 1994 Full Professor and Chairman of the Department of Anaesthesiology, Technical University of Munich, Hospital Rechts der Isar; 2005 editor of the journal »Anesthesiology«; 2010 President Elect of the European Society of Anaesthesiology.

When Kolb stepped down as Chairman in December 1991 Professor Gunter Tempel became interim Chairman until February 1994. On 1 March 1994 Professor Eberhard Kochs (Hamburg) was appointed Full Professor and Chairman of the Department. When he took over chairmanship general or regional anaesthesia was provided to 13,500 patients. Due to the development of the Hospital and its surgical units this number increased to 25,000 patients in 2009 of whom 25% were treated with regional anaesthesia (1994: approximately 8%). In 2004 the pain clinic of the Department was transferred into the Centre of Interdisciplinary Pain Medicine jointly run by the Departments of Anaesthesiology, Neurology and Psychosomatic Medicine. In 2007 the ICUs of the Departments of Anaesthesiology and Surgery were merged under the leadership of the Department of Anaesthesiology in cooperation with the Departments of Surgery and Neurosurgery. Both units taken together provide facilities for the treatment of 35 critically ill patients, i.e. about 3,200 patients annually. Since 1954, more than 700,000 patients have received anaesthesia care and more than 15,000 patients been treated in the ICU. The Department has established a simulation centre equipped with 2 simulation units for training in emergency medicine and anaesthesia for students, nurses, residents, and faculty members.

The following topics are the current clinical and experimental research priorities initiated by Kochs: determination of depth of anaesthesia using electrophysiologic monitoring; quantification of analgesia in anaesthetized and sedated patients, assessment and modulation of nociception by analgesics and hypnotics; investigations of cerebral physiology, including cerebral autoregulation, perfusion, CO_2 reactivity, ischaemia, neuroprotection; experimental and clinical studies on cognitive deficits following anaesthesia and surgery; effect of cardiopulmonary bypass on cerebral function and inflammation; receptor studies of anaesthetic actions on nACh and GABA receptors and long-term potentiation; septic encephalopathy; organ perfusion in sepsis; muscle relaxants (pharmacokinetics, pharmacodynamics, interactions with the NO system); postoperative pain management; assessment of intraoperative workload on anaesthetists.

Qualification as Lecturers in Anaesthesiology

Eckart, Joachim (1974); Tempel, Gunter (1977); Landauer, Bernd (1977); Jelen-Essenborn, Sabine (1981); Abbushi, Walid (1983); von Hundelshausen, Burkhard (1985); Rust, Meinhard (1987); Schneck, Hajo (1988); Eisler, Klaus (1990);Hipp, Rudolf (1991); Hargasser, Stefan (1993); Entholzner, Elmar (1996); Blobner, Manfred (1997); Tassani-Prell, Peter M. (2000); Detsch, Oliver (2001); Mielke, Lars (2002); Hapfelmeier, Gerhard (2004); Engelhard, Kristin (2005); Mackensen, Burkhard G. (2005); Scheller, Michaela (2005); Schneider, Gerhard (2005); Fink, Heidrun (2008); Wagner, Klaus (2008); Jungwirth, Bettina (2010)

Professors of Anaesthesiology
Full Professors

Prof. Dr. Christian Werner (2004), University of Mainz
Prof. Dr. Gerhard Schneider (2010), Hospital Wuppertal, University of Witten-Herdecke (Chair I)

Associate Professors

Prof. Dr. Bernd Landauer (1978), Technical University of Munich
Prof. Dr. Gunter Tempel (1978), Technical University of Munich
Prof. Dr. Christian Werner (1996), Technical University of Munich
Prof. Dr. Peter M. Tassani-Prell (2002), Technical University of Munich
Prof. Dr. Gerhard Schneider (2009), Technical University of Munich

Adjunct Professors

Prof. Dr. J. Eckart, Prof. Dr. W. Abbushi, Prof. Dr. M. Rust, Prof. Dr. B. von Hundelshausen, Prof. Dr. S. Jelen-Esselborn, Prof. Dr. H. Schneck, Prof. Dr. R. Hipp, Prof. Dr. St. Hargasser, Prof. Dr. M. Blobner, Prof. Dr. Elmar Entholzner, Prof. Dr. Patrick Friederich

For further information:

www.med.tu-muenchen.de/de/gesundheitsversorgung/kliniken/anaesthesiologie/index.php

3.2.32   University of Münster

Department of Anaesthesiology and Intensive Care Medicine

H. Van Aken

In 1964 Professor Paul Sunder-Plasssmann, Chairman of the Department of Surgery, University of Münster, established a Division of Anaesthesia which was led by Dr.

Georg-Heinrich Menges. Some years later the Faculty of Medicine decided to provide a Chair of Anaesthesiology.

1976–1995 Chairmanship of Professor Peter Lawin

Prof. Dr. med. Dr. h.c. Peter Lawin, FCCM

Born 20 January 1930 in Königsberg, deceased 27 June 2002 in Le Tignet (France); 1950–1956 student of medicine in Munich; 1956 doctorate in medicine; 1958–1962 Resident, Department of Surgery and Division of Anaesthesia, University Hospital of Hamburg-Eppendorf; 1962 Specialist in Anaesthesiology and head of the newly founded Division of Anaesthesia at Altona General Hospital, Hamburg; 1970 Lecturer in Anaesthesiology, University of Hamburg; 1972 Adjunct Professor; 1976 Full Professor of Anaesthesiology and Chairman of the Department of Anaesthesiology and Intensive Care Medicine at the University of Münster; 1983 honorary doctorate from the Medical Academy of Krakow, Poland; 1987–1992 Medical Director, Medical Institutions of the University of Münster; 1990 Fellow in Critical Care Medicine (FCCM), American College of Critical Care Medicine; 1993 Honorary Member of the German Interdisciplinary Association of Critical Care and Emergency Medicine; 1995 Professor Emeritus; 1998 Honorary Member of the German Society of Anaesthesiology and Intensive Care Medicine.

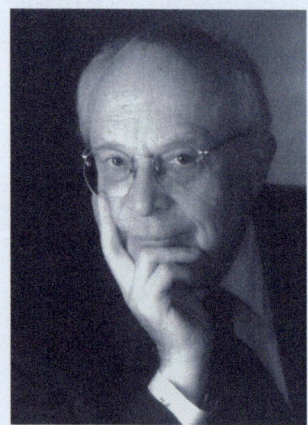

Professor Peter Lawin (Hamburg) was appointed as the first Chairman of the Department of Anaesthesiology and Intensive Care Medicine at the University of Münster on 1 June 1976. He started with a team of 40 physicians, 61 nurses, 3 secretaries, 3 medical laboratory technicians, 1 photo laboratory assistant and 1 biomedical engineer – the first to be employed in an anaesthesiological department in Germany. One of the new Department's central duties was to provide continuing and structured education and training for young physicians, due to the growing demand for anaesthesia consultants in Germany. Training facilities for specialized nursing in anaesthesia and ICM were also established. An outpatient pain clinic to care for patients with chronic pain was established as early as 1981. The treatment approach used in the pain clinic was supplemented with a day care unit in which not only physicians and nurses, but also psychologists, social workers, physiotherapists and art therapists collaborated in caring for some 1,000 patients per year using a multi-modal, integrated approach.

Since 1995 Chairmanship Professor Hugo Van Aken

Prof. Dr. med. Dr. h.c. Hugo Van Aken, FRCA, FANZCA

Born in Mechelen (Belgium) on 2 March 1951; 1969–1976 student of medicine, Catholic University of Leuven, Belgium; 1976 doctorate in medicine, surgery and obstetrics, Leuven; 1976–1980 residencies in anaesthesiology at the Department of Anaesthesiology, Catholic University of Leuven and Department of Anaesthesiology and Intensive Care Medicine, University of Münster; 1980 Specialist in Anaesthesiology in Belgium; 1980–1986 Senior Physician, Department of Anaesthesiology and Intensive Care Medicine, Münster; 1981 doctorate in medicine, Münster; 1983 Lecturer in Anaesthesiology; 1986 Full Professor of Anaesthesiology and Chairman of the Department of Anaesthesia, Catholic University of Leuven, Belgium; 1995 Full Professor of Anaesthesiology and Chairman of the Department of Anaesthesiology and Surgical Intensive-Care Medicine, University of Münster; 1994 Fellow by election of the Royal College of Anaesthetists (FRCA); 1998 Fellow by election of the Australian and New Zealand College of Anaesthetists (FANZCA); Honorary Member of the American Society of Anesthesiologists; honorary doctorate from the Georgian State Medical Academy; Member of the German National Academy of Sciences Leopoldina; 2000–2003 President, European Academy of Anaesthesiology.

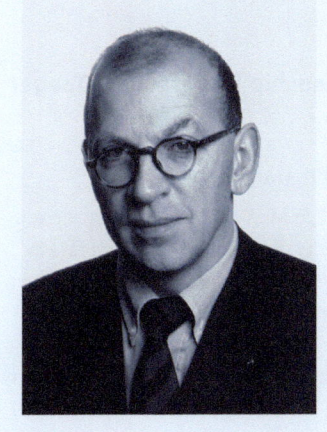

Professor Hugo Van Aken (Leuven) succeeded Peter Lawin on 1 August 1995. Two major new focuses were established under the new director: an acute pain service was established, and scientific and research activities were considerably intensified. Using individualized and differentiated anaesthetic procedures, modern observational techniques, and combined anaesthetic techniques, it is nowadays possible for many patients to undergo surgery in whom it would not previously have been possible due to limited vital functions. A code of procedure for the operating room was passed by the clinical board in 1999 in order to optimize perioperative processes. The Department is one of only six in Germany that have been certified since 1998 by the European Academy of Anaesthesiology and the European Board of Anaesthesiology of the UEMS as European Training Centres for young anaesthetists. As one of the first anaesthesia departments in Germany, Münster has achieved recognition from the German Society of Anaesthesiology and Intensive Care as a centre for skilled training in transoesophageal echocardiography. A total of 2,200 patients are treated annually in the Department's three ICUs. An acute pain service was established in 1995. Each year 2,500 patients receive treatment with continuous patient-controlled analgesia.

Under Van Aken's chairmanship the research activities were systematically expanded. Key aspects of research involve experimental and clinical haemostaseology, postischaemic myocardial dysfunction (myocardial stunning), sepsis, spinal mechanisms of postoperative pain, intravital microscopy of microcirculation, mesenteric perfusion dysfunction and the pharmacology of anaesthetic agents. The Department's scientific achievements are evident from the more than 1,100 Medline-listed articles it has published since 1995.

Qualification as Lecturers in Anaesthesiology

Menges, Georg-Heinrich (1963); Stellpflug, Heiko (1979); Van Aken, Hugo (1983); Paravicini, Dietrich (1983); Puchstein, Christoph (1983); Scherer, Ralf (1984); Reinhold, Paul (1984); Wendt, Michael (1984); Baum, Jan

(1987); Hannich, Hans-Joachim (1988); Hansen, Jochen (1988); Hartenauer, Ulrich (1988); Prien, Thomas (1989); Anger, Christian (1991); Hachenberg, Thomas (1990); Theissen, Joseph (1990); Möllhoff, Thomas (1993); Brüssel, Thomas (1993); Zander, Josef (1993); Möllmann, Michael (1993); Gralow, Ingrid (1996); Rolf, Norbert (1997); Booke, Michael (1997); Berendes, Elmar (1998); Marcus, Abraham Emanuel (1998); Knichwitz, Gisbert (1998); Hinder, Frank (1999); Bürkle, Hartmut (1999); Bone, Hans-Georg (2000); Brodner, Gerhardt (2001); Sielenkämper, Andreas (2001); Meißner, Andreas (2001); Goeters, Christiane (2002); Weber, Thomas (2003); Zahn, Peter (2003); Theilmeier, Gregor (2003); Pogatzki, Esther (2003); Enk, Dietmar (2004); Gogarten, Wiebke (2004), Strümper, Danja (2005); Fischer, Lars (2005); Weber, Frank (2005); Singbartl, Kai (2005); Westphal, Martin (2006); Schmidt, Christoph (2006); Hahnenkamp, Klaus (2007); Stubbe, Henning (2008); Hönemann, Christian (2008); Ellger, Björn (2008); Lange, Matthias (2009); Freise, Hendrik (2009); Zarbock, Alexander (2009)

Professors of Anaesthesiology
Full Professors

Prof. Dr. Hugo Van Aken (1986), Catholic University of Leuven, Belgium
Prof. Dr. Christoph Puchstein (1987), St. Mary's Hospital Herne, University of Bochum
Prof. Dr. Michael Wendt (1993), University of Greifswald
Prof. Dr. Hans-Joachim Hannich (1994) Professor of Medical Psychology, University of Greifswald
Prof. Sabina De Geest (2000), Professor of Nursing, University of Basel, Switzerland
Prof. Dr. Thomas Brüssel (2001), Medical School, College of Medicine and Health Sciences, Australian National University, Canberra, Australia.
Prof. Dr. Hartmut Bürkle (2010), University of Freiburg
Prof. Dr. Peter Zahn (2011), University Hospital Bergmannsheil, Bochum

Associate Professors

Prof. Dr. Thomas Hachenberg (1994), University of Greifswald
Prof. Dr. Esther Pogatzki-Zahn (2006), Münster

Adjunct Professors

Prof. E. Götz, Prof. H. Stellpflug, Prof. D. Paravicini, Prof. H. Schoeppner, Prof. R. Scherer, Prof. J. Baum, Prof. U. Hartenauer, Prof. T. Prien, Prof. J. Theissen, Prof. T. Brüssel, Prof. T. Möllhoff, Prof. M. Loick, Prof. J. Meyer, Prof. B. Kehrel, Prof. P. Reinhold, Prof. N. Rolf, Prof. M. Booke, Prof. E. Berendes, Prof. M. Möllmann, Prof. H. Bürkle, Prof. M. Marcus, Prof. H.G. Bone, Prof. F. Hinder, Prof. G. Knichwitz, Prof. A. Sielenkämper, Prof. G. Brodner,

Prof. T. Weber, Prof. A. Meissner, Prof. L. Fischer, Prof. I. Gralow, Prof. W. Gogarten, Prof. P. Zahn, Prof. B. Ellger.

For further information:

www.klinikum.uni-muenster.de/index.php?id=anaesthesie

3.2.33 University of Regensburg

Department of Anaesthesiology
K. Taeger, B.M. Graf

The University of Regensburg has a short history. Its foundation dates back to a decision of the Bavarian Parliament taken in 1962. In 1967, the first students of medicine began to attend courses in basic sciences. Clinical specialties were established in 3 phases. In the first one the premises to be used by the Department of Dentistry and Maxillo-Facial Surgery were constructed and put into operation in 1984. In a second step the University Hospital was built up and put into operation in 1992 and then extended in a third phase until 1998 now comprising more than 800 beds, 25 operating theatres and 84 ICU beds. The chairs of urology, gynaecology and obstetrics and paediatrics were established in affiliated hospitals. The Faculty of Medicine first convened in 1985 and began to assess the candidates for the new chairs. The elected candidates were appointed in 1991 so that they still could exert some influence on the new facilities, establish functioning structures and select their teams.

When the Department of Dentistry and Maxillo-Facial Surgery took up its activities in 1984 the anaesthesia service was provided by the Department of Anaesthesiology of the University of Munich. In 1988 a Division of Anaesthesia and Intensive Care Medicine was created and headed by Dr. Ernil Hansen. Three years later, Professor Kai Taeger (Munich) was appointed to the new Chair of Anaesthesiology.

1991–2008 Chairmanship Professor Kai Taeger

Prof. Dr. med. Kai Taeger

Born 5 October 1942 in Munich; 1965–1970 student of medicine, University of Munich; 1970 doctorate in medicine; 1971–1975 Research Associate, Department of Pharmacology, University of Munich; 1975–1991, Resident and Senior Physician, Department of Anaesthesiology, University of Munich, 1979 Specialist in Anaesthesiology; 1986 Lecturer in Anaesthesiology; 1987

Adjunct Professor; 1991 Full Professor and Chairman of the Department of Anaesthesiology, University of Regensburg; 2001 German Order of Merit; 2008 Professor Emeritus.

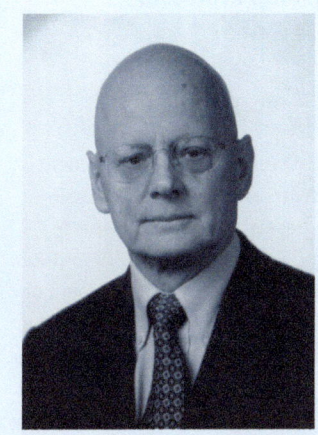

In his function as Full Professor and Chairman of the Department of Anaesthesiology Taeger recruited and formed a team of anaesthetists from the whole of Germany that could take the full responsibility for all aspects of clinical anaesthesiology including ICM, emergency services and pain therapy within one year. In addition, he was appointed Medical Director of the Hospital and as such played a pivotal role in the process of integrating the new Departments. A pain plinic was established in 1992. Since 1993 the mobile life support unit was preferably equipped with doctors of the Department. In 1998 the anaesthesiological ICU increased from 10 to 14 beds. The neurosurgical ICU with 10 beds was jointly run with the Department of Neurosurgery. The annual number of anaesthetics increased to 15,000, that of ICU patients to 1,400. For the preoperative assessment of patients a preanaesthetic clinic was established. Tumour, cardiovascular and transplant surgery and care of patients with multiple injuries developed to the main fields of surgical activities.

For the scientific activities of the Department a research lab with an area of 110 m^2 was established and a large number of experimental methods introduced, e.g. cell separation, cell cultures, flow cytometry, measurement of plasma concentrations. Professor Jonny Hobbhahn was mainly involved in the encouragement and supervision of young clinical and experimental researchers. Several young scientists took fellowships abroad, e.g. in England, Sweden and Switzerland. Main fields of research were pharmacokinetics and mechanisms of action of anaesthetics, toxicity and safety action of volatile anaesthetics, platelet and granulocyte function in anaesthesia and intensive care, circulatory regulation, impact of tumour

cells for autologous transfusion, severe lung injuries, postoperative nausea, vomiting and cognitive deficits.

Since 2008 Chairmanship Professor Bernhard M. Graf

Prof. Dr. med. Berhard M. Graf, MSc.

Born 29 March 1960 in Riedenburg; 1980–1086 student of medicine in Regensburg and Würzburg; doctorate in medicine, University of Würzburg; Resident and Medical Officer in Bad Zwischenahn; 1988–1991 Resident, Department of Anaesthesiology, University of Heidelberg; 1992 Specialist in Anaesthesiology; 1992–1995 Assistant Professor, Medical College of Wisconsin and Children's Hospital, Milwaukee, USA; 1995–2003 Senior Physician, Department of Anaesthesiology, University of Heidelberg; 1997 Lecturer in Anaesthesiology; 2003 Vice Chairman; 2004 Adjunct Professor; 2005 Full Professor and Chairman of the Centre of Anaesthesiology, Emergency and Intensive Care Medicine, University of Göttingen; 2008 Full Professor and Chairman of the Department of Anaesthesiology, University of Regensburg.

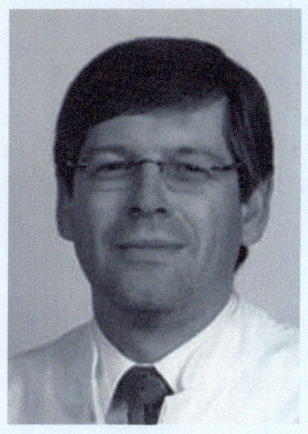

In September 2008, Professor Bernhard Graf (Göttingen) was appointed to the Chair of Anaesthesiology. The helicopter rescue service of Regensburg was put under the medical responsibility of the Department. In addition to the already existing competencies the Department shares the responsibility for the ICUs of the Departments of Surgery (30 beds) and Cardio-thoracic and Vascular Surgery (14 beds) with the respective surgeons. Existing research projects are continued and a number of new ones established, among them toxicity of local anaesthetics, extracorporeal support of heart and lung functions, septic cardiac myopathies, various aspects of cerebral

3

stroke, toxic effects of anaesthetics on the developing brain, point-of-care testing.

Qualification as Lecturers in Anaesthesiology

Hansen, Ernil (1995); Bein, Thomas (1996); Fröhlich, Dieter (1999); Rödig, Gabriele (2000); Metz, Christoph (2001); Funk, Wolfgang (2001); Bucher, Michael (2003); Ittner, Karl-Peter (2007); Schmidt, Christoph (2009); Pawlik, Michael (2010)

Professors of Anaesthesiology
Full Professors

Prof. Dr. Michael Bucher (2009) University of Halle-Wittenberg

Associate Professors

Prof. Dr. Jonny Hobbhahn (1992), Regensburg
Prof. Dr. Michael Bucher (2009), Regensburg

Adjunct Professors

Prof. Dr. Thomas Bein; Prof. Dr. Michael Bucher; Prof. Dr. Dr. Ernil Hansen; Prof. Dr. Wolfgang Zink

For further information

www.uniklinikum-regensburg.de/kliniken-institute/Anaesthesiologie/index.php

3.2.34   University of Rostock

Department of Anaesthesiology and Intensive Therapy

G. Benad, G. Noeldge-Schomburg

The first Division of Anaesthesia was founded by Professor Walter Schmitt in 1954 within the University Department of Surgery. It was headed until 1961 by Dr. Horst Blume. Starting in August 1963, the new Head of the Division Dr. Gottfried Benad who had been trained at the University of Halle began to extend the anaesthetic services to the other surgical departments step by step, however, due to Schmitt's strong opposition he did not succeed before 1966 when anaesthesia service was provided for the ENT Department and in 1967 for the Department of Gynaecology. In order to realize his plans, Benad invited a number of internationally renowned anaesthesiologists to Rostock, what was very important. The exposure to distiguished experts proved to be very fruitful for the otherwise isolated East German anaesthesiology. In 1969 the so-called 3rd university reform in the German Democratic Republic (East Germany) resulted in the acknowledgement of anaesthesiology as an inde-

pendent academic speciality. Consequently, the Division of Anaesthesia became an institution of the Faculty of Medicine of the University and Benad was appointed Director and University Lecturer as of 1st September 1969.

1969–1998 Chairmanship Professor Gottfried Benad

Prof. Dr. med. habil. Gottfried Benad, FRCA

Born 15 March 1932 in Dresden, 1950–1956 student of medicine at Halle-Wittenberg; 1956 doctorate in medicine; 1956–1958 Research Associate, Department of Pharmacology, University of Halle; 1958–1963; Resident, Division of Anaesthesiology, Department of Surgery; University Hospital of Halle; 1962 Specialist in Anaesthesiology; 1963–1969 Senior Physician and Head of the Division of Anaesthesia, Department of Surgery, University of Rostock; 1967 Lecturer in Anaesthesiology; 1969–1981 Head, Division of Anaesthesia, University of Rostock; 1969 University Lecturer; 1972 Full Professor of Anaesthesiology; 1981 Chairman, Department of Anaesthesiology and Intensive Care, University of Rostock; 1985 Member of the German National Academy of Sciences Leopoldina and Honorary Member of the Bulgarian and *Czechoslovakian* Societies of Anaesthesiology; 1988 Corresponding Member of the Austrian Society of Anaesthesiology, Reanimation and Intensive Medicine; 1991 Fellow by election of the Royal College of *Anaesthetists* (FRCA); 1998 Professor Emeritus; 1998 Professor Emeritus; 1999 Honorary Member, German Society of Anaesthesiology and Intensive Care Medicine.

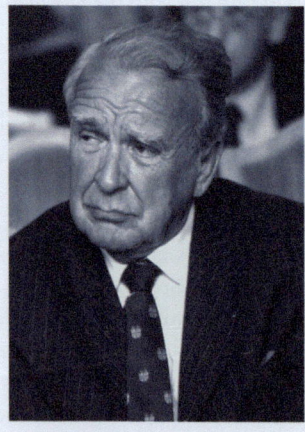

In 1972 a Chair was created and Benad was appointed Full Professor of Anaesthesiology. An ICU was established in 1978, at first with 2 beds which were gradually increased to 11 beds in 1995. In 1981 the Division became the Department of Anaesthesiology and Intensive Therapy. During Benad's chairmanship the Department evolved into a central institution providing anaesthetic services for all surgical departments and units of the University Hospital. Benad also established facilities for emergency medicine (1968-1969) in cooperation with the City of Rostock. Research was focussed on experimental and clinical aspects of muscle relaxants The merit of his chairmanship was not only the establishment of a central unit for anaesthesia and intensive care medicine but also the successful adaptation to the requirements elicited by the German reunification in 1989.

Since 1999 Chairmanship Professor Gabriele Nöldge-Schomburg

Prof. Dr. med. Gabriele Nöldge-Schomburg

Born 19 August 1951 in Neustadt an der Weinstraße; 1971–1976 student of medicine, University of Freiburg; 1976–1977 internship, University Hospital of Freiburg; 1977 doctorate in medicine; 1978–1986 Resident, Department of Anaesthesiology, University of Freiburg; 1982 Specialist in Anaesthesiology; 1987 Senior Physician; 1993 Lecturer in Anaesthesiology; 1999 Adjunct Professor; 1999 Full Professor and Chairperson of the Department of Anaesthesiology and Intensive Care Medicine, University Hospital of Rostock; 2004-2006 Dean of the Faculty of Medicine.

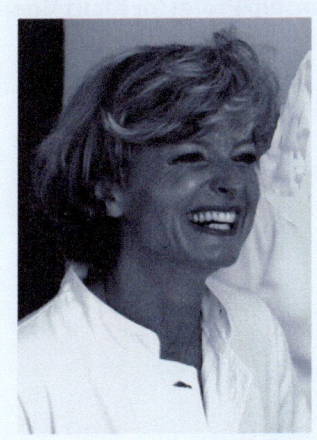

After a brief period of interim chairmanship by Professor Günter Lange, Professor Gabriele Nöldge-Schomburg was appointed Full Professor and Chairperson of the Department of Anaesthesiology on 1st September 1999 being Germany's first female Full Professor of Anaesthesiology. A new organisational responsibility for all surgical ICUs led to an extensive renovation of intensive care medicine facilities (1999/2004). The preanaesthetic clinic and the PACUs

were extended and responsibility for two emergency ambulance locations in Rostock was assumed. Since 2000 a perioperative pain service was established. The main areas of scientific activities are muscle relaxation, oxygenation, ischemia as well as regional and global reperfusion of splanchnic organs and breathing gas analyses. For the development of education, a full scale anaesthesia simulator (ROSANA) to train medical students, residents, medical staff and laymen was acquired. For further enhancement of medical quality and patient safety a critical incident reporting system was established in 2002. Since 2001 the Department has been responsible for the organisation and scientific program of the annual »International Symposium on Anaesthesia, Intensive Therapy, Emergency Medicine and Pain Therapy«, held in St. Anton, Austria. All these activities went along with further increases in staff.

Qualification as Lecturers in Anaesthesiology

Benad, Gottfried (1967); Borchert, Klaus (1973); Lange, Günter und Wilms, Karl-Heinz (1985); Güthenke, Hennrich (1985); Hergert, Matthias (1986); Hinsenbrock, Klaus-Peter (1987); Jacobi, Klaus (1987); Wiegand, Karl (1989); Egerer, Karl (1989); Hofmockel, Rainer (1997); Schubert Jochen (2003); Vagts, Dierk (2004); Mencke,Thomas (2007); Iber, Thomas (2008); Roesner, Jan-Patrick (2010).

Professors of Anaesthesiology
Full Professors
Prof. Dr. Klaus Borchert (1977), University of Greifswald

Associate Professors
Prof. Dr. Günter Lange (1992), Rostock
Prof. Dr. Thomas Scheeren (2004), Rostock

Adjunct Professors
Prof. Dr. Rainer Hofmockel, Prof. Dr. Dipl.-Chem. Jochen Schubert, Prof. Dr. Dierk A. Vagts

For further information:
www.kpai.med.uni-rostock.de

3.2.35   University of Tübingen

Department of Anaesthesiology and Intensive Care Medicine
K. Unertl

The history of anaesthesia at the University of Tübingen is characterized by ups and downs. Viktor von Bruns, Professor of Surgery, started administering ether in 1847, later switched to chloroform and is said to have carried

3

out endotracheal intubations with a silver tube as early as 1873. Around 1930, one of his successors, Professor Martin Kirschner, inaugurated »high pressure regional anaesthesia« and »air sealing spinal anaesthesia« and installed units particularly destined for the care of patients immediately after surgery. As Theodor Naegeli became Professor of Surgery in 1946 he soon strived to establish anaesthesia in his Department. He chose Dr. Jochen Bark who in 1954 became head of the anaesthesia service. But when Walter Dick was appointed Professor of Surgery in 1955 he made every endeavour to prohibit autonomy of anaesthesia until 1968. Bark had been trained in England, served as Founding President of the German Society of Anaesthesia and passed away due to an airplane accident already in 1963. He was followed by Dr. Gerhard Clauberg. In 1968 Professor Rudolf Schorer, Head of the Anaesthesia Division of the Municipal Hospital Augsburg, was appointed Full Professor and Chairman of the new University Department of Anaesthesiology.

1968–1992 Chairmanship Professor Rudolf Schorer

Prof. Dr. med. Rudolf Schorer

Born 27 June 1926 in Weilheim; 1948–1953 student of philosophy at the University of Munich, 1953–1958 student of medicine; 1958 doctorate in medicine; 1959–1961 internship; 1961–1962 Resident at the Surgical Department, University of Göttingen; 1962–1964 Research Associate at the Max Planck-Institute of Physiology in Göttingen; 1964 Lecturer in Anaesthesiology; 1964–1967 Resident and Senior Physician at the Department of Anaesthesiology; 1967–1968 Head of the Anaesthesia Department at the Municipal Hospital Augsburg; 1968 Full Professor and Chairman of the Central Department of Anaesthesiology, University of Tübingen; 1992 Professor Emeritus.

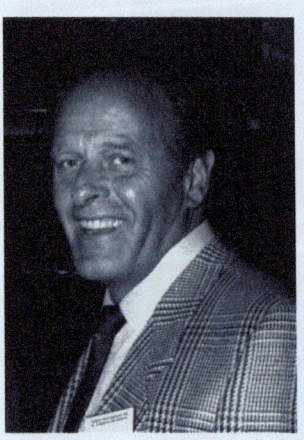

Rudolf Schorer efficiently developed the Department to an institution capable of meeting all requirements in anaesthesia, ICM, research and teaching. He established recovery rooms, a shock room, a technical division, and labs for ECG, blood gas analysis and lung function testing. A preanaesthetic and a pain clinic well as a unit for autologous blood donation and plasmapheresis followed in the 1980s. As various surgical, orthopaedic, radiologic and neurologic departments moved into a new common building together with the Department of Anaesthesiology in 1989, the latter acquired own experimental and clinical labs.

1992–1994 Interim Chairmanship Professor Gunther Lenz

Prof. Dr. med. Gunther Lenz

Born 16 September 1952 in Singen/Htwl.; 1971–1977 student of medicine in Tübingen; 1977 doctorate in medicine; Resident at the Department of Anaesthesiology, University of Tübingen; 1982 Specialist in Anaesthesiology; 1985 Senior Physician; 1988 Lecturer in Anaesthesiology; 1990 Senior Consultant; October 1992 to February 1994 Interim Chairman; 1995 Adjunct Professor; 1996 Director of the Department of Anaesthesiology and Intensive Care Medicine, Hospital Ingolstadt.

Since 1994 Chairmanship Professor Klaus Unertl

Prof. Dr. med. Klaus Unertl

Born 8 September 1945 in Aschaffenburg; 1967–1973 student of medicine at the University of Munich; 1975 doctorate in medicine; 1975–1994 Resident,

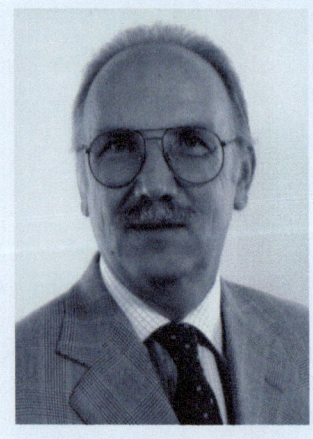

then Senior Physician at the Department of Anaesthesiology, University of Munich; 1981 Specialist in Anaesthesiology; 1987 Lecturer in Anaesthesiology; 1988 Adjunct Professor; 1994 Full Professor and Chairman of the Central Department of Anaesthesiology and Intensive Care Medicine, University Hospital of Tübingen; 2006–2010 Vice-Dean of the Faculty of Medicine.

Professor Klaus Unertl (Munich) was appointed Full Professor and Chairman of the Department of Anaesthesiology and Intensive Care Medicine in 1994. In order to cope with the needs given by the growing number of workplaces and more complex procedures he completely reorganized and optimized the cliniical services. By solving the problems resulting from recurrent manpower shortage the number of intensive care patients could constantly be increased and, in addition, the number of beds of the interdisciplinary surgical ICU gradually be expanded to 34. Main areas of research were infection and inflammation, molecular basis of the action of anaesthetics on the CNS, mechanisms of pain perception, simulation and human error management in anaesthesia. Activities of the Department with supraregional impact are related to the Pain Centre and the Tübingen Patient Safety and Simulation Centre (TÜPASS). In 2002 Unertl established a Section of Experimental Anesthesiology. The group is headed by Professor Bernd Antkowiak. Field of research: In the past decade the knowledge about the molecular mechanisms underlying general anesthesia has been revolutionized by genetic approaches. Translating these achievements into improvements in clinical anesthesia is central to the mission of the Experimental Anesthesiology Section.

Qualification of Lecturers in Anaesthesiology

Bark, Heinz Joachim (1956); Clauberg, Gerhard (1966); Kronschwitz, Helmut (1967); Stolz, Christian (1970); Unseld, Hans (1973); Braun, Ulrich (1974); Junger, Hermann (1975); Voigt, Edgar (1975); Hausdörfer, Juergen (1976); Hempel, Volker (1977);
Rothe, Karl-Friedrich (1980); Heuser, Dieter (1983); Guggenberger, Heinz (1988); Klöss, Thomas (1988); Lenz, Gunther (1988); Schimek, Franz (1988); Fretschner, Reinhold (1996); Bissinger, Ulrich (2000) Eltzschig, Holger (2004); Krüger, Wolfgang (2005); Dieterich, Hans-Jürgen (2006); Nohè, Boris (2006); Schröder, Torsten (2006); Heininger, Alexandra (2007); Häberle, Helene (2008); Reutershan, Jörg (2008); Eckle, Tobias (2008); Grasshoff, Christian (2008); Rosenberger, Peter (2008).

Professors of Anaesthesiology
Full Professors

Prof. Dr. rer. nat. Bernd Antkowiak (2002), Full Professor of Experimental Anaesthesiology, Tübingen

Associate Professors

Prof. Dr. Ulrich Braun (1978), University of Göttingen
Prof. Dr. Jürgen Hausdörfer (1979), Medical University of Hannover

Adjunct Professors

Prof. Dr. Holger Eltzschig, Prof. Dr. Volker Hempel, Prof. Dr. Dieter Heuser, Prof. Dr. Hermann Junger, Prof. Dr. Wolfgang Krüger, Prof. Dr. Gunther Lenz, Prof. Dr. Karl Friedrich Rothe, Prof. Dr. Torsten Schröder, Prof. Dr. Edgar Voigt.

For further information:

http://www.med.uni-tuebingen.de/Presse_Aktuell/Einrichtungen+A+bis+Z/Kliniken/Anaesthesiologie+und+Intensivmedizin.html

3.3.36 University of Ulm

Department of Anaesthesiology
M. Georgieff

The University of Ulm was founded in 1967. Until then there was only a small number of anesthesiologists in the Surgical Division of the Municipal Hospital Ulm. On 1st January 1968 Dr. Friedrich Wilhelm Ahnefeld, Lecturer of at the Department of Anaesthesiology, University of Mainz, was appointed Professor at the University of Ulm and, simultaneously, Chairman of the Divisions of Anaesthesiology of both the Municipal Hospital and Bundeswehrkrankenhaus (Federal Armed Forces Hospital). In 1971 he established an anaesthesiological ICU with 8 beds and a Section of Special Anaesthesia. The latter was headed by Professor Wolfgang Dick (Mainz). Starting with gynaecology all clinical divisions of the Municipal Hospital were gradually transferred under the umbrella of the University. Ahnefeld was consequently advanced to Full Professor and Chairman of the University Department of Anaesthesiology in 1974.

1974–1992 Chairmanship Professor Friedrich Wilhelm Ahnefeld

Prof. Dr. med. Dr. h.c. Friedrich Wilhelm Ahnefeld
Born 12 January 1924 in Woldenberg (Neumark); 1946–1951 student of medicine in Poznan, Münster

3

and Düsseldorf; 1951–1952 doctorate in medicine and Research Associate in Pharmacology (H. Weese); 1952–1958 Resident in Surgery; 1957 Specialist in Surgery; 1959-1965 Resident in Anaesthesiology, University of Mainz; 1962 Specialist in Anaesthesiology; 1964 Lecturer in Anaesthesiology; 1964–1967 Department of Anaesthesiology, University of Mainz, and Head of the Department of Burns at the Federal Armed Forces Hospital, Koblenz; since 1968 forming of a Department of Anaesthesiology at the newly founded University of Ulm; 1974 Full Professor and Chairman of the Department; 1992 Professor Emeritus; honorary doctorate of the Semmelweis University Budapest; 1996 Honorary Member of the German Society of Anaesthesiology and Intensive Care Medicine.

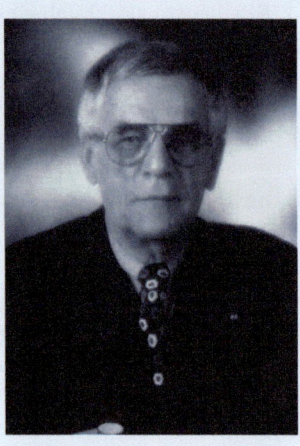

Since 1992 Chairmanship Professor Michael Georgieff

Prof. Dr. med. Dr. h.c. Michael Georgieff

Born August 24 1951 in Hargeisa (Somalia); 1972–1978 student of medicine at the Universities Düsseldorf and Heidelberg/Mannheim; 1978 doctorate in medicine; 1983 Specialist in Anaesthesiology; 1983–1985 Postdoctoral Fellow Harvard Medical School Boston (USA) and Massachusetts Institute of Technology, Department of Applied Biology, Cambridge (USA); 1986 Lecturer in Anaesthesiology, University of Heidelberg; 1987–1989 Lecturer in Anesthesia, Harvard Medical School, Boston (USA); 1988 Adjunct Professor of Anaesthesiology, Department of Anaesthesiology, University of Erlangen-Nuremberg; 1992 Full Professor and Chairman, Department of Anaesthesiology, University of Ulm.

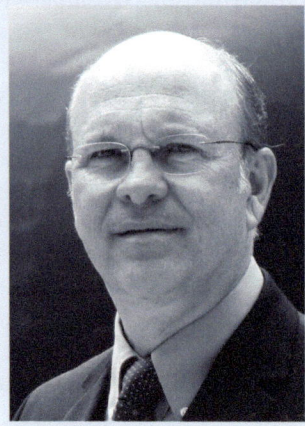

In addition to the two existing clinical sections a Section of Experimental Anaesthesia was brought into existence in 1976 and led by Professor Adolf Grünert. During Ahnefeld's chairmanship his coworkers developed and followed up a large number of scientific projects pertaining to all fields of the speciality. Ahnefeld was one of the pioneers of resuscitation and emergency medicine in Germany and as from 1971 made Ulm to the leading centre in this respect. In 1980 a pain clinic was opened to which 4 inpatient beds were added in 1991 In 1989 a Section of Technology and Process Development was created (Professor Wolfgang Friesdorf). Ahnefeld was an excellent teacher, organized a large number of seminars, workshops and national meetings, published textbooks and proceedings, and rendered outstanding services to the German Society of Anaesthesiology and Intensive Care Medicine.

With the appointment of Michael Georgieff as Professor and Chairman in 1992 the three existing Divisions were unified. The Department of Anaesthesiology provides anaesthesia in 33 operating theatres distributed over different locations and additionally in specialties like radiology, paediatrics, internal and dental medicine. The Department carries the responsability for 36 ICU beds. Appproximately 12 emergency cases are daily taken care of by the emergency medical service within the City of Ulm and its broader suburbs. On the average the Section of Pain Therapy treats 1,200 outpatients and 100 inpatients per year. The teaching of students was extended by the inauguration of practical clinical days and courses for practical skills with dummies. Further more full-scale anaesthesia simulators are offered for resident as well as student training. Georgieff introduced the stable isotope technique to anaesthesia research in Germany.

Associate Professorship for Anaesthesiological Process Development and Pathophysiology

Prof. Dr. med. Dr. h.c. Peter Radermacher

Born March 20 1959 in Düsseldorf; 1977–1984 student of medicine, University of Düsseldorf; 1984–1991 Resident at the Department of Anaesthesiology, University of Düsseldorf; 1991 Specialist in Anaesthesiology; 1991 Lecturer in Anaesthesiology; 1994 Associate Professor of Anaesthesiology, Department of Anaesthesiology, University of Ulm; 1997 Head, Section of Anaesthesiological Process Development and Pathophysiology.

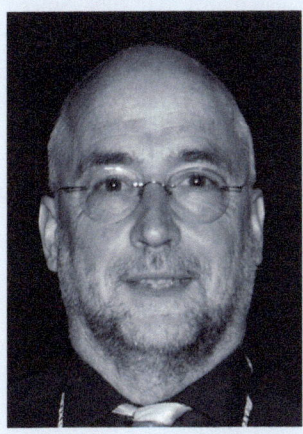

The main areas of research are experimental shock, ischaemia and reperfusion, oxidative DNA damage, stable isotope research; single nucleotide polymorphism, hyperinflammation and haemophagocytosis.

Qualification as Lecturers in Anaesthesiology

Kilian, Jürgen (1973); Borst, Reiner (1974); Reineke, Henner (1974); Dölp, Reiner (1975); Milewski, Peter (1976); Lotz, Peter (1977); Bock, Karl-Heinz (1978); Mehrkens, Hans-Hinrich (1980); Spilker, Diethelm (1981); Seeling, Wulf (1981); Altemeyer, Karl-Heinz (1983); Schmitz, Jürgen (1984); Heinrich, Helmut (1987); Pfenninger, Ernst (1987); Wiedeck, Heidemarie (1988); Lindner, Karl-Heinz (1989); Konrad, Franz Xaver (1993); Ensinger, Hermann (1994); Lampl, Lorenz (1994); Friesdorf, Wolfgang (1995); Goertz, Axel Walter (1995); Weiß, Manfred (1997); Prengel, Andreas (1997); Schricker, Thomas (1998), Schwilk, Bernhard (1998); Schirmer, Uwe (1998); Marx, Thomas (1999); Brinkmann, Alexander (1999); Rockemann, Michael (1999); Weigt, Henry (1999); Geldner, Götz (2000); Schraag, Stefan (2000); Calzia, Enrico (2002); Träger, Karl (2002); Kiefer, Peter (2002); Schütz, Wolfram (2002), Bothner, Ulrich (2003); Gauß, Albrecht (2003); Senftleben, Uwe

(2003); Meierhenrich, Rainer (2005); Steffen, Peter (2005); Fröba, Gebhard (2007); Albuszies, Gerd (2008); Muth, Claus-Martin (2008), Maybauer, Dirk (2008); Maybauer, Marc (2008); Barth, Eberhard (2009); Bracht, Hendrik (2009); Adolph, Oliver (2010); Klingler, Werner (2010)

Professors of Anaesthesiology
Full Professors

Prof. Dr. Wolfgang F. Dick (1982), Ulm; (1983), University of Mainz
Prof. Dr. Dr. Adolf Grünert (1991), Full Professor of Clinical Chemistry, Ulm
Prof. Dr. Karl-Heinz Lindner (1997), University of Innsbruck
Prof. Dr. Dr. Wolfgang Friesdorf (1997) Department for Human Factors Engineering and Product Ergonomics, Technical University of Berlin

Associate Professors

Prof. Dr. Wolfgang Dick (1971), Ulm
Prof. Dr. Dr. Adolf Grünert (1976), Associate Professor of Experimental Anaesthesiology, Ulm
Prof. Dr. med. Dr. h. c. Peter Radermacher (1994), Ulm
Prof. Dr. E. Marion Schneider (1997), Associate Professor of Experimental Anaesthesiology, Ulm

Associate and Adjunct Professors

Prof. Dr. Karl-Heinz Bock, Prof. Dr. Reiner Dölp, Prof. Dr. Helmut Heinrich, Prof. Dr. Franz Konrad, Prof. Dr. Jürgen Kilian, Prof. Dr. Lorenz Lampl, Prof. Dr. Peter Lotz, Prof. Dr. Hans-Hinrich Mehrkens, Prof. Dr. Peter Milewski, Prof. Dr. Ernst Pfenninger, Prof. Dr. Henner Reineke, Prof. Dr. Jürgen-Erik Schmitz, Prof. Dr. Diethelm Spilker, Prof. Dr. Heidemarie Suger-Wiedeck, Prof. Dr. Alexander Brinkmann, Prof. Dr. Manfred Weiß, Prof. Dr. Enrico Calzia, Prof. Dr. Karl Träger

For further information:

www.uniklinik-ulm.de/struktur/kliniken/anaesthesiologie.html

3.2.37   University of Witten/Herdecke

Centre of Anaesthesia, Emergency Medicine and Pain Therapy (Chair I), Helios Hospital Wuppertal Department of Anaesthesiology and Surgical Intensive Care Medicine (Chair II), Hospital Cologne-Merheim

L. Brandt, F. Wappler

The Private University of Witten/Herdecke was founded in 1982. One year later the education of medical stu-

3

dents was started by the Faculty of Medicine. In contrast to other German universities pregradute teaching of students in all disciplines was performed exclusively at teaching hospitals affiliated to the University. The first appointment for a Chair in Anaesthesiology was made on 31st January 1995, when Professor Ludwig Brandt (Mainz) became Professor and Chairman of the University Department of Anaesthesiology, Intensive Care Medicine and Pain Therapy at the Hospital Wuppertal.

1995–2010 Chairmanship Professor Ludwig Brandt

Prof. Dr. med. Ludwig Brandt

Born 23 September 1948 in Heidelberg; 1968–1974 student of medicine in Heidelberg; 1974 doctorate in medicine; 1976–1978 Resident at the Department of Anaesthesiology University Hospital Steglitz, Free University of Berlin; 1978–1980 Resident at the Department of Anaesthesiology, University Hospital Eppendorf, Hamburg; 1980 Specialist in Anaesthesiology; 1984 Lecturer in Anaesthesiology; 1984 Senior Physician, Department of Anaesthesiology, University of Mainz; 1985 Adjunct Professor; 1990 Director, Department of Anaesthesia, Hospital Wuppertal; 1995 Full Professor of Anaesthesiology, Intensive Care Medicine and Pain Therapy, University of Witten/Herdecke; 2010 Professor Emeritus.

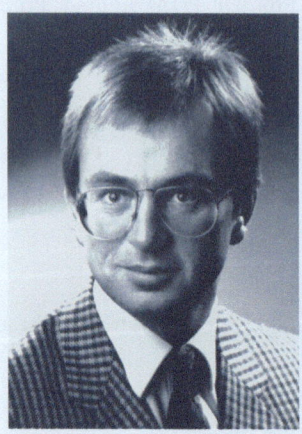

Pursuant to the ideas of the founders of the University the attention of the Faculty of Medicine was focussed on teaching of students and support of so-called alternative methods of medicine. Accordingly, Professor Brandt immediately established teaching courses in the practice of anaesthesiology including pain therapy for students which were expanded when a new curriculum began in 2000. In addition, students could attend courses in acupuncture and traditional Chinese medicine. These were developed into a

3-year university-based educational programme for both pre- and post-graduate students since 1996. Brandt's main scientific interest was the history of anaesthesia. After his retirement in 2010 Professor Gerhard Schneider (Munich) was appointed his successor as Professor of Anaesthesiology (Chair I) at the University of Witten/Herdecke and Chairman of the Centre of Anaesthesia, Emergency Medicine and Pain Therapy, Helios Hospital Wuppertal.

In order to improve the quality of teaching and to comply with the increasing numbers of medical students, the University of Witten/Herdecke had started a cooperation with the Hospital in Cologne-Merheim in 2003, where three new clinical chairs (general and transplantation surgery, traumatology and orthopaedics as well as anaesthesiology) were created on 1 May 2004. Since then, the Professor of Anaesthesiology at the Helios Hospital Wuppertal held the Chair I and the Professor at the Hospital Cologne-Merheim the Chair II of the University.

Since 2004 Chairmanship Professor Frank Wappler

Prof. Dr. med. Frank Wappler

Born 25 July 1960 in Bremerhaven; 1980–1984 student of biology and chemistry, University of Hamburg; 1984–1989 student of medicine; 1989 doctorate in medicine; 1989-1990 Resident, Department of Cardiovascular Surgery, University Hospital Hamburg-Eppendorf; 1990–1996 Resident, Department of Anaesthesiology; 1996 Specialist in Anaesthesiology; 1998 Lecturer in Anaesthesiology; 2000 Senior Physician; 2002 Adjunct Professor; 2004 Full Professor at the University of Witten/Herdecke and Chairman of the Department of Anaesthesiology and Intensive Care Medicine, Hospital Cologne-Merheim; 2008 Chairman of the Department of Paediatric Anaesthesia, Children's Hospital Cologne.

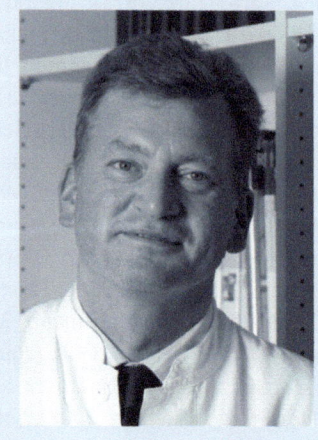

The new Department at the Hospital Cologne-Merheim under the Chairmanship of Professor Frank Wappler started medical education of students in the same year, introducing innovative educational concepts like »problem-based learning« and »objective structured long examination record (OSLER)« for small groups of 4–6 students. In the following year a full-scale anaesthesia simulator (METI) was incorporated in clinical training programmes for students. With the start of Wappler's chairmanship in 2004, a reorganization of the Department of Anaesthesiology was needed due to a steep increase of surgical procedures. Since that time, the number of anaesthesias performed per year increased from 11,000 to 19,000. Additionally, the Department of Paediatric Anaesthesia at the Children's Hospital of Cologne (6,500 anaesthesias/year) was put under Wappler's chairmanship. Thus a comprehensive education could be provided. Furthermore, the surgical ICM was restructured, the neurosurgical and surgical ICUs extended from 19 to 32 beds in 2007, then forming an interdisciplinary surgical ICU under anaesthesiological leadership. One year later a professional pain service was introduced for treatment of patients with acute (postoperative) and chronic pain syndromes. Recently a cooperation with the Fire Department of the City of Cologne was initiated in order to take part in pre-hospital emergency care.

Since the start as a University Department special focus was put on research in patient safety, pain treatment (pharmacology, concepts of regional analgesia etc.), sepsis, monitoring in anaesthesia and intensive care medicine, and, as main topic, in malignant hyperthermia. Research in paediatric anaesthesia was directed on concepts for diagnosis and treatment of inborn as well as acquired malformations of the respiratory tract.

Qualification as Lecturers in Anaesthesiology

Müller-Busch, Christoph (1996); Stuttmann, Ralph (1999); Lampert, Reinhard (2002); Mark U. Gerbershagen (2007); Dirk Knüttgen (2008)

Professors of Anaesthesiology
Adjunct Professor

Prof. Dr. Samir G. Sakka (2008)

For further information:

www.uni-wh.de/gesundheit/
Chair I:
www.helios-kliniken.de/klinik/wuppertal/fachabteilungen/anaesthesie/anaesthesie.html
Chair II:
www.kliniken-koeln.de/krankenhaeuser/Krankenhaus-Merheim/Anaesthesie/

3.2.38 University of Würzburg

Department of Anaesthesiology

J. Mildenberger, C.-A. Greim, N. Roewer, C. Wunder

The first documented anaesthetic in Würzburg was given on 3 February 1847 by Cajetan von Textor, Professor of Surgery at the Juliusspital, the 270 years-old University Hospital, probably with the aid of Robert Ritter von Welz who had carried out experiments with ether since January 1847. Later the gynaecologist Carl Joseph Gauss markedly contributed to the development of anaesthesia. Together with the pharmacologist Hermann Wieland (Heidelberg) he introduced narcylen in 1923 and developed in cooperation with Dräger Company an anesthesia machine for the safe application of this gas resulting in the first circle system containing a carbon dioxide absorber. As of 1927 he began to administer barbiturates like Pernocton and Eunarcon and in 1940 nitrous oxide in oxygen for labour analgesia. Gauss and Wieland were founding editors of the first German anaesthesia journal *Der Schmerz (Pain)*.

A Division of Anaesthesia was established at the Department of Surgery in 1954 and headed by Franz Becker. In 1961 he was succeeded by Kai Rehder who qualified as Lecturer in Anaesthesiology in 1963, but went back to the Mayo Clinic (Rochester, MN) already in 1965. One year later Karl-Heinz Weis, Staff Physician and Lecturer at the Department of Anaesthesiology, University of Mainz, became head of the Division.

1969–1995 Chairmanship Professor Karl-Heinz Weis

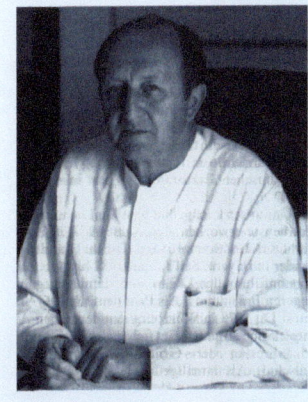

Prof. Dr. med. Dr. Karl-Heinz Weis

Born 23 July 1927 in Rottweil; 1948–1954 student of medicine in Mainz; 1954-1956 internship; 1955 doctorate in medicine; 1957–1959 Resident in surgery and anaesthesia; 1957–1958 Research Associate; Department of Pharmacology, University of Mainz; 1959 Senior Physician at the Department of Anaesthesiology, University of Mainz; 1961 Specialist in Anaesthesiology; 1964 Lecturer in Anaesthesiology; 1966 Senior Physician at the Surgical Department, University of Würzburg, and Head of the Anaesthesia Unit; 1968 Associate Professor of Anaesthesiology and Chairman of the Department of Anaesthesiology; 1969 Full Professor of Anaesthesiology; 1995 Professor Emeritus; 1996 Honorary Member of the European Academy of Anaesthesiology.

at the Department of Physiology, University of Freiburg; 1979–1981 Resident at the Department of Anaesthesia and Intensive Care Medicine, Federal Armed Forces Hospital Hamburg; since 1980 in addition external Research Fellow at the Department of Physiology, University Hospital Eppendorf, Hamburg; 1981–1983 residency in cardiology, University Hospital Eppendorf, Hamburg; 1983–1986 Resident, Department of Anaesthesiology; 1986 Specialist in Anaesthesiology; 1989 Lecturer in Anaesthesiology; 1990 Senior Physician; 1994 Visiting Professor, University Hospital Vienna; 1995 Adjunct Professor; 1995 Full Professor and Chairman of the Department of Anaesthesiology, University of Würzburg.

Weis soon extended the responsibility of the Division to all operative departments of the University and paved the way for a new intensive care unit which was opened in 1967. In 1969 he was appointed to the first Bavarian Chair of Anaesthesiology. He enlarged the ICU, instituted a Section of Emergency Medicine, an outpatient clinic for malignant hypothermia and a pain clinic and continuously supported successful research groups. As from 1987 he organized and hosted the annual Scientific Working Days of the German Society of Anaesthesiology and Intensive Care Medicine (DGAI) in Würzburg and it is worth mentioning that he substantially contributed to the development of the German Society of Anaesthesiology and Intensive Care Medicine.

Since 1995 Chairmanship Professor Norbert Rudolf Roewer

Prof. Dr. med. Norbert Rudolf Roewer

Born 22 February 1951 in Cologne; 1970–1976 student of medicine in Göttingen; 1977 doctorate in medicine; 1977–1978 internship; 1978–1979 Research Associate

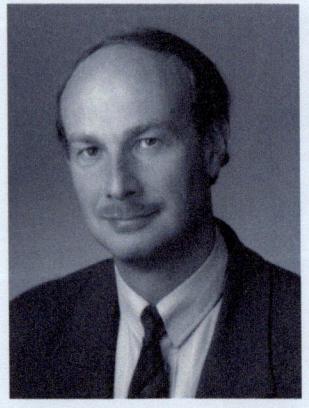

In December 1995 Norbert Roewer was appointed Full Professor and Chairman of the Department of Anaesthesiology. He stuck up for the expansion of the medical staff, the acquisition of new anaesthesia machines and monitoring equipment, the complex renovation of the ICU and the extension of scientific activities. In 2004 the Department moved into the new Centre of Operative Medicine of the University Hospital what enabled the provision of the majority of anaesthesiological services within one area.

An intensive care patient data management system was started in 1998. Special emphasis was laid on the treatment of patients with severe ARDS and ALI eventually resulting in the establishment of an ARDS/ECMO centre which is part of the German ADRS network. A Working Group Chronic Pain was established in 1999 additionally to the pain clinic headed by Professor Günter Sprotte since 1983. Peter Sefrin, Associate Professor and Head of the Section of Preclinical Emergency Medicine, retired in 2006. For his untiring commitment to teaching emergency medicine to both students and doctors he was honoured by a great number of awards. Main areas of clinical and experimental research are malignant hyperthermia, nociception and neuronal actions of anesthetics, blood-brain barrier, molecular mechanisms of pain, anaesthetic depth, use of ultrasound in anesthesia, cardiac preconditioning and protection, mechanisms of organ protection during anaesthesia and intensive care, ARDS, microcirculation, prevention of emesis, simulation in anaesthesia, airway management, evidence-based medicine and clinical economics, and other topics. One or two courses on transoesophageal echocardiography in anaesthesiology and intensive care medicine are held every year.

Qualification as Lecturers in Anaesthesiology

Rehder, Kai (1963); Rietbrock, Ingrid (1973); Cunitz, Günther (1973); Sefrin, Peter (1978); Homann, Barbara (1980); Lazarus, Günter (1980); Sprotte, Günter (1981);

Plötz, Jürgen (1982); Rothhammer, Anton (1984); Sold, Markus (1988); Kress, Hans-Georg (1988); Blumenberg, Detlef (1990); Tas, Petrus W.L. (1993); Engelhardt, Wolfram (1995); Hartung, Edmund Josef (1996); Herbert, Michael (1996); Greim, Clemens (1999); Anetseder, Martin (2003); Eichelbrönner, Otto (2003); Kehl, Franz (2003); Kuhnigk, Herbert (2005), Wunder, Christian (2006), Schwemmer, Ulrich (2007), Brack, Alexander (2007), Rittner, Heike (2008); Lange, Markus (2009); Muellenbach, Ralf (2009); Schuster, Frank (2009); Wurmb, Thomas (2009); Broscheit, Jens (2010)

Professors of Anaesthesiology
Full Professors

Prof. Dr. Klaus Eyrich (1978), University Hospital Steglitz, Free University of Berlin
Prof. Dr. Günter Cunitz (1983), University of Bochum
Prof. Dr. Hans Georg Kress (1992), University of Vienna

Associate Professors

Prof. Dr. Peter Sefrin (1996), Associate Professor of Preclinical Emergency Medicine, Würzburg
Prof. Dr. Clemens Greim (2002), Würzburg
Prof. Dr. Franz Kehl (2004), Würzburg
Prof. Dr. Carola Förster (2007), Associate Professor of Experimental Anaesthesiology, Würzburg
Prof. Dr. Peter Kranke (2009), Würzburg
Prof. Dr. Christian Wunder (2009), Würzburg

Adjunct Professors

Prof. Dr. Günter Cunitz; Prof. Dr. Michael Herbert; Prof. Dr. Franz Kehl; Prof. Hans-Georg Kress; Prof. Günter Lazarus; Prof. Dr. Ingrid Rietbrock; Prof. Dr. Anton Rothhammer; Prof. Dr. Peter Sefrin; Prof. Dr. Markus Sold; Prof. Dr. Günter Sprotte.

For further information:

www.anaesthesie.uk-wuerzburg.de

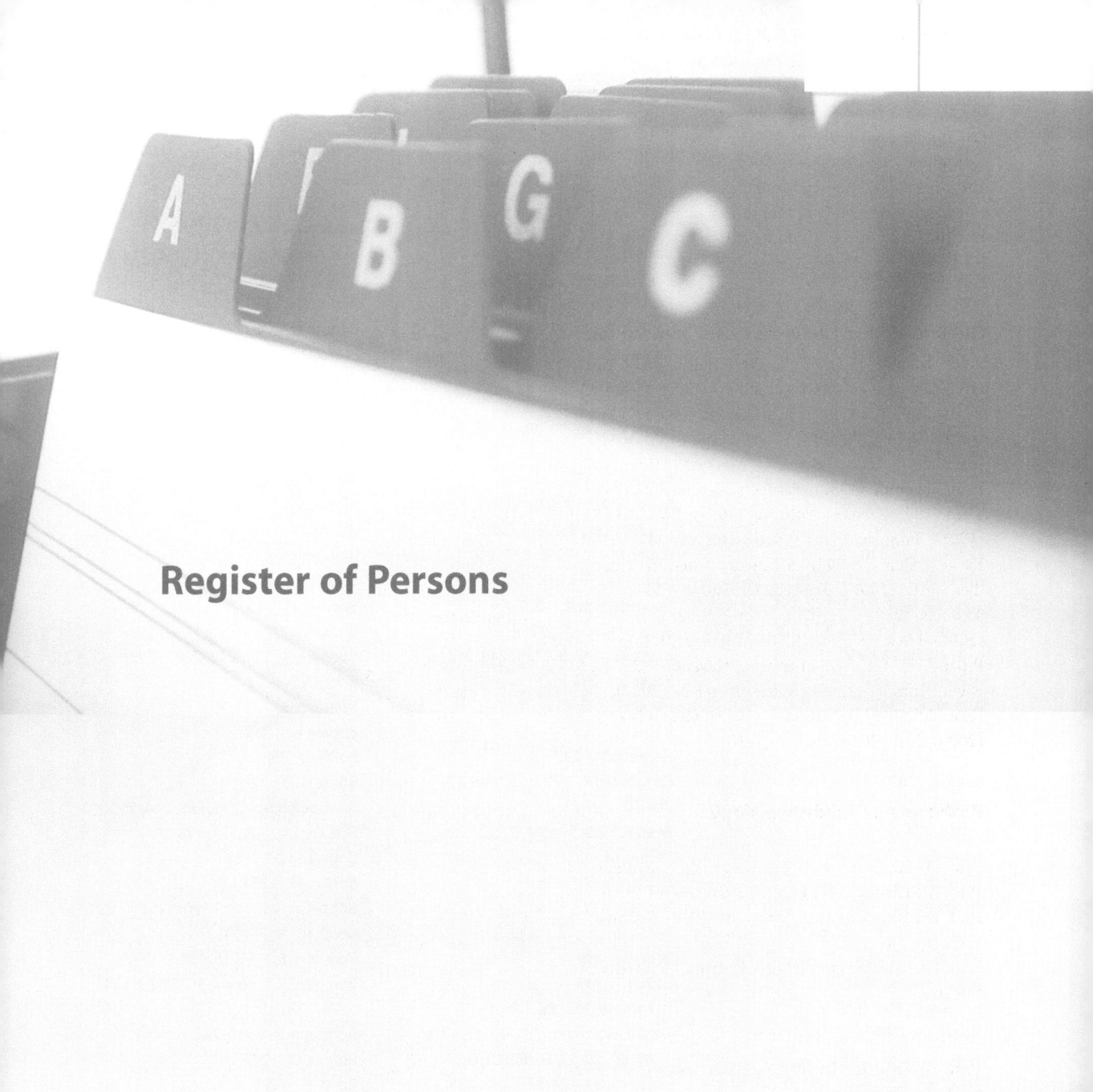

Register of Persons

Table of Figures

Printing: Ten Brink, Meppel, The Netherlands
Binding: Stürtz, Würzburg, Germany

GPSR Compliance

The European Union's (EU) General Product Safety Regulation (GPSR) is a set of rules that requires consumer products to be safe and our obligations to ensure this.

If you have any concerns about our products, you can contact us on ProductSafety@springernature.com

In case Publisher is established outside the EU, the EU authorized representative is:

Springer Nature Customer Service Center GmbH
Europaplatz 3
69115 Heidelberg, Germany

Batch number: 09640709

Printed by Printforce, the Netherlands